# Instructor's Manual to accompany

## Medical Assisting
### Administrative and Clinical Competencies
### Seventh Edition

**Michelle Blesi, MBA, CMA(AAMA)**
Program Director, Medical Assisting
Century College – East Campus
White Bear Lake, MN

**Barbara A. Wise, RN, BSN, MA(Ed)**

**Cathy Kelley-Arney, CMA(AAMA), MLTC, BSHS**

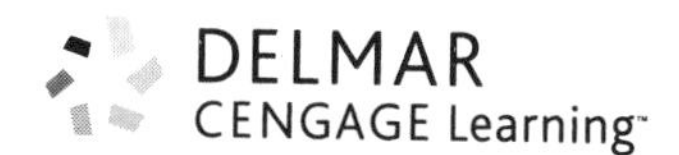


Australia • Brazil • Japan • Korea • Mexico • Singapore • Spain • United Kingdom • United States

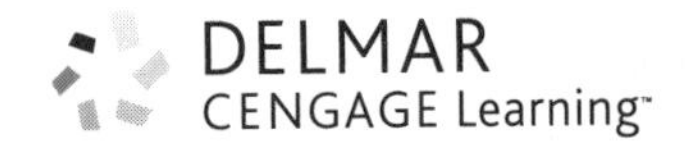

**Instructor's Manual to accompany Medical Assisting: Administrative and Clinical Competencies, Seventh Edition**
**Michelle Blesi, Barbara A. Wise, Cathy Kelley-Arney**

Vice President, Editorial: Dave Garza

Director of Learning Solutions: Matthew Kane

Executive Editor: Rhonda Dearborn

Managing Editor: Marah Bellegarde

Senior Product Manager: Sarah Prime

Editorial Assistant: Lauren Whalen

Vice President, Marketing: Jennifer Baker

Marketing Director: Wendy E. Mapstone

Senior Marketing Manager: Nancy Bradshaw

Senior Production Director: Wendy A. Troeger

Production Manager: Andrew Crouth

Content Project Manager: Thomas Heffernan

Senior Art Director: Jack Pendleton



Library of Congress Control Number: 2011926859
ISBN-13: 978-1-111-13513-3
ISBN-10: 1-111-13513-4

**Delmar**
5 Maxwell Drive
Clifton Park, NY 12065-2919
USA

Cengage Learning is a leading provider of customized learning solutions with office locations around the globe, including Singapore, the United Kingdom, Australia, Mexico, Brazil, and Japan. Locate your local office at:
**international.cengage.com/region**

Cengage Learning products are represented in Canada by Nelson Education, Ltd.

To learn more about Delmar, visit **www.cengage.com/delmar**
Purchase any of our products at your local college store or at our preferred online store **www.cengagebrain.com**

**Notice to the Reader**
Publisher does not warrant or guarantee any of the products described herein or perform any independent analysis in connection with any of the product information contained herein. Publisher does not assume, and expressly disclaims, any obligation to obtain and include information other than that provided to it by the manufacturer. The reader is expressly warned to consider and adopt all safety precautions that might be indicated by the activities described herein and to avoid all potential hazards. By following the instructions contained herein, the reader willingly assumes all risks in connection with such instructions. The publisher makes no representations or warranties of any kind, including but not limited to, the warranties of fitness for particular purpose or merchantability, nor are any such representations implied with respect to the material set forth herein, and the publisher takes no responsibility with respect to such material. The publisher shall not be liable for any special, consequential, or exemplary damages resulting, in whole or part, from the readers' use of, or reliance upon, this material.

Printed in the United States of America
1 2 3 4 5 6 7 15 14 13 12 11

# CONTRIBUTORS

**Yvonne Burbrink, BS, RMA(AMT)**
Curriculum Manager
Medical Assistant Program
Corinthian Colleges
Santa Ana, CA
*Unit 20: Workplace Readiness*

**Virginia Busey Ferrari, BA, MHA**
Adjunct Professor
Business, Computer Science and Career Technical Education
Solano Community College
Fairfield, CA
*Unit 4: Professional Communications*
*Unit 5: Business Communications*
*Unit 10: Managing the Medical Office Environment*

**Cecile R. Favreau, MBA, CPC**
Professional Relations Specialist
UMass Memorial Medical Group
Adjunct Faculty Member at Salter College
West Boylston, MA
*Unit 7: Medical Insurance and Coding*

**Michelle Heller, CMA(AAMA), RMA(AMT)**
Adjunct Faculty Member
Columbus State Community College
Columbus, OH
*Unit 1: Health Care Roles and Responsibilities*

**Brina Hollis, PhD**
Director Healthcare Programs–Cleveland Market
Bryant & Stratton College
Parma, OH
*Unit 16: Minor Surgery Procedures*

**Sherri Mason, RN, BSN, LNCC**
*Unit 6: Beginning the Patient's Record*
*Unit 17: Medication Administration Procedures*

**Michael R. Meacham, JD, MPH**
Associate Professor
Medical University of South Carolina
Charleston, SC
*Unit 3: Medical Law and Ethics*

**Sandra Marmolejo Romero, BSN, RN, CPHQ**
Adjunct Associate Professor
Bilingual Medical Assistant Program
Southwestern Community College District
San Diego, CA
*Unit 2: Medical Terminology*
*Unit 8: Billing and Payment for Medical Services*
*Unit 9: Banking and Accounting Procedures*

**Lynn A. Skafte, BA, CMA(AAMA)**
National Medical Assisting Program Coordinator
School of Health Sciences
Rasmussen College
Bloomington, MN
*Unit 15: Laboratory Procedures*

# CONTENTS

**PART 2: CHAPTER GUIDES WITH LESSON OUTLINES**

# To the Instructor

## Using this Instructor's Manual

The authors sincerely hope the total instructional package assists you with the preparation and presentation of the content to your students. Thank you for selecting *Medical Assisting: Administrative and Clinical Competencies* as the instructional material for your program!

The Instructor's Manual contains three parts:

- Workbook Answers
- Chapter Guides with Lesson Outlines
- Instructor Tools

### PART 1: WORKBOOK ANSWERS

The first part of the Instructor's Manual includes Workbook Assignment Sheets for each chapter, with the answers printed. It correlates exactly to what is printed in the student Workbook.

### PART 2: CHAPTER GUIDES WITH LESSON OUTLINES

The chapter guides are organized as follows:

- References to ABHES and CAAHEP curriculum standards.
- Lesson Outline. Note: This outline correlates with the content and organization of the instructor presentation slides (accessed on the Instructor Resources CD-ROM or Instructor Companion Site).
- Suggested Activities for the chapter.
- Answers to Check Your Knowledge questions from the textbook. These questions are given to students at the end of each textbook chapter.
- Procedure Scenarios, if appropriate. Procedure Scenarios are referenced in some Competency Checklists and provide necessary information so students can complete the procedure. They are optional; instructors may choose to use already developed scenario information. They are provided in this section in the event that this material is needed.

### PART 3: INSTRUCTOR TOOLS

In this part, we have provided mapping tools to ABHES and CAAHEP curriculum standards, as well as instructional tools, including:

- Concepts and principles of learning (included especially for new instructors).
- Ideas for lesson plan design and class activities.
- Notes to help you use the *Competency Challenge 2.0* and *Critical Thinking Challenge 2.0* in your curriculum. These programs are on the Premium Website accompanying the text, and can be used in conjunction with the text.

## Supplements at a Glance

The following Supplements at a Glance table lists all the ancillary materials associated with this text; following, we've provided a brief overview of the instructional features of some of these components.

| SUPPLEMENT: | WHAT IT IS: | WHAT'S IN IT: |
|---|---|---|
| Premium Website | Website | Access at www.cengagebrain.com<br>Media Link library, Procedure Forms, StudyWARE™ Software with quizzes and games, Critical Thinking Challenge 2.0, Competency Challenge 2.0 |
| StudyWARE™ Software | Software program | Access on the Premium Website<br>Chapter Quizzes and Games, Medical Terminology Audio Library, Dosage Calculations Tutorials, Surgical Instruments Review |
| Critical Thinking Challenge 2.0 | Software program | Access on the Premium Website<br>10 video scenarios, with branching options; Scoring, outcomes, and feedback for each decision |

| | | |
|---|---|---|
| Competency Challenge 2.0 | Software program | Access on the Premium Website<br><br>26 video-based case studies focusing on skills, with interactive exercises |
| Mobile Downloads | Mobile Media | Access on the Premium Website<br><br>Spanish-English terms that can be downloaded to a mobile device |
| Workbook | Print | Chapter Worksheets with review and application activities<br><br>Competency Checklists to evaluate performance of text procedures |
| Learning Labs | Web access | Immersive environment with interactive activities which focus on the most difficult concepts of each unit<br><br>Pre-assessment and post-assessment tests |
| CourseMate | Website | Interactive eBook, with highlighting, note-taking, and search<br><br>Interactive learning tools, including quizzes, flash cards, and games<br><br>Engagement Tracker |
| Instructor's Manual | Print | Lesson Planning, curriculum mapping grids, and instructor tools<br><br>Answer key for text and Workbook |
| Instructor Resources | CD-ROM and Web access | Computerized Test Bank, Instructor Presentation Slides in Microsoft Word, Image Library, Customizable Instructor's Manual files |
| Instructor Companion Site | Website | Access at www.cengage.com/login<br><br>Instructor Resources, CourseForward curriculum |
| CourseForward Curriculum | Web access | Access on Instructor Companion Site<br><br>Modular curriculum solution with discussion topics, suggested activities, and homework assignments correlating to key concepts |
| Web Tutor | Web access | Blackboard, WebCT, and Angel platforms<br><br>Content and quizzes corresponding to each chapter |

## Premium Website

The Premium Website contains resources for Students that directly link to the text and Workbook.

### STUDYWARE™ SOFTWARE AND AUDIO LIBRARY

StudyWARE™ is interactive software included with many of Delmar Cengage Learning's products and lets students have fun while increasing knowledge. The StudyWARE™ on the Premium Website includes the following components:

- Medical Terminology Audio Library
- Dosage Calculations Tutorials
- Surgical Instruments Review
- Chapter Quizzes and Games (described below)

Quizzes can be taken in either Quiz Mode or Practice Mode. In Quiz Mode, the test is scored and tracked in the Reports; Practice Mode gives immediate feedback for each question answered and does not report scores.

Games for each chapter include Championship (Jeopardy-style trivia game), Maze, and flash cards. Additionally, chapters within Units 2 (Medical Terminology, chapters 3-4) and 11 (Anatomy & Physiology, chapters 23-35) also include Anatomy image labeling and Spelling Bee games.

### CRITICAL THINKING CHALLENGE 2.0

The Critical Thinking Challenge 2.0 is a game which simulates a 3-month externship in Dr. Conner's medical office. In this game, students will be confronted with a series of situations in which they must use critical thinking skills to select the most correct action in response to the situation.

Part C of this Instructor's Manual includes detailed Synopses, Answer Keys, and Scoring information for the Critical Thinking Challenge 2.0.

### COMPETENCY CHALLENGE 2.0

In the Competency Challenge 2.0, students will simulate a "week in the life" of an externship through 26 activities and a comprehensive patient case study, which are arranged on a Weekly Planner. Each activity corresponds to several general, administrative, and clinical curriculum competencies.

Part C of this Instructor's Manual includes information on using the Competency Challenge 2.0 with the text chapters and Scoring information.

### MEDIA LINKS

Media Link references are included within the textbook to help illustrate a procedure or difficult concept. Media Links may be a *video, animation, or tutorial* and are accessed on the Premium Website:

- Video and animations can be accessed from the left navigation bar.
- Tutorials are launched from within the StudyWARE™ Software. Tutorials are included for the Dosage Calculations unit.

### PROCEDURE FORMS

For the Workbook Competency Checklists, *downloadable Procedure Forms* are provided to complete some of the procedures. If a Procedure Form is required, it is noted on the individual Competency Checklist.

## Workbook

### ABOUT THE WORKBOOK

**Part 1: Chapter Worksheets.** A Worksheet is provided for each chapter in the text, and includes the following features:

- **Words to Know Review** checks vocabulary comprehension of the key terms of the chapter. Each chapter begins with *Spelling* review. Additionally, practice identifying and putting key terms in context with definition *Matching* and *Fill in the blank* activities.
- **Chapter Review** recalls the main Knowledge Base objectives of the chapter. This section features a variety of activities designed to reinforce concepts, including *Short Answer*, *Labeling*, and concept *Matching*, among others.
- **Chapter Application** puts into practice the Skill and Behavior objectives of the chapter. Examples of activity types in this section include *Competency Practice*, *Role-Play* activities, *Case Studies* with critical thinking questions, *Video Case Studies*, and *Research Activities*, among others.

**Part 2: Competency Checklists. Competency Checklists** are printed* for each Procedure in the text, and include the following features:

- Curriculum mapping to *ABHES* and *CAAHEP* programmatic standards.
- *Task*, *Supplies & Conditions*, and *Standards* outlining the purpose and scope of the procedure, and defining the criteria for success for the procedure.
- Some checklists include a listing for *Forms*. Forms indicate a procedure may require the use of documents or scenario information for completion. Students can download Procedure Forms referenced from the Premium Website. Procedure Scenarios are provided in this Instructor's Manual, to be given by the instructor or evaluator when the procedure is to be performed. Procedure Scenarios are included in the Chapter Guide section in this Instructor's Manual.
- When a student has demonstrated competency for the task (Procedure), the instructor or evaluator can sign off in the *Evaluation* space provided.
- *Steps* match up exactly to steps given in the textbook Procedure. Steps printed in *bold/italic* font indicate Behavior competencies.

*Additionally, Competency Checklists are available on the Instructor Companion Site in Microsoft® Word format.

### HOW TO GRADE THE WORKBOOK

You can assign students to complete the **Chapter Worksheets**, tear them out, and turn them in to you for evaluation. The Answer Key for the Chapter Worksheets is included as the first part of this Instructor's Manual.

Some of the exercises in the Chapter Application sections are designed to provide you with student work products for accreditation purposes. (Refer to the ABHES and CAAHEP mapping grids at the end of this Instructor's Manual for specific details.)

### HOW TO GRADE THE COMPETENCY CHECKLISTS

We made every attempt to have a direct link to the required competencies in our Competency Checklists, while still keeping the checklists flexible enough to be tailored to individual program needs. At your discretion, you may determine the required standards based on the actual conditions in your classroom situation. Should you desire to customize the Competency Checklists, they are available on the Instructor Companion Site for this text (www.cengage.com/login). Log in with your Cengage instructor account.

Each checklist offers three attempts for the student to complete the procedure. If the student performs a step of the procedure correctly, the evaluator will place the number of points in the appropriate attempt column. The checklist also includes the actual time the student needed to complete the procedure. During the second and third assessment, the instructor may use his or her discretion regarding scoring. Some instructors choose to divide the scoring by two and three during successive attempts, making the best score possible less than if the student had passed the competency on the first assessment.

The instructor or evaluator can use the Evaluation section to grade student competency for each skill. You may also provide and document suggestions for improving student performance. If a student does not initially achieve competency, he or she must be re-evaluated until competency is achieved. Student competency must be achieved prior to the students being placed in an externship or practicum, where they will be required to perform in the workplace. Because regulations vary from state to state regarding which procedures can be performed by a medical assistant, it will be important to check specific regulations in each state. A medical assistant should never perform any procedure without checking legal responsibilities, without correct instruction, and without proper authorization.

## Instructor Resources CD-ROM

This CD-ROM includes a *computerized test bank* in ExamView. The test bank contains more than 2,600 questions, and each question contains a reference to the text page number and ABHES and CAAHEP curriculum standard. Additionally, access *instructor presentation slides* created in Microsoft® PowerPoint, an *Image Library,* and customizable *Instructor's Manual* files.

## Instructor Companion Site

The Instructor Companion Site is the online home for instructional tools, including:

- Instructor Resources (presentation slides, Test Bank, Image Library, and Instructor's Manual)
- CourseForward Curriculum (described below)
- Access to the student Premium Website

Log on at www.cengage.com/login with your Cengage instructor account. If you are a first-time user, click Create a New Faculty Account and follow the prompts.

### COURSEFORWARD CURRICULUM

CourseForward is a modular curriculum solution that breaks down content into topics for ease of learning and serves as a roadmap for course material. CourseForward is designed for instructors to spend less time planning and more time teaching. Some of the features of CourseForward include equipment lists, homework assignments, in-class discussion topics and suggested responses, individual and group activities, and chapter content mapped to activities and assignments.

# Part 1

# CHAPTER WORKSHEETS

# SECTION 1

# Medical Assisting Foundations

UNIT 1

# Health Care Roles and Responsibilities

CHAPTER 1

# The Medical Assistant

## Words to Know Challenge

**Spelling: Each line contains three spellings of a word. Underline the correctly spelled word.**

| | | |
|---|---|---|
| 1. accreditation | acreditation | accretitation |
| 2. alltruism | alltrueism | altruism |
| 3. inate | innate | innat |
| 4. empathatic | empathic | empathetic |
| 5. addvocate | advocate | advocat |
| 6. confidential | confidental | confidinal |
| 7. generalist | ginerallist | generelist |
| 8. providar | providir | provider |
| 9. partnarship | partnirship | partnership |
| 10. certified | certifeid | cerdified |

**Fill in the Blank: Complete the following sentences with correctly spelled words from the Spelling section.**

1. An unselfish concern for the welfare of others is referred to as altruism.
2. Confidential means being prudent or cautious—especially concerning speech.
3. Accreditation is a process by which an educational institution or program establishes credibility or legitimacy by complying with predetermined standards.
4. A provider oversees the patient's health care and oftentimes is a doctor, NP, or PA.
5. Being empathic means being able to put yourself in another person's shoes.
6. A medical assistant who works as a generalist performs both clinical and administrative functions.
7. Characteristics that are inherent or natural are referred to as innate.

**Matching: Match the term in column I to its definition in column II.**

| | COLUMN I | COLUMN II |
|---|---|---|
| C | 1. Patient-centered medical home | A. Skills necessary regardless of whether working in a clinical or administrative capacity |
| G | 2. Clinical skills | B. When an individual provider makes all the decisions for the practice |
| A | 3. General skills | C. A team-based model of care led by a personal physician who provides continuous and coordinated care throughout a patient's lifetime to maximize health outcomes |
| F | 4. Time management | D. Two or more physicians who have a legal agreement to share in the total business operation of the practice. |
| B | 5. Solo practice | E. Someone who speaks for another person |
| H | 6. Urgent care center | F. An assortment of skills, tools, and practices by which to manage time during daily activities and when accomplishing specific projects |
| D | 7. Partnership | G. Skills that are an extension of the provider's responsibilities and can be divided into fundamental practices, diagnostic procedures, and patient care |
| E | 8. Advocate | H. Ambulatory care centers that take care of patients with acute illness or injury and those with minor emergencies; used quite often when patients cannot see their own provider. |

## Chapter Review

### Short Answer

1. To become a successful medical assistant, you must acquire a specific knowledge base (theory) and skills (procedures) while also demonstrating specific behaviors.
2. What are the three broad areas of medical assisting?
   **a.** General
   **b.** Administrative
   **c.** Clinical
3. What role should the medical assistant take on concerning communications when working with patients?
   Communications liaison
4. The chapter listed eight administrative skills performed by medical assistants; name six.
   Any six of the following: scheduling appointments, performing inpatient and outpatient admissions and procedures, creating and maintaining the patient's medical record, filing medical records and other documents, performing procedural and diagnostic coding for reimbursement, performing billing and collection procedures, performing bookkeeping and financial procedures, preparing submittal (clean) insurance forms
5. The chapter listed twelve clinical skills performed by medical assistants; name any six.
   Any six of the following: applying principles of aseptic technique and infection control; performing vital signs; performing sterilization and minor surgery procedures; collecting and processing specimens; performing lab tests; performing electrocardiograms; administering medications; performing phlebotomy procedures; performing patient screenings; preparing patients for examinations, procedures and treatments; responding to emergencies
6. List four environments in which medical assistants work.
   Any four of the following: doctors' offices, specialty practices, urgent care centers, clinics, hospitals, labs, insurance companies, billing companies, government agencies

7. According to the United States Department of Labor, employment for medical assistants is expected to grow by 34% ________ through 2018.

8. Define professionalism.
   The conduct, aims, or qualities that characterize or mark a professional or a professional person

9. List five traits of a professional medical assistant.
   Any five of the following: accurate; adaptable; courteous; confidential; dependable; empathic; honest; initiative-taking; patient; punctual; respectful; tactful

10. Match the following organizational abbreviations with the responses listed in the chart.

    American Association of Medical Assistants (AAMA)

    American Medical Technologists (AMT)

    National Center for Competency Testing (NCCT)

    National Healthcareer Association (NHA)

    American Academy of Professional Coders (AAPC)

| **Organization Abbreviation** | **Response** |
|---|---|
| AAPC | CPC® |
| AAMA | The only avenue for credentialing with this organization is by graduating from either a CAAHEP- or ABHES-accredited institution. |
| AAMA | Provides the CMA credential with the organization's initials in parenthesis beside it |
| AAPC | Offers training and certification in the areas of medical billing and coding |
| NCCT | Provides the National Certified Medical Assistant (NCMA) credential |
| NHA | Provides the Certified Medical Administrative Specialist (CMAS) credential |
| AAMA | This organization started in 1955 |
| AMT | Provides the Registered Medical Assistant (RMA) credential |
| AAMA | Must take credentialing exam at an approved Prometric center |
| AMT | After receiving the Authorization to Test letter, applicants can take the test at any Prometric center |
| NCCT | Must receive the candidate's application within two weeks of the requested test date |
| NHA | Provides ten certification exams for ten allied health care specialties |

# Chapter Application

## Case Studies with Critical Thinking Questions

### Scenario 1

The following tasks are all occurring at the same time. Prioritize the following tasks by putting numbers 1–4 next to each statement. (1 is the task you will do first, and 4 is the task you will do last.)

1. 3 The doctor asks you to perform an ECG on the patient in room 2 as he goes into room 3.
2. 2 Room 1 is open and ready for a patient.
3. 4 The receptionist calls back to tell you that you have a patient who would like you to call her back regarding lab results.
4. 1 The doctor is going into room 3 to perform a short procedure and needs you to assist him.

### Scenario 2

You are competing with two other candidates for a medical assisting position at a large family practice center. All three of you are new graduates of the same medical assisting program. You all did well in your program and had a good rapport with the other students. Out of the three, you are the only one who is credentialed. During the interview, the supervisor asks you why she should hire you over the other two candidates.

1. What would you say?
   Answers will vary, but the following is an appropriate response: Out of the three of us, I am the only one who is credentialed. Possessing a credential validates my knowledge and right to practice medical assisting. It also shows my initiative and dedication to the profession.

### Role-Play Activity

Bella is a coworker you have grown very fond of. As a matter of fact, she is well respected by everyone in the office. You happen to see her come out of the drug room and slip some drug samples in her purse. You approach her about it, and she says that she received permission from Dr. Castle to take some samples home to her husband. The next week, you see Bella take some more samples; this time she takes several packets of the medicine from the drug cabinet. Once again, you confront her. She states that the doctor told her that it was okay to take as many samples as she wanted because the drug rep always leaves a lot more samples than necessary. The next day, the office manager calls a meeting and states that several samples of the drug that Bella took are missing from the drug cabinet, and she encourages anyone who has knowledge of the disappearance to come forward. Following the meeting, Bella stops you and begs you not to say anything to anyone. Role-play what you would say to Bella.
Answers will vary, but students should state something like the following; I am sorry Bella, but I have no other choice but to go forward and tell the office supervisor. I will allow you to go forward and talk to the office manager; however, I will need to be present when you tell her.

### Competency Practice: Professionalism

1. **Professionalism is a skill you will use daily as a medical assistant**. Write a 1–2 page essay, using the following prompts.
   a. Describe how the patient might associate the medical assistant's poor appearance with a lack of knowledge.
   b. Describe and discuss how being tardy and returning late from breaks will affect your success as a medical assistant.
   c. Discuss the ramifications of not using active listening skills in the field.
   d. Identify tasks that are considered in bounds for a medical assistant and tasks that are considered out of bounds. What are consequences of performing tasks outside of your scope of duty?
   e. How does a poor attitude reflect on you in the work place?
   Answers will vary but should revolve around the professionalism concept.

CHAPTER 2

# The Health Care Team and Medical Environment, Past and Present

## Words to Know Challenge

**Spelling: Each line contains three spellings of a word. Underline the correctly spelled word.**

| | | |
|---|---|---|
| 1. cadoceus | caduceus | caducious |
| 2. docterate | doctorate | doctarate |
| 3. apprenticeship | appretaship | apprentiship |
| 4. epademic | epedemic | epidemic |
| 5. homeopathy | homeopaty | homepathy |
| 6. hospitilist | hospitalist | hospitelist |
| 7. biofeedback | bioofeedback | biofeedbak |
| 8. naturopathy | natropathy | nateropathy |
| 9. plage | plauge | plague |
| 10. receprocity | reciprcety | reciprocity |

**Fill in the Blank: Complete the following sentences with correctly spelled words from the Spelling section.**

1. A hospitalist works with patients admitted to the hospital.
2. An apprenticeship is a period of time during which one is bound by agreement to learn some trade or craft.
3. Reciprocity indicates that one state recognizes the licensing requirements of another state as being similar to its own.
4. Someone who holds a doctorate has attained advanced knowledge through higher education in a discipline such as nursing, mathematics, or education.
5. A medical symbol depicted by a staff with a serpent coiled around its shaft is referred to as a caduceus.
6. A plague is a potentially infectious, life-threatening disease, usually transmitted by bites of rodent fleas.
7. Biofeedback is a method that enables a person, usually with the help of electronic equipment, to learn to control otherwise involuntary bodily functions.
8. Homeopathy is a 200-year-old system based on the Law of Similars.

9. Naturopathy is a multidisciplinary approach to health care based on the belief that the body has power to heal itself.

10. An epidemic is a disease affecting large numbers of individuals in a population.

**Matching: Match the term in column I to its definition in column II.**

| | COLUMN I | COLUMN II |
|---|---|---|
| C | 1. Hippocratic oath | A. A therapy that involves the placement of small magnets close to the skin to correct an imbalance |
| E | 2. Midlevel practitioner | B. Therapy used in addition to traditional therapies |
| H | 3. Ayurvedic medicine | C. A code of behavior that doctors are to follow |
| B | 4. Complementary therapy | D. A professional RN who has had extensive training and experience in labor and development of babies |
| G | 5. Physician assistant | E. Healthcare providers such as an NP or PA |
| D | 6. Nurse midwife | F. Refers to the fact that some people respond favorably to a known ineffective treatment because they believe it is working |
| F | 7. Placebo effect | G. A midlevel practitioner that is able to examine patients, order tests, and prescribe medications. Usually supervised by a physician. |
| A | 8. Magnetic therapy | H. Identifies three types of energy present in all things; imbalance of energies could indicate disease |

## Chapter Review

### Short Answer

1. Physicians now must take all three steps of what exam before being eligible for full licensure as a physician?
   United States Medical Licensing Examination (USMLE)

2. List the members of the three guilds of medicine during the seventeenth century.
   a. Physicians
   b. Surgeons
   c. Apothecaries (pharmacists)

3. List and describe five types of nurses.
   Registered nurse: One who has completed a course of study at a state-approved school of nursing and passed the NCLEX-RN exam
   Nurse Anesthetist: An RN licensed to administer anesthesia
   Nurse Midwife: An RN licensed to care for women in labor and to deliver babies
   Nurse Practitioner: An RN licensed to practice medicine and to work as a midlevel practitioner
   Licensed Practical Nurse: Nurse trained in basic nursing care; usually works under the direction of an RN or a physician

4. Why is it important for medical assistants to know the role of other health care providers?
   Knowing the roles of other health care professionals enables you to direct patients to the right professional and to speak more intelligently with others in the medical field.

5. In ancient civilizations, people thought disease was due to evil spirits and demons brought on as punishment for disobedience to the gods.

6. Egyptians used leeches to remove blood and toxins and produce hirudin, which helps prevent coagulation.

7. The Hindus in India were known for the world's first nurses and hospitals.

8. What did the Romans discover regarding sanitation, and what did they do about it?
They realized that disease was connected to filth and overcrowding and established superior methods of sanitation and water supplies. They drained the marshes, cleaned the streets, and built an extensive underground sewer system and pure water aqueducts capable of bringing drinking water into the city.

9. How did the Christian church feel about illness during medieval history, and what did it suggest for treatment?
It believed that illness was punishment for sin and recommended fasting and prayer.

10. What is a possible theory for the origin of the caduceus symbol?
The priests in the temples of Asklepios used large, nonpoisonous snakes to lick the wounds of patients to aid in healing. The speculation is that this is how the caduceus symbol originated.

11. How did the red and white barber poles originate?
During the medieval time period, barbers not only cut hair but performed minor surgeries, including bloodletting, opening abscesses, and, occasionally, conducting amputations—all with the same razor.

12. In the following table, match the following medical historians with their contributions.

| | | |
|---|---|---|
| Florence Nightingale | Clara Barton | Elizabeth Blackwell |
| Louis Pasteur | Wilhelm Roentgen | Marie Curie |
| George Papanicolaou | Fredrick Banting | Willem Kolff |
| Frank B. Colton | Peter Safar | Robert Jarvik |
| Andreas Versalius | Antony Van Leuwenhoek | Hippocrates |
| Trotula Platearius | Edward Jenner | Rene Laennec |
| Joseph Lister | Sir Alexander Fleming | A. B. Sabin |
| Patrick Steptoe | | |

| Historian | Contribution |
|---|---|
| Robert Jarvik | Designed the first permanently implantable artificial heart |
| Willem Kolff | Invented the first artificial kidney |
| Antony Van Leuwenhoek | Built microscopes, allowing him to see red blood cells for the first time |
| Trotula Platearius | Earliest known female physician |
| Edward Jenner | Known for the first vaccination |
| Rene Laennec | Invented the stethoscope |
| Hippocrates | Known as the father of medicine |
| Florence Nightingale | Founder of modern nursing |
| Joseph Lister | Founder of aseptic technique |
| Wilhelm Roentgen | Discovered X-rays |
| Sir Alexander Fleming | Discovered that mold could stop the growth of bacteria, which later contributed to the discovery of penicillin |
| George Papanicolaou | Originator of the Pap test |
| Peter Safar | Credited for starting the ABCs of CPR |
| Frank B. Colton | Developed the first contraceptive |
| Frederic Banting | Discovered and isolated insulin |

| Historian | Contribution |
|---|---|
| Louis Pasteur | Credited with the pasteurization process |
| Elizabeth Blackwell | First female physician in the United States |
| Clara Barton | Founded the Red Cross |
| A. B. Sabin | Developed the first attenuated vaccine for polio |
| Patrick Steptoe | Credited with the world's first successful in vitro fertilization |
| Marie Curie | First women scientist; discovered radium |
| Andreas Versalius | Anatomist that wrote one of the most influential anatomy books of its kind |

13. Match the patient's symptoms or disease to the type of specialist he or she might see.
Podiatrist, Pediatrician, Chiropractor, Dentist, Ophthalmologist, Pulmonary specialist, Sports medicine specialist, Dermatologist, Allergist, Gynecologist, Optometrist, Nuclear medicine specialist, Plastic surgeon, Otorhinolaryngologist, Anesthesiologist, Urologist, Gerontologist, and Endocrinologist

| Specialist | Symptoms or Disease |
|---|---|
| Chiropractor | Whiplash injury |
| Dentist | Tooth pain |
| Urologist | Impotence or urinary problems |
| Pulmonary specialist | Emphysema patient |
| Sport's medicine specialist | Sports injury |
| Nuclear medicine specialist | Someone who needs radiation treatment for cancer |
| Ophthalmologist | Patient with glaucoma |
| Endocrinologist | Patient with diabetes |
| Allergist | Patient who suffers from hay fever |
| Anesthesiologist | A patient needing an epidural prior to delivery of her baby |
| Gerontologist | An 87-year-old patient |
| Gynecologist | A female with a possible STD |
| Podiatrist | A patient with foot pain |
| Dermatologist | A patient with a suspicious mole |
| Pediatrician | A well-baby check |
| Plastic surgeon | A patient wanting to make facial improvements |
| Otorhinolaryngologist | A patient with persistent hoarseness |
| Optometrist | A patient with vision problems |

14. Match the description with the appropriate organization or legislation.
FDA, NIH, WHO, Medicaid, Medicare, CLIA, Uniform Anatomical Gift Act,
OSHA, Controlled Substances Act, HIPAA, Patient Protection and Affordable Care Act,
Hill–Burton Act, Medicare Part D

| Organization or Legislation | Description |
|---|---|
| Medicare | National insurance for persons over the age of 65, the disabled, or those suffering from end-stage renal disease |
| CLIA | Establishes guidelines for operating laboratories |
| FDA | Regulates the foods we purchase and drugs we consume and is part of the Department of Health and Human Services |
| OSHA | An organization that protects employees in the workplace |
| Uniform Anatomical Gift Act | An act that allows living individuals to indicate their desire for their organs to be gifted at the time of death |
| Patient Protection and Affordable Care Act | An act that expands access to health insurance |
| Medicare Part D | A prescription drug plan for seniors to make drugs more affordable |
| NIH | One of the world's foremost medical research centers |
| Hill–Burton Act | Legislation responsible for improving construction of hospitals |
| WHO | A specialized agency of the United Nations that cooperates to control and eradicate disease worldwide |
| Medicaid | A federal organization that provides for the medical care of the indigent |
| Controlled Substances Act | Legislation that helps control the abuse of drugs |
| HIPAA | Intended to limit health administration costs and provide for patient privacy |

# Chapter Application

## Connecting to the Right Team Member

Connecting patients to the right health care professional is part of the medical assistant's job. Today, you are asked to connect several patients to the correct professional. Fill in the blanks with the appropriate professional.

1. The patient's results to her hearing test were very poor today. The doctor asks you to set up an appointment with Susan Klein, an audiologist for the Orange Valley Speech and Hearing Center.
2. A patient calls on the phone regarding her bill. You connect her to Mike Brown, the clinic's medical biller.
3. Your doctor instructs you to call the EMS for a patient exhibiting chest pain. You will probably need to give the EMT a list of the patient's current medications upon arrival.
4. You send two tubes of blood to the lab. The laboratory technician calls to alert you that the patient's lab results are at a critical level and that the doctor needs to be notified right away.
5. The doctor would like you to set the patient up for an appointment with a physical therapist to assist the patient with walking, following her stroke.
6. The pharmacy technician answered the phone when you called the pharmacy to renew a prescription for Mrs. Wong. She immediately transferred you to the pharmacist.
7. Dr. Prime asked you to contact Missy, the X-ray technician, regarding the last set of X-rays she took on Mr. Hodges.

8. Dr. Smith asks you to call Jason Brown, a respiratory therapist with Visiting Health Professionals, to schedule some breathing tests and treatments on Mrs. Kesterson in her home.

9. Dr. Somadi just completed an exam on Mr. Waterson, who is a diabetic. She would like you to set up an appointment for the patient to see a dietician to educate him about proper food selection.

## Case Study with Critical Thinking Questions

Mrs. Dobson has been struggling with pain over the past six weeks. She was in an automobile accident and suffered some injuries to her back. The patient is tired of the pain and is searching for some alternatives to traditional medicine. She asks whether you are an advocate of acupuncture and goes on to state that a friend had acupuncture for some pain she was having and feels much better now. You know that your physician is not a huge fan of acupuncture but is not totally opposed to it either.

1. How would you respond to the patient's question?
   Answers will vary but might include something like the following: I am not very familiar with acupuncture and am not qualified to give an opinion on the subject; however, I would suggest that you talk to the doctor to get her opinion on the matter.

## Role Play Activities

Delivering messages to other health care professionals is a common responsibility of medical assistants. It is important to have all the details correct. Practice your communication skills by sharing the following message with one of your classmates.

1. The doctor asks you to set up a pelvic ultrasound for Mrs. Jennings, who is pregnant for the first time. The doctor suspects something wrong with the baby because it is measuring at only 12 weeks and should be measuring at 20 weeks. The patient is not scheduled to have an ultrasound today, but the doctor wants the sonographer to skip the patients that are in front of her and perform the ultrasound immediately.

The student should relay the message accurately and in a professional manner.

UNIT 2

# Medical Terminology

CHAPTER 3

# Introduction to Medical Terminology

## Words to Know Challenge

**Spelling: Each line contains three spellings of a word. Underline the correctly spelled word.**

| | | |
|---|---|---|
| 1. phalynxes | phalangis | phalanges |
| 2. appendixes | appendices | apendices |
| 3. atrias | atria | atriums |
| 4. combining form | combinning form | combineing form |
| 5. suffixes | suffices | suffixs |
| 6. singler | cingular | singular |
| 7. pleural | plural | pleral |

**Fill in the Blank: Complete the following sentences with Words to Know from this chapter.**

1. A word part found at the beginning of a medical term is a prefix.
2. Singular means referring to one.
3. *Neur/o*, *cardi/o*, and *cyan/o* are all examples of combining form.
4. *Diagnoses* is the plural form of the word *diagnosis*.
5. A suffix is a word part added to the end of a word to complete the term.
6. A word root is the foundation of a medical term and usually describes part of the body.

## Chapter Review

### Short Answer

1. From which two languages are most medical terms derived?
   Greek and Latin

2. In relation to a medical term:
   a. Does the prefix go on the left or on the right? On the left
   b. Does the suffix go on the left or on the right? On the right

3. Describe the procedure to follow when taking a medical term apart to define it.
   Start with the suffix and determine its meaning and then identify the prefix (if there is one) and determine its meaning; finally, determine the meaning of the word root(s) or combining form(s).

4. What is the difference between a word root and a combining form?
   The difference between combining forms and word roots is simply that a combining form has a vowel added to the word root to help in connecting suffixes or other word roots or combining forms.

5. Explain why spelling is so important in medical terminology.
   Misspelling a term can mean the difference in a diagnosis or treatment.

6. Explain the difference between a singular and a plural term and provide an example of each.
   A singular term applies to one item; the plural refers to multiple items. Examples will vary but could include: vertebra (singular)/vertebrae (plural); apex/apices; appendix/appendices; atrium/atria

**Matching: Determine whether each word in column I is singular (A) or plural (B).**

| | COLUMN I | COLUMN II |
|---|---|---|
| B | 1. bacilli | A. Singular |
| A | 2. vertebra | B. Plural |
| B | 3. diagnoses | |
| B | 4. phalanges | |
| A | 5. atrium | |
| B | 6. vertebrae | |
| A | 7. apex | |
| A | 8. bacillus | |
| B | 9. appendices | |
| A | 10. diagnosis | |
| A | 11. phalanx | |
| B | 12. atria | |
| A | 13. appendix | |
| B | 14. apices | |

# Chapter Application

## Labeling

For each of the following words, identify the word parts. The first one has been filled in for you as an example.

| Word | Prefix | Word Root or Combining Form | Suffix |
|---|---|---|---|
| prenatal | pre- | nat | -al |
| bradycardia | brady- | card | -ia |
| dyspepsia | dys- | (none) | -pepsia |
| leukemia | (none) | leuk | -emia |
| polyneuropathy | poly- | neur/o | -pathy |

## Dissecting and Building Medical Terms

Using Tables 3–1, 3–2, and 3–3 in the text chapter, fill in the missing spaces on this chart. The first one has been filled in for you as an example.

| | |
|---|---|
| leukocyte | white blood cell |
| urology | the study of urine |
| osteotome | instrument used for cutting bone |
| nephrologist | person who studies the kidney |
| cardiomyopathy | disease of the heart muscles |
| apnea | without breathing |
| bradykinesia | slow movement |

## Research Activity

1. Using the Internet or a medical dictionary, find five terms that have Latin or Greek meanings. Explain what the original terms from the original language were and how the ancient physicians assigned such meanings. (Think back to the example in the chapter about the uterus and the word *hysterical*.)

| | Term | Origin |
|---|---|---|
| a. | | |
| b. | | |
| c. | | |
| d. | | |
| e. | | |

2. Make flash cards of the common prefixes and suffixes found in Tables 3–1 and 3–2 in the text. On one side, write the word components and, on the other side, record the meanings of each. Quiz yourself at least once per day with the flash cards to familiarize yourself with this new language.

## Case Study with Critical Thinking Questions

One of your office responsibilities is to schedule patients for procedures. Today, you are working on charts that have been completed by the transcriptionist and need outside referrals. You contact the hospital to schedule a colposcopy for a patient and speak to Sarah. Sarah asks you for the age of the patient, last monthly period, and tentative diagnosis. You tell Sarah the patient is 55 years old, has no record of last monthly period, and the diagnosis is positive occult blood in the stool. Sarah asks you whether you are kidding and says the data you have provided is not a reason for a colposcopy. Then Sarah asks you what the patient's name is, to which you reply, "Jack Kelley." Sarah tells you there must be a mistake because a colposcopy is a procedure performed only on females.

1. Using Tables 3–2 and 3–3 in your text, determine the definition of colposcopy and write it here:
   The direct visual examination of the tissues of the cervix and vagina (colp/o means vagina, and –scopy means direct visual examination)

2. Using Tables 3–2 and 3–3 in your text, determine the definition of colonoscopy and write it here:
   The direct visual examination of the inner surface of the entire colon from the rectum to the cecum (colo/o means colon, and –scopy means visual examination)

3. Based on your answers to the previous question, what is the correct procedure Mr. Jack Kelley should be scheduled for and why? (You may consult the Internet or a medical dictionary if necessary.)
   Mr. Kelley should be scheduled for a colonoscopy because his diagnosis is positive occult blood in the stool (which refers to the gastrointestinal system). A colonoscopy would visualize his colon and possibly reveal the reason for blood in his stools.

CHAPTER 4

# Understanding and Building Medical Terms of Body Systems

## Words to Know Challenge

**Spelling: Each line contains three spellings of a word. Underline the correctly spelled word.**

| | | |
|---|---|---|
| 1. cholecystolithiases | cholecistolithiasis | cholecystolithiasis |
| 2. femural | femeral | femoral |
| 3. alopesia | alopecia | allopesia |
| 4. ascites | acsites | ascitis |
| 5. myacardium | myocardium | miocardium |
| 6. dialysis | dialisis | dyalysis |
| 7. visera | vicsera | viscera |
| 8. superphicial | superficial | superfiscial |
| 9. lukocyte | leukocite | leukocyte |
| 10. hyperglycemia | hyperglicemia | hyperglicymia |
| 11. polineuralgia | polyneuralgia | polynuralgia |
| 12. diafragm | diaphram | diaphragm |
| 13. hystologist | hystoligist | histologist |
| 14. atrium | attrium | atriam |
| 15. septim | septume | septum |
| 16. ventrical | ventricle | ventricall |
| 17. gastroentestinal | gastrointestinil | gastrointestinal |
| 18. jaundise | jandice | jaundice |
| 19. micturition | micturation | micsurition |
| 20. neumonitis | pneumonitis | pnumonitis |

**Matching: Match the terms in column I to their meanings in column II.**

| | COLUMN I | COLUMN II |
|---|---|---|
| F | 1. Feces | A. A red blood cell |
| L | 2. Dermatology | B. Vein that carries deoxygenated blood from the upper half of body |
| N | 3. Alimentary canal | C. A nerve cell |
| T | 4. External | D. Cells and fibers forming a body structure |
| I | 5. Bicuspid | E. Internal organs |
| A | 6. Erythrocyte | F. Stool, bowel movement |
| Q | 7. Chyme | G. Specializes in eye diseases and disorders |
| C | 8. Neuron | H. Pertaining to digestion |
| O | 9. Bolus | I. Mitral valve |
| B | 10. Superior vena cava | J. Inflammation of sebaceous glands, producing pimples |
| S | 11. Inferior vena cava | K. Loss of hair, baldness |
| R | 12. Nephron | L. Study of the skin |
| D | 13. Tissue | M. Specializes in obtaining blood samples |
| P | 14. Pyelonephritis | N. The intestinal tract |
| H | 15. Digestive | O. A mass of masticated food ready to be swallowed |
| M | 16. Phlebotomist | P. Inflammation of the kidney, pelvis, and nephrons |
| K | 17. Alopecia | Q. Mixture of partially digested food and digestive secretions |
| J | 18. Acne vulgaris | R. Structural and functional unit of kidney |
| G | 19. Ophthalmologist | S. Vein that carries deoxygenated blood from the lower half of the body |
| E | 20. Viscera | T. The outermost part of the body |

## Chapter Review

**Fill in the Blank: Complete the following sentences with the correct terms.**

1. Mrs. Holton fell and fractured the thigh bone of her leg. This body part is known as the femur
2. A histologist is a person engaged in the study of the microscopic structure of tissue.
3. The diaphragm is the muscle of breathing that separates the thorax from the abdomen.
4. Mrs. Silva developed a yellowish discoloration of the sclera and skin known as jaundice.
5. High blood sugar is known as hyperglycemia.
6. Cindy is scheduled to see a dermatologist, a physician who specializes in diagnosing and treating disorders and diseases of the skin.
7. Cindy's physician noted her skin condition characterized by inflammation of sebaceous glands that produced pimples and therefore diagnosed her with acne vulgaris.
8. The upper chamber of the heart is known as the atrium.
9. An inflammation of the cervix of the uterus is known as cervicitis.
10. A(n) leukocyte is a white blood cell, and a(n) erythrocyte is a red blood cell.
11. Mr. Romero was found to have inflammation of the lungs and therefore was diagnosed with pneumonitis also known as pneumonia.

12. The muscle layer of the heart is known as the myocardium.
13. Mr. Noto will undergo a valve replacement of his bicuspid, also known as the mitral valve.
14. The membranous wall dividing two cavities, as within the heart, is known as a septum.
15. The functional cells of the nervous system are known as neurons.
16. Mr. Smothers will undergo dialysis, which is the process of removing the products of urine from the blood by passage of the solutes through a membrane.
17. One of the two lower chambers of the heart is known as a ventricle.
18. The skin, hair, nails, and sweat glands comprise the integumentary system.
19. The valve in the right side of the heart, made up of three cusps or leaflets, is known as the tricuspid valve.

**Abbreviations Review: Match the abbreviations in column I to their meanings in column II and write which body system each abbreviation refers to. The first one has been completed for you as a guide.**

| | I | System | II |
|---|---|---|---|
| C | 1. ECG | cardiovascular | A. Chronic obstructive pulmonary disease |
| F | 2. UA | urinary | B. Osteoarthritis |
| H | 3. GU | urinary | C. Electrocardiogram |
| K | 4. TMJ | musculoskeletal | D. Gynecology |
| B | 5. OA | musculoskeletal | E. Electroencephalogram |
| G | 6. OU | the special senses | F. Urinalysis |
| A | 7. COPD | respiratory | G. Each eye |
| J | 8. IV | cardiovascular | H. Genitourinary |
| D | 9. GYN | reproductive | I. Urinary tract infection |
| E | 10. EEG | nervous | J. Intravenous |
| I | 11. UTI | urinary | K. Temporomandibular joint |

# Chapter Application

## Research Activity

Make flash cards of each system's combining forms, word roots, and abbreviations in the text. On one side, write the word components and, on the other side, record the meanings of each. Quiz yourself at least once per day with the flash cards to familiarize yourself with this new language.

## Case Study with Critical Thinking Questions

Mrs. Thornton was referred by her primary care physician to Dr. Laird because of her significantly drooping eyelids. She will likely have surgical repair of her eyelids as indicated by Dr. Laird.

1. What type of specialist is Dr. Laird? ophthalmologist
2. Review the tables in Chapters 3 and 4; what is the term for the eyelid surgery that will be performed on Mrs. Thornton? blepharoplasty

**Building Medical Terms: Using the definitions provided, build the following medical terms.**
(*Hint*: Use the tables from both Chapters 3 and 4 to help you recall all the word parts.)

1. Surgical removal of the appendix: appendectomy

2. Inflammation of the voice box: laryngitis

3. An abnormal condition with bluish discoloration: cyanosis

4. An instrument used to measure breathing: spirometer

5. A condition of gallstones in the gallbladder: cholecystolithiasis

6. The process of making an incision into the skull: craniotomy

7. A condition of scanty urine (production): oliguria

8. Inflammation of the lungs: pneumonitis (or pneumonia)

9. Newborn: neonate

10. Surgical puncture into the chest cavity: thoracocentesis (or thoracentesis)

11. A condition of blood clots: thrombosis

12. Pertaining to the first segment of the small intestine: duodenal

13. A fatty tumor: lipoma

14. The process of viewing the bladder with a lighted instrument: cystoscopy

15. Difficulty speaking: dysphagia

16. A deficiency of white blood cells: leukocytopenia

17. A condition of hardening: sclerosis

18. Pertaining to the kneecap: patellar

19. Inflammation of the eyelid: blepharitis

20. Removal of a testis: orchidectomy

**Defining Medical Terms: Use the definitions of the word parts to define each of the following medical terms. Remember the rules from the text.**

(*Hint*: Use the tables from both Chapters 3 and 4 to help you recall all the word parts.)

1. Myectomy: Removal of a muscle

2. Melanoma: A black tumor (skin cancer)

3. Meningitis: Inflammation of the meninges

4. Phlebotomy: Incision into a vein

5. Atherosclerosis: An abnormal condition of yellow fatty plaque (causing the hardening of the arteries)

6. Pyelonephritis: Inflammation of the renal pelvis of the kidney

7. Brochiectasis: Stretching (dilation) of the bronchi

8. Lymphedema: Abnormal accumulation of fluid in the lymph system

9. Splenomegaly: Enlargement of the spleen

10. Tracheostomy: An opening in the trachea

11. Anencephaly: A condition of having no brain (only a brain stem)

12. Aerobic: Pertaining to air

13. Esophagitis: Inflammation of the esophagus

14. Neuralgia: Pain in a nerve

15. Audiometry: The process of measuring hearing

16. Carcinogenesis: The onset (beginning) of cancer

17. Cardiorrhaphy: Suturing of the heart

18. Polyneuropathy: Disease of many nerves

19. Hematuria: Condition of blood in the urine

20. Hyperthyroidism: Condition of overactive (too much; excessive) thyroid

21. Colonoscopy: Visual examination of the colon by using a lighted instrument

22. Hypoglycemia: Below normal blood sugar

UNIT 3

# Medical Law and Ethics

C H A P T E R **5**

# Legal Issues

## Words to Know Challenge

**Spelling: Each line contains three spellings of a word. Underline the correctly spelled word.**

| | | |
|---|---|---|
| 1. misdeamenor | misdemenor | misdemeanor |
| 2. negligence | negligense | negilgense |
| 3. plantif | plaintiff | plaintif |
| 4. respondeat superior | respondent superior | respondat superior |
| 5. libal | lible | libel |
| 6. gardian | guardian | guardan |
| 7. fellany | fellony | felony |
| 8. jurisdiction | juridiction | juresdiction |

**Matching: Match the term in column I to its definition in column II.**

| | COLUMN I | COLUMN II |
|---|---|---|
| C | 1. Manslaughter | A. Spoken defamation of character |
| G | 2. Compensatory damages | B. Taking money or property belonging to another without the presence of the victim |
| H | 3. Punitive damages | C. The unlawful killing without malice of a human being |
| A | 4. Slander | D. Unlawfully taking money or goods of another from his or her person or in immediate presence by force or intimidation |
| B | 5. Burglary | E. Written defamation of character |
| D | 6. Robbery | F. Having the mental competency to make health care decisions |
| M | 7. Prosecution | G. Damages recovered in payment for actual injury or economic loss |

(continues)

| | | |
|---|---|---|
| L | 8. Felony | H. Damages awarded in a lawsuit as a punishment and example to others for malicious or fraudulent acts |
| J | 9. Statute | I. Legislation enacted by Congress |
| K | 10. Defendant | J. A written federal or state law enacted by Congress or a state legislature |
| I | 11. Federal law | K. The party sued in a civil lawsuit or the party charged with a crime in a criminal prosecution |
| E | 12. Libel | L. Crimes committed by people who intend to do significant harm to others, either through depriving them of their property or injuring them personally |
| F | 13. Capacity | M. In criminal law, the government attorney charging and trying the case against a person accused of a crime |

## Chapter Review

### Short Answer

1. Why is it important for medical assistants to be familiar with the law?
   Understanding the laws that apply to a medical office is important for medical assistants to protect themselves, their employer, and patients. Because medicine is closely regulated by state and federal law, it is necessary to be aware of statutes and regulations that define the procedures they are permitted to perform.

2. What are the four elements that must be present in a given situation to prove that a provider or professional practice is guilty of negligence?
   (1) a *duty* of care owed by the defendant to the plaintiff, (2) a *breach* of that duty by the defendant, (3) harm (*injury*) suffered by the plaintiff, (4) and that harm a result of the defendant's breach of duty (*causation*).

3. A contract may be either implied or express. Define what *implied* and *express* mean.
   An implied contract gives rise to contractual obligations by some action or inaction without verbally expressed terms. An express contract is an actual agreement between the parties, the terms of which are openly stated in distinct and explicit language, either orally or in writing.

4. Explain the difference between medical malpractice and negligence.
   Negligence is defined as not doing something a reasonable person would do or doing something that a reasonable person would not do. Malpractice is associated with professional misconduct and implies a greater duty of care to the injured person than the reasonable-person standard. The term implies that a doctor, nurse, or other licensed health care professional has special knowledge, which raises the expectations of society.

5. Crimes are divided into two categories. Identify and explain the difference between the two.
   A felony is a crime punishable by death or imprisonment in a state prison. A misdemeanor is a crime punishable by imprisonment in jail for less than one year and/or a fine.

6. Explain the concept of "standard of proof" and list the standard of proof in criminal law and civil law.
   The standard of proof in a civil case is the "preponderance of the evidence," whereas the standard of proof in a criminal case is "beyond a reasonable doubt."

7. List and explain the essential elements of a contract.
   A contract comes into being when an offer is made by one part and, accepted by another party, and consideration passes between them.

8. Read the following examples listed. Which are examples of express contracts and which are examples of implied contracts?
   a. A physician treats a patient in the emergency room for a fractured collarbone ______Implied______
   b. You hire your neighbor to clean your house and you confirm the deal with a handshake ______Express______
   c. A patient in your provider's office rolls up his sleeve to have his blood drawn ______Implied______
   d. Written agreement ______Express______
   e. A provider telling a patient that treatment results are guaranteed ______Express______
9. What is the Patient Self-Determination Act?
   The Patient Self-Determination Act, enacted in 1990, requires health care facilities to provide written information to each adult admission concerning patient rights under state law to make decisions concerning the acceptance or refusal of medical or surgical treatment.

# Chapter Application

## Research Activities

1. Visit the website for Caring Connections at www.caringinfo.org. Download a Durable Power of Attorney form from your state and another state. Compare the two forms. Do these forms differ? Take time to read the form from your state and practice (using a fictitious name) filling out the form.
2. Research the advance directives in your state and then write a brief essay, answering each of the following questions.
   a. When do you need to prepare an advance directive?
   b. What is the purpose of the advance directives?
   c. Which of the documents addresses a choice for being kept on life support? Does your state call this document by a different name?
   d. What is the purpose of the power of attorney? Does your state call this document by a different name?
   e. What other documents usually make up the advance directives?
   f. Do you need to have the power of attorney completed by a lawyer for it to be recognized as official?

## Case Studies with Critical Thinking Questions

### Scenario 1

You have just finished seeing Daniel Cho in the office. You are documenting information in his chart. You have accidentally written in some incorrect lab results.

1. Is it appropriate to change the chart entry? In this situation (to correct an erroneous entry), yes.
2. What steps must you take to write in the correct information? If a change is appropriate, the time and date of the change should be noted along with language specifically pointing out the change.

### Scenario 2

You receive samples in your office from pharmaceutical representatives. Rosalee Dunning cannot afford the cost of her blood pressure medication. She comes to you for samples.

1. May you give her samples? Why or why not?
   No, you may not give her samples without the provider's order. Assessing, diagnosing, and treating the patient is beyond your scope of practice. If she is given samples that needs to be recorded in her chart.

## Scenario 3

Mr. Wing has not paid the past-due fees owed your provider. Repeated letters have been sent. The amount owed is now in excess of $1200. You sent a final collection letter stating that he needs to make arrangements with your office to pay on the past-due amount. You receive no monies and no response. Your provider wants to terminate services to Mr. Wing.

1. What steps must you perform so your provider is not responsible for abandonment? The patient must be provided with written notice with reasonable time to find a new provider.

## Critical Thinking

The medical assistant has received a call from a patient. The patient is explaining her symptoms to the assistant, which include fever, chills, nausea, and stomach cramps. The medical assistant explains to the patient that the flu is going around and suggests some over-the-counter medications that might help. Type a one-to-two-page essay responding to the following prompts: Were the medical assistant's actions legal? Why or why not? List some legal implications that can evolve from this encounter.

Answers will vary, but students should demonstrate awareness of the consequences of not working within the legal scope of practice. This medical assistant is practicing medicine, which is not within the scope of practice.

CHAPTER 6

# Ethical Issues

## Words to Know Challenge

**Spelling: Each line contains three spellings of a word. Underline the correctly spelled word.**

| | | |
|---|---|---|
| 1. autonomy | automony | autonnomy |
| 2. vallues | valuse | values |
| 3. extrinics | extrinsic | extinsic |
| 4. benificense | benificence | beneficence |
| 5. intangible | intangeable | intangable |
| 6. distributive justice | distribitive justice | distributative justice |
| 7. morral | morale | moral |
| 8. intrinics | intrinsic | intrinsac |

**Fill in the Blank: Complete the following sentences with correctly spelled words from the Spelling section.**

1. In the context of health care, when we recognize the autonomy ________ of the patient, we are recognizing that the patient has the right to make decisions about his or her life, death, and health.
2. Moral ________ issues stem from a belief system in which one makes judgments about right and wrong.
3. There are a variety of approaches to the concept of distributive justice ; one of the approaches is an egalitarian approach (everyone gets an equal share).
4. Pride in knowing one is upholding the high standards of the organization is an example of an intrinsic ________ reward.
5. Receiving an end-of-year bonus for achieving the highest patient satisfaction scores is an example of an extrinsic ________ reward.
6. Organizational ethics represent the values ________ by which the organization conducts its business.
7. The concept of beneficence ________ requires people to do what is in the best interests of others.
8. The rules of conduct with respect to a particular class of actions are known as ethics ________.

## Chapter Review

**Matching: Match the ethical issues in column I with their descriptions in column II.**

| | COLUMN I | COLUMN II |
|---|---|---|
| G | 1. Cryonics | A. Surgical procedure in which tissue or whole organ is transferred from one species to another |
| F | 2. Human cloning | B. Attempts either to slow down or reverse the processes of aging to maximize life span |
| A | 3. Xenotransplantation | C. Killing an individual so that he or she will not suffer pain |
| H | 4. Suicide | D. Brain surgery carried out to ease the complications associated with mental or behavioral problems |
| B | 5. Life extension | E. Resorting to medical equipment to keep an individual alive |
| I | 6. Eugenics | F. Creating a genetically identical copy of a human |
| C | 7. Euthanasia | G. A process whereby the body of a seriously ill or deceased individual is frozen to stop the decomposition of tissues |
| D | 8. Psychosurgery | H. The act of killing oneself |
| J | 9. Surrogacy | I. Improving genetic qualities by means of selective breeding |
| E | 10. Life support | J. A process whereby a woman agrees to carry and deliver a child for a contracted party |

## Chapter Application

### Case Study with Critical Thinking Questions

#### Scenario 1

Jennifer observes one of the other medical assistants taking samples of a narcotic pain reliever and placing them in her pocket. When Jennifer confronts her coworker, the coworker states that everyone else takes samples, so she is taking some, too.

1. Is this a legal, ethical, or moral issue? It is against the law to steal but also a breach of moral and ethical behavior
2. Should Jennifer report this to her supervisor? Yes. Any suspected theft of drugs must be reported.
3. What could be the outcome for the medical assistant who took the samples? She could (and probably will) be fired.

#### Scenario 2

Gabrielle, a medical assistant, sees Roberto in the medical office where she works. Roberto works for Gabrielle's husband. Roberto and his wife Sally are also personal friends of Gabrielle and her husband Mark. Roberto has been out of work for the past few weeks because of severe back problems. That night at dinner, Mark asks her if Roberto will be able to return to work and when.

1. Is this a legal, ethical, or moral issue? It is primarily a legal issue; HIPAA has made it illegal to disclose confidential health information about patients to unauthorized sources.
2. What should Gabrielle do in this situation? Although Roberto is a family friend, it is not appropriate (and a legal violation) to talk about his health information, even to Gabrielle's husband. She should, therefore, not discuss Mark's condition with anyone, even her own husband.

### Scenario 3

You are standing at the time clock and notice another employee not only clocking herself out but also that of a fellow employee. You know for a fact that this other employee was not at work today. You check the time card and notice the other employee has "punched in" at the beginning of the day as well as recorded time for lunch. Because you work for a large company and the time cards are not completed at the facility, there is no way anyone at payroll will know whether this person worked.

1. Is this a legal, ethical, or moral issue? It is all three.
2. Who would you report this to? You should report this to the practice administrator or office manager.

## Critical Thinking

1. **Ethics and diversity:** Medical assistants are reminded to strive to provide the same quality of care to all their patients regardless of race or ethnicity and eliminate biased behavior toward any group of patients different from themselves. In the following space, explain why caring for a culturally diverse clientele is an ethical issue.
   Answers will vary but should include the following ideas: that medical assistants (as well as all medical professionals) have a responsibility to care for all people equally, without regard to race, creed, or color; medical assistants should recognize and respond appropriately to ideas and elements from other ethnic and cultural backgrounds that might be different from their own.
2. **Personal versus professional ethics:** Whatever your personal perspective might be with regard to ethical matters, you must adapt your personal views to comply with the ethical standards of your profession and the organization in which you are employed.
   a. Assess your personal belief system and upbringing. List two sources that have influenced your own personal ethics the most. Answers will vary.
   b. Review the "Ethics Check Questions" presented in this chapter and list the three questions to ask yourself when considering ethical issues: (1) What promotes the right of the patient to make determinations about his or her own health? (2) What is in the best health interests of the patient? (3) Is doing (or not doing) the act in question fair to others?
   c. Now, compare the AAMA Code of Ethics and Creed with the AMT Standards of Practice. What similarities and differences do you see? Answers will vary. Similarities might include focuses on confidentiality, professional advancement, putting patient needs first, and so on. Differences might include more specificity in the AMT Standard of Practice (such as "do not make or offer a diagnosis").
3. **Organizational ethics:** Go online and research a health care organization near you that has some form of a mission, vision, and values statement. In a one- to two-page essay, describe your findings and discuss conduct and action that you would express if you were an employee of that organization. (Some examples might include Northwest Health [www.nwhc.org], Ohio Health, www.ohiohealth.com], or Sutter Health [www.sutterhealth.org].) Answers will vary but typically include compassion, excellence, stewardship, integrity, respect, and so on.
4. **Your view:** Select one of the topics in Table 6–1 (or another ethical issue related to health care of your choosing) and discuss your personal opinion of the topic. Relate the opinion to the concepts discussed in the chapter (autonomy, beneficence, and distributive justice) if possible.

UNIT 4

# Professional Communications

CHAPTER 7

# Verbal and Nonverbal Communications

## Words to Know Challenge

**Spelling: Each line contains three spellings of a word. Underline the correctly spelled word.**

| | | | |
|---|---|---|---|
| 1. | active listening | activ listening | active listining |
| 2. | persepsion | perseption | perception |
| 3. | deniul | denial | danial |
| 4. | empirically | emperically | imperically |
| 5. | contrudict | contredict | contradict |
| 6. | intalectualization | intellectualization | intallectualization |
| 7. | mallinger | malinger | milinger |
| 8. | regresion | regerssion | regression |
| 9. | sublimination | sublimation | sublimation |
| 10. | compinsation | compensation | compensasion |
| 11. | incongruous | encongruos | incongrunous |
| 12. | suppression | supression | suppresion |
| 13. | rashonization | rationisation | rationalization |

**Fill in the Blank: Complete the following sentences with correctly spelled words from the Spelling section.**

1. Active listening is the participation in a conversation with another by means of repeating words and phrases or giving approving or disapproving nods.
2. It is possible to contradict a verbal message by an inappropriate or incongruous facial expression.
3. With rationalization, you justify behavior with socially acceptable reasons and tend to ignore the real reasons underlying the behavior.
4. When you malinger, you deliberately pretend to be sick to avoid dealing with situations that are unpleasant or cause anxiety.

5. Intellectualization is still another means of denying socially unacceptable feelings or strong feelings that cannot be easily expressed.

6. Suppression describes a condition in which the person becomes purposely involved in a project, hobby, or work so that a painful situation can be avoided.

**Matching: Match the term in column I to its definition in column II.**

| | COLUMN I | COLUMN II |
|---|---|---|
| C | 1. Articulate | A. To impart, as an idea; to transfer |
| G | 2. Conceptualize | B. To explain, translate; to determine the meaning |
| A | 3. Convey | C. To join together, as in a joint |
| F | 4. Distort | D. A defense mechanism of trying to blame another for one's own inadequacies |
| B | 5. Interpret | E. To force painful ideas or impulses into the subconscious |
| H | 6. Intuition | F. To misinterpret; to twist out of unusual shape |
| D | 7. Projection | G. To form a concept, thought, notion, or understanding |
| E | 8. Repression | H. The immediate knowing or learning of something without the conscious use of reasoning |

## Chapter Review

### Short Answer

1. Identify and describe the components of the standard communication model.
   The message originates with the sender. The encoder is the means of transmitting the communication. The message is then encoded and transmitted by the medium. The decoder is the means of deciphering the message into a form the receiver understands. The receiver is the intended target of the message.

2. There are several styles and types of verbal communication. In general, people process and communicate information in three basic ways. Identify and describe the three ways.
   (1) Visual – Visual people need to see pictures or see the information in writing; (2) Auditory – Auditory people learn by hearing; (3) Kinesthetic – Kinesthetic people think in terms of sensations or feeling, often move their hands when talking, and respond physically as well as verbally.

3. List six examples of nonverbal communication.
   Any six of the following: Perception, body language, facial expression, eye contact, gestures, distance, silence, appearance, attitude, therapeutic touch and relationship, and body language in general.

4. Explain perception and state its importance in communication.
   Perception in the context of communication can be considered as being aware of one's own feelings and the feelings of others. Anticipating the needs of others (patients, providers, coworkers) is part of perception.

5. Why do people use defense mechanisms?
   Defense mechanisms are largely unconscious acts we use to help us deal with unpleasant and socially unacceptable circumstances or behaviors. They help us make an emotional adjustment in everyday situations. We all use various defense mechanisms from time to time.

6. The following chart lists the commonly used behavioral defense mechanisms. Next to each defense mechanism, give an example of each. The first two rows have been filled in for you as examples.

| Defense Mechanism | Example |
|---|---|
| Repression | Not crying at a funeral because you've buried the emotions so deeply in the back of your mind. |
| Displacement | Yelling at your spouse for no reason after having a hard day at the office. |
| Suppression | Student answers will vary; an example is working late hours after the death of a close relative. |
| Projection | An obese patient who has gained a few pounds might blame the medical assistant by saying that the scales were set up or read incorrectly. |
| Rationalization | "I dieted strictly all day; therefore, it's okay to eat a couple of candy bars later in the evening after supper." |
| Intellectualization | Discussing all the facts and information about how to begin caring for an elderly relative to avoid dealing with true feelings of sadness. |
| Sublimation | A 30-year-old father who is a frustrated athlete, forcing his child to excel in a sport. |
| Compensation | A person who can no longer participate in sports because of illness or injury finds satisfaction in coaching. |
| Temporary withdrawal | Watching TV or reading excessively to avoid dealing with an issue are common types of withdrawal. |
| Daydreaming | This is a way to escape momentarily from reality and relax. |
| Malingering | You deliberately pretend to be sick to avoid dealing with situations that are unpleasant or cause anxiety. |
| Denial | A person just diagnosed with terminal illness does not accept the reality of it and believes that a recovery is certain. |
| Regression | During final exam week, a college student eats hot fudge sundaes as she did as a child with her mother whenever problems at school piled up. |
| Procrastination | Defined as "always putting off until tomorrow what you could do today." |

7. Explain what could happen to a person who habitually uses one or more of the defense mechanisms listed in this chapter.
It is detrimental to your character and your workload. Habitual use of defense mechanisms can veil reality and interfere with facing personal issues and crises as well as with open and honest communication with others.

8. List the five stages of understanding needs according to Maslow's hierarchical model. Then, identify which of the stages is the one in which the person tends to be a problem solver and places a great deal of emphasis on family and long-term relationships.
Physiological, safety, belongingness and love, esteem, self-actualization. Self-actualization is the highest stage; these people tend to be problem solvers.

9. Dr. Elisabeth Kübler-Ross described five stages of grieving. List the five stages.
Denial, depression, bribery, anger, and resolution

10. Describe the difference between positive and negative coping skills.
    Positive coping helps you through situations at nearly the same level of effectiveness as those who do not have the disadvantage. Use of negative coping skills can provide short-term relief or distraction but can ultimately worsen the circumstance.

11. List seven adaptive coping skills and seven nonadaptive coping skills.
    a. Adaptive: Any seven of the following: deep breathing, thought changing, diet and exercise, music, stretching, positive affirmations, talking, creating boundaries, journaling, spirituality, planning, humor, sleep, appropriate communications with others
    b. Nonadaptive: Any seven of the following: drinking, drug use, gambling, sex addiction, road rage, holding on to anger, inappropriate boundaries, isolation, obsessions, shopping over credit, over- or under-eating, avoiding responsibilities, "Yes, but . . ."

### Labeling

Identify the sections of the following communication process model.

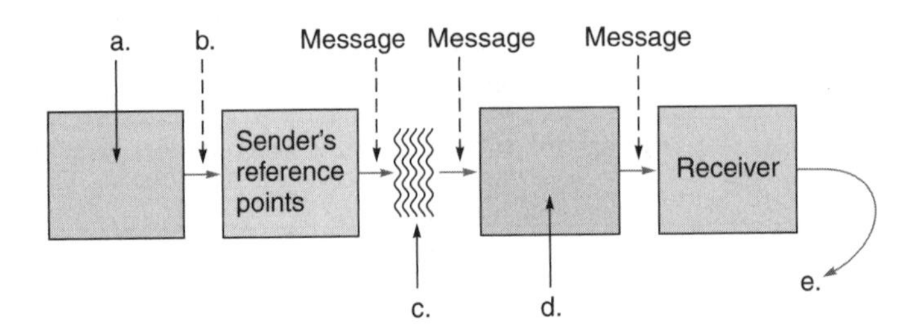


a. Sender

b. Message

c. Possible source of interference

d. Receiver's reference points

e. Feedback loop

## Chapter Application

### Video Case Study

Log on to the Premium Website and view the video for this chapter, "The Importance of Appearance." Develop a one- or two-page paper, responding to the following prompts:

- Discuss how Dee's peers responded to her, based on her appearance and body language.
- If you were sitting in that classroom, how would you have reacted to Dee?
- If Dee was working in an office with patients, how do you think they would have reacted?
- What does a negative appearance say about a person? What does a positive appearance say about a person?
- Why are appearance and personal grooming important, especially for a medical assistant?

## Case Studies with Critical Thinking Questions

### Scenario 1

A middle-aged woman is being seen in the office for insomnia and hot flashes. She says she cannot understand why these things are happening to her. She has always been a good sleeper, and she is always cold. She says that her friends tell her she is going through menopause, but she doesn't think she is old enough for that and refuses to believe them.

a. What type of coping skill is she using? She is using a defense mechanism so that she does not have to deal with the situation.

b. Which of these coping skills is this patient using? Repression and denial.

c. What can you do to help her accept her condition? Provide her with information regarding menopause and ways to help her control her symptoms.

### Scenario 2

You have had an extremely frustrating day at work but have managed to keep your emotions in check and get through the day. You have been very professional with both patients and coworkers even though you wanted to explode. When you get home, your kids ask you what you are making for dinner and you direct all your pent-up anger toward them.

a. Which defense mechanism are you using? Displacement

b. What can you do about reducing the stress at work? Be sure you take breaks during the day and perhaps leave the office for lunch. Find a relaxing hobby or exercise to relieve stress.

c. Which part of you did you use to respond to your children? Your social self

## Role-Play Activities

1. Research the boundaries and customs of several ethnic groups and prepare a brief report of your findings. Choose one of the ethnic groups you researched and, with a partner, demonstrate the correct communication techniques (especially nonverbal ones) you would employ when working with a patient from that ethnic group.

## Competency Practice: Nonverbal Communication

1. Learning to respond to nonverbal communication is a skill you will use daily as a medical assistant. Write a one- to two-page essay, using the following prompts:
   a. Identify systems that should be considered regarding nonverbal communication, such as space, posture, and so on.
   b. Describe and discuss the message perceived during patient interaction when eye contact is maintained, touch occurs, and the medical assistant maintains a smile.
   c. Discuss how important it is to respond to nonverbal communication and demonstrate how nonverbal communication can disrupt communication skills.
   d. Identify barriers to nonverbal communication.

CHAPTER 8

# Applying Communication Skills

## Words to Know Challenge

**Spelling: Each line contains three spellings of a word. Underline the correctly spelled word.**

| | | |
|---|---|---|
| 1. adovocasy | avdocacey | advocacy |
| 2. analitical | analytical | annalytical |
| 3. ascertive | assertive | asertive |
| 4. job description | job descripsion | job discription |
| 5. evalation | evolution | evaluation |
| 6. petty | pettie | pety |

**Matching: Now, using the preceding correctly spelled terms, write each word next to the correct definition.**

1. petty — small, having little value, mean, narrow-minded
2. assertive — confident; BOLD
3. evaluation — assessment; judgment concerning worth, quality, significance, or value of situation, person, or produce
4. advocacy — promoting and protecting the rights of patients, frequently through a legal process
5. analytical — characterized by a method of analysis, a statement of point-by-point contact
6. job description — set of clear expectations or duties to be performed

**Fill in the Blank: Complete the following sentences with Words to Know from this chapter.**

1. Taking a step-by-step approach helps one look realistically and logically at a problem. This method encourages analytical thinking and confident decision making.
2. Petty differences among coworkers should be settled with tact. Sharing enlightening experiences and significant events with other employees is a natural inclination but should be done during non-patient hours to protect the professional office setting.
3. We use many coping skills and defense mechanisms to deal with difficult or stressful situations. Another approach to handle interpersonal problems and concerns is to use critical thinking skills.

4. The tone of your voice goes a long way. Using a genuinely warm and caring tone is referred to as empathy to enhance the meaning of phrases.
5. Patient education in the ambulatory setting keeps patients healthier and medical conditions from worsening and can reduce the need for hospitalization. This can include verbal instructions, printed materials, or electronic format.
6. Reflective communication means to afford the opportunity to examine behaviors and interactions, act as a verbal mirror, and restate what the patient has said for clarification by all parties.

## Chapter Review

### Short Answer

1. What are the steps in applying critical thinking skills to a particular problem?
(1) Determine just what the problem is and write it down. Ask whether there is a contributing problem chain or a series of events. (2) Gather facts and ideas to help you decide what to do about it. (3) List possible decisions and what you think each outcome will be. (4) Prioritize your decisions and begin testing them one by one until results are satisfactory to you and others concerned.
2. Fill in the following grid, identifying resources and adaptations when working with special needs patients.

| | |
|---|---|
| Patients with special needs | Patients with special needs (deaf, blind, etc.) require unique and individually tailored methods to communicate instructions. Reflective (or mirrored) communication can be especially helpful for any patient requiring special attention. |
| Culturally diverse patients | It is critical to understand and respond with sensitivity to the needs and preferences diverse patients present at their health encounter. |
| Pediatric patients | Incorporate use of the four Es: *encouragement, empathy, enlistment,* and *education* to engage the child in health care matters. |
| Geriatric patients | Communication might require additional patience and skill. The normal aging process, involving sensory loss, decline in hearing or memory, retirement from work, and separation from family and friends, affects communication functionality. |
| Difficult or uncooperative patients | The best approach is to hold off any negative judgments and try your best to accommodate the requests. |

3. Often, your doctor will ask you to provide patient education. List three patient education formats.
Patient education can include verbal instructions, printed materials, or electronic formats. Many organizations have an education department or contract with a company to make materials readily available.
4. Describe the steps to follow when providing patient education.
You must first assess the patient's ability to comprehend the instructions. Use reflective (mirror) communication skills, repeating the clear, concise instructions to patient. It is often best to provide a written copy of the educational materials for the patient to take with him or her.
5. What is a patient advocate? Identify situations in which patients might benefit from intervention by a medical assistant.
Advocacy is the promotion and protection of the rights of patients, frequently through a legal process. An advocate can assist patients on any matter affecting their health, legal, or financial status such as medical bills and job discrimination related to the patient's medical condition.
6. What does it mean to be assertive when communicating in the medical office?
Assertive communication is a style by which individuals clearly state their opinions and feelings and firmly advocate for their rights and needs without violating the rights of others. These individuals value themselves, their time, and their emotional, spiritual, and physical needs and are strong advocates for themselves [and others], while being very respectful.

7. Describe relationships among the medical assistant, the employer, and coworkers and how to resolve conflict.
   The relationships must be kept professional and foster a collaborative team approach to health care. Conflict can be resolved by open communication. A great deal of conflict can be nipped in the bud by providing your coworker with a brief and sincere expression of empathy.

8. Explain methods of communicating information in the medical office.
   An intra-office memo is common. Most communications are now sent electronically (email or instant messaging). Some offices use a bulletin board as a means of intra-office communication. Staff meetings and employee evaluations are also methods of communicating.

9. State the purpose of:
   A. A staff meeting: Decisions concerning office policy changes are reached and problems are discussed. New ideas are expressed and exchanged. Allow members of the staff to get to more acquainted with each other. In-service training offered.
   B. An employee evaluation: A time and method for you and your employer to discuss your job performance. Evaluation forms outline the most important qualities and abilities needed for the job and include a section for strengths and weaknesses to be listed.

# Chapter Application

## Video Case Studies

1. Log on to the Premium Website and view the video for this chapter, "Personal Boundaries at Work." Then, develop a one-to-two-page paper, responding to the following questions:
   - What would you do if you had a friend at work with difficulty in his or her personal life?
   - Imagine if Macy was telling her difficulties to a patient with whom she had developed a close relationship. Would that be appropriate and professional? Why or why not?
   - Why is it important to protect your personal boundaries in communicating with others?

2. Log on to the Premium Website and view the video for this chapter, "Cultural Diversity." As a medical assistant, it is important to respect the diversity of all patients. Write a one-to-two-page essay, using the following prompts:
   - Discuss how biases in areas including gender, race, religion, age, and economic status can interfere with patient care.
   - Describe why it is important for medical office staff to assess and address possible biases to ensure quality patient care.
   - Perform a self-assessment of your own possible biases and then describe how each of the biases you identified can be overcome.

## Case Study with Critical Thinking Questions

During the past two weeks, Jennifer has noticed that her coworker, Maryn, has been making some charting errors. Jennifer is very concerned about patient care and does not want any of the patients to suffer because of these errors.

1. Who should Jennifer talk with about her concerns? She should talk to her office manager. The office manager will know the proper way to approach Maryn without implicating Jennifer.

## Competency Practice: Patient Advocacy

Using the Internet, research the process for obtaining a handicap placard in your state. Prepare a memo listing all relevant information regarding the process.

## Competency Practice: Patient Education

1. The provider has asked you to provide patient education on managing diabetes.
   a. Read the following patient education handout on managing diabetes.

**DOUGLASVILLE MEDICINE ASSOCIATES**
**5076 BRAND BLVD**
**DOUGLASVILLE, NY 01234**
**(123)456-7890**

### DIABETES

***Overview:*** Diabetes is a chronic disease of metabolism in which blood glucose levels are elevated. According to a 2005 government study, 20.8 million children and adults, or 7% of the U.S total population, has diabetes. It is estimated that at least 6.2 million of those individuals have yet to be diagnosed.

There are three types of diabetes:

- ***Type 1***: 5-10% of Americans diagnosed have this type of diabetes in which the body does not produce enough insulin. Insulin is a hormone that allows glucose to enter the cells of the body to be used as fuel. This type of diabetes is often seen in children.
- ***Type 2***: This type of diabetes comes from a resistance to insulin. In other words, the body produces enough insulin, but does not use it effectively. Most Americans diagnosed with diabetes have Type 2. This type of diabetes is often seen in adults.
- ***Gestational:*** 4% of all pregnant women develop this type.

There is also a condition called pre-diabetes in which the blood glucose levels are elevated, but not high enough for a diagnosis of Type 2 diabetes. Approximately 41 million Americans have pre-diabetes.

**Possible Complications from Diabetes:**

- Heart attack
- Stroke
- Kidney disease, which can lead to kidney failure and the need for dialysis
- High blood pressure
- Male Impotence

**Treatment**

Type 2 diabetes can often be managed by diet, exercise, oral hypoglycemics, and/or insulin. It is important to maintain good blood pressure control and to lower cholesterol levels.

***What kind of foods should you eat?***

Healthy food choices are important in controlling your glucose levels. The Diabetic Food Pyramid is a helpful tool in determining what to eat. Here are some helpful tips based on the pyramid:

- Eat lots of fruits and vegetables: However, be aware of the sugar content in some fruits.
- Eat whole grains rather than processed grains, like brown rice and whole wheat pasta.

- Eat dried beans.
- Include fish in your diet at least 2-3 times per week.
- Eat lean meats.
- Choose non-fat dairy products.
- Drink lots of water and choose sugar-free "diet" drinks.
- Use liquid oils for cooking.
- Cut down on desserts and high-calorie foods like chips.
- Watch your portion sizes.

***Other Practices to Control Diabetes***

See your physician on a regular basis and consistently monitor your blood glucose. Record results onto a log and share your results with your physician. It is important to keep weight regulated and to alert the physician when symptoms worsen or new symptoms appear. Have regular eye exams and podiatric (foot) exams. Even though diabetes can be a debilitating disease, you can play an active role in delaying the onset of debilitating factors or even the prevention of certain factors.

***Resources:***
**www.diabetes.org** (American Diabetes Association)
**http://diabetes.niddk.nih.gov/index.htm** (National Diabetes Information Clearinghouse)

b. Role-play with a partner a patient education session on managing diabetes. Be sure to use language the patient can understand as well as appropriate techniques of effective verbal and nonverbal communication.
c. Finally, using the following space, document the patient education session in the patient's medical record.

**PROGRESS NOTE**

Patient Name: ______________________ DOB ____________

| DATE/TIME | PROGRESS NOTES ALLERGIES |
|---|---|
| | |
| | |
| | |
| | |
| | |

SECTION 2

# The Front Office

UNIT 5

# Business Communications

CHAPTER 9

# Telephone Communications

## Words to Know Challenge

**Spelling: Each line contains three spellings of a word. Underline the correctly spelled word.**

| | | |
|---|---|---|
| confirmed | confired | confirmd |
| emputhy | empathie | empathy |
| ettiquete | ettiquette | etiquette |
| ecspress | express | escpress |
| fax | facs | facts |
| patient portal | patience portal | patience portle |
| pirsonallity | personallity | personality |
| screening | screaning | skreaning |
| treage | triage | treaje |
| antissipate | anticipate | antisipate |

**Fill in the Blank: Complete the following sentences with correctly spelled words from the Spelling section.**

1. Because the phone call is often the first contact a patient has with the office, your manner of speaking and the empathy you convey are a part of establishing an appropriate image of the practice.
2. An established phone screening manual (sometimes called a triage manual) should be kept near each phone for reference so that each assistant who answers the phone will ask standard questions and give the standard response that has been pre-authorized by the provider.
3. You must anticipate the needs of the patient and provider by asking the proper questions to route accurate information to the appropriate person with the level of urgency required.
4. Appointments should be confirmed by reading the scheduled time back to the patient after it has been recorded in the appointment book or scheduling system.
5. The general rule is that a medical assistant does not give out information or call in a prescription without the express direction of the physician.
6. Professional etiquette dictates that the provider will not keep a colleague waiting unless he or she is involved with an emergency or surgical procedure.

7. Your voice is part of your personality, but over the phone, your voice is you.
8. Messages from the answering service need to be returned in the order of importance within an appropriate and reasonable time period. Remember to check the fax machine and patient portal for other patient-related messages.

## Chapter Review

### Short Answer

1. Explain the proper protocol (steps) for answering the telephone in the medical office, including an example.
Answering each call as soon as possible—at least by the third ring—using customer service skills, with a smile. An example: "Good morning, Central Medical Center, Ellen speaking, how may I help you?"
2. What does screening mean?
Logically proceeding through a preapproved list of questions that will reveal the caller's condition and help determine, if necessary, how soon the patient should be seen by a physician.
3. For each type of call in the following list, identify who it should be routed to: Provider; take a Message for the Provider; Clinical Medical Assistant; or Administrative Medical Assistant.
   a. Critical lab results: Message for Provider; Provider
   b. A patient with a question about insurance: Administrative Medical Assistant
   c. A patient calling for a routine prescription refill: Clinical Medical Assistant
   d. A patient wanting some medical advice: Provider
   e. Another physician: Provider
   f. A patient needing to schedule an appointment: Administrative Medical Assistant
   g. A patient upset about his last visit: Message for Provider
   h. A patient with a question about a statement in the mail: Administrative Medical Assistant
   i. A patient having a heart attack: Provider
4. List at least six pieces of information that should be included in all telephone messages.
Any six of the following: Date, time, name, date of birth, M/F, phone number(s), detailed and accurate message, whether the message is urgent, medical assistant's name or initials
5. Fill in the following chart, identifying four types of telephone calls a medical assistant might have to answer in the medical office; explain how each should be handled. The first one has been filled in for you as an example.

| Type of Phone Call | How It Should Be Handled |
|---|---|
| Appointments | Positively identify the patient (with two identifiers) and confirm the last appointment date. Assess the type of appointment needed and note in the schedule. |
| Prescriptions | Write or document in the EHR the request for prescriptions, in legible handwriting with detailed accuracy. A medical assistant does not give out information or call in a prescription without the express direction of the provider. |
| Lab/Test Results | Observe your office policy for releasing test or lab results. Attach the results of the test, lab result, or consult report for the provider to review along with the message for the provider to call the patient. |
| Personal Calls | When a physician telephones to speak to your provider or employer, politely ask the caller for his or her name and inform the provider. Ask whether the call is regarding a patient and whether you should pull the chart. |
| General Business Calls | Follow provider or employer instructions on how to handle calls from family members, business associates, and salespeople. Calls from attorneys requesting information about a patient must be handled with great caution. |

6. List at least four types of community resources for patients' health care needs and four types of emergency services and how to research current information.
 Answers will vary but can include: CDC, Medicare, Department of Motor Vehicles, Senior Services, Home Health Services, Lab services and locations, Diabetes programs, Women's health center, Osteoporosis center, Research department, Child Protective Services, Emergency Medical Services, Education and training services, and Public Health Services. Locate these resources through such means as office materials and directories, the Internet, intranet, and telephone book.

**Matching: Match the tone of voice in column I to the translation in column II.**

| | COLUMN I | COLUMN II |
|---|---|---|
| C | 1. Monotone flat voice | A. "I don't believe what I'm hearing." |
| E | 2. Slow speed and low pitch | B. "I'm angry and not open to input." |
| D | 3. High-pitched and empathic voice | C. "I'm bored and have absolutely no interest in what you're talking about." |
| B | 4. Abrupt speed and loud tone | D. "I'm enthusiastic about this subject." |
| A | 5. High-pitch combined with drawn-out speed | E. "I'm depressed and want to be left alone." |

# Chapter Application

## Case Studies with Critical Thinking Questions

### Scenario 1

Jennifer, the clinical medical assistant, answers the telephone for the receptionist, who is busy, and encounters a patient who is very upset and anxious. The patient quickly informs Jennifer that her 3-year-old daughter has fallen and is bleeding badly. The patient tells Jennifer her name and phone number but hangs up before Jennifer can find anything to write with or record the message on.

1. How should Jennifer handle this situation? She should obtain a pen and message pad and call the patient back immediately to verify that the information is correct.
2. How can she ensure that this will not happen again? She should make sure always to have a pen and message pad beside each phone in the office and to keep the patient on the phone to obtain all necessary information.
3. What should Jennifer do before answering the phone the next time? She should make sure she has the correct supplies for documenting a telephone message.

### Scenario 2

Several of the telephone lines are ringing at once, and Sarah is already on the line with one patient who needs to have an important question answered immediately.

1. What should Sarah do about answering the other lines? She should place the first caller on hold to answer the second line.
2. Should she continue to talk with the first caller and let the other lines ring? She should attempt to answer all lines as soon as possible and then take care of the calls in the order in which they were received.
3. What device could help in this situation? A telephone message device or a phone menu answering device could help.

## Competency Practice

1. Read the situations in A and B out loud in class and role play how you would handle them.
Answers will vary. You might want to guide the situations or use this as a class activity.

**A. "I Have to See the Doctor—Today!"**

| | |
|---|---|
| Doctor's Identity: | (Use names of local providers or make up) |
| Solo or Group: | Two-provider partnership |
| Specialty | Family practice |
| Time: | 8:30 a.m. |
| Situation: | Both providers are on hospital rounds and are not expected until 10:00 a.m. The appointment book is full. |
| Patient: | (Insert name of student or fictitious name), a patient since infancy |

"I need an appointment today—right away. I'm leaving for college tomorrow, and the doctor just has to see me. Just for a minute. I need a quick physical and a form filled out. It's nothing really. I can't register for class unless the doctor sees me. I just have to have an appointment. I know this is last-minute—but just this once, please. Certainly, you understand; you have to."

**B. Call to Notify Patient**

| | |
|---|---|
| Doctor's Identity: | (Use names of local providers or make up) |
| Solo or Group: | Two-provider partnership |
| Specialty | OB/GYN |
| Time: | 1:00 p.m. |
| Situation: | Both providers have called to say that they will be late in returning to the office. It seems all the babies in town decided to be born today. Dr. A, anticipating a cesarean section, says he might not be in at all. Dr. B says he will be at least one hour late and maybe longer. Office protocol is to notify patients, who have not yet arrived, of the delay. |
| Patient: | (Insert fictitious name) |

You call Mrs. ____________________ and tell her of the delay. She has an appointment for 3:00 p.m., which she made about three weeks ago. You can tell from the tone of her voice that she is upset. The medical assistant knows from past experience that the best thing to do is cancel Mrs. ____________________'s appointment and reschedule her. This cannot be done. About the earliest time that Dr. ____________________ can see Mrs. ____________________ will be 5:00 to 5:30 p.m. Mrs. ____________________ is not enthusiastic about either alternative.

# CHAPTER 10

# *Written Communications*

## Words to Know Challenge

**Spelling: Each line contains three spellings of a word. Underline the correctly spelled word.**

| | | | |
|---|---|---|---|
| 1. | ajective | addjective | adjective |
| 2. | adverb | avderb | advirb |
| 3. | anotate | annotate | anottate |
| 4. | apostrophe | appostrofe | aposstrofee |
| 5. | claws | clausse | clause |
| 6. | conjunction | conjunsion | conjuntion |
| 7. | contracktion | contraction | contration |
| 8. | domestic | domestick | domestik |
| 9. | ellipsis | elypsis | ellypsis |
| 10. | ettiquete | etiquete | etiquette |
| 11. | highfen | hyphen | highphen |
| 12. | misspelled | mispelled | misspeled |
| 13. | postscript | poskript | poscript |
| 14. | proofread | porfread | poorfread |
| 15. | puntcution | punktuation | punctuation |
| 16. | watermarck | waterrmark | watermark |

**Matching: Now, using the correctly spelled terms from the Spelling section, write each word next to the correct definition.**

1. Compose ______ to form by putting together; creating
2. Noun ______ the name of anything, such as a person, a place, or object, an occurrence, or a state
3. Stationery ______ writing materials, especially paper and envelopes
4. Adjective ______ a word that describes, limits, or restricts a noun or pronoun

(continues)

5. Adverb a word that commonly ends in -ly and answesr questions
6. Context the part of a written or spoken statement that surrounds a particular word or passage and can clarify its meaning
7. Conjunction a word that connects words, phrases, and clauses
8. Word processor a system or machine that produces typewritten documents
9. Verb a word or word group that expresses action or a state of being
10. Correspondence communication by the exchange of letters

**Fill in the Blank: Complete the following sentences with Words to Know from this chapter.**

1. A medical assistant should be able to compose (write) the necessary letter after receiving the specific information desired so that all the physician has to do is provide a signature.
2. To make sentences easier to read and to tell a reader when you come to the end of a thought, a variety of marks called punctuation are used.
3. All written communication must be proofread before it is sent. This is a process of carefully reading printed material and marking errors for correction.
4. A watermark appears on bond paper and should read across the paper in the same direction as the typing.
5. For domestic mail, the post office (city), state, and ZIP code or ZIP + 4 should appear, in that order, on the bottom line of the address.
6. Prewritten form letters can be developed and stored electronically on computers. The master of each hardcopy form letter is stored electronically and in a file folder.
7. A template is an electronic file (or preprinted document) with a predesigned, customized, format.

## Chapter Review

### Short Answer

1. List seven types of correspondence medical assistants might need to prepare.
Any seven of the following: Note; IOCs; Form letters; Information sheets; Business letters; Professional letters; Personal letters; Email
2. Name at least four instances when form letters might be indicated.
Any four of the following: (1) Return to work; (2) Annual diagnostic examination reminders; (3) Delinquent account reminder; (4) Office visit verification; (5) Sports participation approval; (6) Information to referred patients
3. Explain the purpose of information sheets and list two examples.
To provide specific written instructions regarding examinations and diagnostic tests performed. They reinforce the explanation and serve as a reminder for patients after they leave the office. Some examples are: cast care, fever control, patient preparation for a particular test, or what to expect when the test is performed
4. List three guidelines to avoid acquiring a virus through email.
(1) Check the sender. Do not open mail from an unfamiliar source. (2) Never open mail with .exe or .vbs suffixes unless you are anticipating them. (3) Use antivirus software but still be vigilant
5. List the pros (at least four) and cons (at least four) of using email.

   a. The pros:
   Any four of the following: (1) Enables communication with many people simultaneously by using multiple addresses; (2) Leaves a trail, so the history of a conversation can be traced; (3) Provides an easy reference to past communications; (4) Doesn't require customers be available to send them a message; (5) Saves time when you need to communicate but don't have time for small talk; (6) Enables you to attach pertinent file without the delay of other mail delivery systems

b. The cons:

Any four of the following: (1) Isn't the best medium for communicating certain emotional or highly charged issues; (2) Often is overused as a substitute for phone and in-person communications; (3) Isn't as secure, private, and confidential as people think; (4) Can be used in court of law as evidence and increases company liability and risk; (5) Can be problematic when dealing with time-sensitive issues that require immediate responses

6. Explain how HIPAA affects correspondence.

   HIPAA rules defined security of patients' personal health information (PHI) as contained in medical records. HIPAA protects the integrity of the information and prevents disclosure to entities that are not directly involved with the provision of health care.

7. Name and give examples of the eight parts of speech.

   a. Noun – The name of anything, such as a person, a place, an object, an occurrence, or a state; examples: bird, house, stethoscope, doctor

   b. Pronoun – A substitute for a noun; examples: I, you, we, she

   c. Verb – A word or word group that expresses action or a state of being; examples: draw, medicate, prescribe

   d. Adjective – Describes, limits, or restricts a noun or pronoun; examples: good, big, orange

   e. Adverb – Modifies a verb, adjective, or another adverb. Adverbs commonly end in -ly and answer questions; examples: softly, well, quickly

   f. Preposition – Shows the relations of an object to some other word in the sentence; examples: above, below, into

   g. Conjunction – Connects words, phrases, and clauses; examples: and, but, or

   h. Interjection – Expresses strong feeling or emotion. These words are usually followed by an exclamation point or a comma; examples: yikes! wow!

8. Name and describe the 12 components of a business letter.

   a. The letterhead: Preprinted name, complete address, and phone number (optional)

   b. Dateline: Date letter is dictated—or composed if not dictated

   c. Inside address: Address of person to whom the letter is being sent

   d. Salutation: The greeting to the recipient

   e. Reference: To identify what or about whom the letter is concerning

   f. Body: The content of the letter

   g. Complimentary closing: Expresses the closing of the letter

   h. Sender's signature: Signature of the writer

   i. Title: Writer's title if appropriate (e.g., Vice President, Director)

   j. Reference initials: Initials of the letter typist

   k. Enclosures: Any identified materials to be sent with the letter

   l. Copies: "cc," meaning "carbon copy," identifies another person or persons to whom a copy of the letter is sent.

9. Explain how to sort, open, and annotate incoming mail.

   a. Sort: Sort into categories, such as mail from patients, physicians, insurance companies, and miscellaneous sources. Other classes of mail, such as magazines, professional journals, and newspapers, should be separated from drug samples and advertisements.

   b. Open: Stack all envelopes so that they are facing in the same direction. Open each letter along the flap edge, being careful to remove all contents from each envelope. Be sure the contents contain the same name and return address shown on the envelope.

   c. Annotate: Follow office policy on whether to keep the envelope with the mail received (keep if needed to help identify the contents). Date-stamp the correspondence and attach any enclosures. If an enclosure is missing, write "None" after the "Encl." notation and circle it to indicate need for follow-up.

10. Describe how mail received during vacation might be handled.
Discuss with provider what to do with urgent mail before he or she leaves. Carefully read all mail and decide how each piece will be handled. Never send an original document by mail; send only copies and comply with HIPAA regulations. Number the envelopes consecutively and keep track of what you send so that you can be sure all the mail is received.

11. List six classifications of mail.
Express; Priority; First-class; Periodicals; Standard mail (A); Standard mail (B)

12. Fill in the following chart, indicating the purpose of each mail service.

| Mail Service | Purpose |
|---|---|
| Certificate of mailing | To show evidence of mailing; for time-sensitive material such as meeting a deadline and for verification of mailing when a return receipt is not necessary |
| Certified mail | Provides proof of mailing and delivery of the mail; the sender receives a mailing receipt when the item is mailed, and a receipt of delivery is kept at the recipient's post office |
| Registered mail | Provides protection for valuables and important mail; insurance up to $25,000 can be purchased for items sent by registered mail |
| Restricted delivery | Mail is delivered only to a specific addressee or someone authorized to receive mail for the addressee |
| Return receipt | Proof of delivery; contains the signature of the receiver and the date |

**Matching: Match the following types of correspondence that would be appropriate for the stated situation.**

Interoffice communication
Informal note
Personal letter
Professional letter
Business letter
Information sheet

Business letter 1. Information sent to a referred patient
Professional letter 2. Correspondence to colleagues on hospital board
Informal note 3. Congratulations to a friend
Information sheet 4. Instructions for a diagnostic procedure
Personal letter 5. Request for membership information at a golf club
Business letter 6. Request to accountant for mid-year status
Intra-office communication 7. Employee memo regarding change in office insurance benefits
Professional letter 8. Request for medical practice reciprocity in another state

## Chapter Application

### Research Activity

The United States Postal Service offers the ability to send mail from the home or office without going to the post office. Go online and research the USPS Website and Stamps.com. Type answers to the following questions

1. What is Stamps.com?
2. What does Stamps.com allow you to print?
3. How much does the service cost per month?
4. Can Stamps.com save money for a medical office?
5. How can you acquire the service?

## Case Studies with Critical Thinking Questions

### Scenario 1

The office manager has asked you to take care of the incoming mail next week while he is gone on vacation. You have never had this responsibility before, but you think you can handle it.

1. Which mail needs to be handled immediately when received? Any mail marked special delivery or special messenger is urgent and should be looked at immediately.

2. What do you do with the provider's personal mail? Office policy will dictate, but usually the provider's unopened personal mail is placed on his or her desk.

3. What kind of categories might your office use to sort mail? Mail from other providers, patient mail, insurance company mail, journal and periodicals. Any drug samples should be separated, logged in, and stored appropriately in a secure area.

### Scenario 2

Your employer has received the consultation on Mr. Green from Dr. Blosser. He asks you to make a copy and send it to Mr. Green. When you look at the consult, you realize it is quite personal in nature.

1. What do HIPAA regulations say about patients' information? The patient's personal information must be protected. Only authorized persons should have access to the information. It might be smart to make a note on the chart that you were instructed by the provider to send the document if you are not authorized to handle this type of information.

2. How can you be sure Mr. Green receives the consult? Using ordinary mail or fax presents the possibility that someone else might get the information. Scanning and attaching it to an email could also expose it to someone else. By using restricted mail, you can be assured that only Mr. Green will receive the letter.

3. What should you check before sending mail to a patient's home? Patients are usually asked to sign a CCP form indicating who may be given information about the patient. This form should be provided in the chart. If a form on file indicates that the spouse, children, or others may receive information, then ordinary mail or fax may be used.

## Competency Practice: Prepare a Letter

Following information in the textbook on style, punctuation, and mailable standards, prepare a letter following the instructions. A letterhead is provided on the next page for use in your printer, or you may enter information on a computer-generated letter. The letter is to Robert Jones, MD, 5000 North High Street, Yourtown, US 43200. The name of the patient is Juan Gomez. Use full block style, as shown in Figure 10–3 A in the textbook, as well as proper capitalization, punctuation, and placement. (Hint: Some words are misspelled, so you will need to use your proofreading skills additionally.) The date is November 15, 20XX.

Dear dr jones

You're patient juan gomez was first seen October 7 complaining of severe tinnitus in both ears.

On physical examination his hearing was 15/20 right ear 13/20 left ear. An audiogram was made which showed considerable hearing loss of high tones. Mr. gomezs complaints of tinnitus and decreased hearing are in accordence with audiometric and clinical findigns of beginning degeneration of his audio nerve. In all probability this condition has been caused by the loud noise he has encountered in his work.

despite treatment his hearing has not increased and tinnitus persists. I believe he should be refered for a hearing asisstance device.

thank you for referring mr gomez.

very truly yours

**SAMUEL E. MATTHEWS, MD**
**100 EAST MAIN STREET, SUITE 120**
**YOURTOWN, US 43200**

CHAPTER 11

# Computers and Office Equipment

## Words to Know Challenge

**Spelling: Each line contains three spellings of a word. Underline the correctly spelled word.**

| | | |
|---|---|---|
| 1. dicktation | dictation | diktation |
| 2. incoder | encorder | encoder |
| 3. faximilie | faxsimilie | facsimile |
| 4. periferral | peripheral | peripherral |
| 5. interface | intraface | interfface |
| 6. erganomic | ergonomic | ergenomic |

**Fill in the Blank: Complete the following sentences with Words to Know from this chapter.**

1. Facsimile machines can be used by hospitals, providers' offices, and clinics to send and receive information regarding patients over telephone lines.
2. Computer hardware includes the hard disk drive, the CPU, the monitor, and the keyboard.
3. Anything you plug into a computer, such as a printer or scanner, is a peripheral.
4. Software refers to the programs containing instructions to the computer that enable it to perform tasks.
5. Ergonomic programs provide a work environment that promotes wellness and minimizes musculoskeletal disorders.
6. Encoder software is available as a powerful application for all CPT®, HCPCS, and ICD-9-CM code sets and Medicare coding guidelines.
7. The hardware and software that enable individual computers and components to interact is known as the interface.
8. An electronic health record (EHR) captures all patient health information harvested from one or more encounters in any health care delivery system (such as a medical office, hospital, urgent care center, and so on).

# CHAPTER REVIEW

## Short Answer

1. Describe the difference between computer hardware and software.
The hardware refers to the hard disk drive, the CPU, the monitor, and the keyboard. Software refers to the programs containing instructions to the computer that enable it to perform tasks. You interact with the software to produce correspondence, maintain records, calculate financial statements, and perform many other tasks.

2. Give two examples of hardware and two examples of software.
Answers will vary but can include: Hardware—CPU, monitor, keyboard, hard disk drive. Software—Word processing (such as Microsoft Word or Apple Pages), spreadsheets (such as Microsoft Excel or Apple Numbers), music (such as iTunes or Windows Media Player), presentation software (such as Microsoft PowerPoint or Apple KeyNote). Other answers are possible.

3. Define application software and application suites. Include examples in your answer.
Software enables users to interact with the computer to perform specific tasks such as word processing, managing databases, preparing spreadsheets, and playing music or videos. An application suite includes multiple applications bundled together, often with related functions. Example suites will vary but can include Microsoft Office® or Apple iWorks®.

4. Explain why caution should be taken when gathering information from the Internet.
The Internet contains a wealth of information, but not all of it is good information. Anyone can create a Web page, so serious problems can be associated with some online sources. Patients should be warned especially about going to Websites to seek medical advice or purchase medications.

5. Describe four guidelines for finding credible information on the Internet.
(1) Check the source for professional affiliations or credentials. (2) Be cautious about personal testimonies from users because they often are receiving monetary compensation for making statements. (3) Watch for dates of the information; the information might be very old and no longer valid. (4) Use analytic and critical thinking to interpret scientific studies or reports.

6. Explain computer term downtime and describe when this term would be used.
A period of lost work time during which a computer is not operating or is malfunctioning because of machine failure. Downtime procedures and forms are critical to keep the practice running smoothly (such as preprinted billing sheets, manual scheduling process, EHR downtime chart note).

7. Fill in the following chart, describing common software applications used in medical offices.

| Software Application | Description/Capabilities |
|---|---|
| Practice management | Manages the operations of a medical practice. The functionality of practice management software varies by program but, typically, enables a medical office to schedule appointments, record patient demographics and insurance information, process claims, perform insurance and billing routines, and generate financial reports. |
| Electronic health records | Captures all patient health information harvested from one or more encounters in a health care delivery system. EHR software enables providers to document all care received by the patient—tests performed, treatments prescribed, patient education given, and so on. Electronic health records (EHR) software often integrates with practice management software. |
| Encoder software | Encoder software is available as a powerful application for all CPT®, HCPCS, and ICD-9-CM code sets and Medicare coding guidelines. |

**Matching: Match the office equipment in column I with the appropriate function in column II.**

| | COLUMN I | COLUMN II |
|---|---|---|
| B | 1. Most machines can be set to use either letter- or legal-sized paper and duplicate a document. | A. Fax machine |
| E | 2. A small electronic device that is activated by a telephone signal. | B. Copy machine |
| D | 3. An electronic device, operating under the control of instructions stored in its own memory unit, which can accept and store data, perform mathematical and logical operations on that data without human intervention, and produce output from the processing. | C. Transcriber |
| A | 4. The machine scans a document and converts the image to electronic impulses that are transmitted over the telephone lines. | D. Computer |
| C | 5. Providers dictate their notes following patients' appointments, and the medical assistant uses this machine for the chart notes. | E. Pager |
| F | 6. The machine produces hard copies from computer files. | F. Printer |

# Chapter Application

## Research Activity

Search the Internet for information regarding Dragon Naturally Speaking® (voice recognition software) and prepare a report on the advantages, disadvantages, and cost to implement.

UNIT 6

# Beginning the Patient's Record

CHAPTER 12

# Scheduling Appointments and Receiving Patients

## Words to Know Challenge

**Spelling: Each line contains three spellings of a word. Underline the correctly spelled word.**

| | | |
|---|---|---|
| 1. matricks | mattrix | matrix |
| 2. unstructured | unstrictured | unstructered |
| 3. waive | wave | weave |
| 4. cloustering | clustering | clustaring |
| 5. modified wave | modified waive | modifide wave |
| 6. streeming | streming | streaming |
| 7. oblitarate | obliterrate | obliterate |
| 8. single-booking | singel-booking | signel-booking |
| 9. open ours | open hours | opin hours |
| 10. double-bookking | duble-booking | double-booking |
| 11. utilization | utilisation | utilazition |

**Matching: Using the correct spellings from the preceding list, enter the correct terms next to the following appropriate description.**

| | |
|---|---|
| Wave | 1. Patients scheduled during first ½ hour, last ½ hour left open for same-day appointments |
| Single-booking | 2. Patient booked for a specific amount of time |
| Streaming | 3. Appointments time allocated based on need |
| Clustering | 4. Scheduling patients for a specific type of visit (physical, new patient, and so on) |
| Modified wave | 5. Scheduled time as a wave, except in the last ½ hour, when appointments are spaced at 10- to 20-minute intervals |
| Double-booking | 6. Same appointment is given to more than one patient |

(continues)

| | |
|---|---|
| Open hours | 7. No appointment is needed; patients seen in order of arrival |
| Unstructured | 8. Open block of time |

## Chapter Review

### Short Answer

1. Name three criteria or pieces of information the medical assistant needs to obtain when making appointments. Any three of the following: Correctly spelled name, reason for visit, contact phone number, morning or afternoon preference, new or existing patient

2. When scheduling an inpatient admission, name at least five items that should be provided to the hospital representative.
Any five of the following: Name, age, date of birth, gender, marital status, Social Security number, address, phone number, insurance information, guarantor information, employer information, referring provider information, diagnosis, plan of care, preadmission testing, special procedures required during hospitalization

3. Describe how the medical assistant should handle a patient who arrives without an appointment.
Explain that appointments are necessary. If a time slot is available and appropriate for the reason for visit, offer it to the patient, being polite but clear that this is not the usual practice. If no time slot is available, offer to schedule the next available appointment.

4. Why should entries in the records or appointment books never be obliterated?
To avoid the appearance of fraudulent entries or attempts at hiding information.

5. Describe how the administrative medical assistant should greet and receive patients.
Introduce self by name and title, address patient with appropriate title (Ms., Mrs., Mr.) and last name unless the patient has previously requested otherwise. Ask the patient for the reason for the visit and whether he or she has brought any materials or information from other doctors or facilities.

6. List the information that should be obtained for every new patient.
Name, address, date of birth, reason for visit, previous medical history, allergies, and current medications being used

7. Explain the importance of discussing general office policies to patients.
Patients should understand what they may expect from the office and what the office expects of patients to provide the most accurate and comprehensive care possible. By ensuring an understanding of policies in advance, such understanding can relieve many of the potential problems encountered in future visits.

8. What benefits can be obtained through assisting patients with payment planning?
Ensure that the practice is paid on time, help the patient make arrangements in advance for bills that will exceed insurance allowances, alleviate stressors during patient's recovery period

**True or False: Identify whether the following statements are true or false. If false, tell why the statement is false.**

1. A computerized appointment scheduling system has increased functionality and flexibility over the handwritten or paper schedule. True

2. All offices should use the same type of appointment matrix to be consistent. False. Each office uses the type of appointment matrix that works best for that office's needs.

3. Patients should be given the next available appointment time without regard to their schedule because employers are required to give them time off from work. False

4. Health insurance providers influence which providers patients can receive services from. True

5. When scheduling a hospital admission, a diagnosis is not required because it will be determined during the patient's stay. False. A diagnosis is required when scheduling a hospital admission.

6. A guarantor is the person who will be responsible for the medical services rendered. True

7. If a patient presents to the office in need of emergency assistance, the provider must first agree to provide services. False. He or she must render reasonable care to stabilize the patient while waiting for 911.

8. A HIPAA release of information authorizes the release of any and all information to the authorized requestor. False. Specific releases are required for mental health, substance abuse, and genetic testing records.

9. Informed consent is a process of explaining a procedure to a patient. True

10. Schedule conflicts can be seasonal. True

# Chapter Application

## Case Studies with Critical Thinking Questions

### Scenario 1

A mother arrives in the office around 11:00 a.m., demanding an appointment immediately for her child who is quiet but alert. The child has been seen before. The mother states that the child has a temperature but denies nausea, vomiting, diarrhea, or other signs or symptoms. The office has been busy all day with several interruptions calling the doctor away. The provider will be seeing patients in the afternoon, and there are a couple of same-day appointments available on your schedule. You offer her an appointment for later that day but she insists that it must be NOW.

1. How do you handle this situation?
   First, remain calm and polite. The mother is most likely concerned about the child even though she may act inappropriately. Let her know that it has been an unusually busy morning and that you are offering her the first available time slot. If she continues to insist, ask her to wait a moment while you call the provider, office manager, or other practitioner. It might be possible to work her in between appointments or no-shows on the schedule. If there is no way in which the child can be seen, offer the next available appointment or advise her that she may seek help at an urgent care or emergency room if the child's illness progresses.
2. What ramifications are possible if you are unable to handle the situation successfully?
   If the child is more ill than he appears at initial glance, failure to treat or diagnose can be a possibility. The practice's reputation might be damaged by an angry mother.

For Scenarios 2 and 3, review the following appointment scheduling guidelines:

- New patients: 50 minutes
- Established patients: 20 minutes
- Physical examinations: 30 minutes
- Immunizations and prescription refills: 10 minutes

## Scenario 2

Elizabeth Jones, age 76, is an established patient in your family practice office. She calls to report that she is out of two of her regular medications, has been running a fever for two days, and has a cough.

1. What type of appointment is needed? This is an established patient who requires medication refills; however, due to her age and suggestion of underlying medical problems, a regular appointment should be scheduled rather than a refill appointment.
2. How much time is required to see this patient? 20 minutes (established patient)

## Scenario 3

Johnny Rodriguez is a 5-year-old who is about to start kindergarten. His mother called to ask for an appointment for a school physical. The family has been without insurance due to a loss of jobs and it is unclear when Johnny was last seen by a medical provider.

1. What type of appointment is most appropriate for this patient?
   This child has an uncertain immunization history and is apparently not an established patient. Whereas other children might be scheduled in a cluster situation, this child should either be scheduled in cluster for school physicals, with additional time allotted, or as a new patient.
2. What information should Ms. Rodriguez be asked to bring to the appointment?
   The mother should bring the last visit notes, if available; prior provider contact information; and any immunization documentation she has.

CHAPTER 13

# The Medical Record, Documentation, and Filing

## Words to Know Challenge

**Spelling: Each line contains three spellings of a word. Underline the correctly spelled word.**

| | | |
|---|---|---|
| 1. awdit | audet | audit |
| 2. ubjective | objective | objetive |
| 3. progress notes | progriss notes | progras notes |
| 4. subjective | sobjective | subjetave |
| 5. docyumentation | documintation | documentation |
| 6. ethnicity | ethincity | ethnicaty |
| 7. privacy | prevasy | prevacy |
| 8. chronalogic | chronologic | kronologic |

**Fill in the Blank: Complete the following sentences with Words to Know from this chapter.**

1. EHR is an acronym for electronic health record.
2. Per HIPAA, each office is required to have a designated privacy officer. This person must keep track of who has access to protected health information within a facility.
3. Progress notes are entered in the chart in chronological order.
4. Three types of charting styles discussed in this chapter include SOAP, HPIP, and CHEDDAR.
5. In the early 1970s, Lawrence L. Weed, M.D., originated a system of recordkeeping for patients called the problem oriented medical record (POMR). Progress notes are organized and entered based on the source from which they come whether from a provider, laboratory, or other source.
6. The chief complaint is the presenting problem and should be recorded in the medical record in the patient's own words.
7. A tickler file can be an expanding file, a card file, or even a portion of a file drawer. It consists of dividers with the names of all the months and dividers numbered from 1 to 31 for the days of the month.
8. Purge means to clean out.

# Chapter Review

## Short Answer

1. What is meant by "meaningful use of EHRs"?
   The manner in which a practice uses the electronic records—whether the system is in place or is actively and consistently used—defines "meaningful use." Meaningful use is evaluated to qualify practices for monetary incentives from the government. Criteria include the percentage of electronic prescriptions and how often patients are given copies of their records within three days of a visit, among others.

2. What types of *non*medical information is kept as part of the medical record?
   Demographics, employer and occupational information, guarantor information, insurance provider information, emergency contact numbers

3. Why is it important to obtain records about new patients from other providers?
   Maintain continuity of care, avoid duplicating tests, avoid duplicating medications, contain expenses for unnecessary testing, decrease time to accurate diagnosis

4. What is an OUTguide used for in filing?
   To keep the place of a chart that has been removed and track who has retrieved or requested it to make locating it later easier and to facilitate quicker filing when returning the chart to the files

5. Describe the necessary steps for pulling a file.
   Find the name of the patient in the alphabetic file; double-check spelling; prepare an OUTguide with date and name of person pulling or requesting file; and replace the file with the OUTguide.

6. Name the steps for filing a record.
   Inspect, index, code, sort, and store

7. What is a tickler file?
   A file used to keep track of future tasks or mailings to be sent to patients, for example, reminders for scheduled or annual appointments

8. What is meant by indexing files?
   Developing a cross-reference of the same file in two or more places, for example, filing a patient's record by name and by primary diagnosis

9. Fill in the blanks in the following chart, telling what each initial of SOAP represents and what the meaning is.

| | Initial Represents | Meaning | Activity That Takes Place in This Phase |
|---|---|---|---|
| S | Subjective | Patient complaint | Patient account of symptoms, sensations, timing, or associated events |
| O | Objective | Provider's examination | Physical exam, vital signs, laboratory testing, radiologic examinations, other diagnostics |
| A | Assessment | Diagnosis | Assimilates subjective and objective data into most likely diagnosis along with other considerations to rule out |
| P | Plan | Methods for treatment or further evaluation | Prescriptions, additional laboratory or radiologic assessment, admissions, therapy, referrals |

**Matching: Tell what each initial of CHEDDAR represents and then match each initial (letter) with its description.**

| | | Initial: | Initial Represents: | Description: |
|---|---|---|---|---|
| E | 1. | C | Chief complaint | A. Medications and amounts |
| F | 2. | H | History | B. Follow-up |
| G | 3. | E | Examination | C. Test results, additional findings |
| C | 4. | D | Details of problems and complaint | D. Diagnosis and plan |
| A | 5. | D | Drugs and dosages | E. Presenting problem |
| D | 6. | A | Assessment | F. Past medical events and problems |
| B | 7. | R | Return visit | G. Objective findings |

**Matching: For each of the following statements, identify whether the statement is subjective or objective.**

|  |  |
|---|---|
| Subjective | 1. I have a burning pain in my chest. |
| Subjective | 2. My daughter has a fever. |
| Objective | 3. The baby is lethargic and has no tears when she cries. |
| Subjective | 4. She looks queasy. |
| Objective | 5. His skin is pale and diaphoretic. |
| Objective | 6. The child's temperature is 38.1°C/100.5°F orally. |

# Chapter Application

## Competency Practice

1. In the course of recording patient information in the chart, it is noticed that an error was made.
   a. Describe the correct procedure for making the correction.
   Verify the information. Cross out the error, clearly annotating it as such, with a single line through. Enter time, date, and initials of the author next to the correction with the reason for the correction
   
   b. On the following progress note entry, use the preceding procedure you described and correct the entry: Ms. Jones called with complaints of right-upper quadrant abdominal pain.

| | |
|---|---|
| 3/2/2010<br>4:15 p.m. | Ms. Jones called regarding complaints of left-upper quadrant abdominal pain that gets worse with eating. She has been using TUMS for relief and feels better when sitting up. Will make appointment with Dr. Anderson for tomorrow. Kelly Taylor, MA |

2. **Filing Steps.** Place the following steps in correct order to file a chart.

| | |
|---|---|
| 4 | SORTING |
| 3 | CODING |
| 1 | INSPECTING |
| 5 | STORING |
| 2 | INDEXING |

3. **Alphabetic Filing.** Place the following patient names in order from 1 to 9.

| Order | Name |
|---|---|
| 6 | Mary Brown |
| 9 | Katherine Browning |
| 8 | Jessie Browning, Sr. |
| 5 | Kelly Brooks |
| 2 | Amy Barnes |
| 4 | Kendra Barrett |
| 1 | Xena Baers |
| 7 | James Browne |
| 3 | Adele Barnet |

UNIT 7

# Medical Insurance and Coding

CHAPTER 14

# Health Insurance

## Words to Know Challenge

**Spelling: Each line contains three spellings of a word. Underline the correctly spelled word.**

| | | |
|---|---|---|
| capitation | capitiation | capitition |
| preauthorisation | preauthoriziation | preauthorization |
| indemity | indemnity | indenmity |
| diductable | deductible | deducteble |
| precertification | precertafication | precertefication |
| quality insurance | quality asurance | quality assurance |

**Matching: Match each definition in column I to the correct term in column II.**

| | COLUMN I | COLUMN II |
|---|---|---|
| E | 1. The person in whose name the insurance policy is written | A. Gatekeeper |
| D | 2. Term used to describe participants in Medicare | B. Fee schedule |
| A | 3. Name used to identify primary care provider in a managed-care arrangement | C. Copayment |
| F | 4. Individual covered by an insurance policy in someone else's name | D. Beneficiary |
| B | 5. List of predetermined payments for services provided to patients | E. Subscriber |
| C | 6. The flat amount some patients pay at every visit | F. Dependent |
| G | 7. The percentage a patient is responsible for paying for each service provided after a deductible has been met | G. Coinsurance |

**ill in the Blank: Complete the following sentences with Words to Know from this chapter.**

1. The deductible ________ is the amount a patient must pay before his or her insurance begins to pay for services.
2. Payment made to providers by insurance carriers on a per-member, per-month basis is known as capitation ________.

3. Precertification is approval obtained from an insurer before services are rendered; preauthorization additionally relates to whether the services are medically necessary.

4. This determines the primary insurance when the patient is a child who has health care coverage through both parents; it is called the birthday rule.

5. When a provider contracts with an insurer and agrees that payment made is payment in full for the services, the provider is said to accept assignment.

6. This form, the advance beneficiary notice (ABN), is provided to Medicare patients when services might not be covered.

7. Reviewing services prior to their provision to determine appropriateness and medical necessity is known as a utilization review.

8. When a patient agrees to allow the provider to submit charges on his or her behalf and for the insurer to send payment directly to the provider, this is known as assignment of benefits.

9. Coordination of benefits refers to procedures used when a patient has more than one insurance to make sure that the responsible insurer pays for the claim.

10. After services are provided and the insurer has been billed, a patient receives a(n) explanation of benefits, a written description of benefits provided to the member by the insurer.

## Chapter Review

### Short Answer

1. What is the purpose of health insurance? A mechanism by which consumers are able to pay for health care coverage prior to obtaining care so that they do not have to pay for the care when they receive it.

2. What was the initial purpose of an HMO? Health care cost containment

3. Identify and define the different types of managed care. Health maintenance organization (HMO) provides coverage for both catastrophic illness and injury and preventive care through a network provider. Patient's care is coordinated through his or her primary care physician. Preferred provider organization (PPO) is a network of physicians and hospitals contracted with insurance companies, employers, or other organizations to provide health care to subscribers and their families for a discounted fee. Point of service (POS) allows patients to seek care outside their network but at a higher out-of-pocket cost. It provides coverage through both a managed care network and indemnity coverage. Consumer-driven health plans allow members to be more involved in the decisions related to their health care by using savings accounts that assist members to pay for out-of-pocket costs associated with that care

4. Define consumer-driven health care and list three types of plans. Health care in which consumers are given more responsibility in the selection of their care and the cost associated with that care. Three types of CDHPs are health savings accounts (HSAs), health reimbursement accounts (HRAs), and flexible spending accounts (FSAs)

5. Describe the concept of primary and secondary coverage and what impact it has on health care coverage. Primary coverage describes the insurance coverage that is first responsible for the payment of services when a patient has coverage through more than one plan. The secondary coverage would be billed for any remaining balance for services provided and/or any out-of-pocket costs the patient has from his or her primary carrier and could possibly pay up to the provider's total charges without exceeding that amount. When a patient has secondary coverage, it is beneficial to the patient in that it can reduce the amount the patient has to pay out of pocket and is beneficial to the provider in that he or she is sometimes able to collect additional reimbursement not otherwise received

6. Why is it necessary for a provider to obtain preauthorization and precertification for some services? Preauthorization and precertification are required for some services so that the insurer can determine the medical necessity for them as well as the cost efficiency prior to the service being rendered.

7. What is a diagnostic-related group (DRG) and in what type of health facility is it used? A prospective payment system developed by Yale University and used by Medicare and other insurers to classify illnesses according to diagnosis and treatment. DRGs group all charges for hospital inpatient services into a single bundle for payment purposes.

**Matching: Identify the types of insurance plans and models from the following list.** (*Hint*: Not all words in the list will be used.)

| | | |
|---|---|---|
| HMO | flexible spending account | Medicare Advantage |
| health savings account | indemnity | Medigap |
| TRICARE | CHAMPVA | Medicaid |
| point-of-service plan | workers' compensation | Fee for service |
| preferred provider organization | Medicare | |

|  |  |  |
|---|---|---|
| Medicaid | 1. | Government program established by the federal government and administered by each individual state. |
| Medicare | 2. | Government insurance program for individuals 65 years of age and older or disabled. |
| TRICARE | 3. | Coverage for military personnel and their dependents. |
| Flexible spending account | 4. | Plan that employee contributes to with pretax dollars; employee must use the funds in the benefit year or lose them. |
| Health savings account | 5. | Type of account in which employees deposit pretax money, and any balance can be used the next year. |
| HMO | 6. | A managed-care plan that requires all members to have a primary care physician who is responsible for all that patient's care. |
| Indemnity | 7. | Insurance coverage that allows subscribers more flexibility in seeking care. This type of plan has the least amount of structural guidelines for patients to follow. |
| Medigap | 8. | Coverage individuals purchase to cover the out-of-pocket expenses of Medicare. |

# Chapter Application

## Research Activities

1. Through the Internet, check your state Medicaid program to see whether it offers managed-care plans and what types of services those plans provide. Create a chart that compares and contrasts the standard Medicaid program benefits and the managed-care plan benefits.
2. Research a local insurance carrier and create a chart that shows what services require prior approval and identify what type of prior approval is required.
3. Go to http://stopmedicarefraud.gov and research the different states that have documented Medicare fraud cases. Create a chart that shows how many claims have been settled in the past two years for the five states that have the largest number of cases and identify the largest settlement.

## Case Studies with Critical Thinking Questions

### Scenario 1

Josephine Robinson is a 65-year-old patient new to Medicare, and she also has a Medigap plan. She was seen in the office recently for her annual physical and has received a bill from the office indicating that Medicare and her Medigap plan did not cover the visit. She would like an explanation because it was her understanding that this was a fully covered service.

1. What could have caused Medicare to reject this service? Medicare does not cover annual physicals, only a one-time "Welcome to Medicare" visit is covered.
2. She doesn't understand why her Medigap plan did not cover this service when Medicare didn't. How would you explain this to her? Medigap coverage pays only for the out-of-pocket expenses Medicare leaves for covered services such as her deductible and 20 percent coinsurance. Medigap plans do not pay for services that Medicare rejects as not covered.

### Scenario 2

Robert Olson was seen two months ago for an ear infection. Robert's mother is on the phone asking why she is receiving a bill for this visit. She indicates during the conversation that Robert is covered by both her insurance and her ex-husband's, so there shouldn't be any balances due.

1. What could have caused her to receive a bill for this service? The office might not have been aware of the secondary insurance and, therefore, did not bill that carrier; the secondary carrier might have denied the service; a deductible might not yet have been met with the secondary carrier.
2. What kind of proactive action can you take to avoid such issues in the future with the Olsons and with other patients? Always verify patients' insurance coverage when they arrive for their appointments. This will avoid unnecessary rework when the information is inaccurate or outdated.

CHAPTER 15

# Procedural and Diagnostic Coding

## Words to Know Challenge

**Spelling: Each line contains three spellings of a word. Underline the correctly spelled word.**

| | | |
|---|---|---|
| 1. specifisity | specificity | spesificity |
| 2. primary diangosis | primary dignosis | primary diagnosis |
| 3. comordibities | comobititys | comorbidities |
| 4. contributory factors | contributary factors | contributery factors |
| 5. key components | key componnents | key componends |
| 6. bundelled | bundled | bundeled |
| 7. medical nessecity | medial necessity | medical necessity |
| 8. modifyer | modifier | modifire |
| 9. sequenced | sequinced | sequeenced |
| 10. reimbersement | reimbursment | reimbursement |

**Fill in the Blank: Complete the following sentences with correctly spelled words from the Spelling section.**

Each E/M code description identifies the key components as well as contributory factors that must be met to report that code.

Codes are sequenced in relation to the intensity and level of service provided; this involves listing the primary reason for the office visit first and other reasons next in order of their importance.

It is important to remember the reason rule, which says that the reason for the patient visit (the primary diagnosis) is coded *first*; any other issues the patient presents with (comorbidities) are coded next in order of importance.

Modifiers are used with HCPCS codes to indicate that something is different about the way the service or procedure was performed.

Use of ICD-9-CM codes establishes the medical necessity for the services or procedures provided to the patient.

6. One of the reasons for the move to ICD-10-CM is that ICD-9-CM lacks sufficient specificity and detail to report morbidity adequately in the twenty-first century.
7. Bundled means it is included in another procedure or service code.
8. It is critical for any codes submitted to an insurance carrier to be accurate; the provider's reimbursement is based upon the codes that are submitted.

# Chapter Review

## Short Answer

1. What are the two main coding systems? Describe what each reports and how the two differ.
   The two main coding systems are HCPCS, which is used to report visits, procedures, and supplies used in the course of a patient encounter; and ICD-9-CM used to report the diagnoses for which the patient was seen by the provider.
2. List the sections of the CPT manual.
   Anesthesia; Surgery; Pathology and Laboratory; Radiology; Medicine; Evaluation and Management.
3. List six of the general CPT coding rules. **Students should list any 6 of these:**
   (1) Never code directly from the index. Always cross-reference codes with actual descriptions. (2) Analyze the description of the procedure performed and isolate the main term. (3) Locate the main term in the index. (4) Check for applicable sub-terms. (5) Make a note of the possible codes. (6) Verify each code description in the appropriate section of CPT. (7) Compare the description of the code selected to the description of the procedure performed. (8) In all cases, review all descriptions of codes listed for main terms and sub-terms to be sure the correct code is selected.
4. Why are modifiers used? What codes are they appended to?
   Modifiers are appended to HCPCS level I and level II codes to indicate that something is significant or significantly different about the performance of this particular procedure.
5. What is the significance of the reason rule and sequencing?
   The reason rule states that the main reason for the patient's visit or encounter must be coded as the primary diagnosis. Sequencing involves listing the diagnoses in a manner that reveals the significance of each condition as it relates to the services provided.
6. List the four general rules for diagnostic coding.
   (1) Code correctly and completely any diagnosis or procedure that affects the care, influences the health status, or is a reason for treatment on that visit
   (2) Code the minimum number of diagnoses that fully describe the patient's care received on that visit
   (3) Code each problem to the highest level of specificity (third, fourth, or fifth digit) available in the classification
   (4) Make sure the diagnosis that represents the main reason for the patient being seen or treated is listed first (primary diagnosis). Then comorbidities should be listed as secondary codes in order of their importance

7. Describe the impact of ICD-10-CM on the health care delivery system.
Answers should include the following: Greater coding accuracy and specificity; Higher-quality information for assessing quality, safety, and efficiency; Improved efficiency of care resulting in lower costs; Reduced coding errors; Ability to recognize the advances in medicine and technology; United States will now be using the same coding system as the rest of the world; Improvement in the ability to track and respond to international public health threats; Enhanced ability to meet HIPAA electronic transaction and code set requirements; Ability to accommodate future expansion of the codes.

8. Identify four types of insurance fraud and why they should be avoided.
Unbundling results in reporting multiple codes for a service that should be reported with one code; upcoding is when a higher-level ICD-9 code is used to report a service to increase reimbursement when the documentation supports a lower code; submitting claims for services that were never provided; or creating a false record. All of these acts of fraud will result in civil penalties and criminal fines and even can result in imprisonment. Sanctions can also be imposed with monetary consequences as well as the provider's exclusion from participation in Medicare, state health programs, or private health insurance plans.

**Matching: Identify the key components and contributory factors in E/M code descriptions.**

B 1. Amount of time physician spent
A 2. Nature of the presenting problem
A 3. Level of history obtained
B 4. Coordination of care
A 5. Degree of medical decision making involved
B 6. Counseling
A 7. Level examination performed

A. Key component
B. Contributory factor

**Labeling: Use the following list to identify each symbol found in the CPT book.**

Modified -51 exempt
Revised guidelines
Revised code description
FDA approval pending
Reinstated code
Code includes moderate sedation
Add-on code
New code

| Symbol | Meaning |
|---|---|
| + | Add-on code |
| ▲ | Revised code description |
| • | New code |
| ▶◀ | Revised guidelines |
| ⊘ | Modifier -51 exempt |
| ⊙ | Code includes moderate sedation |
| ⚡ | FDA approval pending |
| ○ | Reinstated code |

# Chapter Application

## Competency Practice

**ICD-9-CM Coding: Underline the main term in the following diagnostic statements and then find the appropriate ICD-9 CM code.**

1. Senile macular degeneration 362.50
2. Congenital heart block 746.86
3. Corpus luteum hematoma 620.1
4. Genital tract fistula 619.2
5. Onchocerca volvulus infection 125.3
6. Shoulder replacement V43.61
7. Cauda equina syndrome with neurogenic bladder 344.61
8. Idiopathic fibrosing alveolitis 516.3
9. Late effects of skull fracture 905.0
10. Congenital choledochal cyst 751.69

**CPT Coding: Identify the main term you would use to find the following procedures.**

1. Darrach procedure Excision
2. Placement of shunt Insertion
3. New-patient office visit Evaluation & Management
4. ECG, 12-lead w/interpretation and report Electrocardiography
5. Removal of mass, right breast Excision
6. Laparoscopic removal of gallbladder Laparoscopy
7. Suture open wound to left cheek Repair
8. Annual physical Preventive Medicine
9. Hernia repair Repair or Hernia
10. Dead tissue removal Debridement

**CMS-1500 Claim Practice: Complete two CMS-1500 claim forms, including correct code selection. Use the following practice information:**

Practice Information: Angela Dickinson, MD; 890 Medical Center Road, Suite A7, Moontown, US 09876-5432. EIN #11-3456780, Phone (222) 555-0000, NPI #0011223344.

### Case One

- Austin C. Henderson, 7 Penney Lane, Moontown, US 09876, Telephone (222) 555-1111, DOB 9/4/1978. Single.
- Insurance: One Health Plan, ID #239457669. Group Number 887. Employer: Jacobson Paint Supply. Patient is subscriber. Signature on file.
- Office visit for acute bronchitis 3/19/YY
  - Level 4 established patient visit $105.00
  - Chest x-ray, complete $135.00

### Case Two

- Octavia DeFillipo, 90 Elm Street, Moontown, US 09876, Telephone (222) 555-9988, DOB 3/25/1954. Married and employed full time.
- Insurance: Blue Cross Blue Shield US, ID #445590871. Group Number 112. Employer: Applied Jet Technology. Patient is spouse of subscriber: Ernesto P. DeFillipo, DOB 01/18/1952. Signature on file.
- Office visit for annual physical 04/05/YY $236.00
  - Breast and pelvic exam $ 78.00
  - Pap smear $ 49.00

1500

## HEALTH INSURANCE CLAIM FORM

APPROVED BY NATIONAL UNIFORM CLAIM COMMITTEE 08/05

PICA PICA

CARRIER

1. MEDICARE (Medicare #) MEDICAID (Medicaid #) TRICARE CHAMPUS (Sponsor's SSN) CHAMPVA (Member ID#) GROUP HEALTH PLAN (SSN or ID) FECA BLK LUNG (SSN) OTHER (ID)

1a. INSURED'S I.D. NUMBER (For Program in Item 1)

2. PATIENT'S NAME (Last Name, First Name, Middle Initial)

3. PATIENT'S BIRTH DATE MM DD YY SEX M F

4. INSURED'S NAME (Last Name, First Name, Middle Initial)

5. PATIENT'S ADDRESS (No., Street)

6. PATIENT RELATIONSHIP TO INSURED Self Spouse Child Other

7. INSURED'S ADDRESS (No., Street)

CITY STATE

8. PATIENT STATUS Single Married Other

CITY STATE

ZIP CODE TELEPHONE (Include Area Code) ( )

Employed Full-Time Student Part-Time Student

ZIP CODE TELEPHONE (Include Area Code) ( )

9. OTHER INSURED'S NAME (Last Name, First Name, Middle Initial)

10. IS PATIENT'S CONDITION RELATED TO:

11. INSURED'S POLICY GROUP OR FECA NUMBER

a. OTHER INSURED'S POLICY OR GROUP NUMBER

a. EMPLOYMENT? (Current or Previous) YES NO

a. INSURED'S DATE OF BIRTH MM DD YY SEX M F

b. OTHER INSURED'S DATE OF BIRTH MM DD YY SEX M F

b. AUTO ACCIDENT? YES NO PLACE (State)

b. EMPLOYER'S NAME OR SCHOOL NAME

c. EMPLOYER'S NAME OR SCHOOL NAME

c. OTHER ACCIDENT? YES NO

c. INSURANCE PLAN NAME OR PROGRAM NAME

d. INSURANCE PLAN NAME OR PROGRAM NAME

10d. RESERVED FOR LOCAL USE

d. IS THERE ANOTHER HEALTH BENEFIT PLAN? YES NO ***If yes***, return to and complete item 9 a-d.

**READ BACK OF FORM BEFORE COMPLETING & SIGNING THIS FORM.**

12. PATIENT'S OR AUTHORIZED PERSON'S SIGNATURE I authorize the release of any medical or other information necessary to process this claim. I also request payment of government benefits either to myself or to the party who accepts assignment below.

SIGNED ____ DATE ____

13. INSURED'S OR AUTHORIZED PERSON'S SIGNATURE I authorize payment of medical benefits to the undersigned physician or supplier for services described below.

SIGNED ____

PATIENT AND INSURED INFORMATION

14. DATE OF CURRENT: MM DD YY ILLNESS (First symptom) OR INJURY (Accident) OR PREGNANCY(LMP)

15. IF PATIENT HAS HAD SAME OR SIMILAR ILLNESS. GIVE FIRST DATE MM DD YY

16. DATES PATIENT UNABLE TO WORK IN CURRENT OCCUPATION FROM MM DD YY TO MM DD YY

17. NAME OF REFERRING PROVIDER OR OTHER SOURCE

17a.

17b. NPI

18. HOSPITALIZATION DATES RELATED TO CURRENT SERVICES FROM MM DD YY TO MM DD YY

19. RESERVED FOR LOCAL USE

20. OUTSIDE LAB? YES NO $ CHARGES

21. DIAGNOSIS OR NATURE OF ILLNESS OR INJURY (Relate Items 1, 2, 3 or 4 to Item 24E by Line)

1. ____ . ____

2. ____ . ____

3. ____ . ____

4. ____ . ____

22. MEDICAID RESUBMISSION CODE ORIGINAL REF. NO.

23. PRIOR AUTHORIZATION NUMBER

| 24. A. DATE(S) OF SERVICE From MM DD YY To MM DD YY | B. PLACE OF SERVICE | C. EMG | D. PROCEDURES, SERVICES, OR SUPPLIES (Explain Unusual Circumstances) CPT/HCPCS MODIFIER | E. DIAGNOSIS POINTER | F. $ CHARGES | G. DAYS OR UNITS | H. EPSDT Family Plan | I. ID. QUAL. | J. RENDERING PROVIDER ID. # |
|---|---|---|---|---|---|---|---|---|---|
| 1 | | | | | | | | NPI | |
| 2 | | | | | | | | NPI | |
| 3 | | | | | | | | NPI | |
| 4 | | | | | | | | NPI | |
| 5 | | | | | | | | NPI | |
| 6 | | | | | | | | NPI | |

PHYSICIAN OR SUPPLIER INFORMATION

25. FEDERAL TAX I.D. NUMBER SSN EIN

26. PATIENT'S ACCOUNT NO.

27. ACCEPT ASSIGNMENT? (For govt. claims, see back) YES NO

28. TOTAL CHARGE $

29. AMOUNT PAID $

30. BALANCE DUE $

31. SIGNATURE OF PHYSICIAN OR SUPPLIER INCLUDING DEGREES OR CREDENTIALS (I certify that the statements on the reverse apply to this bill and are made a part thereof.)

SIGNED DATE

32. SERVICE FACILITY LOCATION INFORMATION

a. NPI b.

33. BILLING PROVIDER INFO & PH # ( )

a. NPI b.

NUCC Instruction Manual available at: www.nucc.org

APPROVED OMB-0938-0999 FORM CMS-1500 (08/05)

1500

**HEALTH INSURANCE CLAIM FORM**

APPROVED BY NATIONAL UNIFORM CLAIM COMMITTEE 08/05

PICA | PICA | CARRIER

PATIENT AND INSURED INFORMATION

1. MEDICARE (Medicare #) [ ] MEDICAID (Medicaid #) [ ] TRICARE CHAMPUS (Sponsor's SSN) [ ] CHAMPVA (Member ID#) [ ] GROUP HEALTH PLAN (SSN or ID) [X] FECA BLK LUNG (SSN) [ ] OTHER (ID) [ ]

1a. INSURED'S I.D. NUMBER (For Program in Item 1): 239457669

2. PATIENT'S NAME (Last Name, First Name, Middle Initial): HENDERSON, AUSTIN C

3. PATIENT'S BIRTH DATE MM DD YY: 09 04 1978 SEX M [X] F [ ]

4. INSURED'S NAME (Last Name, First Name, Middle Initial): HENDERSON, AUSTIN C

5. PATIENT'S ADDRESS (No., Street): 7 PENNEY LANE

6. PATIENT RELATIONSHIP TO INSURED: Self [X] Spouse [ ] Child [ ] Other [ ]

7. INSURED'S ADDRESS (No., Street): 7 PENNEY LANE

CITY: MOONTOWN STATE: US

8. PATIENT STATUS: Single [X] Married [ ] Other [ ]

CITY: MOONTOWN STATE: US

ZIP CODE: 09876 TELEPHONE (Include Area Code): ( 222 ) 5551111

Employed [X] Full-Time Student [ ] Part-Time Student [ ]

ZIP CODE: 09876 TELEPHONE (Include Area Code): ( 222 ) 5551111

9. OTHER INSURED'S NAME (Last Name, First Name, Middle Initial)

10. IS PATIENT'S CONDITION RELATED TO:

11. INSURED'S POLICY GROUP OR FECA NUMBER: 887

a. OTHER INSURED'S POLICY OR GROUP NUMBER

a. EMPLOYMENT? (Current or Previous) [ ] YES [X] NO

a. INSURED'S DATE OF BIRTH MM DD YY: 09 04 1978 SEX M [X] F [ ]

b. OTHER INSURED'S DATE OF BIRTH MM DD YY SEX M [ ] F [ ]

b. AUTO ACCIDENT? [ ] YES [X] NO PLACE (State)

b. EMPLOYER'S NAME OR SCHOOL NAME: JACOBSON PAINT SUPPLY

c. EMPLOYER'S NAME OR SCHOOL NAME

c. OTHER ACCIDENT? [ ] YES [X] NO

c. INSURANCE PLAN NAME OR PROGRAM NAME: ONE HEALTH PLAN

d. INSURANCE PLAN NAME OR PROGRAM NAME

10d. RESERVED FOR LOCAL USE

d. IS THERE ANOTHER HEALTH BENEFIT PLAN? [ ] YES [X] NO *If yes,* return to and complete item 9 a-d.

READ BACK OF FORM BEFORE COMPLETING & SIGNING THIS FORM.

12. PATIENT'S OR AUTHORIZED PERSON'S SIGNATURE I authorize the release of any medical or other information necessary to process this claim. I also request payment of government benefits either to myself or to the party who accepts assignment below.

SIGNED SOF DATE

13. INSURED'S OR AUTHORIZED PERSON'S SIGNATURE I authorize payment of medical benefits to the undersigned physician or supplier for services described below.

SIGNED SOF

PHYSICIAN OR SUPPLIER INFORMATION

14. DATE OF CURRENT: ILLNESS (First symptom) OR INJURY (Accident) OR PREGNANCY(LMP) MM DD YY: 03 19 YYYY

15. IF PATIENT HAS HAD SAME OR SIMILAR ILLNESS. GIVE FIRST DATE MM DD YY

16. DATES PATIENT UNABLE TO WORK IN CURRENT OCCUPATION FROM MM DD YY TO MM DD YY

17. NAME OF REFERRING PROVIDER OR OTHER SOURCE

17a.

17b. NPI

18. HOSPITALIZATION DATES RELATED TO CURRENT SERVICES FROM MM DD YY TO MM DD YY

19. RESERVED FOR LOCAL USE

20. OUTSIDE LAB? [ ] YES [X] NO $ CHARGES

21. DIAGNOSIS OR NATURE OF ILLNESS OR INJURY (Relate Items 1, 2, 3 or 4 to Item 24E by Line)

1. 466 0

2.

3.

4.

22. MEDICAID RESUBMISSION CODE ORIGINAL REF. NO.

23. PRIOR AUTHORIZATION NUMBER

| | 24. A. DATE(S) OF SERVICE From MM | DD | YY | To MM | DD | YY | B. PLACE OF SERVICE | C. EMG | D. PROCEDURES, SERVICES, OR SUPPLIES (Explain Unusual Circumstances) CPT/HCPCS | MODIFIER | E. DIAGNOSIS POINTER | F. $ CHARGES | G. DAYS OR UNITS | H. EPSDT Family Plan | I. ID. QUAL. | J. RENDERING PROVIDER ID. # |
|---|---|---|---|---|---|---|---|---|---|---|---|---|---|---|---|---|
| 1 | 03 | 19 | YY | | | | 11 | | 99214 | 25 | 1 | 105 00 | 1 | | NPI | |
| 2 | 03 | 19 | YY | | | | 11 | | 71030 | | 1 | 135 00 | 1 | | NPI | |
| 3 | | | | | | | | | | | | | | | NPI | |
| 4 | | | | | | | | | | | | | | | NPI | |
| 5 | | | | | | | | | | | | | | | NPI | |
| 6 | | | | | | | | | | | | | | | NPI | |

25. FEDERAL TAX I.D. NUMBER: 113456780 SSN [ ] EIN [X]

26. PATIENT'S ACCOUNT NO.

27. ACCEPT ASSIGNMENT? (For govt. claims, see back) [X] YES [ ] NO

28. TOTAL CHARGE: $ 240 00

29. AMOUNT PAID: $

30. BALANCE DUE: $

31. SIGNATURE OF PHYSICIAN OR SUPPLIER INCLUDING DEGREES OR CREDENTIALS (I certify that the statements on the reverse apply to this bill and are made a part thereof.)

ANGELA DICKINSON MD

SIGNED DATE MM DD YY

32. SERVICE FACILITY LOCATION INFORMATION

ANGELA DICKINSON MD
890 MEDICAL CENTER ROAD
MOONTOWN US 09876-5432

a. 0011223344 b.

33. BILLING PROVIDER INFO & PH # ( 222 ) 5550000

ANGELA DICKINSON MD
890 MEDICAL CENTER ROAD
MOONTOWN US 09876-5432

a. 0011223344 b.

NUCC Instruction Manual available at: www.nucc.org

APPROVED OMB-0938-0999 FORM CMS-1500 (08/05)

1500

**HEALTH INSURANCE CLAIM FORM**

APPROVED BY NATIONAL UNIFORM CLAIM COMMITTEE 08/05

PICA | PICA

CARRIER

1. MEDICARE (Medicare #) MEDICAID (Medicaid #) TRICARE CHAMPUS (Sponsor's SSN) CHAMPVA (Member ID#) GROUP HEALTH PLAN (SSN or ID) FECA BLK LUNG (SSN) OTHER (ID)

1a. INSURED'S I.D. NUMBER (For Program in Item 1)

2. PATIENT'S NAME (Last Name, First Name, Middle Initial)

3. PATIENT'S BIRTH DATE MM DD YY SEX M F

4. INSURED'S NAME (Last Name, First Name, Middle Initial)

5. PATIENT'S ADDRESS (No., Street)

6. PATIENT RELATIONSHIP TO INSURED Self Spouse Child Other

7. INSURED'S ADDRESS (No., Street)

CITY STATE

8. PATIENT STATUS Single Married Other

CITY STATE

ZIP CODE TELEPHONE (Include Area Code) ( )

Employed Full-Time Student Part-Time Student

ZIP CODE TELEPHONE (Include Area Code) ( )

9. OTHER INSURED'S NAME (Last Name, First Name, Middle Initial)

10. IS PATIENT'S CONDITION RELATED TO:

11. INSURED'S POLICY GROUP OR FECA NUMBER

a. OTHER INSURED'S POLICY OR GROUP NUMBER

a. EMPLOYMENT? (Current or Previous) YES NO

a. INSURED'S DATE OF BIRTH MM DD YY SEX M F

b. OTHER INSURED'S DATE OF BIRTH MM DD YY SEX M F

b. AUTO ACCIDENT? YES NO PLACE (State)

b. EMPLOYER'S NAME OR SCHOOL NAME

c. EMPLOYER'S NAME OR SCHOOL NAME

c. OTHER ACCIDENT? YES NO

c. INSURANCE PLAN NAME OR PROGRAM NAME

d. INSURANCE PLAN NAME OR PROGRAM NAME

10d. RESERVED FOR LOCAL USE

d. IS THERE ANOTHER HEALTH BENEFIT PLAN? YES NO *If yes*, return to and complete item 9 a-d.

**READ BACK OF FORM BEFORE COMPLETING & SIGNING THIS FORM.**

12. PATIENT'S OR AUTHORIZED PERSON'S SIGNATURE I authorize the release of any medical or other information necessary to process this claim. I also request payment of government benefits either to myself or to the party who accepts assignment below.

SIGNED ______ DATE ______

13. INSURED'S OR AUTHORIZED PERSON'S SIGNATURE I authorize payment of medical benefits to the undersigned physician or supplier for services described below.

SIGNED ______

PATIENT AND INSURED INFORMATION

14. DATE OF CURRENT: MM DD YY ILLNESS (First symptom) OR INJURY (Accident) OR PREGNANCY(LMP)

15. IF PATIENT HAS HAD SAME OR SIMILAR ILLNESS. GIVE FIRST DATE MM DD YY

16. DATES PATIENT UNABLE TO WORK IN CURRENT OCCUPATION FROM MM DD YY TO MM DD YY

17. NAME OF REFERRING PROVIDER OR OTHER SOURCE

17a.

17b. NPI

18. HOSPITALIZATION DATES RELATED TO CURRENT SERVICES FROM MM DD YY TO MM DD YY

19. RESERVED FOR LOCAL USE

20. OUTSIDE LAB? YES NO $ CHARGES

21. DIAGNOSIS OR NATURE OF ILLNESS OR INJURY (Relate Items 1, 2, 3 or 4 to Item 24E by Line)

1. ___ . ___

2. ___ . ___

3. ___ . ___

4. ___ . ___

22. MEDICAID RESUBMISSION CODE ORIGINAL REF. NO.

23. PRIOR AUTHORIZATION NUMBER

| | 24. A. DATE(S) OF SERVICE From MM DD YY To MM DD YY | B. PLACE OF SERVICE | C. EMG | D. PROCEDURES, SERVICES, OR SUPPLIES (Explain Unusual Circumstances) CPT/HCPCS MODIFIER | E. DIAGNOSIS POINTER | F. $ CHARGES | G. DAYS OR UNITS | H. EPSDT Family Plan | I. ID. QUAL. | J. RENDERING PROVIDER ID. # |
|---|---|---|---|---|---|---|---|---|---|---|
| 1 | | | | | | | | | NPI | |
| 2 | | | | | | | | | NPI | |
| 3 | | | | | | | | | NPI | |
| 4 | | | | | | | | | NPI | |
| 5 | | | | | | | | | NPI | |
| 6 | | | | | | | | | NPI | |

25. FEDERAL TAX I.D. NUMBER SSN EIN

26. PATIENT'S ACCOUNT NO.

27. ACCEPT ASSIGNMENT? (For govt. claims, see back) YES NO

28. TOTAL CHARGE $

29. AMOUNT PAID $

30. BALANCE DUE $

31. SIGNATURE OF PHYSICIAN OR SUPPLIER INCLUDING DEGREES OR CREDENTIALS (I certify that the statements on the reverse apply to this bill and are made a part thereof.)

SIGNED DATE

32. SERVICE FACILITY LOCATION INFORMATION

a. NPI b.

33. BILLING PROVIDER INFO & PH # ( )

a. NPI b.

PHYSICIAN OR SUPPLIER INFORMATION

NUCC Instruction Manual available at: www.nucc.org

APPROVED OMB-0938-0999 FORM CMS-1500 (08/05)

1500

**HEALTH INSURANCE CLAIM FORM**

APPROVED BY NATIONAL UNIFORM CLAIM COMMITTEE 08/05

PICA

1. MEDICARE (Medicare #) | MEDICAID (Medicaid #) | TRICARE CHAMPUS (Sponsor's SSN) | CHAMPVA (Member ID#) | [X] GROUP HEALTH PLAN (SSN or ID) | FECA BLK LUNG (SSN) | OTHER (ID)

1a. INSURED'S I.D. NUMBER (For Program in Item 1): 445590871

2. PATIENT'S NAME (Last Name, First Name, Middle Initial): DEFILLIPO, OCTAVIA

3. PATIENT'S BIRTH DATE MM DD YY: 03 25 1954 SEX M [ ] F [X]

4. INSURED'S NAME (Last Name, First Name, Middle Initial): DEFILLIPO, ERNESTO P

5. PATIENT'S ADDRESS (No., Street): 90 ELM STREET

6. PATIENT RELATIONSHIP TO INSURED: Self [ ] Spouse [X] Child [ ] Other [ ]

7. INSURED'S ADDRESS (No., Street): 90 ELM STREET

CITY: MOONTOWN STATE: US

8. PATIENT STATUS: Single [ ] Married [X] Other [ ]; Employed [X] Full-Time Student [ ] Part-Time Student [ ]

CITY: MOONTOWN STATE: US

ZIP CODE: 09876 TELEPHONE (Include Area Code): (222) 5559988

ZIP CODE: 09876 TELEPHONE (Include Area Code): (222) 5559988

9. OTHER INSURED'S NAME (Last Name, First Name, Middle Initial)

a. OTHER INSURED'S POLICY OR GROUP NUMBER

b. OTHER INSURED'S DATE OF BIRTH MM DD YY SEX M [ ] F [ ]

c. EMPLOYER'S NAME OR SCHOOL NAME

d. INSURANCE PLAN NAME OR PROGRAM NAME

10. IS PATIENT'S CONDITION RELATED TO:

a. EMPLOYMENT? (Current or Previous) [ ] YES [X] NO

b. AUTO ACCIDENT? [ ] YES [X] NO PLACE (State)

c. OTHER ACCIDENT? [ ] YES [X] NO

10d. RESERVED FOR LOCAL USE

11. INSURED'S POLICY GROUP OR FECA NUMBER: 112

a. INSURED'S DATE OF BIRTH MM DD YY: 01 18 1952 SEX M [X] F [ ]

b. EMPLOYER'S NAME OR SCHOOL NAME: APPLIED JET TECHNOLOGY

c. INSURANCE PLAN NAME OR PROGRAM NAME: BLUE CROSS BLUE SHIELD US

d. IS THERE ANOTHER HEALTH BENEFIT PLAN? [ ] YES [X] NO *If yes,* return to and complete item 9 a-d.

READ BACK OF FORM BEFORE COMPLETING & SIGNING THIS FORM.

12. PATIENT'S OR AUTHORIZED PERSON'S SIGNATURE I authorize the release of any medical or other information necessary to process this claim. I also request payment of government benefits either to myself or to the party who accepts assignment below.

SIGNED SOF DATE

13. INSURED'S OR AUTHORIZED PERSON'S SIGNATURE I authorize payment of medical benefits to the undersigned physician or supplier for services described below.

SIGNED SOF

14. DATE OF CURRENT: MM DD YY ◀ ILLNESS (First symptom) OR INJURY (Accident) OR PREGNANCY(LMP)

15. IF PATIENT HAS HAD SAME OR SIMILAR ILLNESS. GIVE FIRST DATE MM DD YY

16. DATES PATIENT UNABLE TO WORK IN CURRENT OCCUPATION FROM MM DD YY TO MM DD YY

17. NAME OF REFERRING PROVIDER OR OTHER SOURCE 17a. 17b. NPI

18. HOSPITALIZATION DATES RELATED TO CURRENT SERVICES FROM MM DD YY TO MM DD YY

19. RESERVED FOR LOCAL USE

20. OUTSIDE LAB? [ ] YES [X] NO $ CHARGES

21. DIAGNOSIS OR NATURE OF ILLNESS OR INJURY (Relate Items 1, 2, 3 or 4 to Item 24E by Line)

1. V70.0
2. V72.31
3. V76.0
4. .

22. MEDICAID RESUBMISSION CODE ORIGINAL REF. NO.

23. PRIOR AUTHORIZATION NUMBER

| | 24. A. DATE(S) OF SERVICE From MM DD YY | To MM DD YY | B. PLACE OF SERVICE | C. EMG | D. PROCEDURES, SERVICES, OR SUPPLIES (Explain Unusual Circumstances) CPT/HCPCS | MODIFIER | E. DIAGNOSIS POINTER | F. $ CHARGES | G. DAYS OR UNITS | H. EPSDT Family Plan | I. ID. QUAL. | J. RENDERING PROVIDER ID. # |
|---|---|---|---|---|---|---|---|---|---|---|---|---|
| 1 | 04 05 YY | | 11 | | 99396 | 25 | 1 | 236 00 | 1 | | NPI | |
| 2 | 04 05 YY | | 11 | | G0101 | | 2 | 78 00 | 1 | | NPI | |
| 3 | 04 05 YY | | 11 | | Q0091 | | 3 | 49 00 | 1 | | NPI | |
| 4 | | | | | | | | | | | NPI | |
| 5 | | | | | | | | | | | NPI | |
| 6 | | | | | | | | | | | NPI | |

25. FEDERAL TAX I.D. NUMBER: 113456780 SSN [ ] EIN [X]

26. PATIENT'S ACCOUNT NO.

27. ACCEPT ASSIGNMENT? (For govt. claims, see back) [X] YES [ ] NO

28. TOTAL CHARGE: $ 363 00

29. AMOUNT PAID: $

30. BALANCE DUE: $

31. SIGNATURE OF PHYSICIAN OR SUPPLIER INCLUDING DEGREES OR CREDENTIALS (I certify that the statements on the reverse apply to this bill and are made a part thereof.)

ANGELA DICKINSON MD

SIGNED DATE MM DD YY

32. SERVICE FACILITY LOCATION INFORMATION

ANGELA DICKINSON MD
890 MEDICAL CENTER ROAD
MOONTOWN US 09876-5432

a. 0011223344 b.

33. BILLING PROVIDER INFO & PH # (222) 5550000

ANGELA DICKINSON MD
890 MEDICAL CENTER ROAD
MOONTOWN US 09876-5432

a. 0011223344 b.

NUCC Instruction Manual available at: www.nucc.org

APPROVED OMB-0938-0999 FORM CMS-1500 (08/05)

CARRIER | PATIENT AND INSURED INFORMATION | PHYSICIAN OR SUPPLIER INFORMATION

UNIT 8

# Billing and Payment for Medical Services

# CHAPTER 16

# *Patient Accounts*

## Words to Know Challenge

**Spelling: Each line contains three spellings of a word. Underline the correctly spelled word.**

| | | |
|---|---|---|
| 1. debbit | debt | debit |
| 2. bookkeeper | bookeeper | bookkeepper |
| 3. jurnalizing | journalizing | journelizing |
| 4. ledger | leger | legger |
| 5. ascets | assets | asets |
| 6. ajustment | adjusment | adjustment |
| 7. incouter | encouter | encounter |
| 8. posting | posteing | poasting |
| 9. creddit | credit | credibt |

**Fill in the Blank: Complete the following sentences with correctly spelled words from the Spelling section.**

1. A charge slip is also known as the encounter form.
2. A bookkeeper is one who records the financial transitions of a business.
3. The pegboard system uses an actual board as a base with pegs that attach the daysheet, the ledger, and the encounter form.
4. When an entry is made on the daysheet, it is called journalizing.
5. Posting means to transfer information from one record to another.
6. A debit is a charge added to existing balance; a credit is a payment, subtracted from existing balance.
7. In the double-entry bookkeeping system, the two entries allow for balance in the accounting equation: Assets = Liabilities + Owner's Equity.
8. Professional courtesy discounts, write-offs, or amounts not paid by insurance are examples of adjustments.

**Matching: Match each term in column I to its meaning in column II.**

| | COLUMN I | COLUMN II |
|---|---|---|
| E | 1. Accountant | A. Reflects that amount paid is less than total due |
| C | 2. Accounts receivable | B. Each transaction is recorded in two accounts |
| F | 3. Business associate agreement | C. All the outstanding accounts, amounts due to the office |
| G | 4. Trial balance | D. Reflects that the amount paid is greater than was due, or the account is being paid in advance of service provided |
| D | 5. Credit balance | E. Analyzes financial transactions and prepares reports |
| A | 6. Debit balance | F. Signed by an outside company that provides bookkeeping services to a medical office |
| H | 7. Single-entry bookkeeping system | G. Bookkeeping strategy to confirm accuracy in debits and credits in ledger |
| B | 8. Double-entry bookkeeping system | H. Similar to a checkbook register |

## Chapter Review

### Short Answer

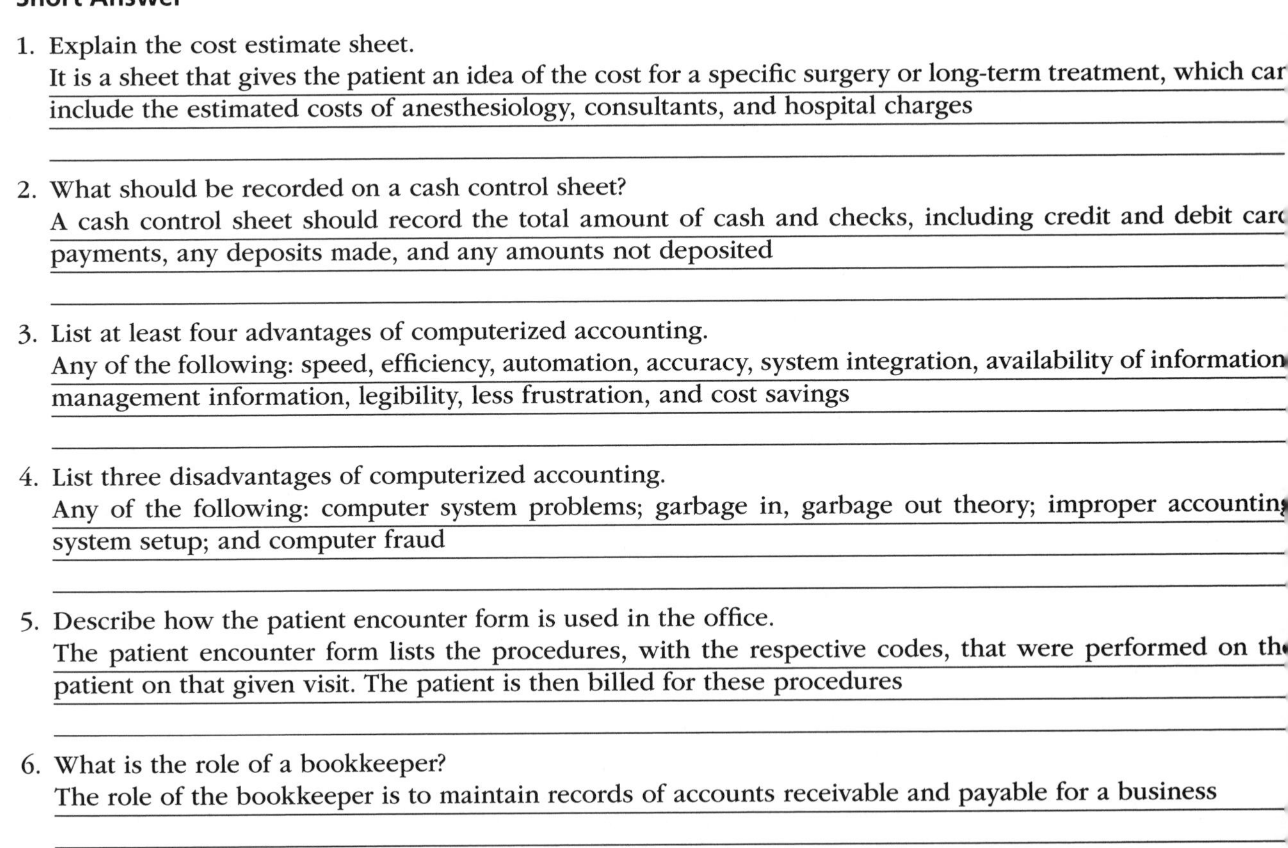

1. Explain the cost estimate sheet.
   It is a sheet that gives the patient an idea of the cost for a specific surgery or long-term treatment, which can include the estimated costs of anesthesiology, consultants, and hospital charges

2. What should be recorded on a cash control sheet?
   A cash control sheet should record the total amount of cash and checks, including credit and debit card payments, any deposits made, and any amounts not deposited

3. List at least four advantages of computerized accounting.
   Any of the following: speed, efficiency, automation, accuracy, system integration, availability of information, management information, legibility, less frustration, and cost savings

4. List three disadvantages of computerized accounting.
   Any of the following: computer system problems; garbage in, garbage out theory; improper accounting system setup; and computer fraud

5. Describe how the patient encounter form is used in the office.
   The patient encounter form lists the procedures, with the respective codes, that were performed on the patient on that given visit. The patient is then billed for these procedures

6. What is the role of a bookkeeper?
   The role of the bookkeeper is to maintain records of accounts receivable and payable for a business

7. Why would you use a Business Associate Agreement (BAA)?
   A BAA is an agreement between your company and another company. This agreement ensures that the second company understands your expectations of what it will be allowed to do with privileged information it will have access to from your company.

8. What are daysheets and patient ledgers?
   A daysheet, or daily journal, holds recorded patient charges and receipts for the day. A patient ledger is a record of all charges or services rendered, any payments made by the patient or the insurance carrier, and any adjustments.

**Matching: Identify whether the statements describe a single-entry bookkeeping system or a double-entry bookkeeping system.**

__A__ 1. Only the revenues and expenses are totaled, not individual values of each one.

__B__ 2. For each debit there is an equal and opposite credit, and the total of all debits must equal the total of all credits.

__A__ 3. Undetected errors can occur and might only be discovered through bank statement reconciliation.

__B__ 4. Two entries are made for each transaction.

__A__ 5. There is no direct link between income and the balance sheet.

__B__ 6. Ability to prepare financial statements directly from the accounts

__B__ 7. The bookkeeping system most often used in the large and busy medical setting

A. Single-entry bookkeeping system

B. Double-entry bookkeeping system

# Chapter Application

## Research Activity

Search the Internet to find *two* company websites that provide information on their computerized medical office accounting software systems. Print out the basic information the companies offer regarding computerized accounting systems.

## Case Study with Critical Thinking Questions

A young mother checks in at the front desk and is asked to fill out a new patient form. Her husband recently left her with two children to raise and no income. She is enrolled in a job training program, but she will be on a state aid program until she can finish her training. The young mother is embarrassed about the fact that she must be on a welfare program, even for a short time. After reviewing the form, the administrative medical assistant calls to the patient across the waiting area and announces to everyone that she will need a copy of her Medicaid card.

1. How could the administrative medical assistant have handled this situation in a more professional manner?
   She should have called the young mother to the front desk and discreetly asked her for her insurance card (Medicaid card)
   .

2. How do you think the patient felt?
   The patient likely felt embarrassed, angry, and humiliated and might not want to return for future services
   .

## Competency Practice

1. **Recording Charges and Credits on a Patient Ledger.** Record the following charges and credits on the Patient Ledger form (Workbook Form 16–1); note that some entries already exist on the form. Use yourself as the patient and your provider's name as the doctor. Use today's date.
   - Insurance information: Insurance Company – Health Care One; Insurance ID – 123-45-6789-A; Coverage Code A – Group II; office visit copayment ($20); this is your own health insurance through your job. You pay with a credit card.
   - Description: You are an established patient requiring a problem-focused exam (99212, $75), throat culture (87060, $60), antibiotic injection (90788, $40), ECG (93000TB, $40), spirometry (94010TB, $40), and chest X-ray review (76140-26, $25).
   - Diagnoses: Acute bronchitis (493.9), pneumonia (486). The doctor wants to see you in two weeks.
   - Insurance payments: On 06/01/20XX, your insurance company made a $50 payment for the problem-focused exam and, on 07/01/20XX, your insurance company made a $200 payment for the office procedures performed on the limited exam date.

WORKBOOK FORM 16–1

## PATIENT LEDGER

**Date:**

**MR#:** **Address:** **Provider:**

**Name:** **City/State/Zip:** **Date of Birth:** **Sex:**

**Charges**

| *Date of Service:* | *Procedure:* | *Description:* | *Diagnosis Codes:* | *Amount* |
|---|---|---|---|---|
| 2/1/20XX | 70373 | X-Ray | 052.9 354.0 503 847.2 | $75.00 |
| 2/1/20XX | 29130 | App. of Finger Splint | 052.9 354.0 503 847.2 | $30.00 |
| 2/1/20XX | 99204 | Office Visit New | 052.9 354.0 503 847.2 | $75.00 |
| 3/1/20XX | J1820 | Inj, Insulin, Up to 100 Units | 052.9 354.0 503 847.2 | $20.00 |
| | | | | |
| | | | | |
| | | | | |
| | | | | |
| | | | | |
| | | | | |
| | | | **Total:** | **$_____** |

**Insurance Payments**

| *Date of Payment:* | *Payment Code:* | *Line Description:* | *Transaction Description:* | *Amount* |
|---|---|---|---|---|
| 2/1/20XX | XP | XYZ Insurance Payment | XYZ | ($40.00) |
| 2/1/20XX | XP | XYZ Insurance Payment | XYZ | ($20.00) |
| | | | | |
| | | | | |
| | | | **Total:** | **($_____)** |

**Insurance Adjustments**

| *Date of Payment:* | *Payment Code:* | *Line Description:* | *Transaction Description:* | *Amount* |
|---|---|---|---|---|
| 5/1/20XX | MED ADJ | Medicare Writeoff | Adjustment | ($10.00) |
| 5/1/20XX | MED ADJ | Medicare Writeoff | Adjustment | ($10.00) |
| | | | **Total:** | ($20.00) |

**Patient Payments**

| *Date of Payment:* | *Payment Code:* | *Payment Description:* | *Transaction Description:* | *Amount* |
|---|---|---|---|---|
| 2/1/20XX | COCHECK | Copay Check Payment | | ($20.00) |
| 3/1/20XX | CCARDCOP | Credit Card Copay | | ($20.00) |
| | | | | |
| | | | **Total:** | **($_____)** |
| | | | **Total Payments** | **($_____)** |
| | | | **Amount Due:** | **$_____** |

## PATIENT LEDGER

**Date:**

**MR#:** **Address:** **Provider:**

**Name:** **City/State/Zip:** **Date of Birth:** **Sex:**

**Charges**

| *Date of Service:* | *Procedure:* | *Description:* | *Diagnosis Codes:* | *Amount* |
|---|---|---|---|---|
| 2/1/20XX | 70373 | X-Ray | 052.9 354.0 503 847.2 | $75.00 |
| 2/1/20XX | 29130 | App. of Finger Splint | 052.9 354.0 503 847.2 | $30.00 |
| 2/1/20XX | 99204 | Office Visit New | 052.9 354.0 503 847.2 | $75.00 |
| 3/1/20XX | J1820 | Inj, Insulin, Up to 100 Units | 052.9 354.0 503 847.2 | $20.00 |
| X/X/20XX | 99212 | Problem-focused exam | 493.9 486 | $75.00 |
| X/X/20XX | 90788 | Injection, antibiotic | 493.9 486 | $40.00 |
| X/X/20XX | 87060 | Throat culture | 493.9 486 | $60.00 |
| X/X/20XX | 93000YB | ECG | 493.9 486 | $40.00 |
| X/X/20XX | 94010YB | Spirometry | 493.9 486 | $40.00 |
| X/X/20XX | 76140-26 | X-ray, review | 493.9 486 | $25.00 |
| | | | **Total:** | $480.00 |

**Insurance Payments**

| *Date of Payment:* | *Payment Code:* | *Line Description:* | *Transaction Description:* | *Amount* |
|---|---|---|---|---|
| 2/1/20XX | XP | XYZ Insurance Payment | XYZ | ($40.00) |
| 2/1/20XX | XP | XYZ Insurance Payment | XYZ | ($20.00) |
| 6/1/20XX | | Health Care One Payment | Problem-focused exam | ($ 50.00) |
| 7/1/20XX | | Health Care One Payment | Procedures | ($200.00) |
| | | | **Total:** | ($370.00) |

**Insurance Adjustments**

| *Date of Payment:* | *Payment Code:* | *Line Description:* | *Transaction Description:* | *Amount* |
|---|---|---|---|---|
| 5/1/20XX | MED ADJ | Medicare Writeoff | Adjustment | ($10.00) |
| 5/1/20XX | MED ADJ | Medicare Writeoff | Adjustment | ($10.00) |
| | | | **Total:** | ($20.00) |

**Patient Payments**

| *Date of Payment:* | *Payment Code:* | *Payment Description:* | *Transaction Description:* | *Amount* |
|---|---|---|---|---|
| 2/1/20XX | COCHECK | Copay Check Payment | | ($20.00) |
| 3/1/20XX | CCARDCOP | Credit Card Copay | | ($20.00) |
| X/X/20XX | CCard Visa | Credit Card Copay | | ($ 20.00) |
| | | | **Total:** | ($ 60.00) |
| | | | **Total Payments** | ($450.00) |
| | | | **Amount Due:** | $ 30.00 |

CHAPTER 17

# Preparing Insurance Claims and Posting Insurance Payments

## Words to Know Challenge

**Spelling: Each line contains three spellings of a word. Underline the correctly spelled word.**

| | | |
|---|---|---|
| 1. reimbursement | rembursement | rembursment |
| 2. cleeringhouse | clearinghose | clearinghouse |
| 3. career | carrier | carrere |
| 4. secondery | secondary | secondarry |
| 5. identifier | identifire | identifeir |

**Matching: Match the abbreviations in column I to their meanings in column II.**

| | COLUMN I | COLUMN II |
|---|---|---|
| E | 1. NPI | A. Centers for Medicare and Medicaid Services |
| A | 2. CMS | B. Electronic claims sent to CMS |
| G | 3. EOB | C. Specifies reasons a provider may submit paper claims |
| F | 4. EDI | D. Standard claim form filed by provider's office for reimbursement |
| H | 5. ECT | E. Unique 10-digit identifier for covered health care providers |
| C | 6. ASCA | F. Electronic system required for filing electronic claims to CMS |
| B | 7. EMC | G. Document explaining payments made by the insurance company |
| D | 8. CMS-1500 | H. Method for monitoring the status and payment of insurance claims |

**Fill in the Blank: Complete the following sentences with Words to Know from this chapter.**

1. Electronic claims tracking is the most common way to monitor insurance claims today.
2. The CMS-1500 form may be filed electronically for provider Medicare and Medicaid reimbursement and is the standard claim form used in provider offices.
3. An explanation of benefits (EOB) is received by the patient and shows what the insurance company has paid.

4. A clearinghouse is a company that provides a service between providers and payers, running a claims scrub on all claims to check for missing or invalid data.

5. The phrase third-party reimbursement was coined to indicate payment of services rendered by someone other than the patient.

6. In many instances, a(n) secondary insurance will pay most, if not all, of the balance left over from the primary insurance to the provider.

7. Use of electronic data interchange transactions allow a medical facility or a provider's office to submit transactions faster and therefore be paid for claims faster.

## Chapter Review

### Short Answer

1. What two things should the office claims processor have before processing a patient's claim?
   The claims processor should have a copy of the patient's insurance coverage card and have secured the patient's signature on a form to permit release of information.

2. Explain the differences between manual and electronic tracking systems.
   Manual tracking systems require use of a log with several columns of information; they are time-consuming and frequently cause payment delays, whereas an electronic tracking system is computerized and allows for quick claims processing, quick electronic transmittals, and quick provider reimbursement turnaround times.

3. List five pieces of information found on an EOB.
   Information found on an EOB includes patient name, insured ID number, claim number, provider name, type of service, date of service, charges, not covered amount, total patient cost, payment made to the patient's provider, and how much of the annual deductible met by the patient.

4. Explain the history of claim forms.
   The claim form is a fairly recent development; with the new industry of health insurance came the third-party reimbursement, with which came the need for a form to report the health care provided to the source of payment.

5. List four pieces of information to have before calling to follow up on a delinquent insurance claim.
   Information to have before calling on a delinquent insurance claim includes practice tax ID number, patient's name, ID number, group name or number, and the insured's name (if not the patient's name).

**Matching: Look at a copy of a CMS-1500 form and match the following information in column I with the claim form's numbered sections listed in column II.**

| | COLUMN I | COLUMN II |
|---|---|---|
| E | 1. Health care coverage being billed | A. Section 4 |
| G | 2. Patient's name | B. Section 10a |
| A | 3. Insured's name | C. Section 11d |
| B | 4. Patient's condition is result of employment | D. Section 21 |
| C | 5. Indicate there is another health plan | E. Section 1 |
| D | 6. Diagnosis code | F. Section 24d |
| H | 7. Insured's policy group | G. Section 2 |
| F | 8. Procedure code | H. section 11 |
| J | 9. Name of referring provider | I. section 25 |
| I | 10. Federal tax ID number | J. section 17 |

**True or False: Place a T for True or an F for False beside each statement.**

1. F A clearinghouse contract is a free service offered to the provider by the federal government.
2. T Medicare will accept a stamped signature on the CMS-1500 form.
3. T When filing a CMS-1500 claim form, use of an incorrect place of service code will suspend a claim.
4. F The NPI is a unique 8-digit number identification for covered health care providers.
5. T Use of EDI transactions allows a provider's office to submit transactions faster with quicker reimbursement.
6. T ECT advantages greatly outweigh those of a manual system.
7. T EOBs may be sent to the patient by mail or email.
8. F Applying insurance payments and adjustments to patient accounts are most commonly done with a manual log system.
9. T Billing a secondary insurance company is fairly similar to billing a primary insurance company.
10. F The office claims processor has the option to file a paper claim or an electronic claim at any given time.

# Chapter Application

## Research Activity

Search the Internet to find *two* company Websites that sell electronic claims tracking (ECT) software systems for the medical office. Print out the services the companies offer and choose which would be best suitable for a large medical office as well as an ECT best suitable for a small practice.

## Competency Practice

Complete the following five insurance forms, using the following information: Code 11, office, for places of service (24B). The provider is Samual E. Matthews, MD, Suite 120, 100 E. Main Street, Yourtown, US 98765-4321. His SS# is 987-65-4321. Phone number (222) 789-0123. NPI 7654321. The patients all live in Yourtown, US 98765.

1. Juan Gomez, 293 West High Street 98765
   Medicare, ID# 29116696A. Phone (222) 263-5538. DOB 2/17/31. Male, single. Patient is insured person signature on file. Abdominal pain and diabetes mellitus. (Consult code book for code numbers needed for procedures.) Seen in office.

| | | |
|---|---|---|
| 5/18/XX | Office visit, Est. Pt., Level 2 | 65.00 |
| | Test stool for blood | 30.00 |
| | Automated hemogram | 30.00 |
| | Venipuncture | 30.00 |

2. LaChar Holley, 4567 Charcoal Lane 98765
   Travelers Insurance, ID# 505209821. Phone (222) 122-7768. DOB 10/7/60. Female. Patient is insured person. No other insurance. Not related to employment or accident. Signature on file. Arthritis, acute back pain. Seen in office.

| | | |
|---|---|---|
| 6/15/XX | Office visit, Est. Pt., Level 2 | 65.00 |
| | X-ray lumbar spine, AP & lat. | 200.00 |
| | Venipuncture | 30.00 |
| | Automated hemogram | 30.00 |

3. Tina Schmidt, daughter. DOB 12/27/07. Phone (222) 891-7145. Insured George Schmidt, 1249 E. Remington Road 98769. Self-employed. BC and BS Insurance, ID# 888207777. DOB 10/6/79. No other insurance. Phone (222) 441-0050. Signature on file. Impetigo. Seen in office.

| | | |
|---|---|---|
| 6/20/XX | Office visit, Est. Pt., Level 1 | 40.00 |

4. Joan Moriarty, wife. DOB 12/19/62. Insured Patrick Moriarty, 397 North Tony Road 98768. Self-employed. Metropolitan-Insurance, ID# 887105566. DOB 11/14/60. Phone (222) 431-6943. No other insurance. Signature on file. Cervicitis, cystitis, acute edema. Patient seen in office.

| | | |
|---|---|---|
| 9/20/XX | Office visit, Est. Pt., Level 3 | 80.00 |
| | Catheterization, urethra | 120.00 |
| | Endometrial biopsy | 300.00 |
| | Urinalysis | 25.00 |

5. Boris Kostrevski 1493 S. James Road 98765. Aetna Insurance, ID# 505208800-A.
   DOB 7/14/32. Phone (222) 298-6483. Signature on file. Diabetes mellitus, coronary atherosclerosis. Seen in office.

| | | |
|---|---|---|
| 9/24/XX | Office visit, Est. Pt., Level 2 | 65.00 |
| | Glucose screen | 25.00 |
| | Venipuncture | 30.00 |

1500

## HEALTH INSURANCE CLAIM FORM

APPROVED BY NATIONAL UNIFORM CLAIM COMMITTEE 08/05

PICA　　　　PICA

CARRIER

1. MEDICARE (Medicare #) MEDICAID (Medicaid #) TRICARE CHAMPUS (Sponsor's SSN) CHAMPVA (Member ID#) GROUP HEALTH PLAN (SSN or ID) FECA BLK LUNG (SSN) OTHER (ID)

1a. INSURED'S I.D. NUMBER (For Program in Item 1)

2. PATIENT'S NAME (Last Name, First Name, Middle Initial)

3. PATIENT'S BIRTH DATE MM DD YY SEX M F

4. INSURED'S NAME (Last Name, First Name, Middle Initial)

5. PATIENT'S ADDRESS (No., Street)

6. PATIENT RELATIONSHIP TO INSURED Self Spouse Child Other

7. INSURED'S ADDRESS (No., Street)

CITY STATE

8. PATIENT STATUS Single Married Other

CITY STATE

ZIP CODE TELEPHONE (Include Area Code) ( )

Employed Full-Time Student Part-Time Student

ZIP CODE TELEPHONE (Include Area Code) ( )

9. OTHER INSURED S NAME (Last Name, First Name, Middle Initial)

10. IS PATIENT'S CONDITION RELATED TO:

11. INSURED'S POLICY GROUP OR FECA NUMBER

a. OTHER INSURED'S POLICY OR GROUP NUMBER

a. EMPLOYMENT? (Current or Previous) YES NO

a. INSURED'S DATE OF BIRTH MM DD YY SEX M F

b. OTHER INSURED'S DATE OF BIRTH MM DD YY SEX M F

b. AUTO ACCIDENT? YES NO PLACE (State)

b. EMPLOYER'S NAME OR SCHOOL NAME

c. EMPLOYER'S NAME OR SCHOOL NAME

c. OTHER ACCIDENT? YES NO

c. INSURANCE PLAN NAME OR PROGRAM NAME

d. INSURANCE PLAN NAME OR PROGRAM NAME

10d. RESERVED FOR LOCAL USE

d. IS THERE ANOTHER HEALTH BENEFIT PLAN? YES NO *If yes,* return to and complete item 9 a-d.

**READ BACK OF FORM BEFORE COMPLETING & SIGNING THIS FORM.**

12. PATIENT'S OR AUTHORIZED PERSON'S SIGNATURE I authorize the release of any medical or other information necessary to process this claim. I also request payment of government benefits either to myself or to the party who accepts assignment below.

SIGNED ________ DATE ________

13. INSURED'S OR AUTHORIZED PERSON'S SIGNATURE I authorize payment of medical benefits to the undersigned physician or supplier for services described below.

SIGNED ________

PATIENT AND INSURED INFORMATION

14. DATE OF CURRENT: MM DD YY ILLNESS (First symptom) OR INJURY (Accident) OR PREGNANCY(LMP)

15. IF PATIENT HAS HAD SAME OR SIMILAR ILLNESS. GIVE FIRST DATE MM DD YY

16. DATES PATIENT UNABLE TO WORK IN CURRENT OCCUPATION FROM MM DD YY TO MM DD YY

17. NAME OF REFERRING PROVIDER OR OTHER SOURCE

17a.

17b. NPI

18. HOSPITALIZATION DATES RELATED TO CURRENT SERVICES FROM MM DD YY TO MM DD YY

19. RESERVED FOR LOCAL USE

20. OUTSIDE LAB? YES NO $ CHARGES

21. DIAGNOSIS OR NATURE OF ILLNESS OR INJURY (Relate Items 1, 2, 3 or 4 to Item 24E by Line)

1. ___ . ___

2. ___ . ___

3. ___ . ___

4. ___ . ___

22. MEDICAID RESUBMISSION CODE ORIGINAL REF. NO.

23. PRIOR AUTHORIZATION NUMBER

| 24. A. DATE(S) OF SERVICE From MM DD YY To MM DD YY | B. PLACE OF SERVICE | C. EMG | D. PROCEDURES, SERVICES, OR SUPPLIES (Explain Unusual Circumstances) CPT/HCPCS MODIFIER | E. DIAGNOSIS POINTER | F. $ CHARGES | G. DAYS OR UNITS | H. EPSDT Family Plan | I. ID. QUAL. | J. RENDERING PROVIDER ID. # |
|---|---|---|---|---|---|---|---|---|---|
| 1 | | | | | | | | NPI | |
| 2 | | | | | | | | NPI | |
| 3 | | | | | | | | NPI | |
| 4 | | | | | | | | NPI | |
| 5 | | | | | | | | NPI | |
| 6 | | | | | | | | NPI | |

25. FEDERAL TAX I.D. NUMBER SSN EIN

26. PATIENT'S ACCOUNT NO.

27. ACCEPT ASSIGNMENT? (For govt. claims, see back) YES NO

28. TOTAL CHARGE $

29. AMOUNT PAID $

30. BALANCE DUE $

31. SIGNATURE OF PHYSICIAN OR SUPPLIER INCLUDING DEGREES OR CREDENTIALS (I certify that the statements on the reverse apply to this bill and are made a part thereof.)

SIGNED DATE

32. SERVICE FACILITY LOCATION INFORMATION

a. NPI b.

33. BILLING PROVIDER INFO & PH # ( )

a. NPI b.

PHYSICIAN OR SUPPLIER INFORMATION

NUCC Instruction Manual available at: www.nucc.org

APPROVED OMB-0938-0999 FORM CMS-1500 (08/05)

1500

## HEALTH INSURANCE CLAIM FORM

APPROVED BY NATIONAL UNIFORM CLAIM COMMITTEE 08/05

PICA

1. MEDICARE [X] (Medicare #) MEDICAID [ ] (Medicaid #) TRICARE CHAMPUS [ ] (Sponsor's SSN) CHAMPVA [ ] (Member ID#) GROUP HEALTH PLAN [ ] (SSN or ID) FECA BLK LUNG [ ] (SSN) OTHER [ ] (ID)

1a. INSURED'S I.D. NUMBER (For Program in Item 1): 291166966A

2. PATIENT'S NAME (Last Name, First Name, Middle Initial): GOMEZ, JUAN

3. PATIENT'S BIRTH DATE MM DD YY: 02 17 1931 SEX M [X] F [ ]

4. INSURED'S NAME (Last Name, First Name, Middle Initial):

5. PATIENT'S ADDRESS (No., Street): 293 WEST HIGH STREET

6. PATIENT RELATIONSHIP TO INSURED: Self [X] Spouse [ ] Child [ ] Other [ ]

7. INSURED'S ADDRESS (No., Street):

CITY: YOURTOWN STATE: US

8. PATIENT STATUS: Single [X] Married [ ] Other [ ]; Employed [ ] Full-Time Student [ ] Part-Time Student [ ]

CITY STATE

ZIP CODE: 98765 TELEPHONE (Include Area Code): (222) 263-5538

ZIP CODE TELEPHONE (Include Area Code) ( )

9. OTHER INSURED'S NAME (Last Name, First Name, Middle Initial)

10. IS PATIENT'S CONDITION RELATED TO:

11. INSURED'S POLICY GROUP OR FECA NUMBER: NONE

a. OTHER INSURED'S POLICY OR GROUP NUMBER

a. EMPLOYMENT? (Current or Previous) [ ] YES [X] NO

a. INSURED'S DATE OF BIRTH MM DD YY SEX M [ ] F [ ]

b. OTHER INSURED'S DATE OF BIRTH MM DD YY SEX M [ ] F [ ]

b. AUTO ACCIDENT? [ ] YES [X] NO PLACE (State)

b. EMPLOYER'S NAME OR SCHOOL NAME

c. EMPLOYER'S NAME OR SCHOOL NAME

c. OTHER ACCIDENT? [ ] YES [X] NO

c. INSURANCE PLAN NAME OR PROGRAM NAME

d. INSURANCE PLAN NAME OR PROGRAM NAME

10d. RESERVED FOR LOCAL USE

d. IS THERE ANOTHER HEALTH BENEFIT PLAN? [ ] YES [ ] NO *If yes,* return to and complete item 9 a-d.

**READ BACK OF FORM BEFORE COMPLETING & SIGNING THIS FORM.**

12. PATIENT'S OR AUTHORIZED PERSON'S SIGNATURE I authorize the release of any medical or other information necessary to process this claim. I also request payment of government benefits either to myself or to the party who accepts assignment below.

SIGNED SIGNATURE ON FILE DATE

13. INSURED'S OR AUTHORIZED PERSON'S SIGNATURE I authorize payment of medical benefits to the undersigned physician or supplier for services described below.

SIGNED

14. DATE OF CURRENT: MM DD YY ILLNESS (First symptom) OR INJURY (Accident) OR PREGNANCY(LMP)

15. IF PATIENT HAS HAD SAME OR SIMILAR ILLNESS. GIVE FIRST DATE MM DD YY

16. DATES PATIENT UNABLE TO WORK IN CURRENT OCCUPATION FROM MM DD YY TO MM DD YY

17. NAME OF REFERRING PROVIDER OR OTHER SOURCE 17a. 17b. NPI

18. HOSPITALIZATION DATES RELATED TO CURRENT SERVICES FROM MM DD YY TO MM DD YY

19. RESERVED FOR LOCAL USE

20. OUTSIDE LAB? [ ] YES [ ] NO $ CHARGES

21. DIAGNOSIS OR NATURE OF ILLNESS OR INJURY (Relate Items 1, 2, 3 or 4 to Item 24E by Line)

1. 789.00
2. 250.00
3. ___ . ___
4. ___ . ___

22. MEDICAID RESUBMISSION CODE ORIGINAL REF. NO.

23. PRIOR AUTHORIZATION NUMBER

| | 24. A. DATE(S) OF SERVICE From MM | DD | YY | To MM | DD | YY | B. PLACE OF SERVICE | C. EMG | D. PROCEDURES, SERVICES, OR SUPPLIES (Explain Unusual Circumstances) CPT/HCPCS | MODIFIER | E. DIAGNOSIS POINTER | F. $ CHARGES | G. DAYS OR UNITS | H. EPSDT Family Plan | I. ID. QUAL. | J. RENDERING PROVIDER ID. # |
|---|---|---|---|---|---|---|---|---|---|---|---|---|---|---|---|---|
| 1 | 05 | 18 | XX | | | | 11 | | 99212 | | 1 2 | 65 00 | 1 | | NPI | 7654321 |
| 2 | 05 | 18 | XX | | | | 11 | | 82270 | | 1 2 | 30 00 | 1 | | NPI | 7654321 |
| 3 | 05 | 18 | XX | | | | 11 | | 85024 | | 1 2 | 30 00 | 1 | | NPI | 7654321 |
| 4 | 05 | 18 | XX | | | | 11 | | 36415 | | 1 2 | 30 00 | 1 | | NPI | 7654321 |
| 5 | | | | | | | | | | | | | | | NPI | |
| 6 | | | | | | | | | | | | | | | NPI | |

25. FEDERAL TAX I.D. NUMBER: 987654321 SSN [X] EIN [ ]

26. PATIENT'S ACCOUNT NO.

27. ACCEPT ASSIGNMENT? (For govt. claims, see back) [ ] YES [ ] NO

28. TOTAL CHARGE $ 155 00

29. AMOUNT PAID $

30. BALANCE DUE $ 155 00

31. SIGNATURE OF PHYSICIAN OR SUPPLIER INCLUDING DEGREES OR CREDENTIALS (I certify that the statements on the reverse apply to this bill and are made a part thereof.)

SIGNATURE ON FILE

SIGNED DATE

32. SERVICE FACILITY LOCATION INFORMATION
SAMUEL E. MATTHEWS
100 E. MAIN ST., STE 120
YOURTOWN, US 98765-4321
a. 7654321 NPI b.

33. BILLING PROVIDER INFO & PH # (222) 789-0123
SAMUEL E. MATTHEWS
100 E. MAIN ST., STE 120
YOURTOWN, US 98765-4321
a. 7654321 NPI b.

NUCC Instruction Manual available at: www.nucc.org APPROVED OMB-0938-0999 FORM CMS-1500 (08/05)

CARRIER — PATIENT AND INSURED INFORMATION — PHYSICIAN OR SUPPLIER INFORMATION

1500

## HEALTH INSURANCE CLAIM FORM

APPROVED BY NATIONAL UNIFORM CLAIM COMMITTEE 08/05

PICA | PICA

CARRIER

1. MEDICARE (Medicare #) MEDICAID (Medicaid #) TRICARE CHAMPUS (Sponsor's SSN) CHAMPVA (Member ID#) GROUP HEALTH PLAN (SSN or ID) FECA BLK LUNG (SSN) OTHER (ID)

1a. INSURED'S I.D. NUMBER (For Program in Item 1)

2. PATIENT'S NAME (Last Name, First Name, Middle Initial)

3. PATIENT'S BIRTH DATE MM DD YY SEX M F

4. INSURED'S NAME (Last Name, First Name, Middle Initial)

5. PATIENT'S ADDRESS (No., Street)

6. PATIENT RELATIONSHIP TO INSURED Self Spouse Child Other

7. INSURED'S ADDRESS (No., Street)

CITY STATE

8. PATIENT STATUS Single Married Other

CITY STATE

ZIP CODE TELEPHONE (Include Area Code) ( )

Employed Full-Time Student Part-Time Student

ZIP CODE TELEPHONE (Include Area Code) ( )

9. OTHER INSURED S NAME (Last Name, First Name, Middle Initial)

10. IS PATIENT'S CONDITION RELATED TO:

11. INSURED'S POLICY GROUP OR FECA NUMBER

a. OTHER INSURED'S POLICY OR GROUP NUMBER

a. EMPLOYMENT? (Current or Previous) YES NO

a. INSURED'S DATE OF BIRTH MM DD YY SEX M F

b. OTHER INSURED'S DATE OF BIRTH MM DD YY SEX M F

b. AUTO ACCIDENT? PLACE (State) YES NO

b. EMPLOYER'S NAME OR SCHOOL NAME

c. EMPLOYER'S NAME OR SCHOOL NAME

c. OTHER ACCIDENT? YES NO

c. INSURANCE PLAN NAME OR PROGRAM NAME

d. INSURANCE PLAN NAME OR PROGRAM NAME

10d. RESERVED FOR LOCAL USE

d. IS THERE ANOTHER HEALTH BENEFIT PLAN? YES NO ***If yes**, return to and complete item 9 a-d.*

**READ BACK OF FORM BEFORE COMPLETING & SIGNING THIS FORM.**

12. PATIENT'S OR AUTHORIZED PERSON'S SIGNATURE I authorize the release of any medical or other information necessary to process this claim. I also request payment of government benefits either to myself or to the party who accepts assignment below.

SIGNED ______ DATE ______

13. INSURED'S OR AUTHORIZED PERSON'S SIGNATURE I authorize payment of medical benefits to the undersigned physician or supplier for services described below.

SIGNED ______

PATIENT AND INSURED INFORMATION

14. DATE OF CURRENT: MM DD YY ILLNESS (First symptom) OR INJURY (Accident) OR PREGNANCY(LMP)

15. IF PATIENT HAS HAD SAME OR SIMILAR ILLNESS. GIVE FIRST DATE MM DD YY

16. DATES PATIENT UNABLE TO WORK IN CURRENT OCCUPATION FROM MM DD YY TO MM DD YY

17. NAME OF REFERRING PROVIDER OR OTHER SOURCE

17a.

17b. NPI

18. HOSPITALIZATION DATES RELATED TO CURRENT SERVICES FROM MM DD YY TO MM DD YY

19. RESERVED FOR LOCAL USE

20. OUTSIDE LAB? YES NO $ CHARGES

21. DIAGNOSIS OR NATURE OF ILLNESS OR INJURY (Relate Items 1, 2, 3 or 4 to Item 24E by Line)

1. ___ . ___

2. ___ . ___

3. ___ . ___

4. ___ . ___

22. MEDICAID RESUBMISSION CODE ORIGINAL REF. NO.

23. PRIOR AUTHORIZATION NUMBER

| 24. A. DATE(S) OF SERVICE From MM DD YY To MM DD YY | B. PLACE OF SERVICE | C. EMG | D. PROCEDURES, SERVICES, OR SUPPLIES (Explain Unusual Circumstances) CPT/HCPCS MODIFIER | E. DIAGNOSIS POINTER | F. $ CHARGES | G. DAYS OR UNITS | H. EPSDT Family Plan | I. ID. QUAL. | J. RENDERING PROVIDER ID. # |
|---|---|---|---|---|---|---|---|---|---|
| 1 | | | | | | | | NPI | |
| 2 | | | | | | | | NPI | |
| 3 | | | | | | | | NPI | |
| 4 | | | | | | | | NPI | |
| 5 | | | | | | | | NPI | |
| 6 | | | | | | | | NPI | |

25. FEDERAL TAX I.D. NUMBER SSN EIN

26. PATIENT'S ACCOUNT NO.

27. ACCEPT ASSIGNMENT? (For govt. claims, see back) YES NO

28. TOTAL CHARGE $

29. AMOUNT PAID $

30. BALANCE DUE $

31. SIGNATURE OF PHYSICIAN OR SUPPLIER INCLUDING DEGREES OR CREDENTIALS (I certify that the statements on the reverse apply to this bill and are made a part thereof.)

SIGNED DATE

32. SERVICE FACILITY LOCATION INFORMATION

a. NPI b.

33. BILLING PROVIDER INFO & PH # ( )

a. NPI b.

PHYSICIAN OR SUPPLIER INFORMATION

NUCC Instruction Manual available at: www.nucc.org

APPROVED OMB-0938-0999 FORM CMS-1500 (08/05)

1500

**HEALTH INSURANCE CLAIM FORM**

APPROVED BY NATIONAL UNIFORM CLAIM COMMITTEE 08/05

PICA | PICA

CARRIER

1. MEDICARE (Medicare #) [ ] MEDICAID (Medicaid #) [ ] TRICARE CHAMPUS (Sponsor's SSN) [ ] CHAMPVA (Member ID#) [ ] GROUP HEALTH PLAN (SSN or ID) [X] FECA BLK LUNG (SSN) [ ] OTHER (ID) [ ]

1a. INSURED'S I.D. NUMBER (For Program in Item 1): 505209821

2. PATIENT'S NAME (Last Name, First Name, Middle Initial): HOLLEY, LACHAR

3. PATIENT'S BIRTH DATE MM DD YY: 10 07 1960 SEX M [ ] F [X]

4. INSURED'S NAME (Last Name, First Name, Middle Initial):

5. PATIENT'S ADDRESS (No., Street): 4567 CHARCOAL LANE

6. PATIENT RELATIONSHIP TO INSURED: Self [X] Spouse [ ] Child [ ] Other [ ]

7. INSURED'S ADDRESS (No., Street):

CITY: YOURTOWN STATE: US

8. PATIENT STATUS: Single [X] Married [ ] Other [ ]; Employed [ ] Full-Time Student [ ] Part-Time Student [ ]

CITY: STATE:

ZIP CODE: 98765 TELEPHONE (Include Area Code): (222) 122-7767

ZIP CODE: TELEPHONE (Include Area Code): ( )

9. OTHER INSURED S NAME (Last Name, First Name, Middle Initial):

10. IS PATIENT'S CONDITION RELATED TO:

11. INSURED'S POLICY GROUP OR FECA NUMBER: NONE

a. OTHER INSURED'S POLICY OR GROUP NUMBER:

a. EMPLOYMENT? (Current or Previous) [ ] YES [X] NO

a. INSURED'S DATE OF BIRTH MM DD YY SEX M [ ] F [ ]

b. OTHER INSURED'S DATE OF BIRTH MM DD YY SEX M [ ] F [ ]

b. AUTO ACCIDENT? [ ] YES [X] NO PLACE (State)

b. EMPLOYER'S NAME OR SCHOOL NAME:

c. EMPLOYER'S NAME OR SCHOOL NAME:

c. OTHER ACCIDENT? [ ] YES [X] NO

c. INSURANCE PLAN NAME OR PROGRAM NAME:

d. INSURANCE PLAN NAME OR PROGRAM NAME:

10d. RESERVED FOR LOCAL USE

d. IS THERE ANOTHER HEALTH BENEFIT PLAN? [ ] YES [ ] NO *If yes,* return to and complete item 9 a-d.

**READ BACK OF FORM BEFORE COMPLETING & SIGNING THIS FORM.**

12. PATIENT'S OR AUTHORIZED PERSON'S SIGNATURE I authorize the release of any medical or other information necessary to process this claim. I also request payment of government benefits either to myself or to the party who accepts assignment below.

SIGNED SIGNATURE ON FILE DATE

13. INSURED'S OR AUTHORIZED PERSON'S SIGNATURE I authorize payment of medical benefits to the undersigned physician or supplier for services described below.

SIGNED

PATIENT AND INSURED INFORMATION

14. DATE OF CURRENT: MM DD YY ILLNESS (First symptom) OR INJURY (Accident) OR PREGNANCY(LMP)

15. IF PATIENT HAS HAD SAME OR SIMILAR ILLNESS. GIVE FIRST DATE MM DD YY

16. DATES PATIENT UNABLE TO WORK IN CURRENT OCCUPATION FROM MM DD YY TO MM DD YY

17. NAME OF REFERRING PROVIDER OR OTHER SOURCE 17a. 17b. NPI

18. HOSPITALIZATION DATES RELATED TO CURRENT SERVICES FROM MM DD YY TO MM DD YY

19. RESERVED FOR LOCAL USE

20. OUTSIDE LAB? [ ] YES [ ] NO $ CHARGES

21. DIAGNOSIS OR NATURE OF ILLNESS OR INJURY (Relate Items 1, 2, 3 or 4 to Item 24E by Line)

1. 715.9
2. 724.5
3. ___ . ___
4. ___ . ___

22. MEDICAID RESUBMISSION CODE ORIGINAL REF. NO.

23. PRIOR AUTHORIZATION NUMBER

| | 24. A. DATE(S) OF SERVICE From MM DD YY | To MM DD YY | B. PLACE OF SERVICE | C. EMG | D. PROCEDURES, SERVICES, OR SUPPLIES (Explain Unusual Circumstances) CPT/HCPCS | MODIFIER | E. DIAGNOSIS POINTER | F. $ CHARGES | G. DAYS OR UNITS | H. EPSDT Family Plan | I. ID. QUAL. | J. RENDERING PROVIDER ID. # |
|---|---|---|---|---|---|---|---|---|---|---|---|---|
| 1 | 06 15 XX | | 11 | | 99212 | | 1 2 | 65 00 | 1 | | NPI | 7654321 |
| 2 | 06 15 XX | | 11 | | 72100 | | 1 2 | 200 00 | 1 | | NPI | 7654321 |
| 3 | 06 15 XX | | 11 | | 36415 | | 1 2 | 30 00 | 1 | | NPI | 7654321 |
| 4 | 06 15 XX | | 11 | | 85024 | | 1 2 | 30 00 | 1 | | NPI | 7654321 |
| 5 | | | | | | | | | | | NPI | |
| 6 | | | | | | | | | | | NPI | |

25. FEDERAL TAX I.D. NUMBER: 987654321 SSN [X] EIN [ ]

26. PATIENT'S ACCOUNT NO.

27. ACCEPT ASSIGNMENT? (For govt. claims, see back) [ ] YES [ ] NO

28. TOTAL CHARGE $ 325 00

29. AMOUNT PAID $

30. BALANCE DUE $ 325 00

31. SIGNATURE OF PHYSICIAN OR SUPPLIER INCLUDING DEGREES OR CREDENTIALS (I certify that the statements on the reverse apply to this bill and are made a part thereof.)
SIGNATURE ON FILE
SIGNED DATE

32. SERVICE FACILITY LOCATION INFORMATION
SAMUEL E. MATTHEWS
100 E. MAIN ST., STE 120
YOURTOWN, US 98765-4321
a. 7654321 b.

33. BILLING PROVIDER INFO & PH # (222) 789-0123
SAMUEL E. MATTHEWS
100 E. MAIN ST., STE 120
YOURTOWN, US 98765-4321
a. 7654321 b.

PHYSICIAN OR SUPPLIER INFORMATION

NUCC Instruction Manual available at: www.nucc.org

APPROVED OMB-0938-0999 FORM CMS-1500 (08/05)

1500

## HEALTH INSURANCE CLAIM FORM

APPROVED BY NATIONAL UNIFORM CLAIM COMMITTEE 08/05

PICA | PICA

CARRIER

1. MEDICARE (Medicare #) | MEDICAID (Medicaid #) | TRICARE CHAMPUS (Sponsor's SSN) | CHAMPVA (Member ID#) | GROUP HEALTH PLAN (SSN or ID) | FECA BLK LUNG (SSN) | OTHER (ID)

1a. INSURED'S I.D. NUMBER (For Program in Item 1)

2. PATIENT'S NAME (Last Name, First Name, Middle Initial)

3. PATIENT'S BIRTH DATE MM DD YY — SEX M F

4. INSURED'S NAME (Last Name, First Name, Middle Initial)

5. PATIENT'S ADDRESS (No., Street)

6. PATIENT RELATIONSHIP TO INSURED — Self Spouse Child Other

7. INSURED'S ADDRESS (No., Street)

CITY — STATE

8. PATIENT STATUS — Single Married Other; Employed Full-Time Student Part-Time Student

CITY — STATE

ZIP CODE — TELEPHONE (Include Area Code) ( )

ZIP CODE — TELEPHONE (Include Area Code) ( )

9. OTHER INSURED S NAME (Last Name, First Name, Middle Initial)

10. IS PATIENT'S CONDITION RELATED TO:

11. INSURED'S POLICY GROUP OR FECA NUMBER

a. OTHER INSURED'S POLICY OR GROUP NUMBER

a. EMPLOYMENT? (Current or Previous) YES NO

a. INSURED'S DATE OF BIRTH MM DD YY — SEX M F

b. OTHER INSURED'S DATE OF BIRTH MM DD YY — SEX M F

b. AUTO ACCIDENT? YES NO — PLACE (State)

b. EMPLOYER'S NAME OR SCHOOL NAME

c. EMPLOYER'S NAME OR SCHOOL NAME

c. OTHER ACCIDENT? YES NO

c. INSURANCE PLAN NAME OR PROGRAM NAME

d. INSURANCE PLAN NAME OR PROGRAM NAME

10d. RESERVED FOR LOCAL USE

d. IS THERE ANOTHER HEALTH BENEFIT PLAN? YES NO *If yes,* return to and complete item 9 a-d.

**READ BACK OF FORM BEFORE COMPLETING & SIGNING THIS FORM.**

12. PATIENT'S OR AUTHORIZED PERSON'S SIGNATURE I authorize the release of any medical or other information necessary to process this claim. I also request payment of government benefits either to myself or to the party who accepts assignment below.

SIGNED ______ DATE ______

13. INSURED'S OR AUTHORIZED PERSON'S SIGNATURE I authorize payment of medical benefits to the undersigned physician or supplier for services described below.

SIGNED ______

PATIENT AND INSURED INFORMATION

14. DATE OF CURRENT: MM DD YY — ILLNESS (First symptom) OR INJURY (Accident) OR PREGNANCY(LMP)

15. IF PATIENT HAS HAD SAME OR SIMILAR ILLNESS. GIVE FIRST DATE MM DD YY

16. DATES PATIENT UNABLE TO WORK IN CURRENT OCCUPATION — FROM MM DD YY TO MM DD YY

17. NAME OF REFERRING PROVIDER OR OTHER SOURCE — 17a. — 17b. NPI

18. HOSPITALIZATION DATES RELATED TO CURRENT SERVICES — FROM MM DD YY TO MM DD YY

19. RESERVED FOR LOCAL USE

20. OUTSIDE LAB? YES NO — $ CHARGES

21. DIAGNOSIS OR NATURE OF ILLNESS OR INJURY (Relate Items 1, 2, 3 or 4 to Item 24E by Line)

1. ___ . ___ 3. ___ . ___

2. ___ . ___ 4. ___ . ___

22. MEDICAID RESUBMISSION CODE — ORIGINAL REF. NO.

23. PRIOR AUTHORIZATION NUMBER

| | 24. A. DATE(S) OF SERVICE From MM DD YY To MM DD YY | B. PLACE OF SERVICE | C. EMG | D. PROCEDURES, SERVICES, OR SUPPLIES (Explain Unusual Circumstances) CPT/HCPCS MODIFIER | E. DIAGNOSIS POINTER | F. $ CHARGES | G. DAYS OR UNITS | H. EPSDT Family Plan | I. ID. QUAL. | J. RENDERING PROVIDER ID. # |
|---|---|---|---|---|---|---|---|---|---|---|
| 1 | | | | | | | | | NPI | |
| 2 | | | | | | | | | NPI | |
| 3 | | | | | | | | | NPI | |
| 4 | | | | | | | | | NPI | |
| 5 | | | | | | | | | NPI | |
| 6 | | | | | | | | | NPI | |

PHYSICIAN OR SUPPLIER INFORMATION

25. FEDERAL TAX I.D. NUMBER — SSN EIN

26. PATIENT'S ACCOUNT NO.

27. ACCEPT ASSIGNMENT? (For govt. claims, see back) YES NO

28. TOTAL CHARGE $

29. AMOUNT PAID $

30. BALANCE DUE $

31. SIGNATURE OF PHYSICIAN OR SUPPLIER INCLUDING DEGREES OR CREDENTIALS (I certify that the statements on the reverse apply to this bill and are made a part thereof.)

SIGNED DATE

32. SERVICE FACILITY LOCATION INFORMATION — a. NPI b.

33. BILLING PROVIDER INFO & PH # ( ) — a. NPI b.

NUCC Instruction Manual available at: www.nucc.org

APPROVED OMB-0938-0999 FORM CMS-1500 (08/05)

1500

**HEALTH INSURANCE CLAIM FORM**

APPROVED BY NATIONAL UNIFORM CLAIM COMMITTEE 08/05

PICA — PICA — CARRIER

1. MEDICARE (Medicare #) / MEDICAID (Medicaid #) / TRICARE CHAMPUS (Sponsor's SSN) / CHAMPVA (Member ID#) / [X] GROUP HEALTH PLAN (SSN or ID) / FECA BLK LUNG (SSN) / OTHER (ID)

1a. INSURED'S I.D. NUMBER (For Program in Item 1): 888207777

2. PATIENT'S NAME (Last Name, First Name, Middle Initial): SCHMIDT, TINA

3. PATIENT'S BIRTH DATE MM DD YY: 12 27 2007 — SEX M [ ] F [X]

4. INSURED'S NAME (Last Name, First Name, Middle Initial): SCHMIDT, GEORGE

5. PATIENT'S ADDRESS (No., Street): 1249 E. REMINGTON ROAD

6. PATIENT RELATIONSHIP TO INSURED: Self [ ] Spouse [ ] Child [X] Other [ ]

7. INSURED'S ADDRESS (No., Street): 1249 REMINGTON RODA

CITY: YOURTOWN — STATE: US

8. PATIENT STATUS: Single [ ] Married [ ] Other [ ]; Employed [ ] Full-Time Student [ ] Part-Time Student [ ]

CITY: YOURTOWN — STATE: US

ZIP CODE: 98765 — TELEPHONE (Include Area Code): (222) 441-0050

ZIP CODE: 98765 — TELEPHONE (Include Area Code): (222) 441-9959

9. OTHER INSURED S NAME (Last Name, First Name, Middle Initial)

10. IS PATIENT'S CONDITION RELATED TO:

11. INSURED'S POLICY GROUP OR FECA NUMBER

a. OTHER INSURED'S POLICY OR GROUP NUMBER

a. EMPLOYMENT? (Current or Previous) [ ] YES [X] NO

a. INSURED'S DATE OF BIRTH MM DD YY: 10 06 1979 — SEX M [X] F [ ]

b. OTHER INSURED'S DATE OF BIRTH MM DD YY — SEX M [ ] F [ ]

b. AUTO ACCIDENT? [ ] YES [X] NO — PLACE (State)

b. EMPLOYER'S NAME OR SCHOOL NAME

c. EMPLOYER'S NAME OR SCHOOL NAME

c. OTHER ACCIDENT? [ ] YES [X] NO

c. INSURANCE PLAN NAME OR PROGRAM NAME: BLUE CROSS BLUE SHIELD

d. INSURANCE PLAN NAME OR PROGRAM NAME

10d. RESERVED FOR LOCAL USE

d. IS THERE ANOTHER HEALTH BENEFIT PLAN? [ ] YES [X] NO *If yes,* return to and complete item 9 a-d.

**READ BACK OF FORM BEFORE COMPLETING & SIGNING THIS FORM.**

12. PATIENT'S OR AUTHORIZED PERSON'S SIGNATURE I authorize the release of any medical or other information necessary to process this claim. I also request payment of government benefits either to myself or to the party who accepts assignment below.

SIGNED SIGNATURE ON FILE DATE

13. INSURED'S OR AUTHORIZED PERSON'S SIGNATURE I authorize payment of medical benefits to the undersigned physician or supplier for services described below.

SIGNED SIGNATURE ON FILE

PATIENT AND INSURED INFORMATION

14. DATE OF CURRENT: MM DD YY — ILLNESS (First symptom) OR INJURY (Accident) OR PREGNANCY(LMP)

15. IF PATIENT HAS HAD SAME OR SIMILAR ILLNESS. GIVE FIRST DATE MM DD YY

16. DATES PATIENT UNABLE TO WORK IN CURRENT OCCUPATION MM DD YY FROM — TO

17. NAME OF REFERRING PROVIDER OR OTHER SOURCE — 17a. — 17b. NPI

18. HOSPITALIZATION DATES RELATED TO CURRENT SERVICES MM DD YY FROM — TO

19. RESERVED FOR LOCAL USE

20. OUTSIDE LAB? [ ] YES [ ] NO — $ CHARGES

21. DIAGNOSIS OR NATURE OF ILLNESS OR INJURY (Relate Items 1, 2, 3 or 4 to Item 24E by Line)

1. 684 .
2. .
3. .
4. .

22. MEDICAID RESUBMISSION CODE — ORIGINAL REF. NO.

23. PRIOR AUTHORIZATION NUMBER

| | 24. A. DATE(S) OF SERVICE From MM | DD | YY | To MM | DD | YY | B. PLACE OF SERVICE | C. EMG | D. PROCEDURES, SERVICES, OR SUPPLIES (Explain Unusual Circumstances) CPT/HCPCS | MODIFIER | E. DIAGNOSIS POINTER | F. $ CHARGES | G. DAYS OR UNITS | H. EPSDT Family Plan | I. ID. QUAL. | J. RENDERING PROVIDER ID. # |
|---|---|---|---|---|---|---|---|---|---|---|---|---|---|---|---|---|
| 1 | 06 | 20 | XX | | | | 11 | | 99211 | | 1 | 40 00 | 1 | | NPI | 7654321 |
| 2 | | | | | | | | | | | | | | | NPI | |
| 3 | | | | | | | | | | | | | | | NPI | |
| 4 | | | | | | | | | | | | | | | NPI | |
| 5 | | | | | | | | | | | | | | | NPI | |
| 6 | | | | | | | | | | | | | | | NPI | |

25. FEDERAL TAX I.D. NUMBER: 987654321 — SSN [X] EIN [ ]

26. PATIENT'S ACCOUNT NO.

27. ACCEPT ASSIGNMENT? (For govt. claims, see back) [ ] YES [ ] NO

28. TOTAL CHARGE: $ 40 00

29. AMOUNT PAID: $

30. BALANCE DUE: $ 40 00

31. SIGNATURE OF PHYSICIAN OR SUPPLIER INCLUDING DEGREES OR CREDENTIALS (I certify that the statements on the reverse apply to this bill and are made a part thereof.)
SIGNATURE ON FILE
SIGNED DATE

32. SERVICE FACILITY LOCATION INFORMATION
SAMUEL E. MATTHEWS
100 E. MAIN ST., STE 120
YOURTOWN, US 98765-4321
a. 7654321 NPI b.

33. BILLING PROVIDER INFO & PH # (222) 789-0123
SAMUEL E. MATTHEWS
100 E. MAIN ST., STE 120
YOURTOWN, US 98765-4321
a. 7654321 NPI b.

PHYSICIAN OR SUPPLIER INFORMATION

NUCC Instruction Manual available at: www.nucc.org — APPROVED OMB-0938-0999 FORM CMS-1500 (08/05)

1500

# HEALTH INSURANCE CLAIM FORM

APPROVED BY NATIONAL UNIFORM CLAIM COMMITTEE 08/05

PICA — PICA — CARRIER

1. MEDICARE (Medicare #) MEDICAID (Medicaid #) TRICARE CHAMPUS (Sponsor's SSN) CHAMPVA (Member ID#) GROUP HEALTH PLAN (SSN or ID) FECA BLK LUNG (SSN) OTHER (ID)

1a. INSURED'S I.D. NUMBER (For Program in Item 1)

2. PATIENT'S NAME (Last Name, First Name, Middle Initial)

3. PATIENT'S BIRTH DATE MM DD YY SEX M F

4. INSURED'S NAME (Last Name, First Name, Middle Initial)

5. PATIENT'S ADDRESS (No., Street)

6. PATIENT RELATIONSHIP TO INSURED Self Spouse Child Other

7. INSURED'S ADDRESS (No., Street)

CITY STATE

8. PATIENT STATUS Single Married Other

CITY STATE

ZIP CODE TELEPHONE (Include Area Code) ( )

Employed Full-Time Student Part-Time Student

ZIP CODE TELEPHONE (Include Area Code) ( )

9. OTHER INSURED S NAME (Last Name, First Name, Middle Initial)

10. IS PATIENT'S CONDITION RELATED TO:

11. INSURED'S POLICY GROUP OR FECA NUMBER

a. OTHER INSURED'S POLICY OR GROUP NUMBER

a. EMPLOYMENT? (Current or Previous) YES NO

a. INSURED'S DATE OF BIRTH MM DD YY SEX M F

b. OTHER INSURED'S DATE OF BIRTH MM DD YY SEX M F

b. AUTO ACCIDENT? YES NO PLACE (State)

b. EMPLOYER'S NAME OR SCHOOL NAME

c. EMPLOYER'S NAME OR SCHOOL NAME

c. OTHER ACCIDENT? YES NO

c. INSURANCE PLAN NAME OR PROGRAM NAME

d. INSURANCE PLAN NAME OR PROGRAM NAME

10d. RESERVED FOR LOCAL USE

d. IS THERE ANOTHER HEALTH BENEFIT PLAN? YES NO ***If yes***, return to and complete item 9 a-d.

**READ BACK OF FORM BEFORE COMPLETING & SIGNING THIS FORM.**

12. PATIENT'S OR AUTHORIZED PERSON'S SIGNATURE I authorize the release of any medical or other information necessary to process this claim. I also request payment of government benefits either to myself or to the party who accepts assignment below.

SIGNED ____________ DATE ____________

13. INSURED'S OR AUTHORIZED PERSON'S SIGNATURE I authorize payment of medical benefits to the undersigned physician or supplier for services described below.

SIGNED ____________

PATIENT AND INSURED INFORMATION

14. DATE OF CURRENT: MM DD YY ILLNESS (First symptom) OR INJURY (Accident) OR PREGNANCY(LMP)

15. IF PATIENT HAS HAD SAME OR SIMILAR ILLNESS. GIVE FIRST DATE MM DD YY

16. DATES PATIENT UNABLE TO WORK IN CURRENT OCCUPATION MM DD YY FROM TO MM DD YY

17. NAME OF REFERRING PROVIDER OR OTHER SOURCE 17a. 17b. NPI

18. HOSPITALIZATION DATES RELATED TO CURRENT SERVICES MM DD YY FROM TO MM DD YY

19. RESERVED FOR LOCAL USE

20. OUTSIDE LAB? YES NO $ CHARGES

21. DIAGNOSIS OR NATURE OF ILLNESS OR INJURY (Relate Items 1, 2, 3 or 4 to Item 24E by Line)

1. ___ . ___ 3. ___ . ___

2. ___ . ___ 4. ___ . ___

22. MEDICAID RESUBMISSION CODE ORIGINAL REF. NO.

23. PRIOR AUTHORIZATION NUMBER

| | 24. A. DATE(S) OF SERVICE From MM DD YY To MM DD YY | B. PLACE OF SERVICE | C. EMG | D. PROCEDURES, SERVICES, OR SUPPLIES (Explain Unusual Circumstances) CPT/HCPCS MODIFIER | E. DIAGNOSIS POINTER | F. $ CHARGES | G. DAYS OR UNITS | H. EPSDT Family Plan | I. ID. QUAL. | J. RENDERING PROVIDER ID. # |
|---|---|---|---|---|---|---|---|---|---|---|
| 1 | | | | | | | | | NPI | |
| 2 | | | | | | | | | NPI | |
| 3 | | | | | | | | | NPI | |
| 4 | | | | | | | | | NPI | |
| 5 | | | | | | | | | NPI | |
| 6 | | | | | | | | | NPI | |

25. FEDERAL TAX I.D. NUMBER SSN EIN

26. PATIENT'S ACCOUNT NO.

27. ACCEPT ASSIGNMENT? (For govt. claims, see back) YES NO

28. TOTAL CHARGE $

29. AMOUNT PAID $

30. BALANCE DUE $

31. SIGNATURE OF PHYSICIAN OR SUPPLIER INCLUDING DEGREES OR CREDENTIALS (I certify that the statements on the reverse apply to this bill and are made a part thereof.)

SIGNED DATE

32. SERVICE FACILITY LOCATION INFORMATION

a. NPI b.

33. BILLING PROVIDER INFO & PH # ( )

a. NPI b.

PHYSICIAN OR SUPPLIER INFORMATION

NUCC Instruction Manual available at: www.nucc.org

APPROVED OMB-0938-0999 FORM CMS-1500 (08/05)

1500

# HEALTH INSURANCE CLAIM FORM

APPROVED BY NATIONAL UNIFORM CLAIM COMMITTEE 08/05

PICA | PICA | CARRIER

1. MEDICARE (Medicare #) [ ] MEDICAID (Medicaid #) [ ] TRICARE CHAMPUS (Sponsor's SSN) [ ] CHAMPVA (Member ID#) [ ] GROUP HEALTH PLAN (SSN or ID) [X] FECA BLK LUNG (SSN) [ ] OTHER (ID) [ ]

1a. INSURED'S I.D. NUMBER (For Program in Item 1): 887105566

2. PATIENT'S NAME (Last Name, First Name, Middle Initial): MORIARTY, JOAN

3. PATIENT'S BIRTH DATE MM DD YY: 12 19 1962 SEX M [ ] F [X]

4. INSURED'S NAME (Last Name, First Name, Middle Initial): MORIARTY, PATRICK

5. PATIENT'S ADDRESS (No., Street): 397 NORTH TONY ROAD

6. PATIENT RELATIONSHIP TO INSURED: Self [ ] Spouse [X] Child [ ] Other [ ]

7. INSURED'S ADDRESS (No., Street): 397 NORTH TONY ROAD

CITY: YOUR TOWN STATE: US

8. PATIENT STATUS: Single [ ] Married [X] Other [ ]

CITY: YOUR TOWN STATE: US

ZIP CODE: 98765 TELEPHONE (Include Area Code): (222) 431-6943

Employed [ ] Full-Time Student [ ] Part-Time Student [ ]

ZIP CODE: 98765 TELEPHONE (Include Area Code): (222) 431-6943

9. OTHER INSURED S NAME (Last Name, First Name, Middle Initial)

10. IS PATIENT'S CONDITION RELATED TO:

11. INSURED'S POLICY GROUP OR FECA NUMBER

a. OTHER INSURED'S POLICY OR GROUP NUMBER

a. EMPLOYMENT? (Current or Previous) [ ] YES [X] NO

a. INSURED'S DATE OF BIRTH MM DD YY: 11 14 1960 SEX M [X] F [ ]

b. OTHER INSURED'S DATE OF BIRTH MM DD YY SEX M [ ] F [ ]

b. AUTO ACCIDENT? [ ] YES [X] NO PLACE (State)

b. EMPLOYER'S NAME OR SCHOOL NAME

c. EMPLOYER'S NAME OR SCHOOL NAME

c. OTHER ACCIDENT? [ ] YES [X] NO

c. INSURANCE PLAN NAME OR PROGRAM NAME: METROPOLITAN-INSURANCE

d. INSURANCE PLAN NAME OR PROGRAM NAME

10d. RESERVED FOR LOCAL USE

d. IS THERE ANOTHER HEALTH BENEFIT PLAN? [ ] YES [X] NO *If yes*, return to and complete item 9 a-d.

**READ BACK OF FORM BEFORE COMPLETING & SIGNING THIS FORM.**

12. PATIENT'S OR AUTHORIZED PERSON'S SIGNATURE I authorize the release of any medical or other information necessary to process this claim. I also request payment of government benefits either to myself or to the party who accepts assignment below.

SIGNED SIGNATURE ON FILE DATE

13. INSURED'S OR AUTHORIZED PERSON'S SIGNATURE I authorize payment of medical benefits to the undersigned physician or supplier for services described below.

SIGNED SIGNATURE ON FILE

PATIENT AND INSURED INFORMATION

14. DATE OF CURRENT: MM DD YY ILLNESS (First symptom) OR INJURY (Accident) OR PREGNANCY(LMP)

15. IF PATIENT HAS HAD SAME OR SIMILAR ILLNESS. GIVE FIRST DATE MM DD YY

16. DATES PATIENT UNABLE TO WORK IN CURRENT OCCUPATION MM DD YY FROM TO

17. NAME OF REFERRING PROVIDER OR OTHER SOURCE 17a. 17b. NPI

18. HOSPITALIZATION DATES RELATED TO CURRENT SERVICES MM DD YY FROM TO

19. RESERVED FOR LOCAL USE

20. OUTSIDE LAB? [ ] YES [ ] NO $ CHARGES

21. DIAGNOSIS OR NATURE OF ILLNESS OR INJURY (Relate Items 1, 2, 3 or 4 to Item 24E by Line)

1. 616.0
2. 595.0
3. 782.3
4.

22. MEDICAID RESUBMISSION CODE ORIGINAL REF. NO.

23. PRIOR AUTHORIZATION NUMBER

| | 24. A. DATE(S) OF SERVICE From MM DD YY | To MM DD YY | B. PLACE OF SERVICE | C. EMG | D. PROCEDURES, SERVICES, OR SUPPLIES (Explain Unusual Circumstances) CPT/HCPCS | MODIFIER | E. DIAGNOSIS POINTER | F. $ CHARGES | G. DAYS OR UNITS | H. EPSDT Family Plan | I. ID. QUAL. | J. RENDERING PROVIDER ID. # |
|---|---|---|---|---|---|---|---|---|---|---|---|---|
| 1 | 09 20 XX | | 11 | | 99213 | | 123 | 80 00 | 1 | | NPI | 7654321 |
| 2 | 09 20 XX | | 11 | | 53670 | | 123 | 120 00 | 1 | | NPI | 7654321 |
| 3 | 09 20 XX | | 11 | | 58100 | | 123 | 300 00 | 1 | | NPI | 7654321 |
| 4 | 09 20 XX | | 11 | | 81000 | | 123 | 25 00 | 1 | | NPI | 7654321 |
| 5 | | | | | | | | | | | NPI | |
| 6 | | | | | | | | | | | NPI | |

25. FEDERAL TAX I.D. NUMBER: 987654321 SSN [X] EIN [ ]

26. PATIENT'S ACCOUNT NO.

27. ACCEPT ASSIGNMENT? (For govt. claims, see back) [ ] YES [ ] NO

28. TOTAL CHARGE: $ 525 00

29. AMOUNT PAID: $

30. BALANCE DUE: $ 525 00

31. SIGNATURE OF PHYSICIAN OR SUPPLIER INCLUDING DEGREES OR CREDENTIALS (I certify that the statements on the reverse apply to this bill and are made a part thereof.)

SIGNATURE ON FILE

SIGNED DATE

32. SERVICE FACILITY LOCATION INFORMATION
SAMUEL E. MATTHEWS
100 E. MAIN ST., STE 120
YOURTOWN, US 98765-4321
a. 7654321 b.

33. BILLING PROVIDER INFO & PH # (222) 789-0123
SAMUEL E. MATTHEWS
100 E. MAIN ST., STE 120
YOURTOWN, US 98765-4321
a. 7654321 b.

PHYSICIAN OR SUPPLIER INFORMATION

NUCC Instruction Manual available at: www.nucc.org

APPROVED OMB-0938-0999 FORM CMS-1500 (08/05)

1500

# HEALTH INSURANCE CLAIM FORM

APPROVED BY NATIONAL UNIFORM CLAIM COMMITTEE 08/05

PICA | PICA

CARRIER

1. MEDICARE (Medicare #) MEDICAID (Medicaid #) TRICARE CHAMPUS (Sponsor's SSN) CHAMPVA (Member ID#) GROUP HEALTH PLAN (SSN or ID) FECA BLK LUNG (SSN) OTHER (ID)

1a. INSURED'S I.D. NUMBER (For Program in Item 1)

2. PATIENT'S NAME (Last Name, First Name, Middle Initial)

3. PATIENT'S BIRTH DATE MM DD YY SEX M F

4. INSURED'S NAME (Last Name, First Name, Middle Initial)

5. PATIENT'S ADDRESS (No., Street)

6. PATIENT RELATIONSHIP TO INSURED Self Spouse Child Other

7. INSURED'S ADDRESS (No., Street)

CITY STATE

8. PATIENT STATUS Single Married Other

CITY STATE

ZIP CODE TELEPHONE (Include Area Code) ( )

Employed Full-Time Student Part-Time Student

ZIP CODE TELEPHONE (Include Area Code) ( )

9. OTHER INSURED S NAME (Last Name, First Name, Middle Initial)

10. IS PATIENT'S CONDITION RELATED TO:

11. INSURED'S POLICY GROUP OR FECA NUMBER

a. OTHER INSURED'S POLICY OR GROUP NUMBER

a. EMPLOYMENT? (Current or Previous) YES NO

a. INSURED'S DATE OF BIRTH MM DD YY SEX M F

b. OTHER INSURED'S DATE OF BIRTH MM DD YY SEX M F

b. AUTO ACCIDENT? PLACE (State) YES NO

b. EMPLOYER'S NAME OR SCHOOL NAME

c. EMPLOYER'S NAME OR SCHOOL NAME

c. OTHER ACCIDENT? YES NO

c. INSURANCE PLAN NAME OR PROGRAM NAME

d. INSURANCE PLAN NAME OR PROGRAM NAME

10d. RESERVED FOR LOCAL USE

d. IS THERE ANOTHER HEALTH BENEFIT PLAN? YES NO ***If yes,*** return to and complete item 9 a-d.

**READ BACK OF FORM BEFORE COMPLETING & SIGNING THIS FORM.**

12. PATIENT'S OR AUTHORIZED PERSON'S SIGNATURE I authorize the release of any medical or other information necessary to process this claim. I also request payment of government benefits either to myself or to the party who accepts assignment below.

SIGNED ________ DATE ________

13. INSURED'S OR AUTHORIZED PERSON'S SIGNATURE I authorize payment of medical benefits to the undersigned physician or supplier for services described below.

SIGNED ________

PATIENT AND INSURED INFORMATION

14. DATE OF CURRENT: MM DD YY ILLNESS (First symptom) OR INJURY (Accident) OR PREGNANCY(LMP)

15. IF PATIENT HAS HAD SAME OR SIMILAR ILLNESS. GIVE FIRST DATE MM DD YY

16. DATES PATIENT UNABLE TO WORK IN CURRENT OCCUPATION FROM MM DD YY TO MM DD YY

17. NAME OF REFERRING PROVIDER OR OTHER SOURCE

17a.

17b. NPI

18. HOSPITALIZATION DATES RELATED TO CURRENT SERVICES FROM MM DD YY TO MM DD YY

19. RESERVED FOR LOCAL USE

20. OUTSIDE LAB? YES NO $ CHARGES

21. DIAGNOSIS OR NATURE OF ILLNESS OR INJURY (Relate Items 1, 2, 3 or 4 to Item 24E by Line)

1. ___ . ___ 3. ___ . ___

2. ___ . ___ 4. ___ . ___

22. MEDICAID RESUBMISSION CODE ORIGINAL REF. NO.

23. PRIOR AUTHORIZATION NUMBER

| | 24. A. DATE(S) OF SERVICE From MM DD YY To MM DD YY | B. PLACE OF SERVICE | C. EMG | D. PROCEDURES, SERVICES, OR SUPPLIES (Explain Unusual Circumstances) CPT/HCPCS MODIFIER | E. DIAGNOSIS POINTER | F. $ CHARGES | G. DAYS OR UNITS | H. EPSDT Family Plan | I. ID. QUAL. | J. RENDERING PROVIDER ID. # |
|---|---|---|---|---|---|---|---|---|---|---|
| 1 | | | | | | | | | NPI | |
| 2 | | | | | | | | | NPI | |
| 3 | | | | | | | | | NPI | |
| 4 | | | | | | | | | NPI | |
| 5 | | | | | | | | | NPI | |
| 6 | | | | | | | | | NPI | |

PHYSICIAN OR SUPPLIER INFORMATION

25. FEDERAL TAX I.D. NUMBER SSN EIN

26. PATIENT'S ACCOUNT NO.

27. ACCEPT ASSIGNMENT? (For govt. claims, see back) YES NO

28. TOTAL CHARGE $

29. AMOUNT PAID $

30. BALANCE DUE $

31. SIGNATURE OF PHYSICIAN OR SUPPLIER INCLUDING DEGREES OR CREDENTIALS (I certify that the statements on the reverse apply to this bill and are made a part thereof.)

SIGNED DATE

32. SERVICE FACILITY LOCATION INFORMATION

a. NPI b.

33. BILLING PROVIDER INFO & PH # ( )

a. NPI b.

NUCC Instruction Manual available at: www.nucc.org

APPROVED OMB-0938-0999 FORM CMS-1500 (08/05)

1500

## HEALTH INSURANCE CLAIM FORM

APPROVED BY NATIONAL UNIFORM CLAIM COMMITTEE 08/05

PICA — PICA — CARRIER

1. MEDICARE (Medicare #) [ ] MEDICAID (Medicaid #) [ ] TRICARE CHAMPUS (Sponsor's SSN) [ ] CHAMPVA (Member ID#) [ ] GROUP HEALTH PLAN (SSN or ID) [X] FECA BLK LUNG (SSN) [ ] OTHER (ID) [ ]

1a. INSURED'S I.D. NUMBER (For Program in Item 1): 505208800A

2. PATIENT'S NAME (Last Name, First Name, Middle Initial): KOSTREVSKI, BORIS

3. PATIENT'S BIRTH DATE MM DD YY: 07 14 1932 SEX M [X] F [ ]

4. INSURED'S NAME (Last Name, First Name, Middle Initial)

5. PATIENT'S ADDRESS (No., Street): 1493 S. JAMES ROAD

6. PATIENT RELATIONSHIP TO INSURED: Self [X] Spouse [ ] Child [ ] Other [ ]

7. INSURED'S ADDRESS (No., Street)

CITY: YOURTOWN STATE: US

8. PATIENT STATUS: Single [X] Married [ ] Other [ ]; Employed [ ] Full-Time Student [ ] Part-Time Student [ ]

CITY STATE

ZIP CODE: 98765 TELEPHONE (Include Area Code): (222) 298-6483

ZIP CODE TELEPHONE (Include Area Code) ( )

9. OTHER INSURED S NAME (Last Name, First Name, Middle Initial)

10. IS PATIENT'S CONDITION RELATED TO:

11. INSURED'S POLICY GROUP OR FECA NUMBER

a. OTHER INSURED'S POLICY OR GROUP NUMBER

a. EMPLOYMENT? (Current or Previous) [ ] YES [X] NO

a. INSURED'S DATE OF BIRTH MM DD YY SEX M [ ] F [ ]

b. OTHER INSURED'S DATE OF BIRTH MM DD YY SEX M [ ] F [ ]

b. AUTO ACCIDENT? [ ] YES [X] NO PLACE (State)

b. EMPLOYER'S NAME OR SCHOOL NAME

c. EMPLOYER'S NAME OR SCHOOL NAME

c. OTHER ACCIDENT? [ ] YES [X] NO

c. INSURANCE PLAN NAME OR PROGRAM NAME

d. INSURANCE PLAN NAME OR PROGRAM NAME

10d. RESERVED FOR LOCAL USE

d. IS THERE ANOTHER HEALTH BENEFIT PLAN? [ ] YES [X] NO *If yes*, return to and complete item 9 a-d.

READ BACK OF FORM BEFORE COMPLETING & SIGNING THIS FORM.

12. PATIENT'S OR AUTHORIZED PERSON'S SIGNATURE I authorize the release of any medical or other information necessary to process this claim. I also request payment of government benefits either to myself or to the party who accepts assignment below.

SIGNED SIGNATURE ON FILE DATE

13. INSURED'S OR AUTHORIZED PERSON'S SIGNATURE I authorize payment of medical benefits to the undersigned physician or supplier for services described below.

SIGNED

PATIENT AND INSURED INFORMATION

14. DATE OF CURRENT: MM DD YY ILLNESS (First symptom) OR INJURY (Accident) OR PREGNANCY(LMP)

15. IF PATIENT HAS HAD SAME OR SIMILAR ILLNESS. GIVE FIRST DATE MM DD YY

16. DATES PATIENT UNABLE TO WORK IN CURRENT OCCUPATION FROM MM DD YY TO MM DD YY

17. NAME OF REFERRING PROVIDER OR OTHER SOURCE 17a. 17b. NPI

18. HOSPITALIZATION DATES RELATED TO CURRENT SERVICES FROM MM DD YY TO MM DD YY

19. RESERVED FOR LOCAL USE

20. OUTSIDE LAB? [ ] YES [ ] NO $ CHARGES

21. DIAGNOSIS OR NATURE OF ILLNESS OR INJURY (Relate Items 1, 2, 3 or 4 to Item 24E by Line)

1. 250.00
2. 414.0
3. ___ . ___
4. ___ . ___

22. MEDICAID RESUBMISSION CODE ORIGINAL REF. NO.

23. PRIOR AUTHORIZATION NUMBER

| | 24. A. DATE(S) OF SERVICE From MM DD YY | To MM DD YY | B. PLACE OF SERVICE | C. EMG | D. PROCEDURES, SERVICES, OR SUPPLIES (Explain Unusual Circumstances) CPT/HCPCS | MODIFIER | E. DIAGNOSIS POINTER | F. $ CHARGES | G. DAYS OR UNITS | H. EPSDT Family Plan | I. ID. QUAL. | J. RENDERING PROVIDER ID. # |
|---|---|---|---|---|---|---|---|---|---|---|---|---|
| 1 | 09 24 XX | | 11 | | 99212 | | 1 2 | 65 00 | 1 | | NPI | 7654321 |
| 2 | 09 24 XX | | 11 | | 82947 | | 1 2 | 25 00 | 1 | | NPI | 7654321 |
| 3 | 09 24 XX | | 11 | | 36415 | | 1 2 | 30 00 | 1 | | NPI | 7654321 |
| 4 | | | | | | | | | | | NPI | |
| 5 | | | | | | | | | | | NPI | |
| 6 | | | | | | | | | | | NPI | |

25. FEDERAL TAX I.D. NUMBER SSN EIN: 987654321 [X] [ ]

26. PATIENT'S ACCOUNT NO.

27. ACCEPT ASSIGNMENT? (For govt. claims, see back) [ ] YES [ ] NO

28. TOTAL CHARGE $ 120 00

29. AMOUNT PAID $

30. BALANCE DUE $ 120 00

31. SIGNATURE OF PHYSICIAN OR SUPPLIER INCLUDING DEGREES OR CREDENTIALS (I certify that the statements on the reverse apply to this bill and are made a part thereof.)
SIGNATURE ON FILE
SIGNED DATE

32. SERVICE FACILITY LOCATION INFORMATION
SAMUEL E. MATTHEWS
100 E. MAIN ST., STE 120
YOURTOWN, US 98765-4321
a. 7654321 b.

33. BILLING PROVIDER INFO & PH # (222) 789-0123
SAMUEL E. MATTHEWS
100 E. MAIN ST., STE 120
YOURTOWN, US 98765-4321
a. 7654321 b.

PHYSICIAN OR SUPPLIER INFORMATION

NUCC Instruction Manual available at: www.nucc.org

APPROVED OMB-0938-0999 FORM CMS-1500 (08/05)

CHAPTER 18

# Patient Billing, Posting Patient Payments, and Collecting Fees

## Words to Know Challenge

**Spelling: Each line contains three spellings of a word. Underline the correctly spelled word. Identify the following correctly spelled Words to Know.**

| | | |
|---|---|---|
| 1. bankrupcy | bankruptcy | bankurptcy |
| 2. idol | idel | idle |
| 3. outsourcing | outsourching | outsorcing |
| 4. termination | ternimation | terminiation |
| 5. vibility | viabality | viability |
| 6. expanded | expender | expended |

**Matching: Match each term in column I to its meaning in column II.**

| | COLUMN I | COLUMN II |
|---|---|---|
| E | 1. Bankruptcy | A. Seeking a name by entering in a system the first few letters of the name |
| L | 2. Viability | B. Accounts due from the provider's patients to the practice |
| P | 3. Account history | C. Date of service |
| Q | 4. Termination | D. Practice management software |
| A | 5. Alpha search | E. Legal petition to the courts if one is unable to pay creditors |
| K | 6. Expended | F. Harmless, ineffectual, meaningless |
| M | 7. Third-party | G. Contracting work out |
| B | 8. Accounts receivable | H. Patient who has moved to avoid payments |
| O | 9. YTD | I. An act enforced by the FTC |
| D | 10. PMS | J. At the time of service |
| F | 11. Idle | K. Used up or spent |
| N | 12. Aging of accounts | L. Capable of success or continuing effectiveness; practicable |

(continues)

| | | |
|---|---|---|
| C | 13. DOS | M. One other than the individuals involved in an account |
| H | 14. Skip | N. System used to analyze A/Rs on past due |
| G | 15. Outsourcing | O. A period starting January 1 of the current year and ending today (example) |
| I | 16. Truth in Lending | P. Computer term for a patient ledger |
| J | 17. ATOS | Q. End in time or existence |

# Chapter Review

## Short Answer

1. What are the typical results of outsourcing physician office work?
Outsourcing usually results in cost savings and higher quality

2. Describe practice management software.
PMS is a category of software that provides the medical office the electronic components to deal with day-to-day financial operations of a practice

3. What types of services do PMS systems offer?
PMS can offer electronic claims posting, statistics, and monthly or YTD billing information

4. What is a third-party check?
A third-party check is generally one made out to the patient by someone unknown to the medical office

5. Describe the use of an alpha search.
An alpha search involves typing the first few letters of the name with the screen automatically listing all names of patients starting with those letters

6. List the three forms of payment described in this chapter.
Cash, credit card, or check are forms of payment

7. What should you do when a credit balance is discovered on a patient account?
When a credit balance is identified, the medical assistant should issue a refund check to the patient

8. List both the positive and negative terms that should or should not be used in a collection letter.
Positive collection letter terms are missed, overlooked, and forgotten; negative terms to avoid are neglected, ignored, and failure

## B. Matching: Match each item in column I to its meaning in column II.

| | COLUMN I | COLUMN II |
|---|---|---|
| I | 1. Cycle billing | A. Billing method more efficient in small practices |
| G | 2. Patient payments | B. Computer terminology for a patient ledger |
| D | 3. Antagonizing terms | C. NSF |
| E | 4. Truth in Lending Act | D. Neglect, ignored, failure |

H 5. Fair Debt Collection Practices Act

A 6. Monthly billing

F 7. Statutes of limitation

B 8. Account history

J 9. Proper collection letter terms

C 10. Nonsufficient funds

E. Specifies agreement between patient and doctor regarding installments and finance charge disclosure

F. Establishes number of years during which legal collection procedures may be filed against a patient

G. Vital for the financial success of a medical facility

H. Prohibits debt collectors from abusive, unfair, or deceptive collection practices

I. Billing commonly used in large practices

J. Missed, overlooked, forgotten

**True or False: Place a T for True or an F for False beside each statement.**

1. F Collection letters should include words such as *neglected*, *ignored*, or *failure*.
2. F An estate claim involves sending a bill owed by a deceased patient to the address of any known next of kin.
3. T Written communication is the least effective means of collecting patient fees.
4. F The best collection opportunity after face-to-face contact is by an email.
5. T A patient's check marked NSF returned to the office by a bank indicates that there are insufficient funds to cover the amount of the check.
6. F The Truth in Lending Act enforces fair debt collection practices.
7. T The monthly billing cycle is typically more efficient in smaller medical practices.
8. T An accurate patient account statement is a required document in the patient billing process.
9. T The violation of any credit law can invite an opportunity for the patient to sue the provider.
10. F The collection agency generally comes into play when a bill is delinquent for more than three months.

# Chapter Application

## Case Study with Critical Thinking Questions

Chris, the billing person at Bonita Medical Clinic, is responsible for all patient billing and bookkeeping. He has fallen behind on his daily posting and is having trouble catching up. His totals are not balancing for accounts receivable, and he is frustrated.

1. When should posting be done? Posting should be done daily as the payments are received within the office.
2. In what order should the entries be placed? The entries should be placed in date order with the oldest date first.
3. What could be the possible outcome of sloppy bookkeeping practices? The outcome could show inaccuracies, jeopardize the practice's viability, and demonstrate skewed numbers in statistical data.
4. What should Chris do in this situation? Chris should report his situation to the office manager and request assistance by other staff or overtime to catch up on his work if allowed by the office. He can also request an assessment of the need to hire a second person in the billing department.

UNIT 9

# Banking and Accounting Procedures

CHAPTER **19**

# Banking Procedures

## Words to Know Challenge

**Spelling: Each line contains three spellings of a word. Underline the correctly spelled word.**

| | | |
|---|---|---|
| 1. reconcilling | reconciling | recountciling |
| 2. negotiable | negoshiable | necotible |
| 3. denomanation | demonination | denomination |
| 4. withdralle | withdrawl | withdrawal |
| 5. endorsement | endorcement | endorsment |
| 6. currensy | currency | currancy |
| 7. deposite | diposit | deposit |
| 8. registre | register | registir |
| 9. transaction | trensaction | transacion |

**Matching: Match the terms in column I to their meanings in column II.**

| | COLUMN I | COLUMN II |
|---|---|---|
| G | 1. Agent | A. An amount of money (cash or checks) placed in a bank account |
| I | 2. Endorser | B. A check generally made out to the patient by someone unknown to you |
| F | 3. Deposit slip | C. An amount beyond what is currently in the account |
| H | 4. Withdrawal | D. A fee charged by the bank for services rendered |
| B | 5. Third-party check | E. Used when an error is made on a check |
| J | 6. Outstanding | F. An itemized list of cash and checks deposited into an account |
| A | 7. Deposit | G. A person authorized to act for another person |
| E | 8. VOID | H. Removal of funds from an account |
| D | 9. Service charge | I. Payee |
| C | 10. Overdraft | J. A check that has been written but that does not appear on the bank statement |

# Chapter Review

## Short Answer

1. Explain the handling of currency in the office.
All cash should be placed out of sight as soon as received, in a cash box, file drawer, or some other secure (locked) location. Care should be taken that your money storage place is not in view of patients in the reception area. Usually, all daily proceeds are either locked in a safe or deposited at the close of the day.

2. List the seven components of a check you must examine to ensure that it is valid.
(1) The date; (2) Words of negotiability; (3) The payee; (4) The numeric amount; (5) The written amount; (6) The drawee financial institution; (7) The signature.

3. List five pieces of information a bank needs to stop payment on a check. For what reasons may a payment be stopped?
(1) Check number, (2) Date issued, (3) Name of payee, (4) Amount of check, and (5) Reason for stopping payment. Reasons include: Lost check or disagreement regarding product or service rendered.

4. Name the two types of endorsements and explain what each means.
(1) Blank endorsement: a signature only. This type of endorsement should be used only when immediately cashing a check. Otherwise, if the check is stolen, it could be endorsed by someone else and cashed. (2) Restrictive endorsement: limits the payment to the bank and physician's account only.

5. Briefly describe a bank statement.
A bank statement is a record of all financial activity that occurred on a specific account, usually in a month's time period. Bank statements may be offered by mail or by online banking services.

## Labeling: Identify each component on the following check.

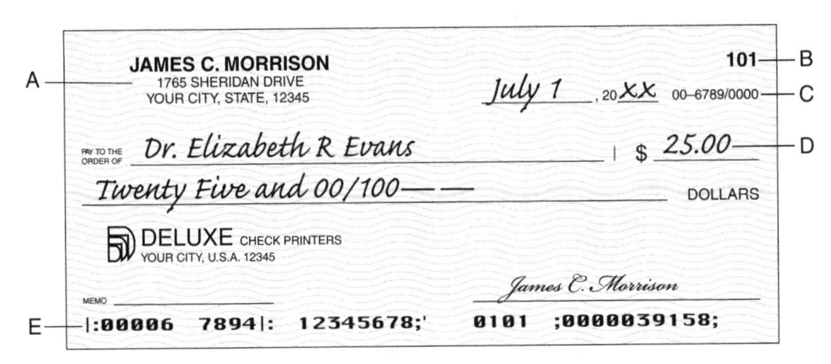


a. Name and address of maker

b. Chronologic check number

c. ABA number

d. Numeric amount of check

e. MICR numbers

# Chapter Application

## Competency Practice: Writing Checks

Use the following information to write a check to Physician's Supply, Inc., for $125.50, using the sample check provided in Work Product 19–1. Use the current date and sign the checks with the physician's name provided with your name below the line. Complete the stub end, subtracting each subsequent check with the initial total starting balance of $8480.64. *Work product forms are provided at the end of the chapter.*

## Competency Practice: Preparing a Deposit

Use the following list of cash and check payments to prepare a bank deposit slip, provided in Work Product 19–2. Use today's date as the deposit date. *Work product forms are provided at the end of the chapter.*

| | |
|---|---|
| Currency/coin | 1 – $50.00 bill; 6 – $20.00 bills; 15 – $10.00 bills; 17 – $5.00 bills; 14 – $1.00 bills; 4 – quarters |
| Checks | Smith, check #1458: $40.00<br>Manolo, check #501: $425.00<br>Vronski, check #998: $220.00<br>Leu, check #4010: $25.00<br>Wallace, check #1155: $150.00 |
| Money orders | Jones: $15.00 |

## Competency Practice: Reconciling a Bank Statement

Use the information below to reconcile the bank account on Work Product 19–3. (You may assume the opening balance agrees with the previous statement.) *Work product forms are provided at the end of the chapter.*

### CHECKBOOK (REGISTER)

Ending balance: $3173.71

Checks written during the month:

| Check # | Amount | √ | Check # | Amount | √ |
|---|---|---|---|---|---|
| 201 | 25.00 | | 217 | 785.00 | |
| 202 | 600.00 | | 218 | 28.37 | |
| 203 | 75.00 | | 219 | 60.00 | |
| 204 | 37.54 | | 220 | 36.30 | |
| 205 | 30.00 | | 221 | 115.45 | |
| 206 | 95.94 | | 222 | 35.00 | |
| 207 | 73.87 | | 223 | 95.94 | |
| 208 | 44.00 | | 224 | 19.00 | |
| 209 | 130.00 | | 225 | 75.00 | |
| 210 | 95.94 | | 226 | 400.00 | |
| 211 | 500.00 | | 227 | 78.37 | |
| 212 | 18.22 | | 228 | 95.94 | |
| 213 | 133.28 | | 229 | 200.00 | |
| 214 | 57.50 | | 230 | 33.60 | |
| 215 | 38.60 | | 231 | 1200.00 | |
| 216 | 500.00 | | 232 | 100.00 | |

Deposits made during the month:

| Deposit Date | Amount | √ |
|---|---|---|
| 6-02 | 500.00 | |
| 6-03 | 750.00 | |
| 6-06 | 350.00 | |
| 6-07 | 700.00 | |
| 6-09 | 335.00 | |
| 6-12 | 500.00 | |
| 6-14 | 440.50 | |
| 6-15 | 180.00 | |
| 6-18 | 175.00 | |
| 6-19 | 520.00 | |
| 6-20 | 522.50 | |
| 6-22 | 720.00 | |
| 6-25 | 600.00 | |
| 6-27 | 662.00 | |
| 6-30 | 191.00 | |

**Account Statement**

*THE NEVER FAIL BANK*

*NEVER FAIL ACCOUNT*

ANYWHERE BRANCH
0000 THIS STREET
ANYTOWN, STATE 00000-0000

CUSTOMER SERVICE 24 HOURS A DAY, 800-000-0000

ACCOUNT
12345-678910
STATEMENT PERIOD
6-1-20xx TO 7-1-20xx

JANE D. CUSTOMER
1234 HOME STREET
ANYTOWN, STATE 00000-0000

**ACCOUNTS SUMMARY**

| CHECKING | | SAVINGS |
|---|---|---|
| BEGINNING BALANCE | 1840.57 | |
| DEPOSITS | 6955.00 | |
| CHECKS PAID | 3715.32 | |
| ATM & DEBIT CARD WITHDRAWALS | 0.00 | |
| SERVICE CHARGES/FEES | 3.27 | |
| ENDING BALANCE | 5076.98 | |

**CHECKING ACTIVITY**

| DEPOSITS POSTED | AMOUNT | DESCRIPTION |
|---|---|---|
| 6-03 | 500.00 | ATM DEPOSIT |
| 6-04 | 750.00 | ATM DEPOSIT |

| | | |
|---|---|---|
| 6-07 | 350.00 | DEPOSIT |
| 6-08 | 700.00 | DEPOSIT |
| 6-10 | 335.00 | DEPOSIT |
| 6-13 | 500.00 | ATM DEPOSIT |
| 6-15 | 440.50 | ATM DEPOSIT |
| 6-16 | 180.00 | DEPOSIT |
| 6-19 | 175.00 | DEPOSIT |
| 6-20 | 520.00 | DEPOSIT |
| 6-21 | 522.50 | DEPOSIT |
| 6-23 | 720.00 | DEPOSIT |
| 6-26 | 600.00 | DEPOSIT |
| 6-28 | 662.00 | ATM DEPOSIT |

| **CHECKS PAID CHECK #** | **AMOUNT** |
|---|---|
| 201 | 25.00 |
| 202 | 600.00 |
| 203 | 75.00 |
| 205 | 30.00 |
| 206 | 95.94 |
| 207 | 73.87 |
| 208 | 44.00 |
| 209 | 130.00 |
| 210 | 95.94 |
| 211 | 500.00 |
| 212 | 18.22 |
| 213 | 133.28 |
| 214 | 57.50 |
| 215 | 38.60 |
| 216 | 500.00 |
| 218 | 28.37 |
| 219 | 60.00 |
| 220 | 36.30 |
| 221 | 115.45 |
| 222 | 35.00 |
| 223 | 95.94 |
| 224 | 19.00 |
| 226 | 400.00 |
| 227 | 78.37 |
| 228 | 95.94 |
| 229 | 200.00 |
| 230 | 33.60 |
| 232 | 100.00 |

**CHECKING SERVICES CHARGE AND FEE SUMMARY**

| **AMOUNT** | **DESCRIPTION** |
|---|---|
| 3.27 | MONTHLY SERVICE CHARGE |

# Work Product Forms

## Work Product 19–1

1490 BAL. BRO'T FOR'D

20

TO

DEPOSITS

FOR

TOTAL

THIS CHECK

BALANCE

**ELIZABETH R. EVANS, M.D.**
SUITE 205 100 E. MAIN ST.
YOURTOWN, US 98765-4321

1490

20

25-64/440

PAY TO THE ORDER OF $

DOLLARS

THE NEVER FAIL BANK
ANYWHERE, U.S.A 00000

7-88-25

FOR

|:00006 7894|: 12345678;' 01491 ;0000039158;

## Work Product 19–2

I.M. Healthy, M.D.
101 Fitness Lane
Anywhere, U.S.A. 00000

DATE 20

The Never Fail Bank
Anywhere, U.S.A.

| CASH | CURRENCY | | |
|---|---|---|---|
| | COIN | | |
| LIST CHECKS SINGLY | | | |
| | | | |
| | | | |
| TOTAL FROM OTHER SIDE | | | |
| TOTAL | | | |
| LESS CASH RECEIVED | | | |
| NET DEPOSIT | | | |

USE OTHER SIDE FOR ADDITIONAL LISTING

BE SURE EACH ITEM IS PROPERLY ENDORSED

⑆044000024⑆ 02894110861⑈

CHECKS AND OTHER ITEMS ARE RECEIVED FOR DEPOSIT SUBJECT TO THE PROVISIONS OF THE UNIFORM COMMERCIAL CODE OR ANY APPLICABLE COLLECTION AGREEMENT

| CHECKS LIST SINGLY | DOLLARS |
|---|---|
| 1 | |
| 2 | |
| 3 | |
| 4 | |
| 5 | |
| 6 | |
| 7 | |
| 8 | |
| 9 | |
| 10 | |
| 11 | |
| 12 | |
| 13 | |
| 14 | |
| 15 | |
| 16 | |
| 17 | |
| 18 | |
| 19 | |
| TOTAL | |

ENTER TOTAL ON THE FRONT OF THIS

## Work Product 19–3

RECONCILING THE BANK STATEMENT

Bank Statement Balance $ _____

(+) Plus Deposits not shown

_______

Total _______ $ _____

(–) Less Outstanding Checks

# _______

# _______

# _______

# _______

Total _______ $ _____

| CORRECTED BANK STATEMENT BALANCE $ _____ |
|---|

Checkbook Balance $ _____

(–) Less Bank Charges $ _____

| CORRECTED CHECKBOOK BALANCE $ _____ |
|---|

## Answer Key for Work Product 19–1

**Check stub:**

| 1490 | BAL. BRO'T FOR'D | 8480 | 64 |
|---|---|---|---|
| Current Date 20 | | | |
| TO Physician's Supply Inc. | DEPOSITS | | |
| FOR | | | |
| | TOTAL | 8480 | 64 |
| | THIS CHECK | 125 | 50 |
| | BALANCE | 8355 | 14 |

**Check:**

ELIZABETH R. EVANS, M.D.
SUITE 205 100 E. MAIN ST.
YOURTOWN, US 98765-4321

1489

Current Date 20___ 25-64/440

PAY TO THE ORDER OF Physician's Supply Inc. $ 125.50

One Hundred Twenty Five and 50/100 —— DOLLARS

THE NEVER FAIL BANK
ANYWHERE, U.S.A 00000

7-88-25

FOR ______ Elizabeth R. Evans MD.

|:00006 7894|: 12345678;' 01489 ;0000039158;

## Answer Key for Work Product 19–2

I.M. Healthy, M.D.
101 Fitness Lane
Anywhere, U.S.A. 00000

DATE *Today's date* 20____

| CASH | CURRENCY | 419 | 00 |
|---|---|---|---|
| | COIN | 1 | 00 |
| LIST CHECKS SINGLY | | | |
| | | | |
| | | | |
| TOTAL FROM OTHER SIDE | | 860 | 00 |
| TOTAL | | 1280 | 00 |
| LESS CASH RECEIVED | | | |
| NET DEPOSIT | | 1280 | 00 |

USE OTHER SIDE FOR ADDITIONAL LISTING

BE SURE EACH ITEM IS PROPERLY ENDORSED

The Never Fail Bank
Anywhere, U.S.A.

⑆044000024⑆ 0289411086⑈

CHECKS AND OTHER ITEMS ARE RECEIVED FOR DEPOSIT SUBJECT TO THE PROVISIONS OF THE UNIFORM COMMERCIAL CODE OR ANY APPLICABLE COLLECTION AGREEMENT

| CHECKS LIST SINGLY | DOLLARS |
|---|---|
| 1 *Smith#1458* | 40 0 |
| 2 *Manolo#501* | 425 0 |
| 3 *Vronski#998* | 220 0 |
| 4 *Leu#4010* | 25 0 |
| 5 *Wallace#1155* | 150 0 |
| 6 | |
| 7 | |
| 8 | |
| 9 | |
| 10 | |
| 11 | |
| 12 | |
| 13 | |
| 14 | |
| 15 | |
| 16 | |
| 17 | |
| 18 | |
| 19 | |
| TOTAL | 860 |

ENTER TOTAL ON THE FRONT OF THIS

## Answer Key for Work Product 19–3

RECONCILING THE BANK STATEMENT

Bank Statement Balance $ 5076.98

(+) Plus Deposits not shown

6/30 $191.00

Total $191.00 $ 5267.98

(-) Less Outstanding Checks

\# 204 $37.54

\# 217 $785.00

\# 225 $75.00

\# 231 $1200.00

Total $2097.54 $ 3170.44

| CORRECTED BANK STATEMENT BALANCE | $ 3170.44 |
|---|---|

Checkbook Balance $ 3173.71

(-) Less Bank Charges $ 3.27

| CORRECTED CHECKBOOK BALANCE | $ 3170.44 |
|---|---|

CHAPTER 20

# Accounts Payable and Accounting Procedures

## Words to Know Challenge

**Spelling: Each line contains three spellings of a word. Underline the correctly spelled word.**

| | | |
|---|---|---|
| ecquity | eqity | equity |
| voucher | vowcher | voutcher |
| writ-offs | rite-offs | write-offs |
| cost raetio | cost rashio | cost ratio |
| manegerial | managerial | manigerial |
| account payable | accounts payable | account payabel |
| balence sheet | balanse sheet | balance sheet |

**Fill in the Blank: Complete the following sentences with correctly spelled words from the Spelling section.**

1. Allie took $25 from petty cash to purchase stamps for the office and completed a voucher to account for this action.
2. Managerial accounting is the study and analysis of financial data as it applies to operational issues within a company.
3. Total expenses for one month ÷ total number of procedures for one month = cost ratio.
4. Accounts payable refers to the total amounts owed by the practice to suppliers and other service providers for regular business operating expenses.
5. Net worth or equity demonstrates the value of a business.
6. A statement of financial position is also known as the balance sheet.
7. Bad debts and professional courtesy discounts are considered write-offs for a medical facility.

**Matching: Match the terms in column I to their meanings in column II.**

| | COLUMN I | COLUMN II |
|---|---|---|
| I | 1. A/P | A. Debts or A/P owed by the business |
| H | 2. Expenditure | B. Adjusted collection ratio |
| G | 3. Petty cash | C. Current A/R balance ÷ average monthly gross production |
| F | 4. Net worth | D. Allows for program evaluation |
| J | 5. Assets | E. Document with itemized goods or services |
| B | 6. Net collection ratio | F. Assets – liability |
| E | 7. Invoice | G. Small amount of stored money, ranging from $25–$75 |
| A | 8. Liabilities | H. An acquired material in exchange for money |
| C | 9. A/R ratio | I. Total amounts owed by practice to supplier |
| K | 10. Income statement | J. The money and items of value in a business |
| D | 11. Cost–benefit analysis | K. Demonstrates the profit and expenses for a given time period |

## Chapter Review

### Short Answer

1. Explain why comparing shipments to packing lists or invoices is important.
   Comparing company shipments with invoices is important because payment of the total amount of the invoice would represent payment for all goods received. If something is missing from the shipment when compared to the invoice, not all goods were received, and payment must be corrected.

2. Describe what should be done when a shipment item does not match the invoice.
   When a shipment does not match the invoice, notification of any discrepancy should be brought immediately to the attention of the supplier.

3. For what purpose is a petty cash fund used?
   Petty cash is used when small payments are required, such as for postage stamps, inexpensive office supplies, and small charitable donations.

4. Explain why it is important to know the net worth of a business.
   It is important to know the net worth of a business because it demonstrates the value of a business; little net worth might not hold a business very long.

5. Explain why collection ratios might be important to a doctor's office.
   Collection ratios might be important to a doctor's office because they show the provider how the practice is doing with collections and whether the employees are working to their fullest capacity to enhance business.

6. What are charges considered when deemed uncollectible? Provide two examples.
   Charges deemed uncollectible by a business are considered write-offs. Examples will vary, but many include professional courtesy discounts, insurance adjustments, contractual adjustments, and bad debts.

7. What are the three steps of cost–benefit analysis?
   The three steps to cost–benefit analysis are: identify costs, identify benefits, and compare costs and benefits.

8. Explain what income statements and balance sheets demonstrate to a medical practice.
   An income statement demonstrates the profit and expenses for a given month and includes year-to-date information. A balance sheet reveals the company's assets, liabilities, and owner's equity (net worth)

9. Name the two types of collection ratios most frequently used in a medical office.
   The two types of collection ratios most frequently used are gross collection and net collection.

**Matching: Match the ratios in column I to their formulas in column II.**

| | COLUMN I | COLUMN II |
|---|---|---|
| C | 1. A/R ratio | A. Assets – Liabilities = Net Worth |
| D | 2. Cost ratio | B. Total Payments (A/R) ÷ Total Charges Minus Write-Offs |
| A | 3. Basic accounting formula | C. Current A/R Balance ÷ Average Monthly Gross Production |
| E | 4. Gross collection ratio | D. Total Expenses ÷ Total Number Of Procedures For One Month |
| B | 5. Net collection ratio | E. Total Payments (A/R) ÷ Total Charges |

# Chapter Application

## Case Study with Critical Thinking Questions

Sabrina Holton is the office manager, and Dr. Imel asks her to report back on whether the use of the contracted diabetic educator is cost effective to house in the office. The educator has been teaching patients for one month in a small office space rented by Dr. Imel and, during that month, has taught 20 patients. The educator bills the doctor $30.00 per patient. Additional details: The rental of the office space is $100 per month; electricity and Internet service for the space is $50; office supplies are $15.

1. What ratio formula will MA Sabrina use to calculate this loss or gain and why?
   MA Sabrina will use the cost ratio formula because it demonstrates the cost of a specific procedure or service, and, in this case, the diabetic educator is a service

2. Calculate the answer to the ratio formula you identified.
   $765 (Total Expenses) ÷ 20 (Total Number of Procedures for One Month) = $38.25 (Cost Ratio)

## Competency Practice: Completing a Petty Cash Form

Use Work Product 20–1 and the following amounts to establish and maintain a petty cash fund, which was opened on 9/19 (current year) with an opening balance of $25.00. When the petty cash fund decreases below $5.00, a new check should be written to bring the fund back up to the $25.00 level.

a. Bill: postage $5.00, 9/20
b. Voucher 1: charity donation $10.00, 9/23
c. Bill: envelopes and pens $8.00, 9/24
d. Voucher 2: mileage $5.00, 9/27
e. Bill: postage $8.50, 9/30

**Work Product 20–1**

| PETTY CASH FORM | | | |
|---|---|---|---|
| Date | Bill/Voucher Description | Amount | Balance |
| | | | |
| | | | |
| | | | |
| | | | |
| | | | |
| | | | |
| | | | |
| | | | |
| | | | |

**Answer Key for Work Product 20–1**

| PETTY CASH FORM | | | |
|---|---|---|---|
| Date | Bill/Voucher Description | Amount | Balance |
| 09/19/20XX | Fund established | | $25.00 |
| 09/20/20XX | Bill: Postage | $5.00 | $20.00 |
| 09/23/20XX | Voucher 1: Charity donation | $10.00 | $10.00 |
| 09/24/20XX | Bill: Envelopes and pens | $8.00 | $2.00 |
| 09/24/20XX | New check: replenish petty cash to $25 | $23.00 | $25.00 |
| 09/27/20XX | Voucher 2: Mileage | $5.00 | $20.00 |
| 09/30/20XX | Bill: Postage | $8.50 | $11.50 |
| | | | |
| | | | |

UNIT 10

# Managing the Medical Office Environment

CHAPTER 21

# Facilities Management and Emergency Preparedness

## Words to Know Challenge

**Spelling: Each line contains three spellings of a word. Underline the correctly spelled word.**

| | | |
|---|---|---|
| 1. asault | assault | assoult |
| 2. biohazard | biohazzard | biohazerd |
| 3. environment | enviroment | enviromint |
| 4. extinguisher | extinguischer | extingusher |
| 5. hazzard | hazerd | hazard |
| 6. inventory | invetorie | inventorie |
| 7. irratioshonal | irrational | irationnal |
| 8. reception | reseption | recepsion |
| 9. volatile | volittle | volotile |

**Fill in the Blank: Complete the following sentences with correctly spelled words from the Spelling section.**

1. Physical or sexual assault can also occur when the interior office is accessible from unlocked outside access or the reception area.
2. A safe environment begins at the front door. The reception room requires a safety check every morning to ensure that it presents no hazards for patients and visitors.
3. Atmosphere affects how people experience their environment and can have a relationship to their response to treatment.
4. Chemicals kept in the office for laboratory work must be properly labeled and stored and monitored carefully because they could become volatile when kept beyond their expiration date.
5. If a spill involves bodily fluids such as blood or urine, universal precautions must be observed, and materials should be placed in a biohazard waste bag to be disposed of properly.
6. Careful monitoring of inventory is vital. You do not want to run out of needed supplies, yet you also do not want to over-order items.

**Matching: Match the term in column I to its definition in column II**

| | COLUMN I | COLUMN II |
|---|---|---|
| G | Atmosphere | A. To prevent access; bar passage |
| A | Barrier | B. Withdrawal, to remove, to make empty |
| E | Emergency preparedness | C. Care beforehand; a preventive measure |
| J | Emergency | D. Provide information about working with or handling a particular chemical substance |
| B | Evacuated | E. Preparing for the first and immediate response to any type of emergency or hazard |
| H | Intervention | F. The act of keeping something from coming to pass; to hinder |
| C | Precaution | G. Any surrounding influence |
| F | Prevention | H. Taking action to modify, hinder, or change an effect |
| D | MSDS | I. A minimum amount of supplies to be maintained; also known as par level |
| I | Threshold | J. An unexpected occurrence or situations demanding immediate action |

# Chapter Review

## Short Answer

1. List five things to check in the reception area at the beginning of the day.
   Any five of the following: Temperature, the room's appearance (neat, clean, well lit), reading material (current, clean, appropriate materials), safety check (furniture, flooring, lighting, electrical devices), toys and books (clean, sanitized, and safe), smoking policy is displayed.

2. List five tasks to perform when preparing the front desk at the beginning of the day.
   Any five of the following: Turn on computers, scanners, printers, other electronic equipment; retrieve telephone messages; retrieve faxes; retrieve printed lab and hospital reports; place charts for check-in; prepare sign-in sheets; prepare cash balance forms.

3. List five tasks to perform when preparing an examination room for use.
   Any five of the following: Visually inspect for cleanliness, be certain trash is emptied, check temperature, plug in equipment, restock supplies, keep hazardous material secured, keep prescription pads in a locked area, secure electrical cords.

4. Describe the importance of materials safety data sheets.
   MSDSs ensure that the hazards of all chemicals produced or imported are evaluated and that information concerning their hazards is transmitted to employers and employees.

5. Using the abbreviations OSHA, CDC, and CLIA, indicate which organization has the responsibility for the following:
   a. Protects employees: OSHA
   b. Collects data on diseases: CDC
   c. Certifies physician's laboratory testing: CLIA
   d. Establishes policies to reduce disease transmission: CDC
   e. Develops standard precautions: CDC
   f. Provides employees with safe working conditions: OSHA
   g. Classifies diseases according to method of spread: CDC
   h. Regulates testing of specimens: CLIA
   i. Dictates the use of gloves: OSHA

6. Name three elements necessary for fire.
   Heat, fuel, and oxygen

7. List at least two ways a fire might start.
   Answers will vary but can include: A carelessly discarded match or cigarette; a defective outlet or frayed wires on any electrical appliance or office equipment; coffee pots and water sterilizers boiling dry and causing a fire

8. Explain the PASS acronym.
   The PASS acronym refers to the correct operation of a fire extinguisher: (P)ull the pin at the top of the extinguisher; (A)im at the base of the fire; (S)queeze the handle slowly; (S)weep from side to side until the fire is out.

# Chapter Application

## Research Activity

Research the emergency preparedness plans your community has. Summarize your findings in the following space:

Answers will vary

## Critical Thinking

Identify each safety sign, symbol, or label and then describe methods of complying with each.

| Sign, Symbol, or Label | What It Means | Describe Ways to Comply |
|---|---|---|
|  | Biohazard | Answers will vary |
| 3 0 0 OXY | NFPA Fire Triangle | Answers will vary |
|  | No Smoking Sign | Answers will vary |
|  | Flammable | Answers will vary |

## Video Case Study

1. Log on to the Premium Website and view the video for this chapter on "Stress and Emergency Situations." Develop a 1–2 page paper, responding to the following prompts:
   - What do you think this statement means: "Sometimes [family members'] presence may be a distraction," related to an emergency situation?
   - The video mentioned signs to look for in a family member that indicate that person might not be tolerating the emergency situation well. Think about other emergency situations, such as a natural disaster or a chemical exposure event, and discuss signs or stresses you think someone might experience during these situations.
   - Take an assessment of yourself and how you would respond during an emergency situation.
   - Why is it important to practice and be prepared for an emergency?

## Case Studies with Critical Thinking Questions

### Scenario 1

As Mary Ramirez, the medical assistant, escorts the first patient into the exam room, she notices that the room is disorganized and that there is evidence of the last patient from the day before. Mary needs to take the patient's vitals and notices that the blood pressure cuff is missing, so she leaves the room to find it.

1. What might the patient's impression of the office be? The office might appear as though the employees are careless and do not practice good ethics.
2. What should the medical assistant have done before bringing the patient to the exam room? She should have checked the room to be sure everything was in order.
3. How can this situation be prevented in the future? It can be prevented by assigning one individual each day to check the rooms before seeing patients.

### Scenario 2

While carrying a rack full of tubes containing blood to be discarded into the biohazard container, Jennifer slips and falls. The tubes scatter everywhere, but, fortunately, only three of them break. This accident occurred in the main hallway, so Jennifer needs to think fast and get this mess cleaned up.

1. What PPE should Jennifer apply? Safety glasses or goggles, face shield, gloves, apron, hair and shoe covers.
2. Describe the steps Jennifer should use to clean up the spilled blood. After donning appropriate PPE, locate and apply the prepared spill kit. Clean the area with a 10 percent bleach solution. Bag contaminated clothing and materials in a leak-proof biohazard bag. Place a second bag around the first and dispose of in the proper method (licensed waste disposal service).
3. Where should the tubes be discarded? Tubes should be discarded in a sharps container.

## Competency Practice: Opening and Closing the Office

Using the information in your book, create typed checklists to use when opening and closing the medical office. In the checklists, be sure to include items to be observed for safety as well as any environmental considerations and other precautions that should be taken.

## Competency Practice: Perform an Office Inventory

Perform an inventory of the school laboratory supplies listed on the following inventory sheet. Accurately count and record number and amount of each item. Indicate if reordering is necessary, following the protocol for the exact inventory that should be available.

| Item | Amount on Hand | Minimum Needed | Place Order? | Date |
|---|---|---|---|---|
| Urine reagent strips | | 2 bottles | | |
| Urine specimen cups | | 25 | | |
| Microhematocrit tubes | | 2 bottles | | |
| Sealing clay | | 2 | | |
| ESR kits | | 1 | | |
| Rapid strep kits | | 2 | | |
| Glass slides | | 10 boxes | | |
| Cover slips | | 3 boxes | | |
| Pregnancy test kits | | 2 | | |
| Lens paper | | 5 tablets | | |

## Competency Practice: Develop a Personal Safety Plan

Start developing your personal safety plan for yourself and your family by answering the following prompts:

- Teach children to call 911 and to know what information should be given to the 911 operator. The information to be given to the operator is: Name, address, telephone number, brief description of the emergency ______________________________________________.
- Create a list of emergency numbers and information. Some of the information to include on this list is:
  a. Police: Answers will vary
  b. Fire department: Answers will vary
  c. Poison control center: 1-800-222-1222
  d. The closest hospital to my house is: Answers will vary

## Competency Practice: Evaluate the Work Environment to Identify Safe vs. Unsafe Working Conditions

To practice for this competency, evaluate a personal living space (your apartment, your home, your parents' home, your workplace, and so on) for safe and unsafe conditions. Write down five safe conditions and five unsafe conditions present.

Place of evaluation: Answers will vary

| | Safe Conditions Present | Unsafe Conditions Present |
|---|---|---|
| 1. | | |
| 2. | | |
| 3. | | |
| 4. | | |
| 5. | | |

## Competency Practice: Explain an Evacuation Plan for a Medical Office

Discuss how to evacuate patients during a fire alarm in the following situations and then role-play each scenario with a partner.

1. Hearing-impaired patients in the waiting room
2. Sight-impaired patient with an escort in an exam room
3. Personnel working in the laboratory
4. Wheelchair-bound patient in an exam room

CHAPTER 22

# Managing the Office

## Words to Know Challenge

**Spelling: Each line contains three spellings of a word. Underline the correctly spelled word.**

1. acounttant | accountant | accowntant
2. benefits | benifits | bennefits
3. complimentary | complamentary | complimentry
4. dissability | disability | disabbility
5. expendature | expenditure | expendichure
6. fring benafits | fringe bennefits | fringe benefits
7. Internal Revenue Service | Internal Revinue Service | Internal Revanue Service
8. profit shareing | profit sharing | profut sharing
9. berevement | bearevement | bereavement

**Fill in the Blank: Complete the following sentences with Words to Know from this chapter.**

1. Employees can be paid an hourly wage (a varying amount, depending on hours worked) or a salary (a fixed amount paid on a regular basis for a prescribed period of time).
2. Full-time medical office employees can expect benefits in addition to their wages. These are sometimes known as fringe benefits.
3. Bereavement time is when an employee can take time off when a family member dies.
4. Sometimes medical care is offered to employees (referred to as complimentary health care); however, some practices prohibit employee–physician relations due to potential conflicts of interest.
5. All invoices for purchases, checks (banking), and disbursement records are examples of expenditures of a medical office, which must be carefully accounted for and entered in the bookkeeping system.
6. When an accountant, management firm, or payroll (or HR) department is employed to prepare payroll, office records must be provided by a designated date each pay period (weekly, bi-weekly, or monthly) so that payroll can be prepared in a timely manner and records maintained on file.

7. Profit sharing is a form of retirement or pension plan for employees who meet certain requirements, such as being at least 21 years old, working a minimum of 1,000 hours in a year, and remaining employed for at least a year to establish eligibility.

**Matching: Match the term in column I to its definition in column II.**

| | COLUMN I | COLUMN II |
|---|---|---|
| J | 1. Site review | A. Freed from or not liable for something to which others are subject |
| D | 2. Deductions | B. A long duration of life; lasting a long time |
| A | 3. Exemption | C. The amount of work accomplished in a period of time |
| H | 4. Fiscal | D. To deduct or subtract; remove, take away |
| F | 5. Gross | E. Settled; complete; absolute; continuous |
| B | 6. Longevity | F. Exclusive of deductions; total, entire |
| I | 7. Net | G. To pay back or compensate for money spent or losses or damages incurred |
| C | 8. Productivity | H. Of or pertaining to finances in general |
| G | 9. Reimbursement | I. Remaining after all deductions have been made; to clear as profit |
| E | 10. Vested | J. An inspection to ensure compliance with regulations and policies |

## Chapter Review

1. Describe six responsibilities a manager has to employees.
   Any six of the following: Interview, hire, discipline, and terminate employees; Supervise or personally train employees; Conduct staff meetings; Create, implement, and enforce work and vacation schedules; Conduct performance evaluations; Consult providers concerning performance evaluations, salary increases, and benefits.

2. Describe how HIPAA has affected office policy.
   Answers will vary but may include: Check-in process, medical charts, secured fax machine, required confidential phone lines, covering medical information in unsecured areas, computer screen, disposal of documents, reporting a security incident, unique passwords.

3. Explain the purpose of W-4, W-2, and I-9 forms.
   a) W-4: A Withholding Allowance Certificate indicating the number of exemptions claimed by the employee
   b) W-2: A summary of all earnings for the year and all deductions withheld for federal, state, and local taxes, provided to each employee by January 31 of each year
   c) I-9: Issued by the Department of Justice, Immigration and Naturalization Service to ensure that all employed persons are United States citizens, lawfully admitted aliens, or aliens authorized to work in the United States

4. Differentiate between gross and net salary.
   Net pay is the actual amount of the paycheck after deductions. Gross salary is the total amount of pay (number of hours work multiplied by salary per hour)

5. Describe the office manager's role in staff meetings.
   The office manager is responsible for setting staff meeting schedules and the agenda and conducting the meetings. Staff meetings should last from 30 minutes to one hour, and be held at least once a month

6. Describe the office manager's role in employee evaluation and review.
   The role of the manager in employee evaluations is vital, conducted in a private meeting setting, to discuss personal goals, performance, expectations, wage adjustments, and educational pursuits. Most organizations require employees to have regular, routine, or periodic reviews or evaluations regarding their work performance.

7. Describe the office manager's role in termination employment.
   It is often the responsibility of the manager to terminate support staff after discussion and coordination with provider(s) and HR department. The manager must synchronize the termination with the payroll department to comply with Department of Labor regulations.

8. What are salary benefits? In your answer, identify six examples of benefits an employee might receive.
   Any six of the following: Paid time off (PTO), vacation, holidays, sick time, personal time; bereavement time, jury duty, health insurance, disability insurance, life insurance, profit sharing (retirement).

9. Describe and list at least six responsibilities a manager has to the providers.
   Any six of the following: Assisting in creating or updating business policies; attending professional meetings; updating physicians on insurance changes, fee schedules, and reimbursement rates; ordering and evaluating CPT and ICD books; holding provider meetings to discuss practice concerns; managing staff; maintaining safety and security of patients, office, and staff; ensuring legal compliance; managing the information technology component; monitoring the financial status of the practice.

10. In the following chart, place an X in the column next to items that would be included on a practice information brochure.

| | |
|---|---|
| Lengthy physician biography | |
| After-hours policy | X |
| Missed appointment policy | X |
| Physician specialties | X |
| Smoking policy | |
| Hospital affiliation | X |
| Office hours | X |
| Prescription refill policy | X |

11. List at least four organizations that inspect medical offices during site visits.
    Any four of the following: Insurance companies, CLIA, COLA, OSHA, Local or state board of health, DEA, fire department.

**Matching: For each item listed in column I, identify whether it is considered an office POLICY (A) or PROCEDURE (B). (*Note*: Answers in column II may be used more than once.)**

| | COLUMN I | COLUMN II |
|---|---|---|
| A | 1. Absenteeism | A. Policy |
| A | 2. Paid time off | B. Procedure |
| B | 3. Opening and closing the office | |
| A | 4. Harassment | |
| B | 5. OSHA and CLIA requirements | |
| A | 6. Confidentiality | |
| B | 7. Laboratory tests | |

(continues)

B 8. Emergency procedures

A 9. Employment evaluations

A 10. Information technology

**Matching: For each item listed in column I, identify whether it is considered the manager's responsibility to EMPLOYEE (A), PHYSICIAN (B), or FACILITY (C). (*Note*: Answers in column II may be used more than once.)**

| | COLUMN I | COLUMN II |
|---|---|---|
| C | 1. Subscriptions to magazines | A. Responsibility to employee |
| A | 2. Conduct staff meetings to inform, discuss, and exchange information | B. Responsibility to physician |
| B | 3. Assist in creating/updating business policies to increase efficiency | C. Responsibility for facility |
| C | 4. Monitor and pay utilities | |
| C | 5. Security (locks, alarms), privacy (HIPAA) | |
| B | 6. Order CPT and ICD books annually to review for deleted or added codes | |
| A | 7. Create, implement, and enforce work schedules | |
| B | 8. Manage staff in most efficient and effective manner for provider productivity | |
| C | 9. Information technology support | |
| A | 10. Conduct performance evaluations | |

# Chapter Application

## Case Studies with Critical Thinking Questions

### Scenario 1

A job applicant for the position of clinical medical assistant has passed the first interview and is handed a stack of paperwork to be filled out to ensure that she is eligible to work in this capacity and in this country. She is hired for the job, but at the end of the first two-week pay period, the person responsible for payroll in the office sends the clinical supervisor a note stating that the applicant cannot be paid.

1. Can you think of a reason the employee cannot be able to be paid? Answers will vary, but it is likely that all paperwork was not completed.

2. Which form must be filled out before anyone can begin working in the United States? All employees in the United States must complete an I-9 form to be eligible for employment.

### Scenario 2

Maryn Leonard, a single mother of three, has just been hired to work as a medical assistant at the Downtown Clinic. She has completed all required documents for employment and has started working. Her first paycheck seems to be lower than what she expected, and she wants to know why.

1. How many dependent deductions can she claim? Four

2. On which form would you check to ensure that the correct number of dependent deductions are claimed to raise her pay? W-4

### Scenario 3

You have just been hired at Downtown Clinic as a clinical medical assistant. The office manager tells you that although the office carries liability insurance, you personally are not covered under the policy. You ask another medical assistant about whether she has insurance, and she tells you she does not. She says she hasn't looked into it, but she thinks it might be expensive. She says she's been working there for five years, and it's not a big deal whether you get the insurance. What should you do?

If liability is not offered by the practice, medical assistants should purchase their own coverage to protect their personal assets.

### Scenario 4

While a patient was leaving the exam room at the Downtown Clinic, she slipped and fell on a wet surface. You helped her up and discovered a large gash on her forehead. You contact the treating physician to attend to the patient and then immediately notify the practice manager of the incident and prepare an incident report. Why is office liability insurance important?

It protects the employee's personal and professional assets if he or she is found liable for some action or lack of action (commonly referred to as malpractice insurance).

### Research Activity

1. Go to the IRS Website (www.irs.gov) and locate an I-9 form. Locate "Section 2. Employer Review and Verification" on the form and the "List of Acceptable Documents." In the following chart, identify which types of documents are included in lists A, B, and C and then identify three documents within each category.
   Documents in List A are documents that establish both identity and employment authorization.
   Documents in List B are documents that establish identity.
   Documents in List C are documents that establish employment authorization.

| | List A | List B | List C |
|---|---|---|---|
| 1. | Answers will vary but can include any of the answers below: U.S. passport, permanent resident card, foreign passport with temporary i-551 stamp, employment authorization document with photo, foreign passport with Form I-94/I-94A | Answers will vary but can include any of the answers below: (other answers exist) Driver's license, federal, state, and local ID card, school ID card with photo voter's registration card; U.S. military card or draft record, Military dependent ID card | Answers will vary but can include any of the answers below: (other answers exist) Social Security card, birth certificate, certificate of birth abroad (from state dept.) Native American tribal document, U.S. citizen ID card |
| 2. | | | |
| 3. | | | |

2. Go online and search for free employee evaluation form templates. Compare several forms and print out the form you think is the best. With a partner, complete the evaluation form based on your partner's performance in the classroom.

## Competency Practice

1. Using a travel site such as Kayak (www.kayak.com), Expedia (www.expedia.com), or Travelocity (www.travelocity.com), search for the cheapest flights meeting the criteria provided. Search for a flight three months from the current day.
   - Search for a round-trip flight to Chicago (O'Hare airport); select the airport closest to your town or city. The flight should be in the morning and have no more than one connecting flight (if possible from your airport). *Note*: If you live in the greater Chicago area, choose another destination city of your choice.
   - Search for a nonstop, round-trip flight from New York City (JFK airport) to Denver, Colorado. The flight can be at any time.
2. Payroll activity. An employee has worked 32 hours for the week of August 1 to August 7. Her hourly rate is $16.50 per hr. She has claimed four exemptions on her W-4.
   - What is her GROSS pay?
   - What is her NET pay?

# SECTION 3

# Structure and Function of the Body

UNIT 11

# Anatomy and Physiology of the Human Body

# Anatomical Descriptors and Fundamental Body Structure

## Words to Know Challenge

**Spelling: Each line contains three spellings of a word. Underline the correctly spelled word.**

| | | |
|---|---|---|
| 1. antonomy | anotomy | anatomy |
| 2. anterior | aunterior | antieror |
| 3. cavitie | cavity | cavety |
| 4. conective | connective | conneckdtive |
| 5. cranial | craneal | cranal |
| 6. doorsal | dursal | dorsal |
| 7. edama | edema | edemma |
| 8. epigastric | epagastric | epaghastric |
| 9. epatheleal | epathelial | epithelial |
| 10. jean | geen | gene |
| 11. illiac | iliac | illac |
| 12. lateral | latarel | laterel |
| 13. lumbar | lumber | lambar |
| 14. midlane | mildline | midline |
| 15. muscelle | muscel | muscle |
| 16. orgen | organ | organne |
| 17. posterior | posteror | posterear |
| 18. smoothe | smooth | smouth |
| 19. vantral | ventril | ventral |

**Matching: Match the term in column I to its description in column II.** (Note: Not all descriptions will be used.)

| | COLUMN I | COLUMN II |
|---|---|---|
| D | 1. Cardiac | A. Groin area |
| H | 2. Cranial | B. A nerve cell |
| P | 3. Cytoplasm | C. A covering on a nerve |
| S | 4. Diaphragm | D. Heart tissue |
| Y | 5. Dorsal | E. Toward the midline |
| W | 6. Epigastric | F. Change in the genetic code |
| R | 7. Homeostasis | G. Part of extremity nearest the body |
| CC | 8. Hypochondriac | H. Above the body's tranverse line |
| A | 9. Inguinal | I. Midline |
| T | 10. Lateral | J. Muscle tissue in organs |
| E | 11. Medial | K. Abdominal area around navel |
| C | 12. Myelin | L. Stores hereditary material of the cell |
| B | 13. Neuron | M. Consists of like cells |
| G | 14. Proximal | N. Skeletal muscle tissue |
| J | 15. Smooth | O. Below the body's tranverse line |
| N | 16. Striated | P. Cellular fluid |
| X | 17. Thoracic | Q. Part of extremity farthest away from body |
| M | 18. Tissue | R. State of normal functioning |
| K | 19. Umbilical | S. Muscle that divides anterior cavity |
| V | 20. Ventral | T. Away from the midline |
| F | 21. Mutation | U. Carried by X chromosome |
| L | 22. Chromosome | V. The anterior section |
| U | 23. X-linked gene | W. Pertaining to the abdominal area above umbilical |
| I | 24. Midsagittal | X. Chest area |
| O | 25. Caudal | Y. Of or pertaining to the posterior section |
| | | Z. The abdominal area below the umbilical |
| | | AA. The cell nucleus |
| | | BB. Swelling in the tissues |
| | | CC. Abdominal area below ribs |

## Chapter Review

**Fill in the Blank: Use information from the chapter to complete the sentence.**

1. In anatomical position, the patient's right side is across from your left side.
2. Something toward the midline is said to be medial; if it is away from the midline it is lateral.
3. Arms and legs are known as extremities.

4. The front of the body is called the anterior or ventral section.
5. The back section is called the dorsal or posterior side.
6. The body has two main cavities. The anterior cavity is further divided into an upper thoracic and a lower abdominopelvic cavity.
7. The posterior body section has a(n) cranial cavity and a(n) spinal cavity.

## Short Answer

1. Describe the meaning of the phrase "anatomical position." Refers to the universally accepted means of describing the location of structures based on the body standing erect, facing you, with arms down at sides, and the palms of the hands facing forward.
2. List the organs within each body cavity.
   a. Thoracic: Heart, lungs
   b. Abdominal: Stomach, small intestine, large intestine, liver, spleen, pancreas, gall bladder
   c. Pelvic: Urinary bladder, internal reproductive organs
   d. Cranial: Brain
   e. Spinal: Spinal cord
3. The abdomen can be divided into four sections for reference purposes. Name the sections.
   a. Right upper quadrant
   b. Left upper quadrant
   c. Right lower quadrant
   d. Left lower quadrant
4. List the structures of a cell.
   a. Cell membrane
   b. Cytoplasm
   c. Nucleus
   d. Centrioles
   e. Endoplasmic reticulum
   f. Mitochondria
   g. Golgi apparatus
   h. Lysosomes
   i. Pinocyte vesicles
   j. Ribosomes
5. List three things that may cause a mutation to occur.
   a. DNA has been lost
   b. rearranged
   c. paired in error
6. Name three types of inheritance patterns and explain how they affect an individual's inherited traits.
   a. Dominant—results in structural defects
   b. Recessive—if paired with similar mutated gene, produces a recessive disorder
   c. X-linked—is carried by the X chromosome and depends on which parent carries the defect and whether the child is male or female
7. List the six processes by which materials pass through cell membranes.
   a. Diffusion
   b. Osmosis

c. Filtration
d. Active transport
e. Phagocytosis
f. Pinocytosis

8. What is the name of the project that sequenced genes? The Human Genome Project

9. Explain the term "DNA fingerprinting" and how it can be used. It is a detection and identification method based on DNA code. It permits positive identification because it is based on DNA molecules, which are unique to each individual.

10. List the four types of tissues. Identify three places in the body where the tissue can be found.
    a. Epithelial
        1. Skin
        2. Cavity linings
        3. Organs (also glands, organ linings)
    b. Connective
        1. Fat
        2. Tendons
        3. Ligaments
    c. Nerve
        1. Nerves
        2. Brain
        3. Spinal cord
    d. Muscle
        1. Skeletal muscles
        2. Organ walls
        3. Eye (heart)

11. List the 10 systems of the body.
    a. Nervous
    b. Integumentary
    c. Skeletal
    d. Muscular
    e. Circulatory
    f. Respiratory
    g. Digestive
    h. Urinary
    i. Endocrine
    j. Reproductive

## Labeling

1. Label the nine anatomical divisions and one reference point of the abdomen on the following illustration. Refer to Figure 23–7 in the textbook.

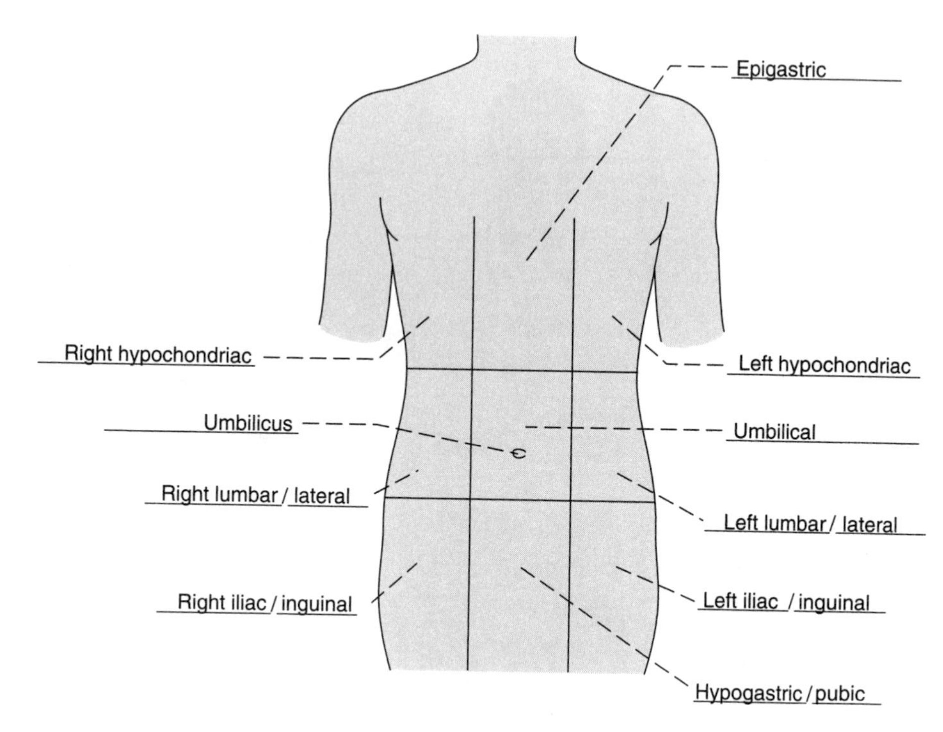

2. Label the directional reference terms on the illustrations of anatomical position. Refer to Figure 23–1 in the textbook.

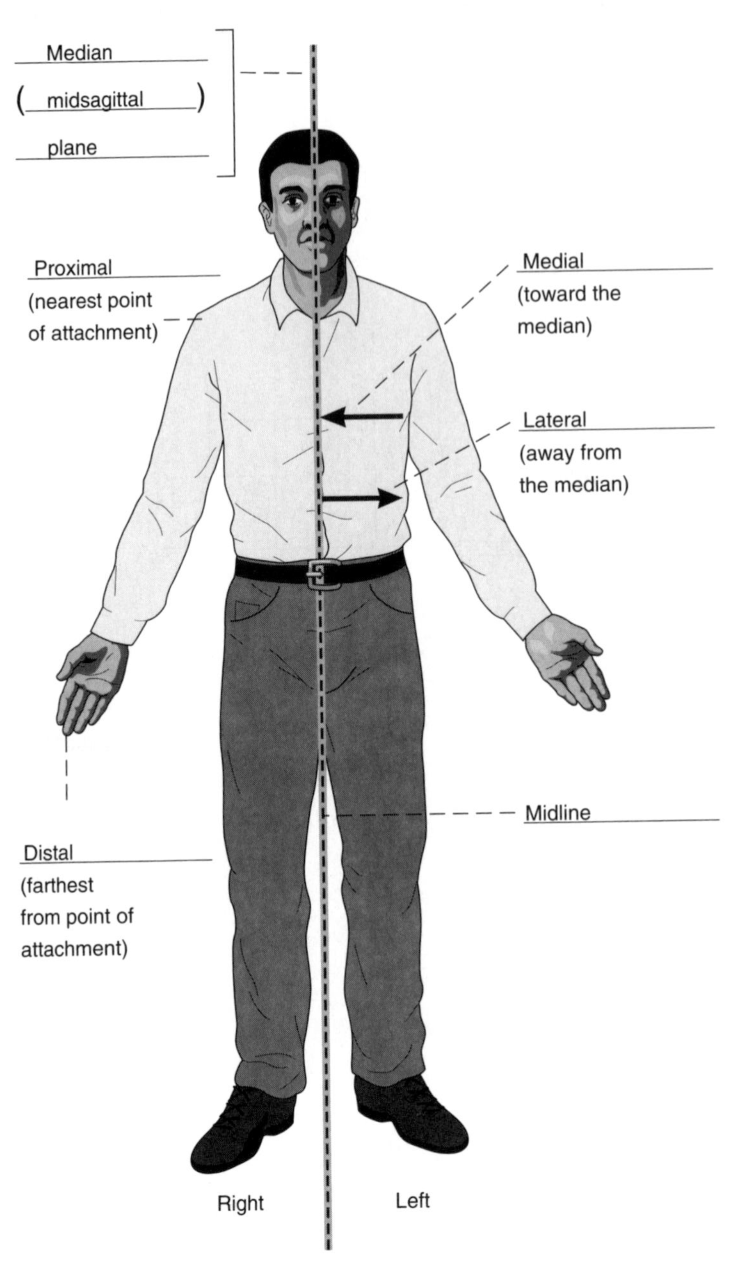

3. Label the directional reference terms on the illustration of anatomical position. Refer to Figure 23–3 in the textbook.

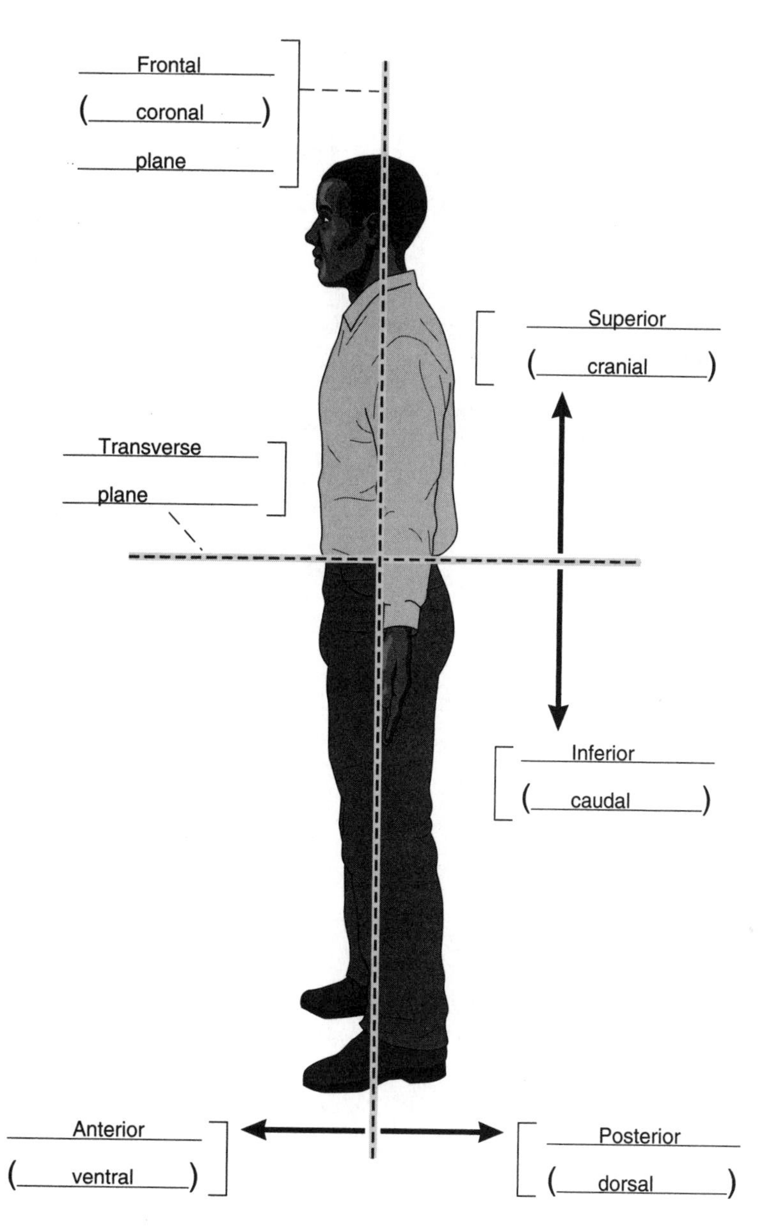

4. Label the eight body cavities on the following illustration. Refer to Figure 23–4 in the textbook.

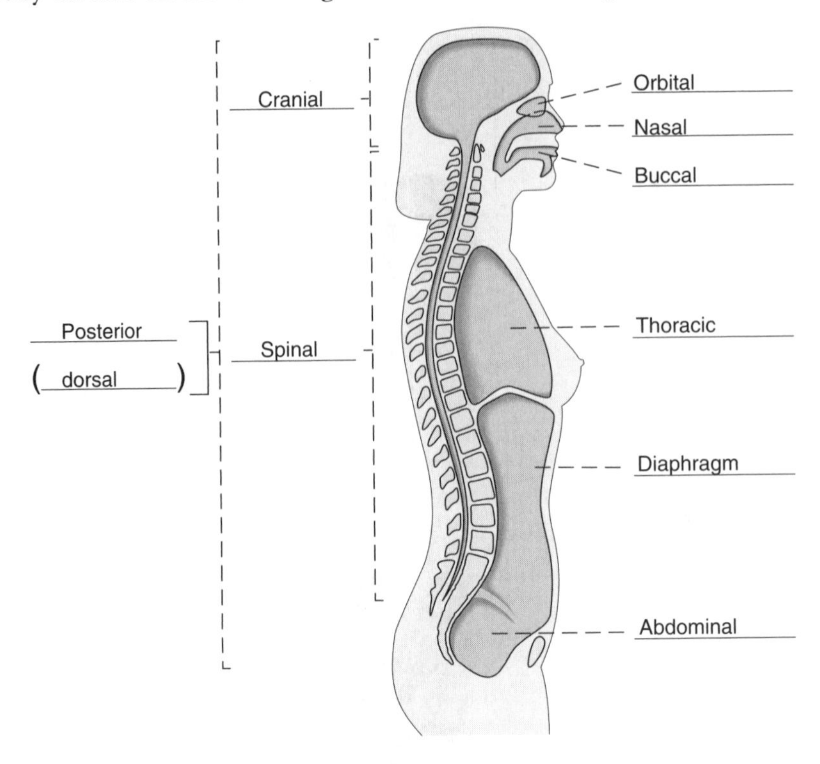


5. Label the thoracic and abdominal organs. Refer to Figure 23–5 in the textbook.

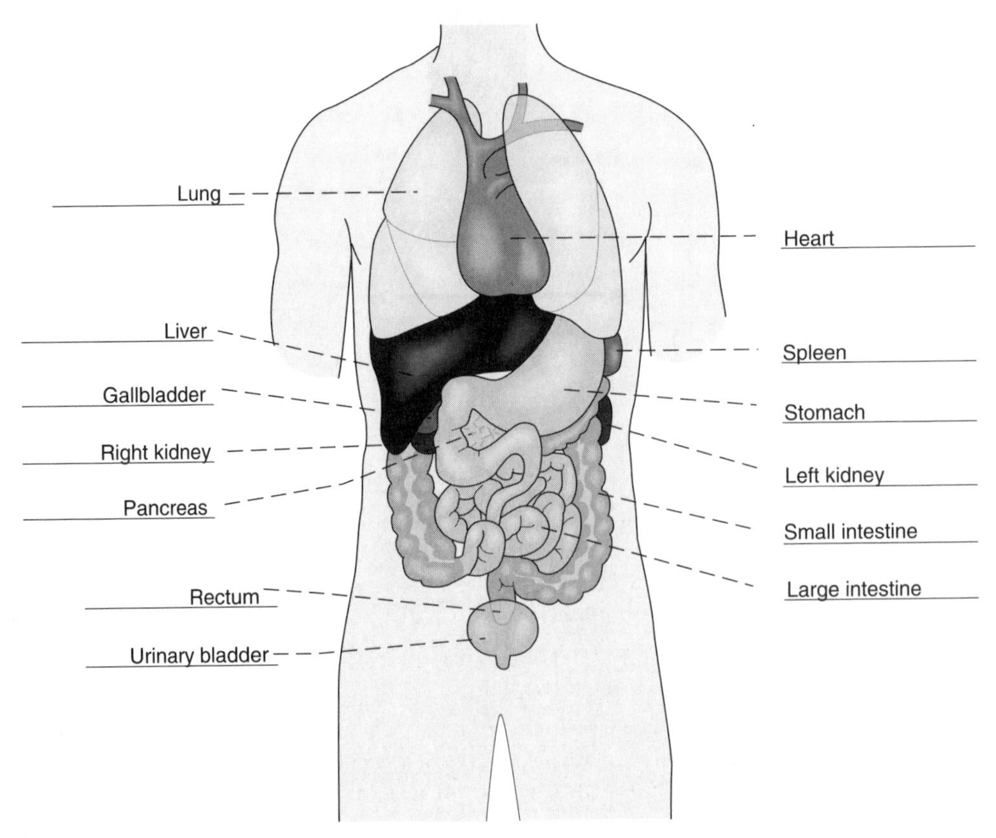

## Matching

**1. Match the acid or base in column I with its possible material in column II.**

| | COLUMN I | COLUMN II |
|---|---|---|
| D | 1. Acetic acid | A. Batteries |
| F | 2. Boric acid | B. Household liquid cleaners |
| E | 3. Hydrochloric acid | C. Lye |
| A | 4. Sulfuric acid | D. Vinegar |
| B | 5. Ammonium hydroxide | E. The stomach |
| G | 6. Magnesium hydroxide | F. Weak eyewash |
| C | 7. Sodium hydroxide | G. Milk of Magnesia |

**2. The following genetic conditions have visible abnormal characteristics that make them readily recognized. Match the condition in column I to its visible sign in column II.**

| | COLUMN I | COLUMN II |
|---|---|---|
| C | 1. Cleft lip | A. Male with long legs and short, obese trunk |
| E | 2. Cleft palate | B. Malformation of one or both feet |
| F | 3. Down syndrome | C. Vertical split in upper lip |
| G | 4. Spina bifida | D. Female with webbing of the neck |
| A | 5. Klinefelter's syndrome | E. Opening in the top of mouth |
| B | 6. Talipes | F. Small head and slanting eyes |
| D | 7. Turner's syndrome | G. A malformation of the back |

# Chapter Application

## Case Studies with Critical Thinking Questions

### Scenario 1

Your best friend shares with you that she is trying to become pregnant. You know that she is 39 years old and has a younger brother with Down syndrome. She tells you she has not talked to a physician about pregnancy.

1. What type of physician does she need to see? She needs to see her primary care, if a referral is required by her insurance or an obstetrician before she becomes pregnant. She may also need to be referred to a genetic specialist. You need to encourage her to seek medical advice as soon as possible.

2. How do you feel about asking her if she considered the risks of this pregnancy? If you feel comfortable in your friendship and have adequate knowledge to discuss her risks of age and a family history, you could at least bring up the subject. Since she has a brother with Down syndrome, she is probably quite comfortable discussing it. Again, she needs to discuss this aspect with a medical professional.

3. How would you determine if it might be appropriate to talk with her about how she would deal with it if she learned she was having a Down child? Again, this depends on your relationship. Since she was mostly likely closely involved with her brother, she may not be too concerned if she has a Down infant; it depends on her experience. If the experience has not been good, then she may need to discuss available options. You need to encourage her to consider her true feelings and discuss them without judging. Again, a professional needs to be consulted.

### Scenario 2

A neighbor confides in you that her 15-year-old son has not shown any signs of sexual maturity, even though he is in high school and almost 6 feet tall. You know from previous discussions that he has had some difficulty in school. She has asked you what you think.

1. What kind of questions do you need to ask to determine what she means by sexual maturity? Is the mother referring to physical or social characteristics? If physical, he should have evidence of masculine changes in his penis and scrotum, as well as the distribution of pubic and facial hair. His voice would also show signs of deepening. If social, perhaps he has trouble talking to girls, feels he is not macho or popular enough, or feels self-conscious for some perceived imperfection.
2. What could you tell her if it sounds like he might have a hormone deficiency? After determining he is not developing physically, you need to suggest that she discuss her concerns with his pediatrician or her primary care physician, who might refer him to an endocrinologist if the situation warrants it. Explain to her that a lack of male hormone needs to be ruled out. You probably should not mention you suspect he might have a genetic disorder, since that diagnosis is very serious.
3. How can you help her to identify a physician for her to consult? If the son does not have a pediatrician and she does not have a primary care physician, you might suggest she get one, since this is where she should start. You may want to discuss the situation with your employer and set up an appointment or get a recommendation.

### Research Activity

Select one of the congenital disorders discussed in the text. Do an Internet search to learn more about the condition. Find out about the causes and treatment. Is there a support group for people and families dealing with the condition? Is there a national, state, or local association supporting the disorder? (You may need to refer to your phone directory for local information.) Prepare a short written report of your findings.

As an alternative to a disorder search, find out more about gene therapy, genetic engineering, or genetic counseling. Look for new techniques or options for genetic conditions.

### Role Play Activity

Working in a group of three, one is the model, one is the medical assistant, and one asks the questions. Using the textbook Figures 23–1, 23–2, 23–3, 23–4, 23–6, and 23–7, the questioner asks the medical assistant to show on the model 10 of the directional terms, body cavities, or abdominal regions. Then, the group changes roles and continues the identification. Repeat as long as desired.

CHAPTER 24

# The Nervous System

## Words to Know Challenge

**Spelling: Each line contains three spellings of a word. Underline the correctly spelled word.**

| | | | |
|---|---|---|---|
| 1. angiography | angiografie | angeography | angiographe |
| 2. aracknoid | arachnoid | arachenoid | arachnoyd |
| 3. autonomech | autanomic | autonomic | autenomic |
| 4. cerebellam | ceribellum | cerabellum | cerebellum |
| 5. hypothalamous | hypothalamus | hypathalmus | hypethalmous |
| 6. mininges | menegies | maninges | meninges |
| 7. periferal | peripherel | peripheral | peripharel |
| 8. sciatika | sciatica | siaticka | sciateca |
| 9. sympathetic | synpethetic | synpathitic | synpathic |
| 10. ventrickle | vantricle | ventracle | ventricle |

**Matching: Match each word in column I with its definition in column II.**

| | COLUMN I | COLUMN II |
|---|---|---|
| E | 1. Meninges | A. The skull |
| C | 2. Motor | B. Nerve that causes action or movement |
| H | 3. Occipital | C. Small brain part at top of brain stem |
| A | 4. Cranium | D. Contains sensory nerve cell bodies |
| G | 5. Autonomic | E. Membranes covering the central nervous system |
| J | 6. Frontal | F. Nerve of vision |
| B | 7. Motor | G. Part of the peripheral nervous system |
| D | 8. Ganglion | H. Posterior lobe of cerebrum |
| F | 9. Optic | I. Cavity within the brain |
| I | 10. Ventricle | J. Portion of cerebrum behind forehead |

## Chapter Review

**Matching: For each symptom, write the letter of the appropriate disease or disorder.**

D 1. Sudden, acute onset of fever, headache, and vomiting, which progresses to a stiff neck and back, drowsiness, and eventual coma

K 2. Blurred or double vision with sensations of tingling or numbness; periods of attacks and remission characterized by tremor, muscular weakness, and paralysis

N 3. Severe muscle rigidity, drooling, tremor, and a bent-forward position when walking

R 4. Temporary double vision, slurred speech, dizziness, staggering, and falling

G 5. Loss of sensation with paralysis of one side of the body

P 6. Sharp, piercing pain in the back of the thigh extending down the side of the leg

B 7. Weakness and paralysis on one side of the face causing drooping mouth, drooling, and inability to close the affected eye

F 8. Fluid-filled vesicles on the skin associated with fever, severe pain, itching, and abnormal skin sensations

E 9. Seizures of varying duration, possible loss of consciousness, loss of body function control, and convulsions

H 10. Abnormally large head, distended scalp veins, shiny scalp skin, irritability, vomiting

C 11. Hyperactive tendon reflexes, underdeveloped affected extremities, muscular contractions; may also have seizures, mental retardation, and impaired speech

I 12. High fever, chills, headache, positive Brudzinski's and Kernig's signs

L 13. Severe pain along the course of a nerve anywhere in the body

S 14. Excruciating facial pain upon stimulation of a trigger zone

M 15. Paralysis with loss of sensation and reflexes in lower extremities

A 16. Muscular weakness and atrophy; problems with speech, chewing, and swallowing; respirations may be affected; choking and drooling

J 17. Prodromal symptoms of fatigue, visual disturbances, tingling of face and lips, sensitivity to light, nausea, and vomiting

Q 18. Incomplete closure of one or more vertebra, bladder and bowel control problems, hydrocephalus, weakness or paralysis of legs, often includes mental retardation

O 19. Vomiting, lethargy, liver dysfunction, hyperventilation, delirium and coma, with eventual respiratory arrest

A. Amyotrophic lateral sclerosis
B. Bell's palsy
C. Cerebral palsy
D. Encephalitis
E. Epilepsy
F. Herpes zoster
G. Hemiplegia
H. Hydrocephalus
I. Meningitis
J. Migraine headache
K. Multiple sclerosis
L. Neuralgia
M. Paraplegia
N. Parkinson's disease
O. Reye's syndrome
P. Sciatica
Q. Spina bifida
R. Transient ischemic attack
S. Trigeminal neuralgia

## Short Answer

1. List the two main divisions of the nervous system.
   a. Central nervous system (CNS)
   b. Peripheral nervous system
2. What is a synapse? A minute space between the axon of one cell and the dendrite of another, over which nerve impulses must jump chemically.
3. Identify two types of peripheral nerves.
   a. Cranial
   b. Spinal
4. List the two types of spinal nerves and describe their functions.
   a. Motor nerves, which provide for movement by innervating muscles or causing organs to function
   b. Sensory nerves, which pick up and transmit messages from receptor cells to the spinal cord and brain
5. What is the purpose or function of the autonomic nervous system? Unconscious regulation of body functions
6. Name the two divisions of the autonomic nervous system, explaining their actions.
   a. Sympathetic—accelerates activity in the smooth, involuntary muscles of the body's organs
   b. Parasympathetic—reverses the action of the sympathetic and slows down activity
7. List the five divisions of the brain and identify what function each division provides.
   a. Cerebrum—controls sensory and motor function (including emotions, personality, the senses, skin sensors, movement of hands, feet, etc.)
   b. Cerebellum—responsible for smooth muscle movement, muscle tone, equilibrium, walking, and dancing
   c. Medulla oblongata—influences heart, lungs, stomach secretions, and size of blood vessel openings
   d. Pons—helps regulate breathing and is the reflex center for chewing, tasting, and secreting saliva
   e. Midbrain—controls reflex movements of eyes and conducts impulses between parts above and below it
8. List the lobes of the cerebrum and their associated functions.
   a. Frontal—emotions, personality, moral traits, and intellectual functions; voluntary muscle movements and speech
   b. Occipital—vision
   c. Parietal—speech, receives impulses from hands, feet, tongue and sends impulses to cause movement; receives impulses for pain, heat, cold, and touch
   d. Temporal—senses of hearing and smell
9. List the two structures between the cerebrum and the midbrain, describing their functions.
   1. Thalamus—Relay station for impulses going to and from or within brain.
   2. Hypothalamus—Autonomic nervous control; Controls blood pressure; Maintains body temperature; Stimulates antidiuretic hormone; Assists in appetite regulation; Increases intestinal secretions and motility; Involved with emotions; Helps maintain wakefulness.
10. List the three meninges, describing their characteristics as given in the text.
    a. Pia mater—innermost layer; contains blood vessels to nourish
    b. Arachnoid—middle layer, lacelike membrane
    c. Dura mater—outer layer; protects the CNS from damage from bones

11. What are the spaces called between the (a) dura mater and the arachnoid and (b) the arachnoid and the pia?

    Subdural and Subarachnoid

12. Name the fluid within the cavities of the CNS and describe its function. Cerebrospinal—acts as a cushion or shock absorber and transports nutrients

**Matching: Match the diagnostic tests in column I with their purposes in column II.**

| | COLUMN I | COLUMN II |
|---|---|---|
| G | 1. Arteriography | A. Detects abnormal electrical impulses in the brain |
| I | 2. Brain scan | B. Detects tumors, bleeding, clots, brain size, and edema |
| J | 3. Glasgow Coma Scale | C. Measures cerebrospinal fluid pressure or obtains a sample of fluid |
| B | 4. CAT scan | D. Images enhanced with color |
| A | 5. EEG | E. Detects cranial fractures or dense cerebral areas |
| H | 6. Electromyography | F. Instills a dye or air to show irregularities in the CNS |
| C | 7. Lumbar puncture | G. Detects cerebral hemorrhage, aneurysm, or CVA |
| F | 8. Myelography | H. Detects neuromuscular disorders or nerve damage |
| E | 9. Skull x-ray | I. Radioisotopes are measured to detect abnormal masses or blood vessel lesions |
| D | 10. Position emission tomography | J. Describes the level of consciousness |

**Fill in the Blank: Use information from the chapter to fill in the blank space in the sentence.**

1. Simple reflex actions involve an impulse traveling along a nerve to the spinal cord and back.
2. A common test used to illustrate this action is called the knee jerk test.
3. Complex reflex actions involve an impulse traveling from its source through nerve cells to the spinal cord and up to the brain. The message is interpreted and the motor nerves carry the response message back to the spinal cord and out the appropriate nerve.

### Labeling

Label the illustration using the following terms. Refer to Figure 24-10A in the textbook.

| | | |
|---|---|---|
| Brainstem | Medulla | Sulci |
| Cerebellum | Midbrain | Temporal lobe |
| Cerebrum | Occipital lobe | |
| Convolutions | Parietal lobe | |
| Frontal lobe | Pons | |

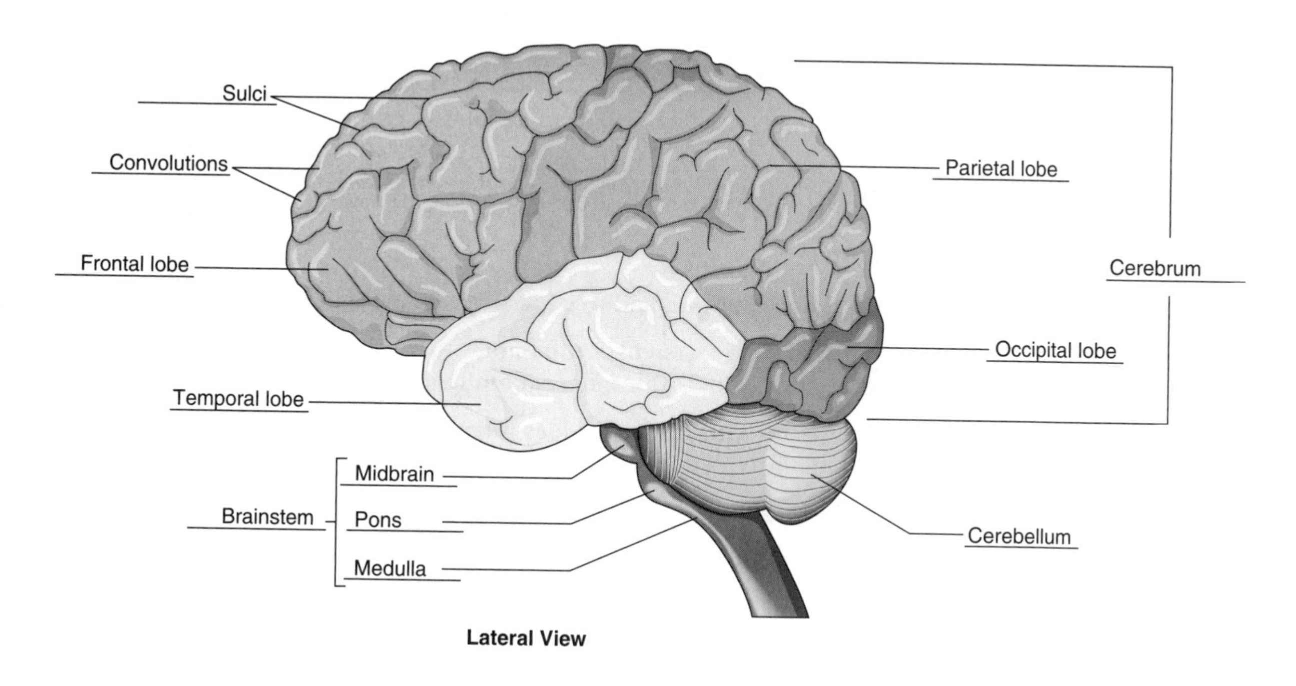


**Lateral View**

# Chapter Application

## Case Studies with Critical Thinking Questions

### Scenario 1

Yesterday your nephew was severely injured in a motorcycle accident. The physician believes there is a fracture in the thoratic spine but needs to have a radiological workup to determine the extent of the injury. Your brother is very concerned because his son has no sensations or control of his body from the waist down. He has asked you what you think of his condition.

1. Is it important to ask what the nephew's physician has told your brother? You need to determine what your brother has been told by the physician so you do not treat the situation either too lightly or unnecessarily grave. Try to elaborate on what the doctor has said and explain why he has the symptoms and that they may improve after initial swelling has subsided.
2. How would you answer your brother if he asks if the paralysis may be permanent? If the physician has not explained the fact that paralysis is permanent, it may not be anticipated. Often, after swelling decreases, some level of function will return; however, it is highly unlikely full recovery will be anticipated.
3. How much encouragement for recovery should you give him? Do not give unrealistic hope but explain no one knows for sure at this point how much function will return. It will be atleast two years before the extent of recovery can be determined.

### Scenario 2

A male patient phoned the office to request the doctor to call the pharmacy to order some cream to apply on a rash that the patient has on the right side of his chest. He said it started a couple days ago and is getting worse.

1. What do you need to know about the appearance of the rash? Ask the patient to describe the rash, its extent, how it is distributed, and when it began. Was he exposed to any poison ivy or oak? Does it look like insect bites?.
2. What subjective symptoms would you want to ask the patient about? Itching, pain, or other systemic symptoms.
3. Does this patient need to be seen? Explain that the physician cannot diagnose over the phone and he will need to be seen. If you think he may have shingles, explain to him that treatment may require an injection of medication to limit its progression and topical ointment will not be effective.

### Role-Play Activities

Choose a partner to participate in some nerve testing and to experience some neurological responses.

1. Following instruction from your teacher, use a percussion hammer to perform the knee-jerk test on your partner. Do it on both legs. Is the reaction equal? Does it seem too reactive or under-responsive?
2. With your partner lying on an exam table with his or her legs relaxed and shoes off, stroke the bottom of each foot, from the heel to the toes, with the hammer handle. What happened?
3. Try to perform the Brudzinski and Kernig's tests.
4. Experience hemiplegia: For 15 minutes, refrain from using your dominant hand and arm. Try to not use your dominant leg except to support you; you cannot make it move. Try to get up from a sitting position without the use of your dominant hand or leg.
5. If possible, spend at least one hour in a wheelchair during lab time when you should be moving about. Can you express your feelings about not being able to perform routine tasks?

CHAPTER 25

# The Senses

## Words to Know Challenge

**Spelling: Each line contains three spellings of a word. Underline the correctly spelled word.**

| | | |
|---|---|---|
| 1. acqueous | acquous | aqueous |
| 2. tinnitus | tinitis | tinnitis |
| 3. staples | stappes | stapes |
| 4. chorhoid | choroid | chorid |
| 5. cochlea | choclea | cocklea |
| 6. cataraxt | cattaract | cataract |
| 7. lacramal | lacrimal | lacramil |
| 8. vittreous | vitreous | vitrious |

**Fill in the Blank: Complete the following sentences with Words to Know from this chapter.**

1. Myopia, commonly called nearsightedness, is a defect in vision so that objects can only be seen when very near. The opposite of this is hyperopia, or farsightedness.
2. Amblyopia is a condition known commonly as "lazy eye."
3. Within the middle ear, sound waves vibrate the membrane and the malleus (hammer) attached to its inner surface. This in turn "strikes" the incus (anvil), which moves the stapes (stirrups).
4. The middle ear is connected to the throat via the Eustachian tube.
5. The gradual loss of hearing that occurs normally as part of the aging process is known as presbycusis.
6. Otitis causes pain and hearing loss; two types include externa and media.
7. The most common cause of conductive deafness is otosclerosis.

## Chapter Review

### Short Answer

1. List the five senses of the human body and identify the organ(s) responsible for the perception.
   a. Sight/vision/seeing—eyes
   b. Hearing—ears
   c. Smell—nose
   d. Taste—tongue
   e. Touch—skin (and nerves)

2. Name the structures of the eye through which light passes in the process of sight.
   a. Cornea
   b. Aqueous humor
   c. Pupil
   d. Lens
   e. Vitreous humor
   f. Retina

3. Explain the function of the lens and the process of accommodation. The lens focuses the image onto the retina by the process of accommodation. The lens shape is changed by the ciliary body to become rounder for near vision or thinner to focus on distant objects.

4. How does the cornea affect vision? The cornea is curved to correct unclear images that the edge of the lens projects. If the corneal shape becomes abnormal, vision will be blurred.

5. Name the two humors and describe their purpose.
   a. Aqueous
      1. Maintains curvature of the cornea
      2. Assists with refraction
   b. Vitreous
      1. Aids in refraction
      2. Maintains shape of the eyeball

6. Explain how sounds are heard. Vibrations are picked up by the outer ear and directed into the external auditory canal. The sound waves vibrate the tympanic membrane, causing the malleus to strike the incus, which in turn moves the stapes. The stapes pushes against the fluid in the vestibule of the inner ear, causing vibrations to enter the cochlea. Here the organ of Corti transmits the impulses to the auditory nerve, which passes them on to the auditory center of the temporal lobe of the cerebrum and the vibration is interpreted as a sound.

7. How is equilibrium maintained? Hairlike nerve cells embedded in a gelatin-like material in the semicircular canals of the inner ear maintain balance. When the head is moved, the material pushes against the nerve cells, which transmit changes to the brain. Also, small sacs of tiny grains of limestone react to movement of the head, causing impulses.

8. Describe the structure of the olfactory organ and explain how an odor can be detected. The olfactory organ is connected to nerve fibers running through the skull to the olfactory center in the brain. The nerve fibers are connected to a group of hair cells that are the detectors of odors.

9. Define the following terms:
   a. Epistaxis A nosebleed
   b. Allergic rhinitis An allergic reaction to airborne allergens that causes profuse, watery nasal discharge
   c. Nasal polyp A benign growth in the nose

10. Identify the sensations that are perceivable by the skin.
    a. Touch
    b. Pain
    c. Heat
    d. Cold
    e. Pressure
    f. Traction
    g. Tickle

## Matching

**1. Match the disease or disorder of the eye in column II with the major symptoms in column I.**

| | COLUMN I | COLUMN II |
|---|---|---|
| G | 1. Scratch from foreign body or injury to the cornea | A. Age-related macular degeneration |
| D | 2. Red-rimmed, crusted eyelids with scales, itching, and burning | B. Amblyopia |
| J | 3. Aching, loss of peripheral vision, visual halos around lights | C. Arcus senilis |
| P | 4. Visual deviation of the eyeball; blurred or double vision | D. Blepharitis |
| N | 5. Drooping of the upper eyelid | E. Cataract |
| B | 6. Inward turning of one eye with blurred vision | F. Conjunctivitis |
| F | 7. Redness, pain, and occasional discharge caused by an infectious microbe | G. Corneal abrasion |
| E | 8. Painless, gradual visual blurring, and loss of vision | H. Corneal ulcers |
| H | 9. Pain, especially on blinking; excessive tearing; exudate; irregular cornea; blurred vision | I. diabetic retinopathy |
| K | 10. Red, painful swelling of gland of the eyelid | J. Glaucoma |
| M | 11. Inability to accommodate for near vision | K. Hordeolum |
| O | 12. Visual floating spots, light flashes, and gradual vision loss | L. Myopia |
| I | 13. Glare, blurred vision, reduced visual acuity, eventual blindness | M. Presbyopia |
| C | 14. A thin, grayish-white circle at edge of cornea | N. Ptosis |
| A | 15. Gradual loss of central vision | O. Detached retina |
| L | 16. Vision is blurred except close objects due to misshapen eyeball | P. Strabismus |

**2. Match the major symptoms in column II with the diseases and disorders of the ear in column I.**

| | COLUMN I | COLUMN II |
|---|---|---|
| D | 1. Auditory canal obstruction | A. Loss of equilibrium, headache, nausea, and vomiting due to movement |
| E | 2. Ménière's disease | B. Severe, deep, throbbing pain; fever; hearing loss; nausea; and vomiting, dizziness, bulging eardrum |
| A | 3. Motion sickness | C. Slow, progressive conduction hearing loss |
| F | 4. Otitis externa | D. A degree of hearing loss; possible discomfort; may be a foreign body |
| B | 5. Otitis media | E. Severe vertigo, tinnitus, nerve hearing loss, nausea, and vomiting |
| C | 6. Otosclerosis | F. Infection in auditory canal, pain, fever, conduction hearing loss |
| G | 7. Presbycusis | G. Loss of ability to hear high-frequency sounds, tinnitus, possible depression |

## Labeling

1. Add labels to each part of the eye. Refer to Figure 25–1 in the textbook.
   Anterior chamber
   Choroid coat
   Ciliary body
   Conjunctiva
   Cornea
   Fovea centralis
   Iris
   Lens
   Optic nerve
   Path of light
   Posterior chamber
   Pupil
   Retina
   Sclera
   Vitreous body

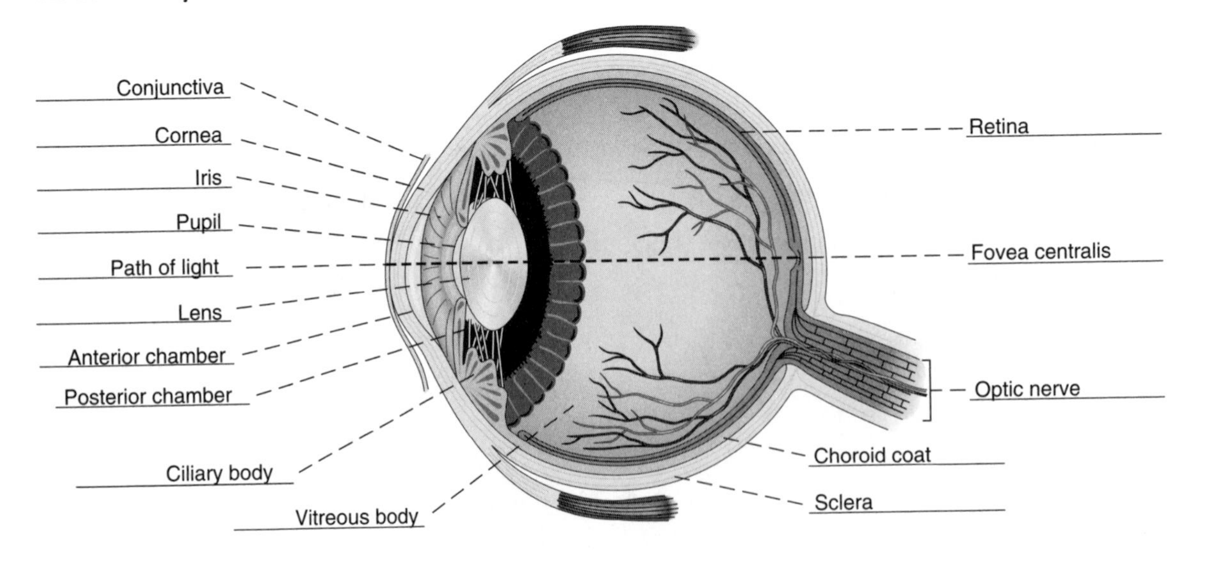

2. Label the illustrations of the outer, middle, and inner ear using the following terms. Refer to Figures 25-11 and 25-12 in the textbook.

**Outer and Middle Ear**

Auricle
Cochlea
Eustachian tube
External auditory canal
Incus
Malleus
Semicircular canals
Stapes
Tympanic membrane
Vestibulocochlear nerve

**Inner Ear**

Cochlea
Cochlear nerve
Lateral semicircular canal
Oval window
Posterior semicircular canal
Superior semicircular canal
Vestibular nerve
Vestibule

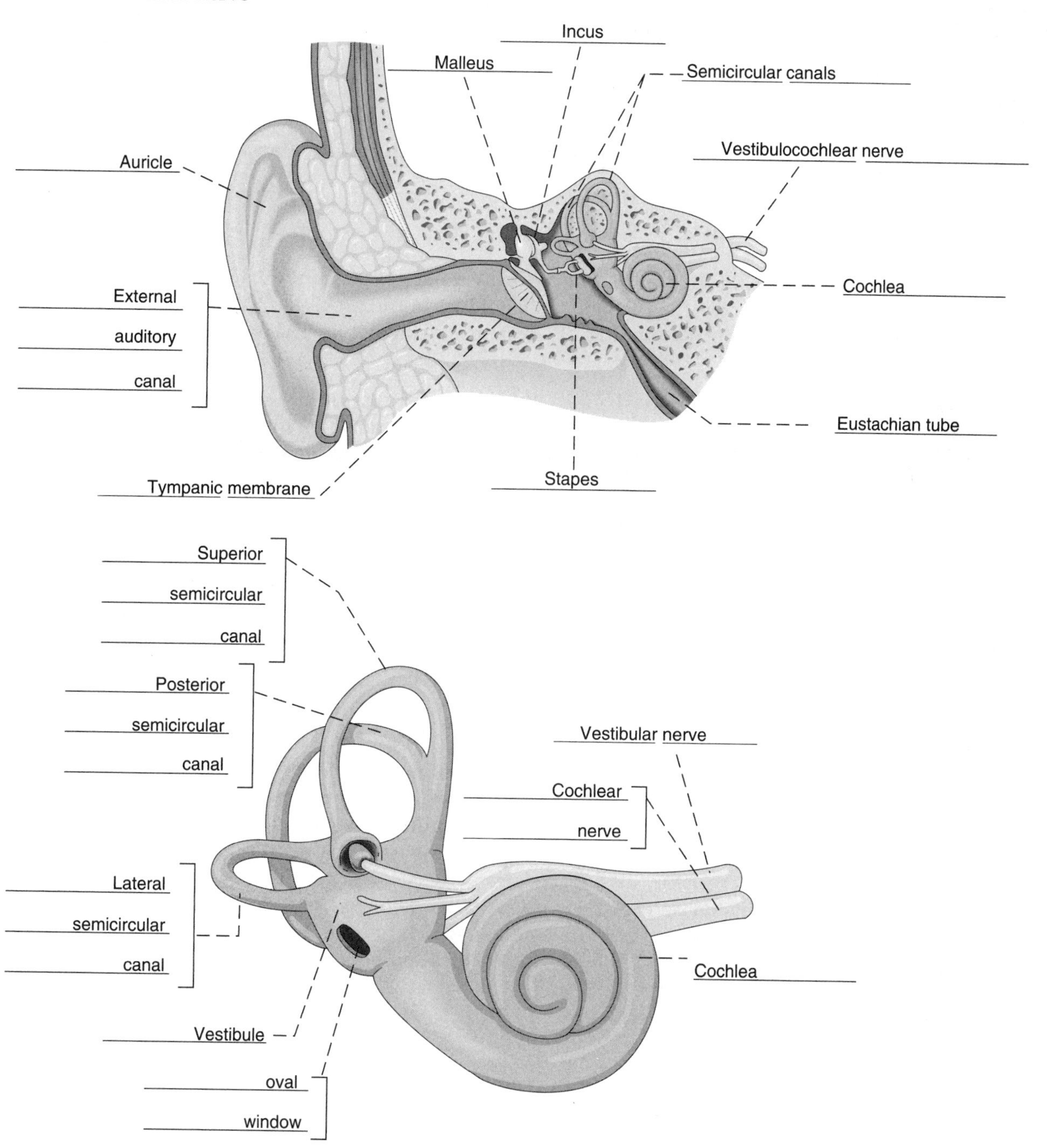

# Chapter Application

## Case Studies with Critical Thinking Questions

### Scenario 1

You notice that a little girl in your daughter's preschool class has one eye that turns inward. You have never seen the child with glasses. You have a chance to talk with the mother at a preschool program. She says she is not worried about it because she thinks her daughter will outgrow it and they don't have any insurance coverage.

1. How far should you go to impress on the mother that the child needs to be evaluated by a pediatric ophthalmologist? The mother needs to understand that an inward eye is not able to focus and may become unusable. The ophthalmologist can determine if a simple patch will treat the situation. The eye will not improve with age; in fact, it will worsen.
2. What could you say to the mother to impress upon her that her daughter's vision might be lost if the eye is not treated? Explain that there is a window of opportunity to correct the situation, and once that passes, nothing can be done to save the vision in that eye. Ask her how she would feel if something should injure her daughter's good eye later, resulting in the child's unnecessary loss of vision.
3. How can you find out if treatment is available without a lot of cost to the parents? Check with your employer if there are any community resources available. Organizations such as the Lions Club, Charity Newsies, The Blind Society, and various others might have assistance available. Children's specialty hospitals usually have clinics that offer services on a graduated able-to-pay scale, which could be helpful for treatment and any surgery that may be needed.

### Scenario 2

A 24-year-old male patient is being seen in the office for treatment of an upper respiratory infection. During your interview he proudly announces that he has quit smoking. In the process of your assessment you notice his teeth are quite stained, especially on one side. He explains to you that he is using a little smokeless tobacco to satisfy his need for nicotine.

1. What should you tell him about his new habit? Impress on him that he has only exchanged one form of cancer for another. The repeated contact from the tobacco on his gums and inner surface of his mouth may cause oral cancer to develop. The disfigurement from excision of oral cancer sites is not something he would want to deal with.
2. Where can you obtain some written materials for him? The American Cancer Society has pamphlets dealing with oral cancer, some especially directed at the use of smokeless tobacco.
3. What should you question about his dental care? Determine if he has seen a dentist lately. A dentist can evaluate the condition of his gums and oral cavity and will certainly reinforce your statements. If he has not seen a dentist in some time, stress the importance of a checkup.

### Research Activity

There are four rather common conditions that may lead to blindness, sometimes unnecessarily. Make a chart that divides a piece of paper horizontally into four sections after saving the top inch for headings. You will need five vertical columns, one small and four of equal size. In the first, smaller column, enter: Age-related macular degeneration, Diabetic retinopathy, Glaucoma, and Retinal detachment, one in each of the horizontal sections. Across the top row enter for titles: Description, Signs/symptoms, Etiology, and Treatment. Referring to the text, enter the information on each condition. When completed, look at the descriptors in each column. Which disorders occur slowly and which are sudden? Which ones require immediate treatment? Which ones can be "cured"? Are there any that could be avoided with good health practices? Which ones cause pain? Which ones are most likely to go unnoticed until some damage has occurred? Your knowledge of these conditions may some day help save someone's vision.

CHAPTER **26**

# The Integumentary System

## Words to Know Challenge

**Spelling: Each line contains three spellings of a word. Underline the correctly spelled word.**

1. dermatitus　　dermatitis　　dermitius
2. epidermis　　epedermis　　epidermus
3. erathema　　erithema　　erythema
4. intagumantary　　integumentory　　integumentary
5. psoriasis　　psariasis　　spsorisis
6. sabeceous　　sebaceous　　sebaceus
7. subcutanous　　subcutaneous　　subcuteneous
8. urticaria　　urtecaria　　urticarea
9. varrucai　　verrucae　　varrucae
10. alopecia　　alopechia　　alepecia
11. egsema　　egzema　　eczema
12. mellonoma　　melanoma　　mellenoma
13. leshion　　lesion　　leishon

**Matching: Match the terms in column I to their definitions in column II.**

| | COLUMN I | COLUMN II |
|---|---|---|
| E | 1. Erythema | A. Color |
| J | 2. Melanin | B. Skin with little or no color |
| F | 3. Pustule | C. Provides lubrication |
| A | 4. Pigment | D. A chronic condition |
| C | 5. Sebaceous | E. Sunburn |
| G | 6. Subcutaneous | F. A lesion with exudates |
| H | 7. Dermis | G. A skin layer |
| K | 8. Vesicle | H. True skin |
| B | 9. Albino | I. Round elevations of skin |
| I | 10. Wheals | J. A pigment |
| D | 11. Psoriasis | K. A blister-like lesion |

# Chapter Review

## Short Answer

1. List the five functions of the skin.
   a. Protection
   b. Perception
   c. Temperature control
   d. Absorption
   e. Excretion
2. How does the skin regulate body temperature? If too warm, the surface vessels dilate to allow heat from the blood to escape. If too cool, the surface vessels constrict to reduce heat loss.
3. How does the body cool its surface? The sweat glands produce sweat, which evaporates from the skin surface, causing the body to cool.
4. List the three layers of skin tissue; identify the characteristic structure of each layer.
   Epidermis is the top layer; it is full of ridges, which make fingerprints on the fingertips and lines on the soles of the feet. The dermis flakes off dead cells as new ones push up to the surface
   Dermis is the middle layer; it contains blood vessels, nerves, hair follicles, oil, and sweat glands. It is also called true skin. The top of the layer is covered with cone-shaped papillae that create an uneven surface
   Subcutaneous is the bottom layer; it contains fat globules, blood vessels, and nerves.
5. What causes wrinkles? The fatty underlying layer of tissue in the skin is absorbed with aging, causing an excess of the outer layer and resulting in the development of folds or wrinkles.
6. Why does exposure to the sun cause the skin to darken? The skin has a dark pigment, called melanin, and another yellow pigment. When exposed to the sun, the melanin pigment moves to the surface to protect the underlying tissue, causing a tan.

7. Why does the skin become red when a person blushes? The blood vessels dilate, which brings more blood into contact with the surface and allows the red color to be seen.

8. What causes birthmarks? A concentration of blood vessels or a patch of pigment

9. What is a mole? A pigmented patch of tissue

10. Define "albinism" and describe the main characteristics of the condition. A condition characterized by the lack of pigment in the skin, hair, and eyes. The hair will be nearly white, the skin extremely light, and the eyes appear red and are very sensitive to light.

11. Define the lesion in column I by placing the number of its correct definition from column II in the space.

| | COLUMN I | COLUMN II |
|---|---|---|
| 3 | Macule | 1. A small, circumscribed lesion filled with exudate and lymph |
| 4 | Papule | 2. A round lesion with a white center and a red periphery that usually itches |
| 1 | Pustule | 3. A variously colored spot that is neither elevated nor depressed |
| 5 | Vesicle | 4. A solid, elevated circular red mass about a pinhead to a pea in size |
| 2 | Wheal | 5. A blisterlike, elevated mass containing serous fluid |

12. Identify the ABCD rules of melanoma.
    Asymmetry—One half does not match the other half
    Border irregularity—The edges are ragged, notched, or blurred
    Color—The pigment is not uniform. Shades of tan, brown, and black are present. Red, white, and blue may add to the mottled appearance
    Diameter—It is greater than 6 millimeters. Any sudden or continuing increase in size is a sign of melanoma.

13. What two words describe the skin in the following age groups?
    a. Infant and child — soft and supple
    b. Teenager — acne and increase oil gland activity
    c. Aging — less elastic and wrinkles
    d. Aged — fragile, thin, increased pigmentation

14. Identify the body systems involved in Lyme disease.
    1. Integumentary
    2. Circulatory
    3. Skeletal/muscular
    4. Nervous

## Matching

**1. Match the primary disease characteristics in column I with the disease or disorder in column II.**

| | COLUMN I | COLUMN II |
|---|---|---|
| D | 1. Dry skin, redness, itching, edema, scaling | A. Scabies |
| G | 2. A small red macule becomes a vesicle and then changes into a pustule with yellow crust and outer rim | B. Psoriasis |
| H | 3. A thickened scar | C. Urticaria |
| B | 4. Itching red papules covered with silvery scales | D. Dermatitis |
| F | 5. Flat lesion that can be dry and scaly or moist and crusty: has characteristic outer ring with clear center | E. Verrucae |
| A | 6. Threadlike red nodules at the inner wrists, elbows, between fingers, and in axilla | F. Ringworm |
| C | 7. Distinct raised wheals surrounded by reddened areas; usually itches | G. Impetigo |
| E | 8. Rough, elevated, rounded surface, especially on the hands and fingers: some forms appear on soles of feet and on genitalia | H. Keloid |
| O | 9. A loss of hair, usually on the scalp | I. Lyme disease |
| M | 10. A lesion exhibiting some of the ABCD characteristics | J. Herpes simplex |
| N | 11. Red, dry, itching, and scaly skin; occurs in both acute and chronic forms, often producing watery discharge | K. Pediculosis capitus |
| J | 12. Cold sores or blisters on the mouth or face | L. Hirsutism |
| P | 13. A deep abscess involving several follicles with multiple drainage points | M. Melanoma |
| I | 14. A bull's eye rash and a bite site | N. Eczema |
| K | 15. Oval, grayish, dandruff-appearing flecks, itching scalp, matted hair | O. Alopecia |
| L | 16. Excessive body hair on females and children, in an adult male growth pattern | P. Carbuncule |

**2. Match the definition in column II with the correct term in column I.**

| | COLUMN I | COLUMN II |
|---|---|---|
| D | 1. Dermis | A. Reddened, flat area with definite edge |
| H | 2. Epidermis | B. Bottom layer of skin |
| J | 3. Keloid | C. Hives |
| A | 4. Macule | D. The middle layer of skin |
| I | 5. Melanin | E. Raised areas surrounded by reddened area |
| G | 6. Pustule | F. Raised lesion containing serous fluid |
| B | 7. Subcutaneous | G. Lesion with purulent material |
| C | 8. Urticaria | H. The top layer of skin |
| F | 9. Vesicle | I. Pigment in the skin |
| E | 10. Wheals | J. An overgrowth of scar tissue |
| M | 11. Whorl | K. The lack of skin pigment |
| | | L. An oil gland |
| | | M. Fingerprints |

# Chapter Application

## Case Studies with Critical Thinking Questions

### Scenario 1

Johnny's mother called the office almost hysterical because he brought home a note from school saying one of his classmates has head lice. She is sure the entire family has lice because they've all started to itch.

1. How can you help her to determine if they actually have lice? Tell her to look for little, grayish, dandruff-like flecks on the hair that cannot be shaken off and to ask the child if he feels "itchy".

2. If a family member does have lice, what steps should be taken besides treating the hair? Family members should refrain from using one another's combs, brushes, hats, towels, and other clothing if the nits are on the body. Body lice require bathing and the washing of bedding, towels, and clothing, as well as treating the infected body areas.

### Scenario 2

You are following a co-worker up a flight of stairs when you notice a very unusually colored mole on the calf of her leg. When you ask her about it she says it's been there for a while and it doesn't bother her. She thinks it's just a mole because she has several on her back and chest area.

1. What could you say to express your concern? You should encourage her to check it out just to make sure. Tell her you are concerned. Ignoring a melanoma could prove fatal.

2. Ask her to describe the signs of a melanoma and if she will see your employer. Do anything you think would convince her to at least have it examined. If she doesn't want your employer to treat her, help her to make an appointment with someone else.

3. When would it be appropriate to schedule an appointment for her with a dermatologist? If a family practice physician is either not consulted or feels he does not see enough lesions to be certain, then by all means get her to see a dermatologist soon. If it is a malignant lesion of any type, a wide excision around the area will be required and radiation or chemotherapy may be indicated with certain types.

## Research Activity

Look in your local phone directory. How many physicians specialize in dermatology? Make a list of the different services or treatments they provide. You will notice they range from cosmetic to serious conditions.

## Role-Play

Choose a partner to explore the skin.

1. Use a magnifying glass to identify the few places on the body where there is no hair.
2. Using fingerpaint or an ink stamp pad, make a page of right thumbprints of all classmates. Look at the differences in the lines and patterns.
3. See how the skin surface reacts to hot or cold. Apply a hot, wet cloth to your partner's forearm for two minutes. Remove it and record what you observe. Now apply a cold, wet cloth wrapped around ice for two minutes. Remove and record your findings. What is the skin trying to do in each situation?
4. Blindfold your partner and see if his or her skin can perceive different stimuli. Have your partner tell you what you are doing; be considerate and do not cause harm.
   a) Touch the skin on the forearm lightly with your fingertip.
   b) Gently pinch the skin.
   c) Press a pencil or pen into the skin.
   d) Press an object that you've held under hot water against the skin.
   e) Press an item that is cold against the skin.
   f) Try to tickle the surface with the edge of a tissue, barely touching the skin.

CHAPTER 27

# The Skeletal System

## Words to Know Challenge

**Spelling: Each line contains three spellings of a word. Underline the correctly spelled word.**

| | | | |
|---|---|---|---|
| 1. | axeal | axyal | axial |
| 2. | carpelle | carpel | carpal |
| 3. | epiphysis | ephiphysis | epyphysis |
| 4. | cocyx | coccyx | coscix |
| 5. | ischium | ishium | ishiem |
| 6. | kyfosis | kiphosis | kyphosis |
| 7. | osteopersis | osteoporosis | osteoperosis |
| 8. | phalancks | phalanx | phalenx |
| 9. | prosthesys | prothesis | prosthesis |
| 10. | synovial | sinovial | sinoval |

**Matching: Match the terms in column I with their definitions in column II.**

| | COLUMN I | COLUMN II |
|---|---|---|
| F | 1. Fracture | A. Sensation after amputation |
| L | 2. Femur | B. Floating mass in blood vessel |
| E | 3. Alignment | C. Incomplete fracture |
| P | 4. Callus | D. To stretch a ligament |
| C | 5. Greenstick | E. To straighten a fracture |
| A | 6. Phantom limb | F. Break |
| K | 7. Ligament | G. Fills long bones |
| N | 8. Vertebrae | H. Bones of the hands and feet |
| O | 9. Ulna | I. Bone in the rib cage |
| M | 10. Humerus | J. Pelvic bone |
| G | 11. Marrow | K. Attaches bone to bone at joints |
| B | 12. Embolus | L. Thigh bone |
| J | 13. Ilium | M. Upper arm bone |
| H | 14. Phalanges | N. Bones of the spine |
| I | 15. Sternum | O. Bone of forearm |
| D | 16. Sprain | P. Bulgy deposit around a new fracture |

## Chapter Review

**Fill in the Blank: Use information from the chapter to fill in the blank space in the sentence.**

1. The skeletal system is divided into sections. The axial skeleton is made up of the spinal column, skull and rib cage. The appendicular skeleton is made up of the arms, hands, feet, legs, shoulders and pelvis.
2. The rib cage consists of 12 pairs of ribs that attach by cartilage strips to the sternum anteriorly and to the thoracic vertebrae posteriorly. The top 10 pairs are attached both anteriorly and posteriorly. The bottom 2 pairs are attached only to the spinal column and are therefore called floating ribs.
3. The rib cage is also classified as having true and false ribs. This division considers the first 7 pairs to be true ribs because of their posterior and direct anterior attachmens. The last 5 pairs are called false ribs because they attach anteriorly to the cartilage of the rib above or have no anterior attachment
4. The primary function of the rib cage is to protect the heart and lungs.

## Labeling

1. Label the skeletal system with these terms. Refer to Figure 27–1 in the textbook.

| | | |
|---|---|---|
| Carpals | Ilium | Sacrum |
| Clavicle | Ischium | Scapula |
| Coccyx | Metacarpals | Sternum |
| Cranium | Metatarsals | Tarsals |
| Facial bones | Patella | Tibia |
| Femur | Phalanges (used twice) | Ulna |
| Fibula | Pubis | Vertebral column |
| Greater trochanter | Radius | |
| Humerus | Ribs | |

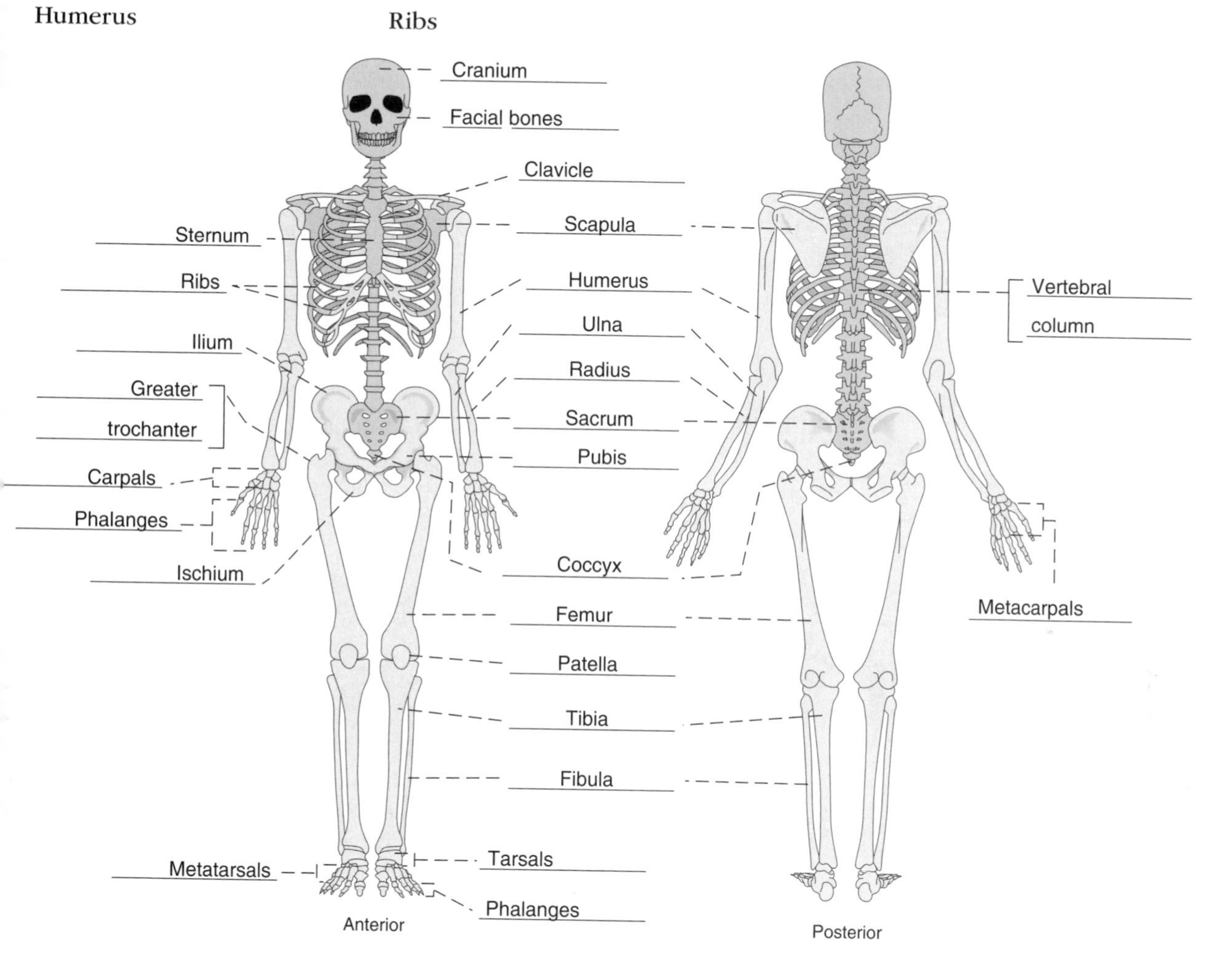

2. Label the illustration of the vertebral column using the following terms. Refer to Figure 27–5 in the textbook.
   Cervical vertebrae
   Coccyx
   Intervertebral disk
   Lumbar vertebrae
   Sacrum
   Thoracic vertebrae
   Vertebral body

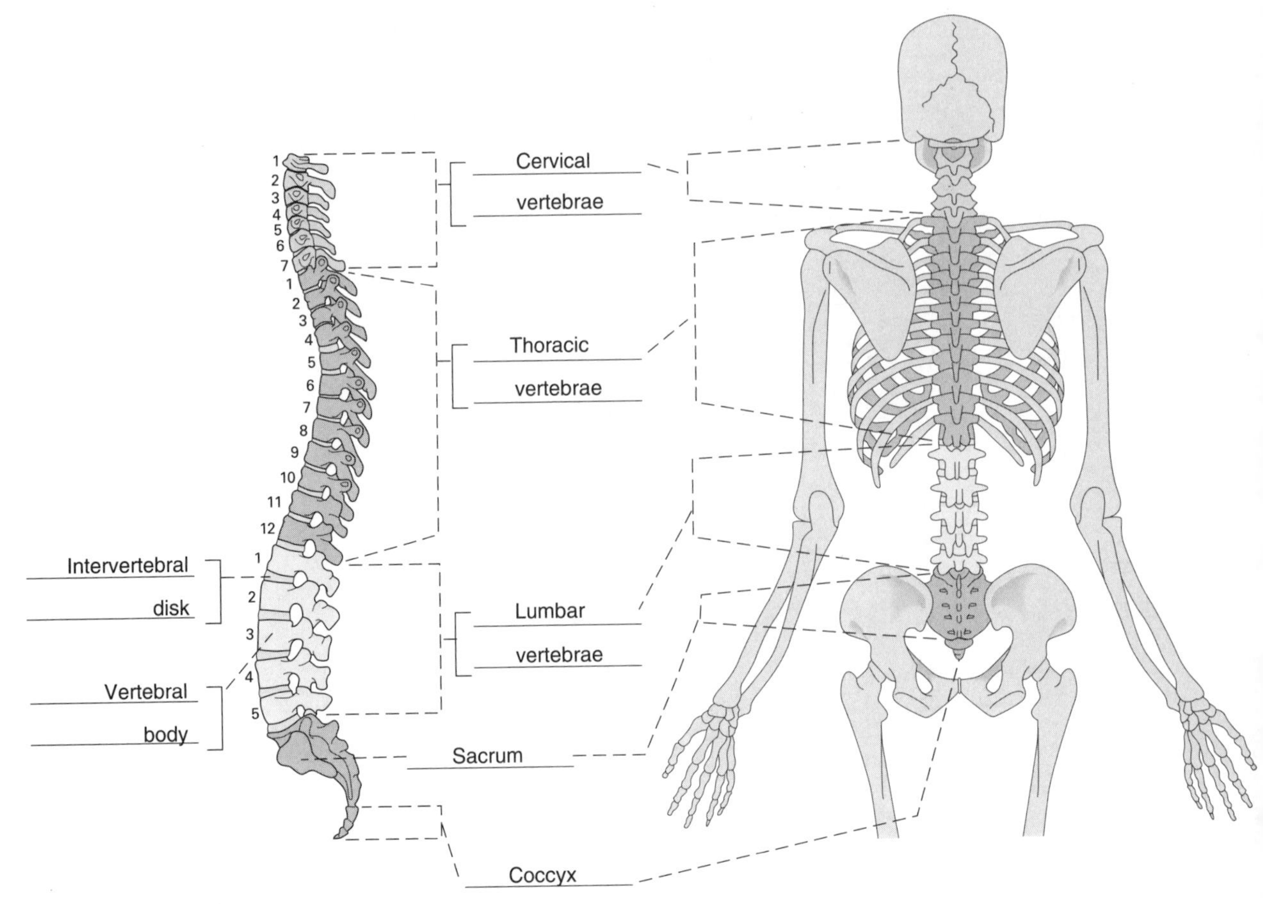

3. Label the illustration of the rib cage with the following terms. Refer to Figure 27–7 in the textbook.
   Clavicle
   Costal cartilage
   False ribs
   Floating ribs
   Manubrium
   Spinal column
   Sternum
   True ribs
   Xiphoid process

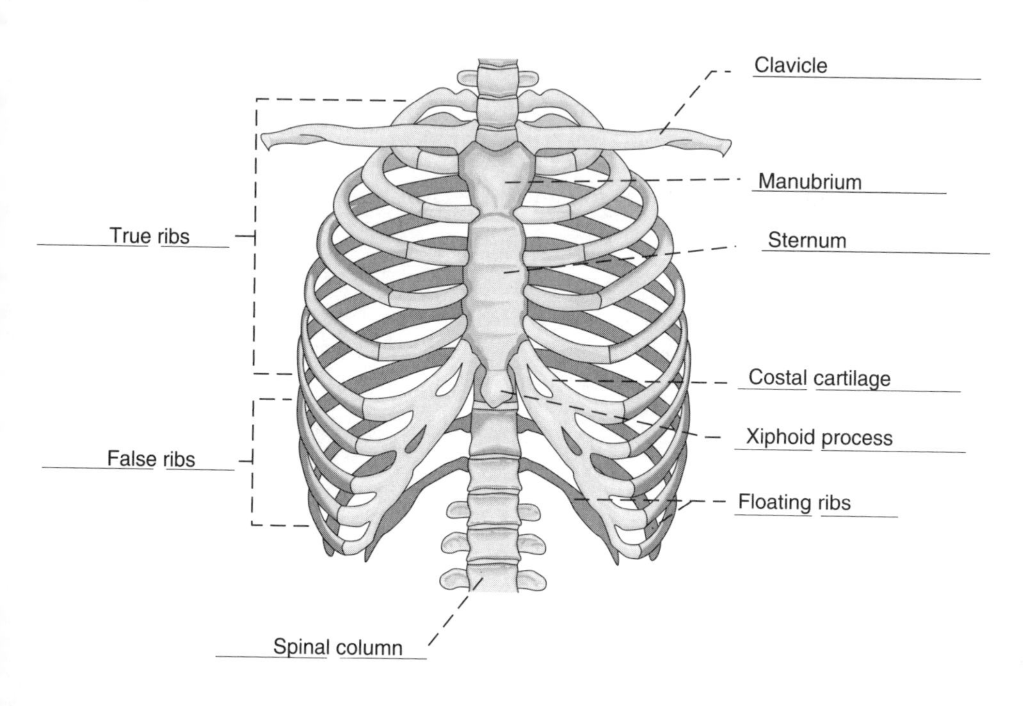


## Short Answer

1. What is bone composed of? The main minerals are calcium, phosphorus, and magnesium. The organic matter is primarily collagen.
2. List six functions of the skeletal system.
   a. Supports body
   b. Protects vital organs
   c. Provides attachments for muscles
   d. Gives support to body
   e. Assists in formation of red blood cells
   f. Stores body calcium
3. Describe the spinal column. The spinal column is a stack of vertebrae separated by cartilage disks. There are 7 cervical, 12 thoracic, 5 lumbar, a saccral, and a coccyx section.
4. How is a long bone constructed? Long bone has a hollow shaft or diaphysis with ends called epiphyses. The ends and part of the shaft contain red and yellow marrow. Bone is covered with a membrane called periosteum.
5. How do long bones grow? The cartilage in the epiphyses is a growth plate that allows long bones to increase in length until maturity.

6. Identify three kinds of synovial joints, giving examples of each.
   a. Ball and socket—hip
   b. Hinge—knee, finger, elbow
   c. Pivot—elbow, wrist
7. List the seven types of fractures, describing the characteristics of each type.
   a. Greenstick—a crack or incomplete fracture
   b. Simple or closed—complete break without penetration of the skin
   c. Compound or open—complete break with penetration of the skin
   d. Impacted—broken ends are jammed together
   e. Comminuted—more than one fracture line and several bone fragments
   f. Depressed—where a piece of fractured bone is driven inward
   g. Spiral—a twisting break that winds around the bone
8. Identify each type of fracture illustrated below. Refer to Figure 27–11 in the textbook.

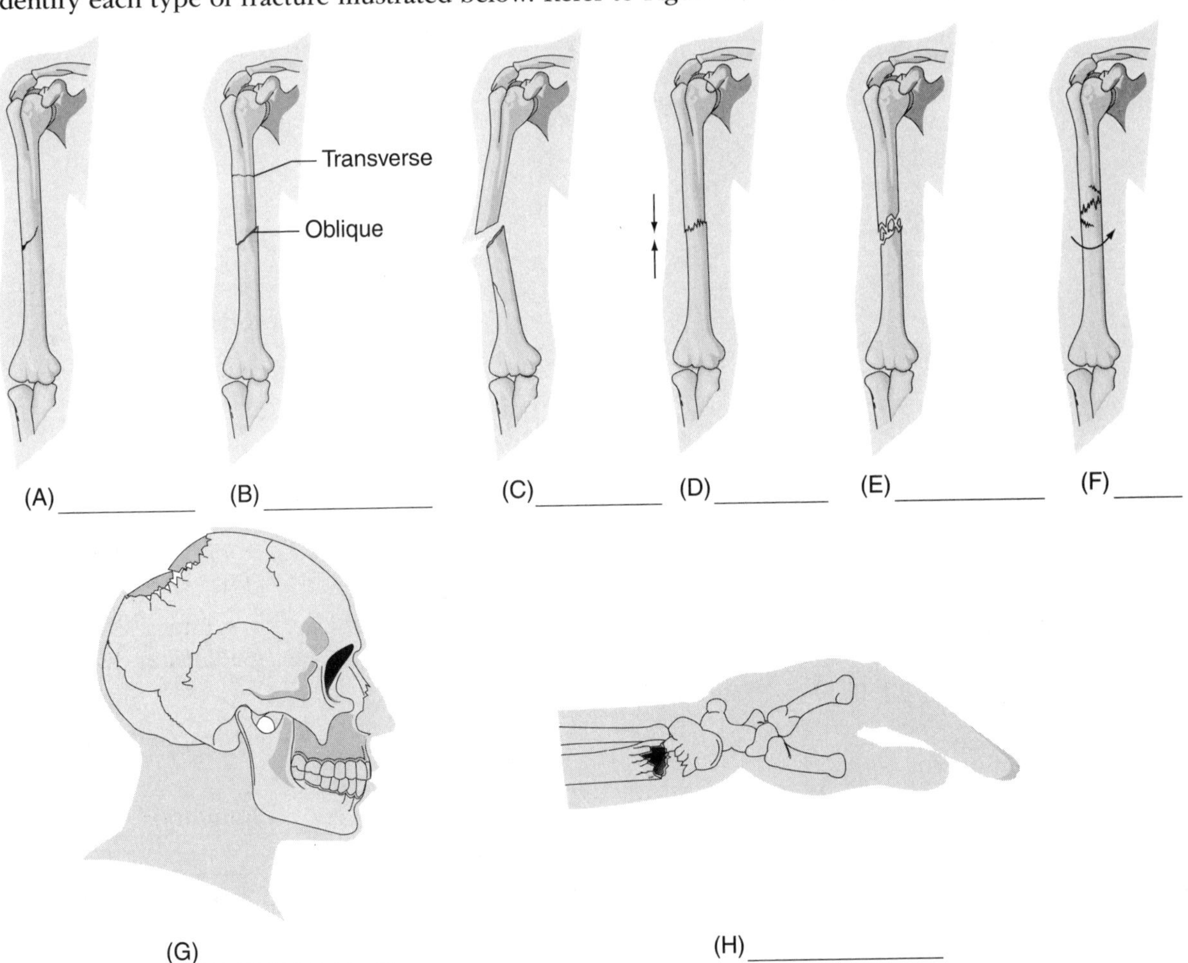


9. Describe the initial and follow-up treatment of fractures. The fractured part is supported and immobilized. Measures are taken to prevent shock. If there is bleeding or external involvement of tissue, the wound i dressed and bleeding is controlled. Long bone fractures must be reduced using traction, either manuall or mechanically, until the bones are in alignment to be splinted or casted. Compound and comminute fractures require surgical treatment of the wound and/or the arrangement of the bone fragments into po sition to heal
10. How does bone heal? A collection of blood (hematoma) forms around the fracture site. The hematoma be gins an inflammatory reaction that initiates the healing process. A fibrous bridge is formed between th fracture fragments. Some of the cells in this fibrous mesh differentiate into cartilage cells and begin to ac cumulate calcium, forming a callus

11. What is a fat embolus and how does it occur? A fat embolus is a mass of foreign material circulating in the blood vessels. It may follow the release of fat droplets from bone marrow or fatty acids activated by catecholamines.

12. What conditions might result in the need for an amputation?
    a. Severe trauma
    b. Malignant tumor
    c. Lack of circulation
    d. Complications from diabetes

13. Explain the condition known as phantom limb. This refers to the sensation of itching or tingling where an extremity was amputated, as if it still existed.

**Matching: Match the disease or disorder in column I with the appropriate symptoms in column II.**

| | COLUMN I | COLUMN II |
|---|---|---|
| E | 1. Osteoarthritis | A. Painful displacement of the bones of the joint, usually fingers, shoulders, knees, often resulting in joint fracture |
| I | 2. Rheumatoid arthritis | B. A metabolic disease resulting in severe joint pain due to deposits of urates |
| L | 3. Bursitis | C. A lateral spinal curvature, usually thoracic, resulting from spinal column rotation |
| F | 4. Congenital hip dysplasia | D. Porous, brittle bones, prone to fracture; caused by metabolic disorder; found primarily in postmenopausal women |
| A | 5. Dislocation | E. Progressive deterioration of joint cartilage, usually hip and knee; joint pain; stiffness; grating; and joint fluid |
| H | 6. Epicondylitis | F. The dislocation of a child's hip joint at birth |
| B | 7. Gout | G. A bowing of the back, usually at the thoracic level |
| M | 8. Hallux valgus | H. Inflammation of forearm extensor tendon at its attachment on the humerus; more painful with twisting of forearm |
| J | 9. Herniated disk | I. Chronic inflammatory disease occurring intermittently; damages synovial membrane, causing edema and congestion, bone atrophy, deformities |
| G | 10. Kyphosis | J. Causes severe low back pain, radiating deep into buttocks and down back of the leg |
| D | 11. Osteoporosis | K. A tear of the ligaments of a joint resulting in pain, swelling, and local bleeding |
| C | 12. Scoliosis | L. Painful inflammation of the joint sac, usually at the knee, elbow, or shoulder |
| K | 13. Sprain | M. Lateral deviation of the great toe with enlarged first metatarsal and the formation of a bunion |
| P | 14. Carpal tunnel syndrome | N. Partial or incomplete dislocation of the articulating surfaces of bones at a joint, causing deformity, pain, and extremity length change |
| O | 15. Bunion | O. An inflamed bursa of the great toe filled with fluid and covered with a callus |
| Q | 16. Lordosis | P. Decreased sensitivity in the first two fingers and thumb, often with atrophy of the thumb muscle on the palm side |
| N | 17. Subluxation | Q. Abnormal anterior convex curvature of the lumbar spine |

# Chapter Application

## Case Studies with Critical Thinking Questions

### Scenario 1

You are alone in the office when the wife of a patient calls to find out what she should do. Her husband suffered a leg fracture at work yesterday, but in the last hour he started perspiring and looks pale. He also seems to be breathing faster and his pulse is above normal. She wonders if this is normal.

1. What should you initially tell the patient's wife? Explain to her that he may be experiencing a serious complication, and you will try to contact the doctor. In the meantime, he should be very quiet and she should get prepared to go to the ER if necessary. Write down her phone number and tell her you will call her back quickly. If her husband's condition should worsen, she should call emergency services immediately and not wait for your call.
2. When is it appropriate for you try to reach the physician? If you know you can reach the physician quickly, make the call and relay the information and follow the physician's directions. If you cannot reach the doctor, call the patient's wife and advise her to call EMS services to transport him to the ER for evaluation. It is better to err on the side of caution than to take a chance.
3. Why might this be a real emergency? With a fracture history along with the symptoms, it is very possible he could be experiencing an embolus, which could rapidly become an emergency and cause death. Even with appropriate care, an embolism is often fatal.

### Scenario 2

Your neighbor calls to tell you he sprained his ankle the night before, but it is a lot more swollen and painful today. He tells you he has been keeping the heating pad on it like his friend told him, but it just seems to be getting worse.

1. What advice should you give him first? Discontinue the heat immediately and instead apply cold to the area for the next 24 to 48 hours. Caution him about ice coming into direct contact with the skin, which could cause frostbite and further difficulties. He should also keep the ankle elevated and avoid bearing weight on it for several days. Ace bandage wrapped in a spiral from the foot toward the leg may provide support and comfort. Remove it if the foot becomes swollen.
2. How can you be certain it's just a sprain? Without X-ray there is no way to positively rule out fracture. With the excess swelling in the area it would even be more difficult to determine by observation and manipulation. Probably no harm would come from a day or two of cold treatment followed by heat to see if the situation improves.
3. When should you recommend medical evaluation? If there is obvious misalignment, then medical evaluation with X-ray and an orthopedic consult is necessary. If his condition does not improve within 48 hours, it might be wise to seek medical attention.

## Role-Play: Bone identification and spelling

A. Practice identifying the bones of the body. With a partner, use a model of a skeleton or a chart without labels and try to identify all the bones of the body. Your partner can say whether you are right or wrong.

B. Choose a partner and play hangman using the Words to Know. Each person makes a list of 10 words and then tries to win against his or her partner.

CHAPTER 28

# The Muscular System

## Words to Know Challenge

**Spelling: Each line contains three spellings of a word. Underline the correctly spelled word.**

| | | |
|---|---|---|
| 1. distrophy | dystrophy | dystraphy |
| 2. pecktoralis | pectoralles | pectoralis |
| 3. extensor | extenser | egtensor |
| 4. gastructnemius | gastrocnemius | gastrocnemious |
| 5. hiccupp | hiccough | hicough |
| 6. intercostal | intracostal | intercoastal |
| 7. spincter | sphinctor | sphincter |
| 8. tortacollis | torticollis | torticolis |
| 9. fibramyositis | fibromyositis | fibromyasitis |

**Matching: Match the term in column I with its description in column II.** (Note: Not all descriptions will be used.)

| | COLUMN I | COLUMN II |
|---|---|---|
| F | 1. Abduction | A. Spasmotic contractions of the diaphragm |
| K | 2. Adduction | B. Excessive stress on a skeletal muscle |
| G | 3. Anchor | C. A doughnut-shaped muscle |
| D | 4. Atrophy | D. A progressive wasting of muscle tissue from lack of use |
| H | 5. Contracture | E. A tough membrane sheath attachment |
| I | 6. Dystrophy | F. To move an extremity away from the body's center |
| E | 7. Fascia | G. The origin of a muscle |
| A | 8. Hiccough | H. Permanent shortening of flexor muscles with bent joints |

(continues)

L 9. Spasm

B 10. Strain

I. Congenital progressive skeletal muscle wasting

J. A state of partial muscle contraction

K. To move an extremity toward the body's center

L. A painful contracted muscle that will not relax

## Chapter Review

### Short Answer

1. What is a motor unit? The group of cells within the muscle tissue and the motor neuron axons that innervate it and cause contraction
2. Why does muscular activity produce heat in the body? The muscles use glycogen, which is stored in the muscles for fuel during activity. As the glycogen is released, it is changed into glucose to make it available for use. Heat is produced as the stored glycogen is used, raising body temperature
3. List six functions of skeletal muscles.
   a. Provide heat
   b. Provide ability to move
   c. Protect blood vessels and nerves
   d. Provide protective padding
   e. Add shape to the body
   f. Aid in the return flow of blood
4. What is the purpose of a muscle team? Give one example. A muscle team consists of a flexor and an extensor to bend and straighten joints. The biceps and triceps of the upper arm are one example
5. What does the term *muscle tone* mean? A constant state of partial muscle contraction
6. Describe the structure and function of a tendon, locating the body's strongest example. A tendon is a fibrous extension of connective tissue sheath of a muscle. It is very strong and will not stretch. The Achilles tendon is the strongest tendon in the body
7. Explain the meaning of the terms *origin* and *insertion*. Origin refers to the attachment of the muscle to an anchor bone. It is the end nearest the center of the body or the proximal end of the muscle. Insertion refers to the attachment of the muscle to a bone to be moved. It is the distal end of the muscle
8. Describe a muscle sheath and bursa; explain their functions. A muscle sheath separates muscle groups to reduce friction with movement and to protect tendons from damage. A bursa is a watery sac that acts as cushion to reduce friction and pressure over bone and under tendons at joints
9. Identify the muscles of respiration and explain their actions. The diaphragm and the intercostal muscles. The diaphragm is the main muscle. When it contracts, air is drawn into the lungs. When it relaxes, air is forced out. The intercostal muscles between the ribs function to enlarge the rib cage during inspiration and allow the ribs to return to normal position upon expiration
10. Explain peristaltic action. Peristalsis is a smooth muscle action resulting from two layers of muscle. The longitudinal contracts to shorten the intestinal tract while the circular layer contracts to narrow it. The alternating contraction and relaxation of the layers moves material through the system

11. Describe the structure and function of a sphincter. A sphincter is a circular-shaped muscle that alternately contracts and relaxes to control openings in blood vessels and in intestines to regulate the flow of blood and food

## Labeling

1. Label the six illustrations below to indicate direction of movement in the muscle teams. Refer to Figures 28–3 and 28–4 in the textbook.

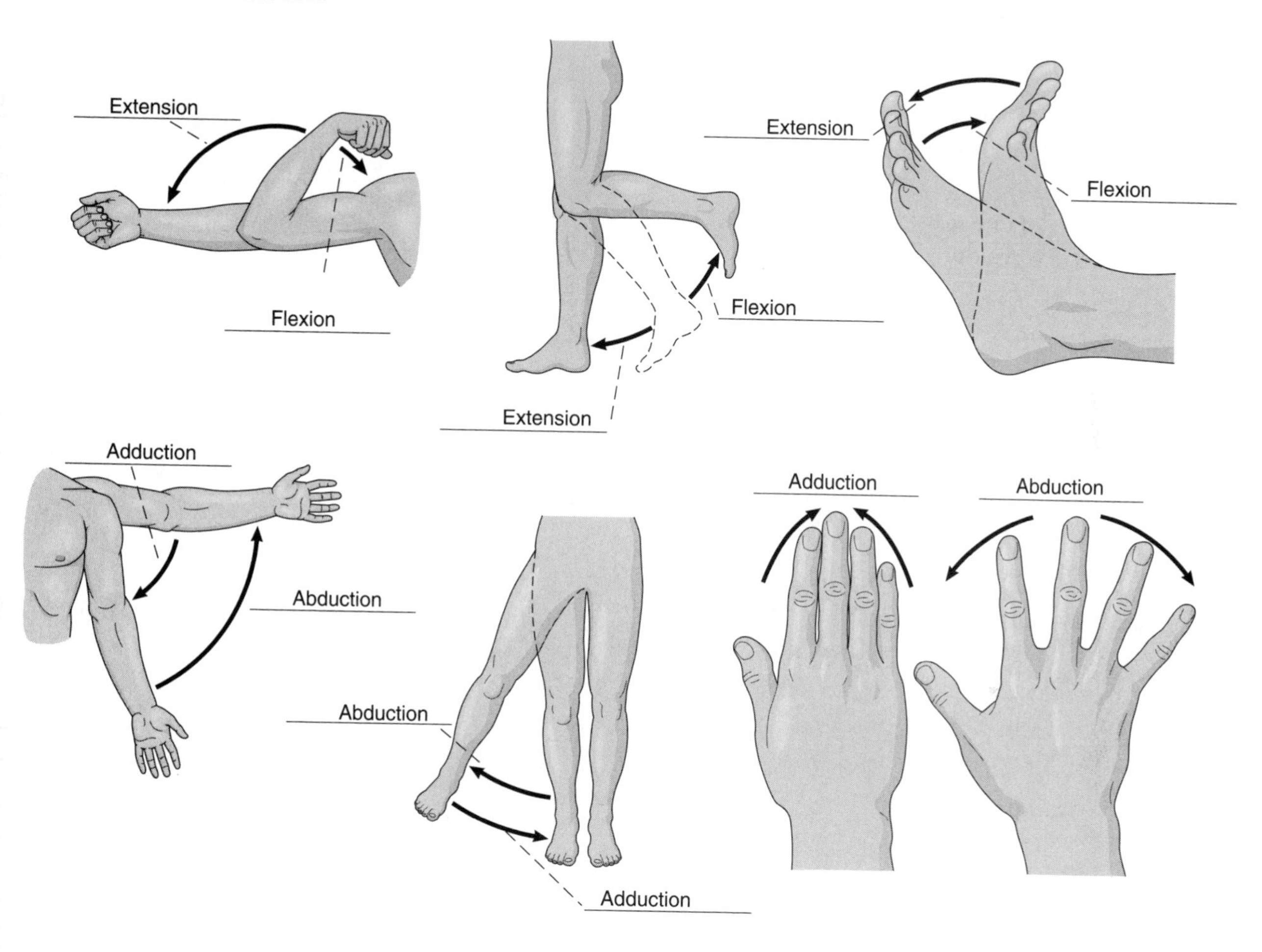

2. Label the illustration with the following major anterior body muscles. Refer to Figure 28–6 in the textbook.
   Bicep brachii
   Deltoid
   External oblique
   Intercostals
   Masseter
   Orbicularis oculi
   Orbicularis oris
   Pectoralis major
   Quadriceps femoris
   Rectus abdominis
   Sartorius
   Soleus
   Tibialis anterior
   Vastus lateralis

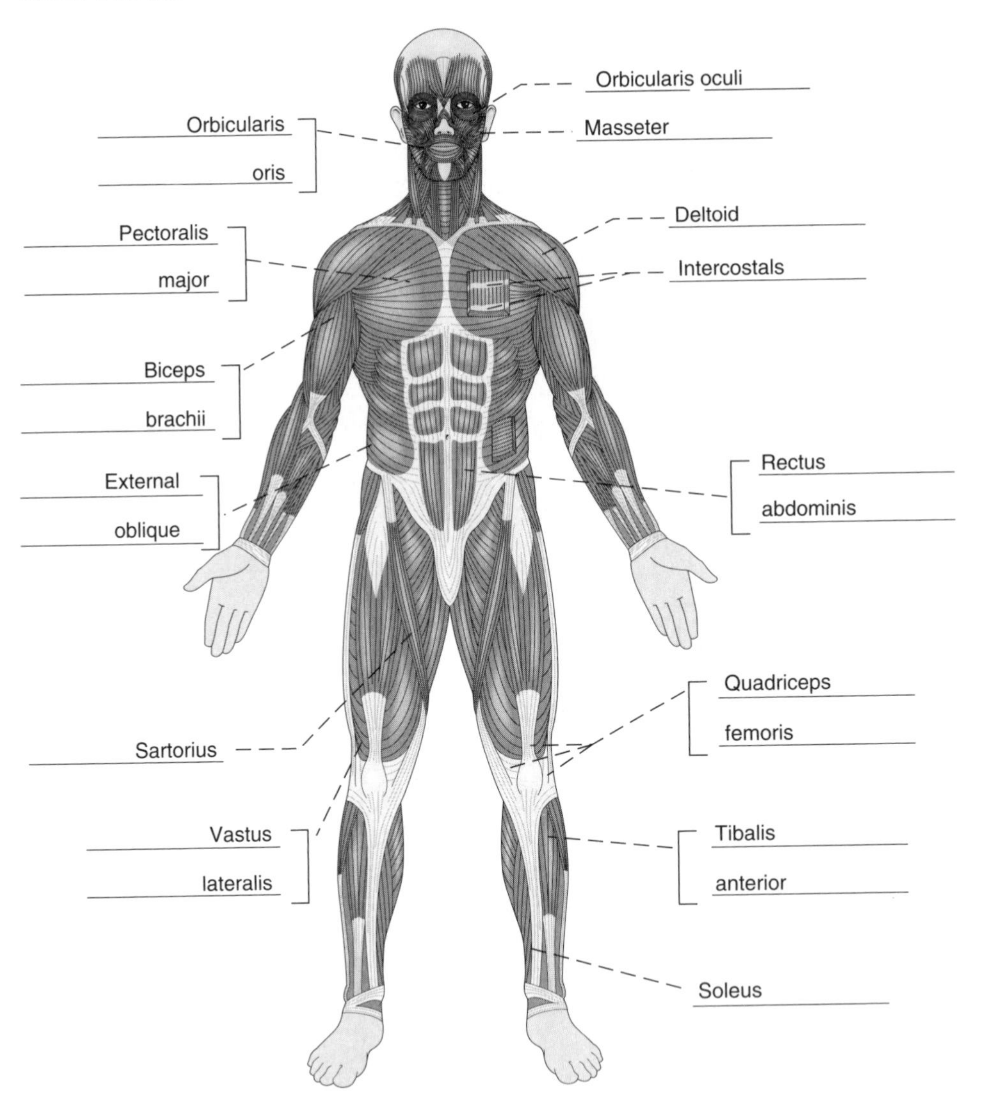

3. Label the illustration with the following major posterior body muscles. Refer to Figure 28–7 in the textbook.
   Achilles tendon
   Biceps femoris
   Deltoid
   Gastrocnemius
   Gluteus maximus
   Gluteus medius
   Hamstring group
   Latissimus dorsi
   Occipitalis
   Semi-membranosus
   Semi-tendinosus
   Sternocleidomastoid
   Trapezius
   Triceps brachii

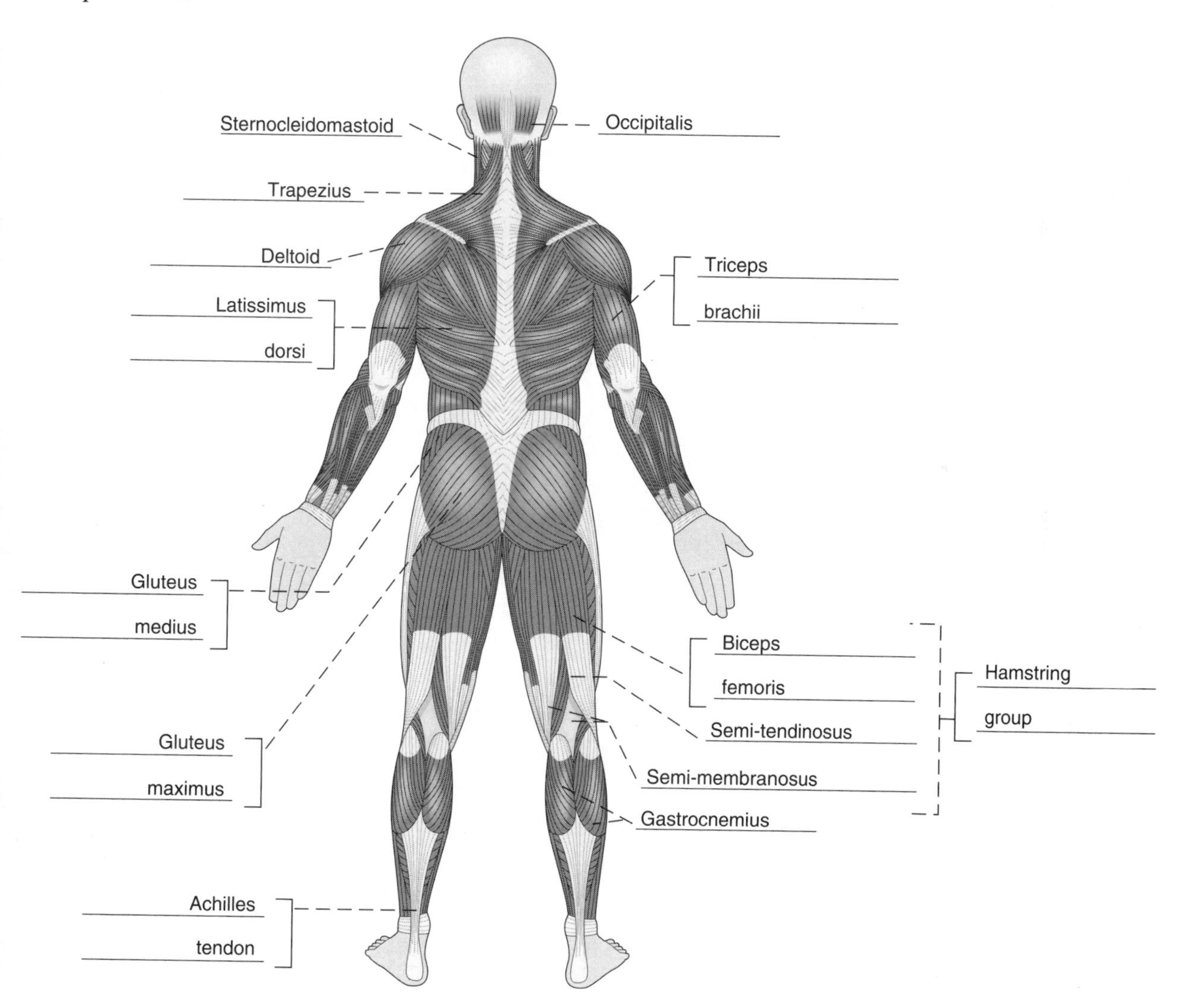

**Design a table: List the three types of muscular tissue, describe the characteristics of each type, the location in the body, and the function performed.**

| TYPE | CHARACTERISTICS | LOCATION | FUNCTION |
|---|---|---|---|
| a. Skeletal (voluntary) | Long, strong in muscle bundles | Attached to bone | Movement |
| b. Smooth (involuntary) | Small, delicate cells | Internal organs | Breathing, peristalsis, pupil of eye, dilate and constrict blood vessels |
| c. Cardiac (involuntary) | Joined in a continuous network, without sheaths | Heart | Contract to produce heartbeat |

## Chapter Application

### Case Studies with Critical Thinking Questions

#### Scenario 1

A male patient has been treated for tendonitis of the elbow. He calls the office to complain that for the past two days he has experienced an increase of pain and feels he is worse than when he was first diagnosed. He has been applying heat like he was advised. He wants to know what to do.

1. What additional information should you get? Question him as to what he means by worse; get a description of symptoms and pain evaluation. Explain you will talk with the doctor and get back to him as soon as possible
2. What advice will the physician likely give him? Suggest he discontinue the heat and apply an ice pack to see if that gives any relief while he is waiting. Also suggest he supports the arm so it is at rest
3. Do you think the physician needs to see him again? Explain that the doctor may need to see him again and that perhaps an X-ray or MRI might be necessary to rule out additional damage

#### Scenario 2

One of your best friends calls you and is very upset. She tells you the doctor thinks she may have fibromyalgia. She has never heard of the condition and is asking you for information. You realize she needs help and support.

1. Why should you question her about her symptoms? Ask her to explain how she feels so that she is accurately and completely describing her symptoms. There is a lot of similarity between some musculoskeletal disorders
2. Why should you determine what the physician has already told her? Determine what the physician has already told her so you know how much she has been informed. Try to elaborate on anything she wants explained further. Do not go into too much depth until the diagnosis is confirmed. There is no point in adding to her anxiety
3. Where else can she go for help? The physician may refer her to a rheumatologist for consultation. After the diagnosis is confirmed, suggest she get involved in a support group to help her adjust to the changes the disorder will cause. These groups can offer many hints and activities to make dealing with the disorder easier. The local Arthritis Association should be able to help her find a group to join if the rheumatologist doesn't identify a source

CHAPTER 29

# The Respiratory System

## Words to Know Challenge

**Spelling: Each line contains three spellings of a word. Underline the correctly spelled word.**

| | | |
|---|---|---|
| 1. alveala | alveola | alveoli |
| 2. cyanosis | cyaniosis | cyinosis |
| 3. emphasema | empfazema | emphysema |
| 4. hickcoughs | hiccoughs | hiccoufs |
| 5. influenza | enfluenza | influensa |
| 6. larengitis | laryngitis | laringitis |
| 7. pnewmonia | pneumonia | pneumonea |
| 8. spontaneus | spontaneous | spauntaneous |
| 9. ventalation | ventelation | ventilation |

**Matching: Match the disorders or diseases in column I with their major symptoms in column II.**

| | COLUMN I | COLUMN II |
|---|---|---|
| I | 1. Allergic rhinitis | A. A progressive, complex disease with marked dyspnea, productive cough, frequent respiratory infections, barrel chest, respiratory failure |
| O | 2. Asthma | B. A nosebleed |
| U | 3. Atelectasis | C. Coldlike symptoms initially, progressing to involve liver, spleen, and lymph glands; productive cough, dyspnea, weakness |
| L | 4. Bronchitis | D. Acute, contagious disease with chills, fever, headache, muscular aches, non-productive cough |
| A | 5. COPD | E. Sharp, stabbing pain with lung respirations, some dyspnea, usually one-sided |
| R | 6. Emphysema | F. Surgical removal of the larynx |

(continues)

| | | |
|---|---|---|
| B | 7. Epistaxis | G. Fluid collection within lung tissue associated with heart disease; causes dyspnea, orthopnea, frothy bloody sputum |
| C | 8. Histoplasmosis | H. Dyspnea, chest pain, rapid heart, productive cough, low-grade fever; caused by blood vessel obstruction |
| P | 9. Respiratory distress syndrome | I. Reaction to airborne allergens causing sneezing, profuse watery nasal discharge, and nasal congestion |
| D | 10. Influenza | J. Prolonged apnea in infants, irregular heart rate, severe lack of oxygen |
| F | 11. Laryngectomy | K. Nodular lesions and patchy infiltration of lung tissue causing fatigue, weakness, lack of appetite, weight loss, night sweats |
| N | 12. Legionnaires' disease | L. An infectious, acute, or chronically developed disease causing wheezing, dyspnea, productive cough |
| V | 13. Paroxysmal nocturnal dyspnea | M. Sore throat, nasal congestion, headache, burning, watery eyes, fever, non-productive cough |
| W | 14. Pleural effusion | N. Diarrhea, lack of appetite, headache, chills, fever that persists, weakness, grayish sputum |
| E | 15. Pleurisy | O. Bronchospasms; an allergic disorder causing wheezing, dyspnea, sputum production |
| T | 16. Pneumonoconiosis | P. Affects infants, causing respiratory distress, rapid and shallow breathing, retracted sternum, flared nostrils, grunting |
| Q | 17. Pneumonia | Q. Acute infection causing coughing, sputum, chills, fever, pleural chest pain; impairs exchange of oxygen and carbon dioxide |
| S | 18. Pneumothorax | R. Inability to exchange oxygen and carbon dioxide, causing chronic cough, pursed-lips breathing, cyanosis, weight loss |
| G | 19. Pulmonary edema | S. Sudden sharp pain, unequal chest wall expansion, may be chest wound; weak rapid pulse, dyspnea, lung collapse |
| H | 20. Pulmonary embolism | T. Environmental disease causing dyspnea, lack of oxygen, bronchial congestion |
| J | 21. SIDS | U. Dyspnea due to collapse of the alveoli |
| K | 22. Tuberculosis | V. Awaken from sleep with feeling of suffocation |
| M | 23. URI | W. Hypoxia due to the presence of excess fluid in the pleural space |

## Chapter Review

**Matching: Match the diagnostic examination from column I with its purpose in column II.**

| | COLUMN I | COLUMN II |
|---|---|---|
| D | 1. Bronchoscopy | A. To evaluate pulmonary emboli |
| C | 2. Chest X-ray | B. To withdraw fluid from the pleural space |

(continues)

| Answer | Item | Description |
|---|---|---|
| A | 3. Lung scan | C. To determine basic condition of the lungs or identify a disease process |
| E | 4. Sputum analysis | D. To observe the trachea and bronchial tree, obtain a sample, or remove a foreign body |
| B | 5. Thoracentesis | E. To diagnose infectious organisms or cancer cells |
| G | 6. Arterial blood gases | F. Aid in diagnosing pulmonary emboli and evaluating pulmonary circulation in certain heart conditions before surgery |
| H | 7. Lung perfusion scan | G. To measure the partial pressures of $O_2$ and $CO_2$ in the lungs by determining the pH of the blood |
| I | 8. Lung ventilation scan | H. To provide a visual image of pulmonary blood flow to diagnose blood vessel obstruction |
| F | 9. Pulmonary angiography | I. To determine the distribution pattern of an inhaled gas to identify obstructed airways |

## Short Answer

1. Where is oxygen produced, and how important is it to the human body? Oxygen is produced by plants on land and in the sea. It is essential to the survival of human cells. A lack of oxygen for a few minutes may be fatal.

2. What causes a breath to be taken? The respiratory center in the brain is triggered and a breath is taken when the level of $CO_2$ in the blood increases.

3. Trace the pathway of oxygen to an internal cell. Oxygen enters the nose, goes to the pharynx, under the epiglottis through the larynx to the trachea, bronchi, and bronchioles into the alveoli. Here it enters a blood capillary, which becomes a venule and then a vein to join the pulmonary veins. The oxygen is carried through the left side of the heart and sent out through the aorta to arteries, arterioles, and capillaries, where it enters an internal cell.

4. How is voice sound produced? Exhaled air vibrates the vocal cords. The pitch of the noice is higher when the cords are stretched tight. Loudness is determined by the amount of force (pressure) of the exhaled air.

5. Explain the difference between external and internal respiration. External respiration is the process of getting oxygen from the nose to the capillaries surrounding the alveolus and picking up carbon dioxide to send to the nose to be exhaled. Internal respiration is the exchange of oxygen and carbon dioxide at the level of the cell.

6. What is surfactant and how does it affect inflation of the lungs? Surfactant is a fatty molecule on the membranes of the respiratory system of newborns. It maintains the inflated alveolus so it does not collapse between breaths.

7. List five instances when a breathing pattern is altered normally.
   a. Coughing
   b. Hiccoughing
   c. Sneezing
   d. Yawning
   e. Crying

8. Describe the pleural coverings of the lungs and explain their purpose. The pleura is a membrane that is divided into two layers: a visceral pleura, which covers the lungs, and a parietal pleura, which lines the thoracic cavity. The space between the layers is called the pleural space. This space contains fluid to allow the lungs to move without causing friction.

**Design a Table: Enter the structure and function of each of the following parts of the respiratory system.**

| PART | STRUCTURE | FUNCTION |
|---|---|---|
| a. Nose | Divided by cartilage septum; has two turbinates on each side, lined with epithelium and cilia | Filters, warms, and moistens incoming air |
| b. Pharynx | Passageway lined with ciliated mucosa | Passageway for air and food |
| c. Epiglottis | A cartilage "lid" sitting on top of the larynx | Closes over larynx when food is swallowed to prevent aspiration |
| d. Larynx | A tube with nine cartilages that keep it open; has mucous membrane lining, which forms the vocal cords | Passageway for air and responsible for production of voice |
| e. Trachea | Has a series of C-shaped cartilage rings; has an elastic wall to permit flexibility | Passageway for air |
| f. Bronchi | Incomplete cartilage rings to maintain opening | Passageway for air |
| g. Bronchioles | Tiny bronchi with muscular walls | Passageway for air |
| h. Alveolus | Grapelike clusters of microscopic air sacs with one-cell-thick membrane walls that are surrounded by blood capillaries | Exchanges oxygen and carbon dioxide with the surrounding capillaries |

## Labeling

Label the illustration of the lungs. Refer to Figure 29–7 in the textbook.

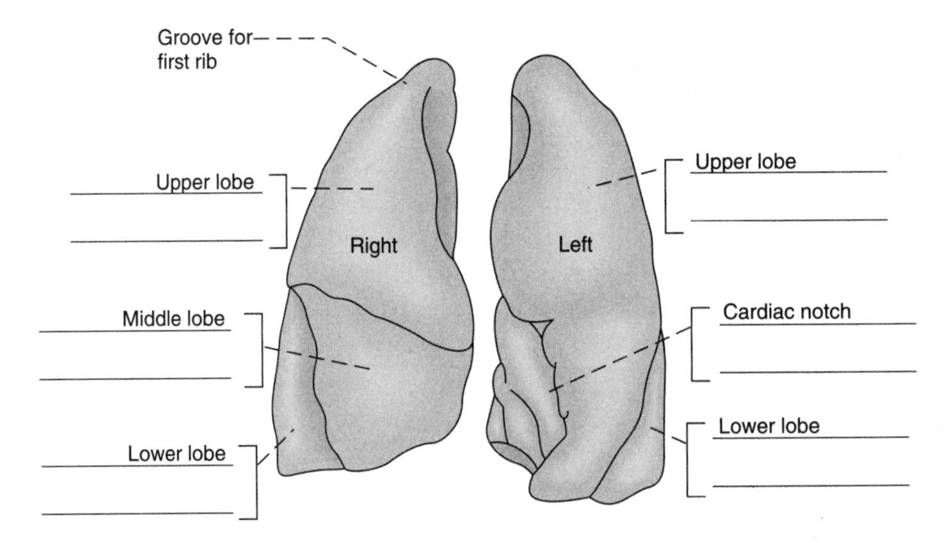

# Chapter Application

## Case Studies with Critical Thinking Questions

### Scenario 1

You are employed in a pediatrician's office. A young, first-time mother calls the office crying because her toddler is having a temper tantrum and is holding his breath until he gets red and then gasps for air. She is afraid he is going to quit breathing and die. She wants to know what to do.

1. What should you ask the mother before responding? Ask her to describe the situation just before the episode began. Confirm there is no chance of toy aspiration or other airway obstruction. Find out how long these episodes last, when they first started, and how often they occur. Find out if giving in to him stops the episode.
2. Is this common for toddlers? Yes, this is common behavior in some children; he cannot voluntarily stop breathing.
3. Should you check with the doctor about referring her to a behavior specialist or child psychiatrist? Tell her to call back if she is unable to change his behavior after a period of time or she feels she wants to talk to the physician. If it continues, the doctor may want to evaluate him and recommend professional assistance.

### Scenario 2

An elderly patient calls to complain of a high fever, muscle aches, a headache, and chills. He thinks he is getting the flu. He stated he had a flu shot about nine months ago, even though he didn't want it, and he is not supposed to get sick.

1. Should you take his self-appraisal of his condition without further question? You need to evaluate what he means by a high fever and the severity of his condition. Review his symptoms, documenting his complaints and determining the severity and length of time of his symptoms.
2. How would you explain to him the nature of the flu vaccine and its effectiveness? Explain to him that after nine months viruses change because they become ineffective. This means the injection he received does not match the current virus he has contracted. Also, the shots are not 100 percent effective. Vaccines are produced upon strain speculation months ahead of an anticipated outbreak and may not be perfectly matched.

### Research Activity

There are four lung diseases or disorders that are very interesting and quite serious that should be further researched. The four conditions are pulmonary fibrosis, respiratory distress syndrome (RDS), sudden infant death syndrome (SIDS), and tuberculosis (TB). Select one and prepare a report to share with the class. Perhaps the instructor could divide the class and each group could work on the assigned report. In your research, determine the cause, the rate of incidence within the population, the age group affected, symptoms, treatment, prognosis, and any other aspect of the disease. RDS and SIDS, for example, each have a profound impact on parents. Discuss this situation. Can you identify any support groups? Tuberculosis was thought to be a thing of the past but it has returned. Why? Pulmonary fibrosis is probably unknown to most people, yet it is not that uncommon.

CHAPTER 30

# The Circulatory System

## Words to Know Challenge

**Spelling: Each line contains three spellings of a word. Underline the correctly spelled word.**

| | | |
|---|---|---|
| 1. excelerator | accelerator | accelerater |
| 2. aneurysm | anurysm | anurism |
| 3. bradicardia | bradycardea | bradycardia |
| 4. endecardium | endocardium | endocardeum |
| 5. erythrocyte | erithrocyte | erythrocite |
| 6. hemaglobin | hemoglobin | hemogloben |
| 7. eschemia | ischemea | ischemia |
| 8. murmer | murrmur | murmur |
| 9. myocardium | myocardeum | myacardeum |
| 10. phelebitis | phlebitus | phlebitis |
| 11. tachycardea | tachycardia | tachicardia |
| 12. varicose | veracose | vericose |
| 13. arrhythmea | arrhythmia | arrhthmya |

**Matching: Match the major symptom or description in column II with the disease or disorder in column I.**

| COLUMN I | COLUMN II |
|---|---|
| J 1. Anemia | A. Sharp, sudden pain at sternum radiating to back of shoulders and arms; decreases when erect or leaning forward |
| M 2. Aneurysm | B. A circulating foreign substance in a blood vessel |
| E 3. Angina | C. Irregular heart rhythm |
| N 4. Arrest | D. Fatty deposits on the lining of blood vessels |
| C 5. Arrhythmia | E. Severe chest pain from a coronary artery spasm |

(continues)

| Answer | Term | Description |
|---|---|---|
| K | 6. Arteriosclerosis | F. Pounding heartbeats after exercise, enlarged heart, slow pulse |
| D | 7. Atherosclerosis | G. Blood pressure consistently above normal |
| F | 8. Athletic heart syndrome | H. Congestion of blood in the circulatory system; edema of extremities and lungs |
| L | 9. CVA | I. Tightness of chest, substernal chest pain radiating down left arm, nausea and vomiting, perspiration, fainting |
| H | 10. CHF | J. Lack of red blood cells and/or hemoglobin |
| I | 11. Coronary artery disease | K. Rigid arterial walls; causes hypertension |
| B | 12. Embolus | l. Confusion, weakness of one side, visual changes, paralysis, personality change |
| P | 13. Endocarditis | M. A bulging arterial wall that may produce palpitations or tear |
| G | 14. Hypertension | N. Complete and sudden cessation of heart action |
| Y | 15. Hypotension | O. Mild chest soreness, fever, dyspnea, palpitations, feeling of pressure |
| S | 16. Leukemia | P. Vegetative growths or inflammation of inner heart structures |
| V | 17. Murmur | Q. Abnormally shaped red blood cells, enlarged liver, pallor, painful crisis periods |
| X | 18. MI | R. Skin breakdown from inadequate circulation |
| O | 19. Myocarditis | S. Excessive WBCs, bruising, fatigue, painful lymph nodes |
| A | 20. Pericarditis | T. Inflamed vein lining with thrombus formation, severe pain, fever, chills, and discoloration of involved extremity |
| W | 21. Phlebitis | U. Dilated, twisted veins, inefficient valves, leg cramps |
| Q | 22. Sickle cell anemia | V. A gurgling or swishing sound heard upon auscultation of the heart |
| R | 23. Stasis ulcer | W. Localized inflammation of a vein |
| T | 24. Thrombophlebitis | X. Severe, crushing pain radiating through chest to neck and jaw and down left arm; nausea, dyspnea |
| U | 25. Varicosities | Y. Consistently low blood pressure |

## Chapter Review

### Short Answer

1. List the four major parts of the circulatory system.
   a. Heart
   b. Blood vessels
   c. Blood
   d. Lymphatic system
2. What is the difference between pulmonary and systemic circulation? Pulmonary circulation refers to the flow of blood from the right ventricle through the right pulmonary artery to the lungs and back to the left atrium. Systemic circulation refers to the flow of blood from the left ventricle through the rest of the body to the right atrium.

3. Describe the heart sounds and what heart action causes the sound. Identify where the sounds may be auscultated.

| Sound | Caused by | Where auscultated |
|---|---|---|
| Lubb | Closing of the bicuspid and tricuspid valves | Apex |
| Dupp | Closing of the semilunar valves | Second intercostal space on each side of the sternum |

4. Describe the location and action of the pacemaker. The pacemaker, or SA node, is located in the right atrium. It initiates the heartbeat. The impulse causes both atria to contract. It also carries over to the AV node, which causes the ventricles to contract due to impulses sent over the bundle of His and through the Purkinje fibers.

5. Explain how the action of the pacemaker is related to the symptoms of heart block and fibrillation. When the impulse from the SA node does not carry over to the AV node, this person has a heart block. The atria beat at a normal rate and the ventricles contract about 40 beats per minute. Fibrillation is caused by the breakdown of rhythm and strength of the contraction due to malfunction of the node. The heartbeat is uncoordinated and ineffective, and the condition is life-threatening.

6. What is the basic cause of arrhythmia? An area of the heart "sparks" and stimulates a contraction of the myocardium. This area is known as an ectopic pacemaker.

7. What purpose does an artificial pacemaker serve and how does it function? It generates the electrical impulse through an electrode catheter connected to an battery-powered pulse generator. It causes a contraction when the SA node fails.

8. Explain how the rate of the heartbeat is basically controlled. The vagus and accelerator nerves affect the rate. The vagus slows the action while the accelerator increases the rate.

9. How does a capillary bed function? It receives blood from an arteriole. A series of sphincters allow only part of the cells to receive blood at a time. The sphincters open and close to control the flow of blood so all cells receive their share.

10. Trace the pathway of blood through the pulmonary and systemic circulation beginning at the vena cava, going to a capillary of the body, and returning to the atrium of the heart. Name the structures of the heart and lungs, and the major vessels. Superior and inferior vena cava to right atrium–through tricuspid valve into right ventricle–through semilunar valve into right and left pulmonary arteries to arterioles and capillaries of the alveoli; to venules then right and left pulmonary veins to left atrium–through bicuspid valve into left ventricle–through semilunar valve to aorta to arterioles and capillaries of the body–into venules and veins to the superior and inferior vena cava and into the right atrium.

11. From where does the blood in the portal circulation come? Where does it go, and why? It comes from single organs such as the stomach, pancreas, large and small intestines, and spleen and goes to the liver to be processed by the liver cells, which perform many life-preserving functions.

12. Name five things that blood transports through the body.
    a. Oxygen
    b. Nutrients
    c. Cell waste
    d. Hormones
    e. Minerals

13. What is plasma? List 17 things that can be found circulating in plasma. It is a straw-colored liquid that makes up over half the volume of blood.

| | | |
|---|---|---|
| a. Water | l. Amino acids | m. Oxygen |
| b. Calcium | g. Vitamins | n. Carbon dioxide |
| c. Sodium | h. Hormones | o. Fibrinogen |
| d. Potassium | i. Enzymes | p. Serum albumin |
| e. Phosphorus | j. Glucose | q. Serum globulin |
| f. Bicarbonates | k. Fatty acids | |

14. List the three types of blood cells, describing the basic function of each.
    a. Red blood cells—have hemoglobin, which carries oxygen to cells
    b. White blood cells—destroy bacteria within the tissue fluid; consume toxic substances and provide immunity
    c. Platelets—clot blood

15. Why is blood typed and crossmatched before being given to a patient? The recipient's blood must match the donor's to be compatible. Agglutins and agglutinogens must be of a different type in order to prevent agglutination of the blood and possible death.

16. Why is the Rh factor especially important with a pregnancy or a transfusion? Rh is an antigen in the blood. If a person does not have the factor and receives blood that is Rh+, the body produces antibodies against the foreign material. If later the person receives Rh blood, the body's antibodies react against the antigen, causing serious complications. With pregnancy, a mother who is Rh– and who delivers an Rh+ baby may get some of the antigen within her bloodstream, causing antibodies to be developed. Subsequent pregnancies will be in danger because the antibodies destroy the baby's RBCs and the baby will be born profoundly anemic.

**Matching: Match the cardiovascular tests in column I with the appropriate purpose for conducting it in column II.**

| | COLUMN I | COLUMN II |
|---|---|---|
| D | 1. Arteriograph | A. To evaluate cardiac function and structure, and to detect defects by means of sound waves |
| G | 2. Cardiac catheterization | B. To detect irregularly occurring symptoms or evaluate status of a recovering cardiac patient |
| E | 3. Doppler ultrasonography | C. Detects condition of deep veins of the legs, especially deep vein thrombosis |
| A | 4. Echocardiograph | D. Injecting dye to indicate the status of blood flow, malformed vessels, aneurysm, or hemorrhage |
| F | 5. Electrocardiograph | E. To evaluate major blood vessels to determine deep vein thrombosis, peripheral aneurysms, and occluded carotid arteries |
| B | 6. Holter monitor | F. To identify heart rhythm, electrolyte imbalance, and conduction abnormalities |
| C | 7. Venogram | G. To visualize by fluoroscope the internal heart structure and activity and to visualize the coronary arteries |
| H | 8. MUGA scan | H. To determine condition of myocardium |

## Labeling

Label the following structures of the heart on the illustration below: apex, right atrium (auricle), left atrium (auricle), right ventricle, left ventricle, aorta, pulmonary semilunar valve, tricuspid valve, inferior vena cava, septum, bicuspid (mitral) valve, aortic semilunar valve, right pulmonary artery, left pulmonary artery, right pulmonary veins, left pulmonary veins, superior vena cava, endocardium, and myocardium. Refer to Figure 30–3 in the textbook.

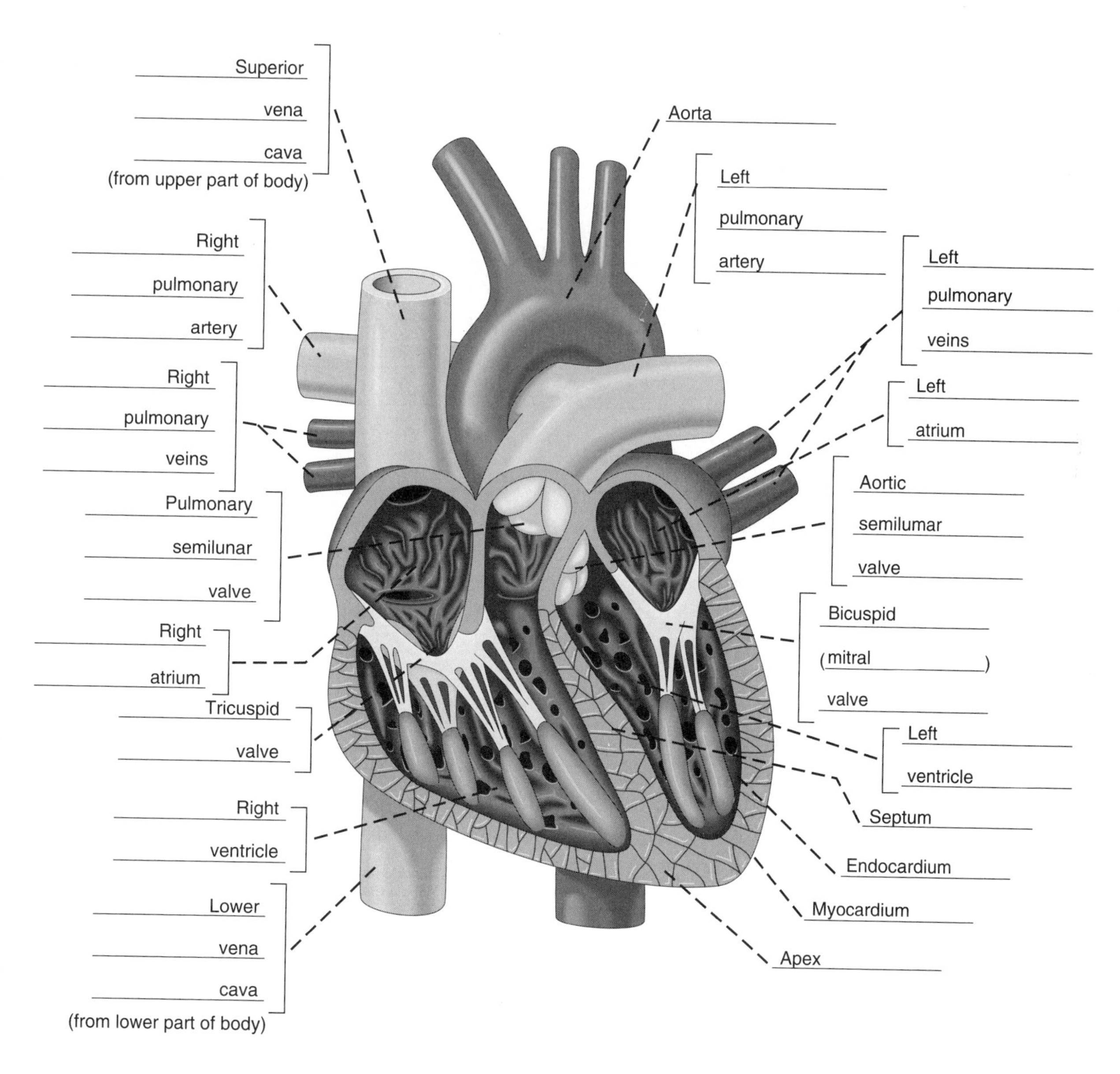


**Fill in the Blank: Use information from the chapter to fill in the blank space in the sentence.**

The lymphatic system consists of lymph vessels, which are located throughout the body. Lymph capillaries absorb fluid ______ and other substances and return them to the circulatory system. The system is a(n) one-way ______ system; there are no vessels bringing lymph ______ to the cells ______. The capillaries join to become small lymph vessels ______, which in turn become larger vessels called lymphatics ______. The lymphatics eventually form two main ducts ______, a right lymphatic ______ duct and a thoracic ______ duct. Lymph nodes ______ are located along lymph vessels at various places in the body. During an infection, the nodes become swollen ______ and tender ______ because of the collection of lymphocytes.

**Design a Table: Make a table of blood vessels in the order in which blood would flow from the heart and back. List the five types of blood vessels, describing the structure and explaining the function of each type.**

| TYPE | STRUCTURE | FUNCTION |
|---|---|---|
| a. Arteries | Have elastic fibers in their walls to expand and recoil to produce a pulse | Carry oxygenated blood away from the heart |
| b. Arterioles | Same as arteries, only smaller | Carry blood from artery to capillary |
| c. Capillaries | One-cell-thick walls, microscopic blood vessels | Exchange of oxygen and carbon dioxide with the cells; permit WBCs to leave to attack bacteria and allow plasma to leave to add to the tissue fluid |
| d. Venules | Small veins | Carry blood from capillary to vein |
| e. Veins | Have thinner walls than arteries and lack an elastic layer; have valves to assist the return flow of blood | Carry deoxygenated blood back to the heart |

# Chapter Application

## Case Studies with Critical Thinking Questions

### Scenario 1

A male patient who has angina calls to report that he has been experiencing fairly severe chest pains off and on for the past few hours. He says he is perspiring and has had constant pain for the last 20 minutes, which has not been relieved by the three nitroglycerin tablets he has taken. Unfortunately, the physician is not in right now so you need to decide what to do.

1. Why should you determine if he is home alone? If he is alone, he may not be able to help himself. Have the patient stay as calm as possible. Question his symptoms and current status. Assure him you will get him help. Ask if someone else is there so you can talk with him or her. Make sure the patient is as comfortable as possible and summon emergency services. Examination is necessary because it sounds like he is experiencing a heart attack.
2. Why should you call for emergency services? If the patient is alone, you should call just in case he should suddenly become unable to do it. With the symptoms he is experiencing, a cardiac emergency may be imminent.

### Scenario 2

A female patient has been under treatment for two years for hypertension. She has lost 50 pounds and is getting regular exercise as well as watching her diet. Last time she was in the office, about three months ago, her blood pressure was normal and had been for about six months. Today it is elevated again, she has gained 15 pounds, and the patient states that she thought she was cured.

1. Why could maintaining her weight be a factor? Additional weight may increase blood pressure if gained in sufficient amount, but this is not likely with a modest gain.
2. Why would determining if she is continuing to watch her intake of fats and sodium be important? If she is no longer eating properly, a diet with excess fats and high sodium intake may also increase blood pressure over time, but probably not this quickly.
3. What else could cause an elevation in her blood pressure? Maybe she is doing something differently or is encountering a very stressful situation. Be sure to question her compliance with her medication. The most suspicious thing may be that since she felt she was "cured," she may have quit taking her medication.

## Research Activity

Observe blood flow. With a partner, observe the back of your hands or the inner surface of your wrist for visible blood vessels. Observe the blood flow and decide if the vessel is an artery or a vein.

1. Using your partner's hand, wrist, or forearm, put pressure on the proximal ends of the visible blood vessels. With the fingers of the other hand, press and slide the fingers distal to the point where the blood flow is shut off.
   a. Observe and explain what happens and why.
2. Now put pressure at the distal end and slide the fingers toward the body.
   a. Observe and explain what happens and why
   b. Did you detect branching vessels? What happened to maintain blood flow?

CHAPTER 31

# The Immune System

## Words to Know Challenge

**Spelling: Each line contains three spellings of a word. Underline the correctly spelled word.**

| | | |
|---|---|---|
| 1. antebody | antibody | antybody |
| 2. compliment | complament | complement |
| 3. humoral | humural | humeral |
| 4. viris | virus | viruss |
| 5. antegin | antegene | antigen |
| 6. benine | benigne | benign |
| 7. biopsy | biospy | biopsie |
| 8. thymus | thymuss | thymas |
| 9. nioplasm | neoplasam | neoplasm |
| 10. metatasis | metastasis | metasastis |
| 11. remmision | remission | remmission |
| 12. chemotherapy | chematherapy | chemitherapy |

**Matching: Match the term in column I with its description in column II.**

| | COLUMN I | COLUMN II |
|---|---|---|
| G | 1. Abstinence | A. Capable of destroying cells |
| J | 2. Anaphylaxis | B. An administered substance to prevent disease |
| L | 3. Autoimmune | C. Protected from disease |
| N | 4. Benign | D. An term to identify the extent of a disease process |
| A | 5. Cytotoxic | E. Can be penetrated; allowing entrance |
| C | 6. Immune | F. A period that is disease- and symptom-free |
| I | 7. Lymphedema | G. Refrain from; avoid; stay away from |

(continues)

K 8. Malignant

O 9. Metastasis

M 10. Mutation

H 11. Neoplasm

E 12. Permeable

F 13. Remission

D 14. Staging

B 15. Vaccine

H. A new growth

I. Tissue swelling due to the presence of lymph fluid

J. A hypersensitive reaction of the body to a foreign protein

K. Pertaining to cancerous growth

L. Relating to the process when person's own antibodies act against their normal tissue

M. A change in the structure of a cell

N. Non-cancerous

O. The movement of cells to another part of the body

## Chapter Review

### Short Answer

1. What are antigens? Things that are non-self
2. List five types of antigens. Foreign material, bacteria, viruses, fungi, and parasites
3. Name five kinds of foreign materials. Cells, tissues, proteins, food items, and particles in the air
4. What are the body's three main lines of defense against antigens? Barriers, inflammation process, and antibodies
5. What is the function of the immune system? Create effective immune responses to continually defend the body against antigens
6. Name the organs of the immune system and their location (see Figure 31–2).
   a. Bone marrow—in bones
   b. Thymus—in the thoracic cavity
   c. Lymph nodes—along lymphatic vessels
   d. Spleen—at splenic flexion of colon
   e. Tonsils—in throat
   f. Adenoids—in throat
   g. Appendix—at end of cecum
   h. Peyer's patches—in small intestine
   i. Blood—within blood vessels
   j. Lymphatic vessels—throughout the body
7. What is MHC and what does it do? Major histocompatibility complex codes cells with "fingerprint" to identify them as "self"
8. Name the four types of T lymphocyte cells. T helper, T suppressor, T memory, and T killer
9. How does a B lymphocyte destroy an antigen? By producing an antibody
10. Why do killer cells cause rejection of an organ transplant? Because the MHC markers of the donor cells are not identified as self
11. What stops an immune response? The suppressor T cells
12. a. How do immunizations and vaccines provide protection against antigens? They cause an antigen-antibody complex and the development of memory cells.
    b. Active immunity means: recipients make their own immunity
    c. Passive immunity means: antibodies from another source are injected to provide temporary immunity

13. Name the body fluids in which the AIDS virus survives the best.
    a. Blood
    b. Semen
    c. Vaginal secretions
14. Identify four early symptoms of HIV infection. Headache, fever, fatigue, and enlarged lymph glands
15. Explain how HIV destroys the immune system. By invading the helper T cells and macrophages, causing the T cells to not make the macrophages act
16. List the three infections that are signs of AIDS.
    a. pneumocystis carinii pneumonia
    b. Kaposi's sarcoma
    c. candidiasis
17. List five ways to acquire HIV.
    a. Unprotected sex
    b. Sharing drug needles
    c. Transmission from mother to fetus
    d. Blood transfusions
    e. Needle sticks, blood, and body fluids
18. What four high-risk behaviors should be avoided?
    a. Unprotected sex with a person with HIV
    b. Using IV drugs and sharing needles
    c. Having many sex partners
    d. Having other STDs
19. What is cancer? Cancer is a group of diseases characterized by uncontrolled growth of abnormal cells.
20. Identify six characteristics of a cancer cell.
    a. Altered cell structure
    b. Lack of normal growth control
    c. Lack of contact inhibition
    d. Does not respond to growth factors that control normal cells
    e. Frequently escapes immune surveillance
    f. Is invasive

    (Also: can metastasize and have increased metabolic rate)
21. Name the four classifications of cancer.
    a. Carcinomas
    b. Sarcomas
    c. Leukemias
    d. Lymphomas
22. What is the basic cause of cancer? Cellular mutation or abnormal activation of cellular genes that control growth and division
23. List four types or categories of carcinogens.
    a. Chemical
    b. Viral
    c. Physical
    d. Familial

24. Name three types of procedures used to diagnose cancer.
    a. Biopsy
    b. Laboratory test
    c. Tumor imaging
25. Briefly describe grading and staging cancer. Grading refers to the degree of differentiation ranging from I to IV. Staging is used to identify the extent of spread of the disease. It uses a system of description that states the size, node involvement, and metastasis. It also has four staging classifications.
26. What are the four major methods of treating cancer?
    a. Surgery
    b. Radiation
    c. Chemotherapy
    d. Biological response modifiers
27. What is a clinical trial? A research study that determines the effectiveness and safety of a cancer treatment regime
28. List five symptoms of chronic fatigue syndrome.
    a. Persistent and overwhelming fatigue
    b. Low-grade fever
    c. Sore throat
    d. Swollen lymph nodes
    e. Headaches

    (Also: lingering fatigue, unexplained muscle weakness, pain in joints, forgetfulness, irritability, confusion, inability to concentrate, depression, sensitivity to light, impaired vision, sleep disturbances)
29. Describe rheumatoid arthritis. It is a chronic systemic autoimmune disease that affects joints and surrounding muscles, tendons, ligaments, and blood vessels.
30. Explain how lupus affects the immune system and name the organs it affects. Lupus causes the production of antibodies that react against the person's own normal tissue. It affects the skin, joints, kidneys, lungs, heart, and nervous system.

**Fill in the Blank: Use information from the chapter to fill in the blank space in the sentence.**

1. The process of antibody-mediated responses and other chemicals also causes a(n) inflammatory response.
2. Basophils and mast cells release histamine, which dilates blood vessels and makes them more permeable. This slows down blood flow and allows fluid to seep into the surrounding tissues. This results in localized warmth, redness, and swelling.
3. Natural killer cells (NK) destroy cancer and virus-infected cells. They contain granules filled with potent chemicals. They are called natural because they do not need to recognize a specific antigen like other T cells to kill the invading antigen. NK cells bind to their targets and deliver a(n) lethal burst of chemicals to produce holes in a cell's membrane, which destroys the cell.
4. There are two branches of immune response: antibody-mediated, which results from B cell activity, and cell-mediated, which results from T cell activity. Response can also be primary, which means the first encounter, or secondary (subsequent encounters).
5. A primary response requires five to six days to develop. Antibody-mediated responses act against bacteria and extracellular viruses, fungi, and parasites. They cannot react against microorganisms already within a cell's cytoplasm; they only react to those in circulation or attached to a cell's surface.

6. Secondary response requires two or three days because of the leftover clonal lymphocytes with memory. Cell-mediated responses attack intracellular viruses, fungi, protozoans, cancer cells, and transplant tissue cells.
7. All blood cells originate in the bone marrow and initially develop from stem cells.
8. Erythrocytes develop from erythroid stem cells and mature in the bone marrow.
9. Granulated white blood cells develop from myeloid stem cells.
10. One type of agranulocyte, the lymphocyte, develops from a lymphocyte stem cell into two major classes: B cells, which mature in the bone marrow, and T cells, which mature in the thymus.
11. Mononuclear phagocyte stem cells become the monocytes, which circulate in the blood and then enter the tissues to become macrophages.
12. Phagocytes are cells that engulf and destroy antigens.
13. Neutrophils carry granules with potent chemicals to destroy microorganisms.
14. Neutrophils attack and destroy invading bacteria, viruses, and other antigens.
15. Eosinophils are produced in large amounts in response to parasitic infections.

# Chapter Application

## Case Studies with Critical Thinking Questions

### Scenario 1

A neighbor has just been diagnosed with lung cancer. He says he is not going to go through chemotherapy or radiation because he will just end up dying anyway. He believes those treatments just make you feel worse while you are waiting for the inevitable. Instead, he is going to take the advice of a friend and send for a cancer cure that's available from Mexico.

1. How can you get him to reconsider his refusal of conventional treatment? Explain that you know this has been a shocking diagnosis and he really needs to think about his decision instead of just taking someone else's word. See if you can get him to research treatments so he can be more informed himself. Explain that almost all nontraditional treatments have been proven ineffective. He is substituting known effective treatment for the unknown, and he may not have a chance at remission or a longer survival. He may not have a second chance.
2. What can you do to help him change his attitude toward the diagnosis? Get him to at least talk with the physician. His treatment may not be as bad as he thinks. His chances of survival may be fairly good. Explain that a positive attitude and a sense of hope are very important to success when treating cancer.
3. Why does he think that chemo and radiation will be used? Question him to see if he has been told what treatments will be used for his type of cancer. He may be making statements based on what he knows about treatment. Various methods are used today, and medications are given to prevent many of the side effects of the treatments.
4. How can you discourage him from taking a so-called "cure"? Explain there are no controls or standards governing the manufacture and sale of these drugs. They also have not been scientifically tested and evaluated for effectiveness.

## Scenario 2

You notice one of your co-workers has looked and acted very tired lately. She has also been losing a lot of weight. She has recently developed flulike symptoms, with headache, fever, and fatigue. When you start to talk with her about it, she breaks down and cries, telling you she is HIV positive and is having a hard time dealing with it. She asks that you do not tell anyone, especially the doctor because she has to work to care of herself and her son. She's afraid she will lose her job.

1. Should you respect her wishes and not tell the doctor? It certainly is not your responsibility to tell the physician; however, she must be encouraged to speak with him because her condition requires certain precautions.
2. Could she putting the patients at danger? There is the chance that while performing certain clinical procedures, an accident could occur that would be of concern, especially if she had an open wound. It would seem appropriate for her to be assigned to nonclinical responsibilities as a precaution.
3. Why should you determine if she has any support system from family or friends to help her? She definitely needs family and friends who can help her. She needs to confide in them. Most people are willing to help when someone needs it. She may have to explain that she is not a threat to them through ordinary day-to-day activities. At work it may be necessary to be flexible with scheduling in order for her to make appointments or to take time off occasionally when treatments or symptoms are a problem.

## Research Activity

Suppose you are the co-worker of the woman in Scenario 2. She is in need of support and perhaps financial assistance. Where in your community could she go for help? Is there an HIV support group? Can you identify community services that might help her?

Check in your local phone directory; you will be surprised at the number of organizations. Choose one or two to call. Inform the organization you are a student medical assistant and you are researching what support groups or assistance might be available to HIV persons in your community. Find out if it sponsors a support group to help people who are HIV positive. Ask what kinds of services it provides. Also ask about the requirements to obtain financial assistance, if available, should a single parent develop AIDS and be unable to work.

CHAPTER 32

# The Digestive System

## Words To Know Challenge

**Spelling: Each line contains three spellings of a word. Underline the correctly spelled word.**

| | | | |
|---|---|---|---|
| 1. | apendix | appendix | appenddix |
| 2. | cirrhosis | cirhosis | cirrosis |
| 3. | collitis | colytis | colitis |
| 4. | diahrrea | diarhea | diarrhea |
| 5. | digestion | digestation | digeshion |
| 6. | dudenum | duodenum | duodunem |
| 7. | esofagus | esophagus | esophegus |
| 8. | hepattitis | hepetitis | hepatitis |
| 9. | iluocecal | illucecal | illuocecal |
| 10. | insalen | insilun | insulin |
| 11. | jaundice | jawndice | jaundace |
| 12. | nasea | nausea | nausae |
| 13. | pancrase | pancrease | pancreas |
| 14. | sigmiod | sigmoid | sigmyod |
| 15. | stenosis | stenasis | stenesis |
| 16. | stomack | stomach | stomache |
| 17. | tong | tungue | tongue |
| 18. | varies | varices | verices |

**Matching: Match the term in column I with its description in column II.**

| | COLUMN I | COLUMN II |
|---|---|---|
| G | 1. Alimentary canal | A. Inability to control bowel elimination |
| J | 2. Bile | B. A backup of stomach contents |
| O | 3. Cholelithiasis | C. The organ between the mouth and stomach |
| P | 4. Cystic duct | D. Smooth muscle action that moves material |
| K | 5. Duodenum | E. Engorged veins |
| C | 6. Esophagus | F. Protrusion of an organ through an opening |
| L | 7. Flatus | G. The chain of organs of the GI system |
| M | 8. Gastric | H. The yellowish discoloration caused by bile in the tissues |
| N | 9. Gastroscopy | I. An instrument to visualize the rectum |
| F | 10. Hernia | J. Stored by the gallbladder |
| A | 11. Incontinent | K. The first section of the small intestine |
| H | 12. Jaundice | L. Intestinal gas |
| D | 13. Peristalsis | M. Refers to the stomach |
| I | 14. Proctoscope | N. An instrument to view the stomach |
| B | 15. Reflux | O. Gallstones |
| E | 16. Varices | P. The drainage tube for the gallbladder |

# Chapter Review

## Short Answer

1. Define "digestion." It is the process by which food is broken down mechanically and chemically in the gastrointestinal tract and is converted into a form that can be absorbed and used by the cells of the body

2. List the raw materials the body requires to promote good health.
   a. Carbohydrates
   b. Proteins
   c. Fats
   d. Minerals
   e. Vitamins
   f. Water
   g. Roughage

3. List, in order, the organs of the alimentary tract through which food passes.
   a. Mouth
   b. Pharynx
   c. Esophagus
   d. Stomach
   e. Small intestine
   f. Large intestine

4. List the accessory digestive organs of the mouth; explain their function in the digestive process.
   a. Teeth—mechanically chop, grind, and crush food into a form suitable for swallowing
   b. Tongue—moves food within the mouth to put in contact with the teeth and pushes it toward the back to be swallowed
   c. Salivary glands—excrete saliva to begin digestion by breaking carbohydrates down into sugar. Also supplies moisture so the taste buds can perceive tastes. Saliva also aids in cleansing the teeth and keeps the surfaces of the mouth moist, which aids in speech.

5. a. What are the initial teeth called? Deciduous
   b. When do they appear? Begins at about 6 months of age
   c. Initial teeth are lost beginning about age 6 and are replaced by permanent teeth.
   d. Identify the four types of "secondary" teeth and their specific duties.
      a) Incisors—bite food
      b) Canines or cuspids—puncture or tear
      c) Premolars or biscupids—grinding and crushing
      d) Molars—grinding and crushing

6. How is swallowing accomplished? The muscles of the mouth work together. The tongue presses upward and back against the palate and the cheek muscles to form a chute and aid in moving food to the pharynx. When food is swallowed, the epiglottis moves across the opening of the larynx, the soft palate closes off the nasal cavity, and the larynx moves upward against the epiglottis to close its opening.

7. How is food moved through the esophagus? Peristalsis moves food through the esophagus. The esophagus wall contains circular and longitudinal muscles that alternately contract and relax to move the food in only one direction.

8. Describe the structure of the stomach and explain its function. The stomach is a 10-inch-long S-shaped organ. It has a cardiac sphincter at the upper end and a pyloric sphincter at the lower end. Its wall has three muscle layers to churn the food and break it down mechanically. The inner lining is full of folds so it can expand during eating. There are mucous and gastric glands that secrete mucus, enzymes, and hydrochloric acid to digest the food chemically. When food approaches the stomach, the cardiac sphincter opens. Once the food has entered, it closes off and the muscles begin to churn their contents while the glands secrete the digestive juices, turning the contents into chyme. When chyme is thoroughly mixed and broken down into a semiliquid state, the pyloric sphincter opens slightly to it chyme to leave.

9. Describe the structure of the small intestine, naming its sections and explaining its function. The small intestine is a tube 20 feet long and about an inch in diameter. It is divided into three sections: the duodenum, the jejunum, and the ileum. Its role is to complete digestion and absorb the nutrients from the chyme. The small intestine completes digestion by secreting intestinal juices and receiving secretions from the accessory organs (liver, gallbladder, and pancreas). It absorbs nutrients through the villi in its lining.

10. What functions does the liver perform, including the relationship with the portal circulation?
    a. Secretes bile
    b. Stores glycogen
    c. Releases glucose
    d. Processes proteins
    e. Burns or stores fat
    f. Manufactures fibrogen and prothrombin to clot blood
    g. Produces antibody
    h. Neutralizes most poisons
    i. Stores large quantities of blood and body fluids. The liver receives blood from all the abdominal organs by way of the portal vein in order to obtain the absorbed nutrients and other substances upon which it rests.

11. What role does the gallbladder play and how is it related to the liver? The gallbladder receives bile from the liver and concentrates and stores it until the body has a need for additional bile beyond what is currently available from the liver. Then it is released through the cystic duct into the common bile duct, which empties into the duodenum.

12. Explain why the duodenum is vital to digestion. The duodenum is the location for the ducts from the liver, gallbladder, and pancreas to empty their secretions into the alimentary canal. It is also the connecting link between the stomach and the remainder of the system.

13. Describe the location and function of the pancreas. The pancreas lies behind and somewhat below the stomach with its head in the curve of the duodenum. The pancreas functions as an exocrine gland, secreting pancreatic digestive juices by way of the pancreatic duct into the duodenum. It is also an endocrine gland, secreting insulin directly into the bloodstream.

14. Where in the body are nutrients absorbed, and how is absorption accomplished? Nutrients are absorbed in the small intestine, mainly in the jejunum. The process is performed by millions of microscopic villi that project from the lining of the small intestine. Each villi has a blood capillary to absorb some fats, carbohydrates, proteins, and water. The lacteals in the villi absorb fats into the lymphatic system for processing and returning to the circulatory system.

15. Explain the function of the colon and name its five sections. The colon absorbs excess liquid from the chyme and eliminates the leftover waste products.
    a. Cecum
    b. Ascending colon
    c. Transverse colon
    d. Descending colon
    e. Sigmoid colon

16. What function does the rectum perform? The rectum collects the remains of digestion and eliminates its contents when an appropriate amount has been accumulated.

17. Describe the structure and function of the anal canal. The anal canal is a one-inch-long passageway with an involuntary internal sphincter and a voluntary external sphincter through which solid waste is eliminated from the body.

## Labeling

1. Label the illustration of the structures involved in swallowing using the following terms. Refer to Figure 32–4 in the textbook.

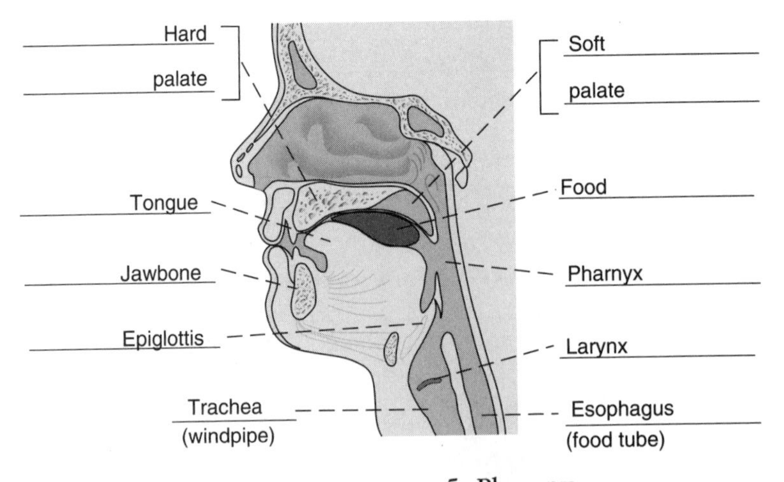


1. Epiglottis
2. Food
3. Hard palate
4. Jawbone
5. Pharynx
6. Soft palate
7. Tongue

2. Label the organs of digestion on the illustration using the following terms. Refer to Figure 32–1 in the textbook.

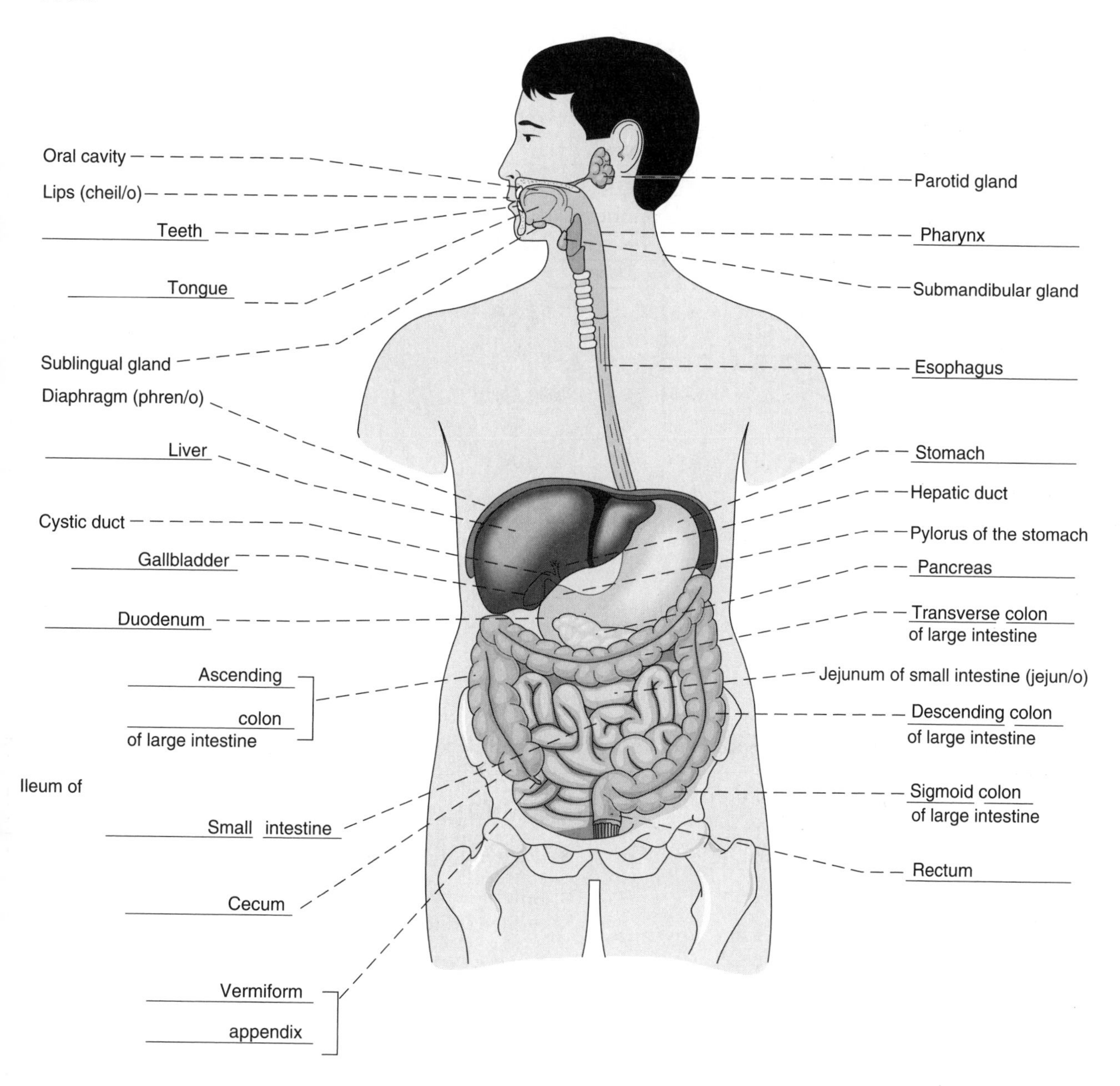


1. Ascending colon
2. Cecum
3. Descending colon
4. Duodenum
5. Esophagus
6. Gallbladder
7. Liver
8. Pancreas
9. Pharynx
10. Rectum
11. Sigmoid colon
12. Small intestine
13. Stomach
14. Teeth
15. Tongue
16. Transverse colon
17. Vermiform appendix

3. Label the illustration using the following terms. Refer to Figure 32–7 in the textbook.

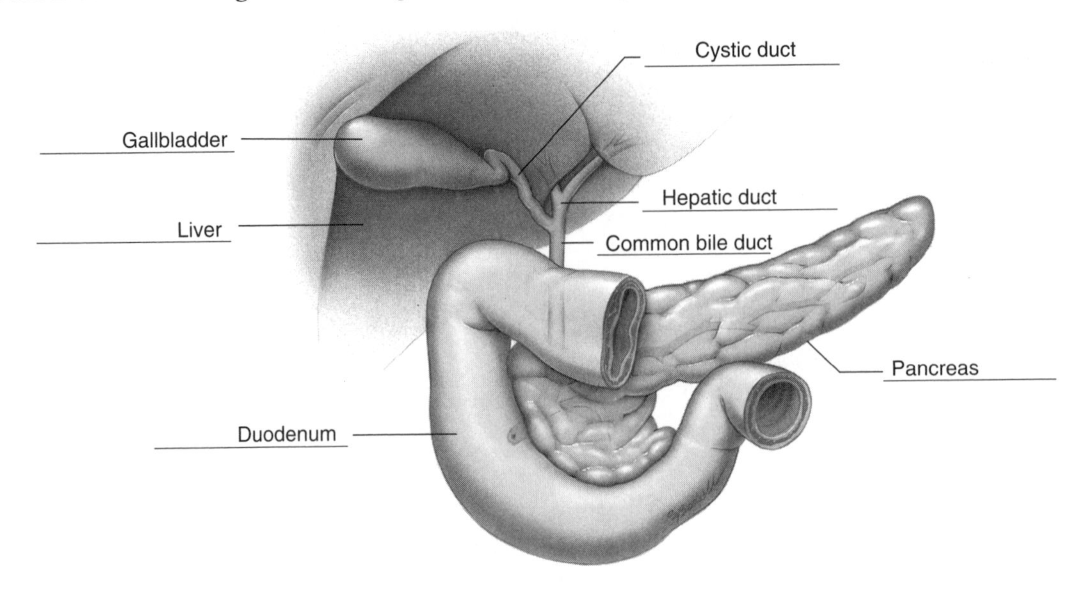


1. Common bile duct
2. Cystic duct
3. Duodenum
4. Gallbladder
5. Hepatic duct
6. Liver
7. Pancreas

**Matching: Match the disease or conditions in column I with the appropriate symptoms or description in column II.**

| | COLUMN I | COLUMN II |
|---|---|---|
| J | 1. Anorectal abscess or fistula | A. Frequent, liquid stools |
| O | 2. Cirrhosis | B. Enlarged spleen, ascites, bloody emesis and stools, reduced platelets |
| E | 3. Colitis | C. Dilated anal veins, painful defecation, bleeding |
| Q | 4. Colostomy | D. Protruding mass at inguinal area or loop of intestine in scrotum |
| A | 5. Diarrhea | E. Tenderness and discomfort of the colon |
| T | 6. Diverticulitis | F. Jaundice, hepatomegaly, loss of appetite, fatigue, clay-colored stools, weight loss |
| B | 7. Esophageal varices | G. Absence of peristalsis, abdominal distention, distress, vomiting |
| U | 8. Anal fissure | H. Severe epigastric pain, not relieved by vomiting; a rigid abdomen, rales, tachycardia, fever, cold, perspiring extremities |
| K | 9. Gastroenteritis | I. Asymptomatic growths protruding from the intestinal lining |
| C | 10. Hemorrhoids | J. Painful, throbbing lump near the anus, with or without drainage |
| F | 11. Hepatitis | K. Fever, nausea and vomiting, abdominal cramps, travelers' diarrhea |

V 12. Hiatal hernia

D 13. Inguinal hernia

S 14. Ileostomy

H 15. Pancreatitis

G 16. Paralytic ileus

R 17. Peptic ulcer

I 18. Polyps

N 19. Pruritus ani

K 20. Pyloric stenosis

P 21. Spastic colon

M 22. Ulcerative colitis

L. Forceful vomiting, dilation of stomach, difficulty emptying contents of stomach into duodenum

M. Recurrent bloody diarrhea with mucus and exudate, weight loss, weakness, anorexia, nausea, vomiting, abdominal pain

N. Itching of anal area, especially following bowel movement, reddened skin, weeping and thickened skin, darkening of tissue

O. Lack of appetite, indigestion, nausea, vomiting, nosebleeds, bleeding gums, enlarged and firm liver, jaundice, ascites

P. Alternating periods of constipation and diarrhea, lower abdominal pain, daytime diarrhea, mucus stools

Q. A single or double opening on the abdomen through which solid fecal material passes

R. Heartburn, epigastric pain relieved by food, weight gain, bubbling hot water sensation

S. Opening of small intestine into the abdomen through which liquid stool is expelled

T. Bulging pouches in the intestine that cause abdominal pain, nausea, flatus, irregular bowel movements, high white blood cell count

U. Burning rectal pain with a few drops of blood with passing of stool, sentinel pile

V. Heartburn, regurgitation, vomiting, fullness, stomach spasms, difficulty swallowing, gastric reflux

# Chapter Application

## Case Studies with Critical Thinking Questions

### Scenario 1

A male patient called to schedule an appointment. He is complaining about what he thinks is an ulcer. Almost every time he eats he gets a feeling of indigestion and discomfort. He usually has heartburn and sometimes brings food up into his throat. The doctor is away on vacation for the next 10 days and you cannot schedule an appointment.

1. How would you decide if this situation is an emergency? Since it occurs after eating, it appears it is due to that activity. You must always be certain to question for any additional symptoms to rule out a possible heart attack.
2. Should he be offered an alternative physician since his current physician is away? Tell him what you think is causing his problems and offer to get him an appointment with another physician. If he elects to wait until the doctor returns, schedule him as soon as an appointment is available.

## Scenario 2

Your neighbor tells you her 14-year-old daughter has not felt well for the past couple days. The neighbor explains that her daughter first had a general discomfort in her abdomen, but then it became more severe and seemed to be located just below her umbilicus on her right side. She was nauseated and couldn't eat. She also had a slight fever. However, she had a good night sleep and the pain has gone away; she is feeling better today. The mother thinks she probably ate something that didn't agree with her.

1. Why do you think she should she be advised to have the daughter examined? Since it sounds like her daughter may have appendicitis that may have now ruptured, she should be seen just to be certain.
2. What else could be causing her symptoms? These symptoms may also be a sign of an ovarian problem. It is important that a physician determines the cause of her pain. A simple blood count will help determine her condition, as will an abdominal examination.
3. What are the possible complications that could develop if nothing is done? When an appendix ruptures, it releases exudate into the abdominal cavity, which can cause a dangerous infection called peritonitis. The patient always feels better at first but then becomes seriously ill.

## Research Activity

The incidence of GERD is very common. Go online to http://digestive.niddk.nih.gov/ddiseases/pubs/gerd to read the article and find the answers to the following questions.

1. What is GERD?
2. What are the symptoms?
3. What causes GERD?
4. How is GERD treated?
5. What if GERD symptoms persist?
6. What are the long term complications of GERD?
7. What is Barrett's esophagus?

CHAPTER 33

# The Urinary System

## Words to Know Challenge

**Spelling: Each line contains three spellings of a word. Underline the correctly spelled word.**

| | | |
|---|---|---|
| 1. noturia | nocturea | nocturia |
| 2. oliguria | oligurea | olliguria |
| 3. pollyurea | polyurea | polyuria |
| 4. calyces | calcyces | callcyces |
| 5. ptosis | tosis | phtosis |
| 6. dialasis | dialysis | dilyasis |
| 7. sectretion | secreton | secretion |
| 8. lithotripsy | lithatripsy | lithotrypsy |
| 9. unuria | auria | anuria |
| 10. glommerulus | glomerulus | glomurelus |

**Matching: Match the term in column I with its description in column II.**

| COLUMN I | COLUMN II |
|---|---|
| D 1. Cystitis | A. Urgency, dysuria, nocturia, hematuria, ammoniac or fishy odor to urine, high fever, chills, flank pain, fatigue |
| H 2. Glomerulonephritis | B. Small stream of urine, prolonged urination time |
| F 3. Nephrotic syndrome | C. Oliguria, azotemia, severe electrolyte imbalance, acidosis, uremia, other body system involvement |
| I 4. Polycystic kidney disease | D. Frequency, dysuria, bladder spasms, sharp stabbing pain upon urination |
| A 5. Pyelonephritis | E. Severe pain beginning in kidney, moving to groin area, nausea, vomiting, chills, and fever |
| C 6. Renal failure | F. Generalized dependent edema, pleural effusion, ascites, lethargy, fatigue, pallor, swollen external sexual organs |

(continues)

| | | |
|---|---|---|
| B | 7. Stricture | G. Urine products in the blood, coma, toxic waste levels in blood, eventual death |
| E | 8. Calculi | H. Moderate edema, proteinuria, hematuria, oliguria, fatigue, urinary casts, hypertension |
| G | 9. Uremia | I. Pointed nose, small chin, floppy low-set ears, inner eyelid folds, eventually widened body, swollen, tender abdomen, life-threatening bleeding, ureteral spasms |

## Chapter Review

### Short Answer

1. List the three main functions of the urinary system, explaining the meaning of each.
   a. Excretion—the removal of waste products and other elements from the blood
   b. Secretion—the production of urine
   c. Elimination—the emptying of urine from the bladder
2. Identify the organs of the urinary system; describe their physical characteristics.
   a. Kidneys—shaped like a kidney bean, 4 1/2 inches long, 2 to 3 inches wide, and about 1 inch thick. They are covered with a fibrous capsule and have a notch called a hilum on the concave border
   b. Ureters—muscular tubes 10 to 12 inches long, extending from the kidneys to the urinary bladder. They widen at the top to join the renal pelvis
   c. Bladder—a collapsable muscular bag lined with a membrane of many folds that allows for expansion. The bladder can hold approximately 1000 cc, but 250 cc cause an urge to void
   d. Urethra—a tube leading from the bladder to the urinary meatus. It is about 1 1/2 inches long in the female and 8 inches long in the male
3. How does the urinary system work with the other body systems to accomplish its job? Food and water are taken into the digestive system, absorbed into the circulatory system, and delivered to the kidneys of the urinary system to be filtered. The urine moves through the ureters by muscular system peristalsis. The nervous system and muscular system cooperate to control elimination. The respiratory and urinary systems cooperate to balance the body's acid–base ratio to control fluid elimination. Endocrine system hormones influence kidney function and the integumentary system works closely with the urinary system in the elimination or retention of body fluid
4. How is the interior of the kidney constructed? It is divided into two sections: an outer layer, the cortex and an inner section, the medulla. The medulla is sectioned into triangular wedges called renal pyramids which empty into the cavities called calyces. The pyramids appear to be striped but the cortex is smooth
5. List the parts of the nephron and describe the function of each part.
   a. Bowman's capsule—surrounds the glomerulus
   b. Glomerulus—filters fluid and other useful substances out of the blood into the Bowman's capsule
   c. Proximal tubule—reabsorbs 80% of the water filtered out plus other substances in relation to the body's needs
   d. Distal tubule—final reabsorption of 10% to 15% of the water according to need
6. Describe kidney dialysis, and identify two major methods. Dialysis is a mechanical process of removing waste products from the blood. The process utilizes a thin, membranous sac and brings blood in contact with one side while a solution circulates on the other. The concentrated waste products in the blood pass through the membrane into the dilute solution on the other side, thereby "filtering" the blood. This typ

of dialysis is called hemodialysis. Another type is known as peritoneal dialysis. With this type, the solution is placed into the peritoneal cavity for approximately six hours and is then drained off. The concentrated waste products in the capillaries within the peritoneal cavity leave the blood and enter the solution to be drained off and discarded.

7. What are the two main categories of diagnostic examinations? Give one example of each type. Noninvasive and invasive. Types of noninvasive tests are intake/ouput, 24-hour specimen, and KUB. Examples of invasive tests are catheterization, IVP, cysourethroscopy, and retrograde ureterpyelography.

8. Name the three types of incontinence.
   a. Stress
   b. Overflow
   c. Urge

9. Name four methods for connecting a patient to hemodialysis.
   a. Intravenous catheter
   b. Arteriovenous fistula
   c. Synthetic graft
   d. Permacath

10. Identify the types of peritoneal dialysis.
    a. Continuous peritoneal
    b. Continuous cycler-assisted peritoneal dialysis
    c. Nocturnal intermittent peritoneal dialysis

## Labeling

1. Label the illustration of the urinary system using the following terms. Refer to Figure 33–1 in the textbook.
   Aorta
   Inferior vena cava
   Hilum
   Left kidney
   Left ureter
   Right kidney
   Urethra
   Urinary bladder

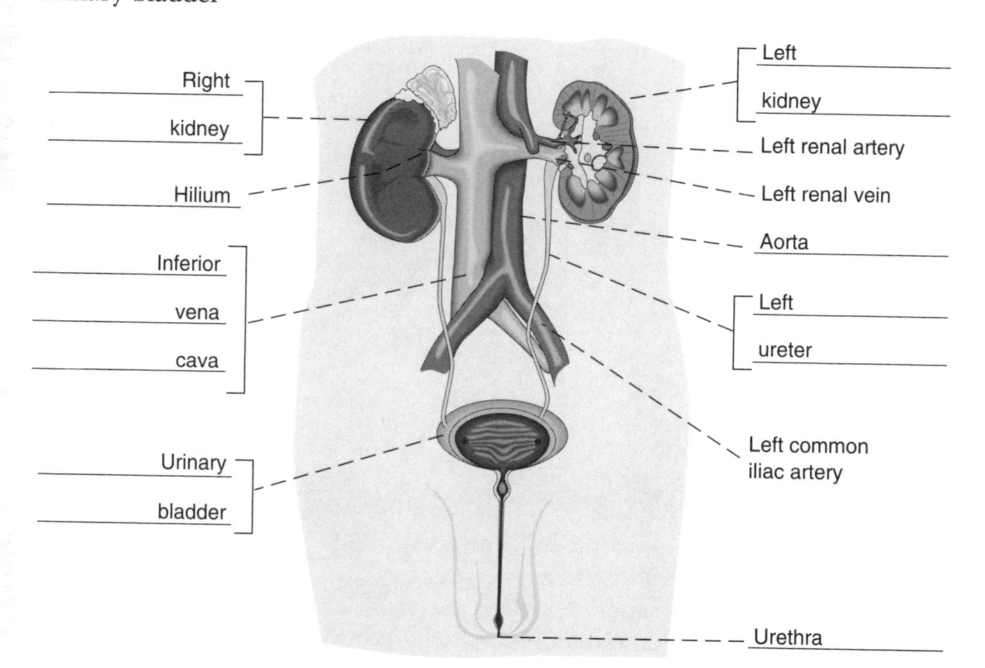

2. Label the illustration of the interior of the kidney with the following terms. Refer to Figure 33–2 in the textbook.
   Cortex
   Hilum
   Medulla
   Renal papilla
   Renal pelvis
   Renal pyramid
   Ureter

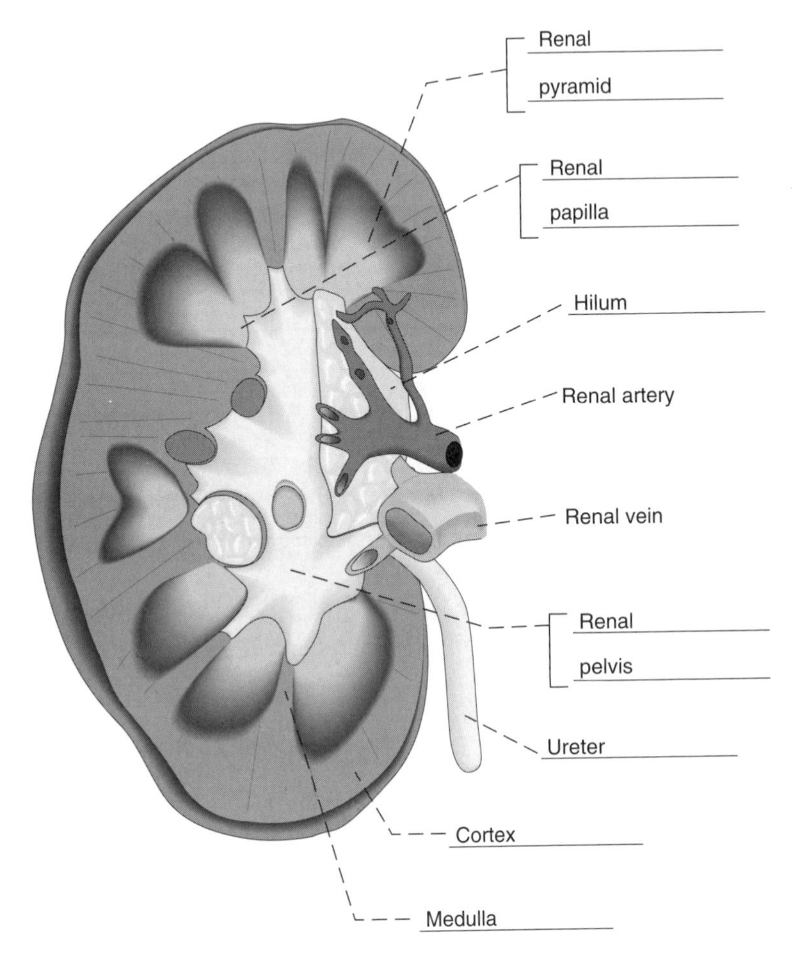

3. Label the illustration of a glomerulus using the following terms. Refer to Figure 33–3 in the textbook.
   Afferent arteriole
   Ascending limb-loop of Henle
   Bowman's capsule
   Collecting tubule
   Descending limb-loop of Henle
   Distal convoluted tubule
   Efferent arteriole
   Glomerulus
   Peritubular capillaries
   Proximal convoluted tubule

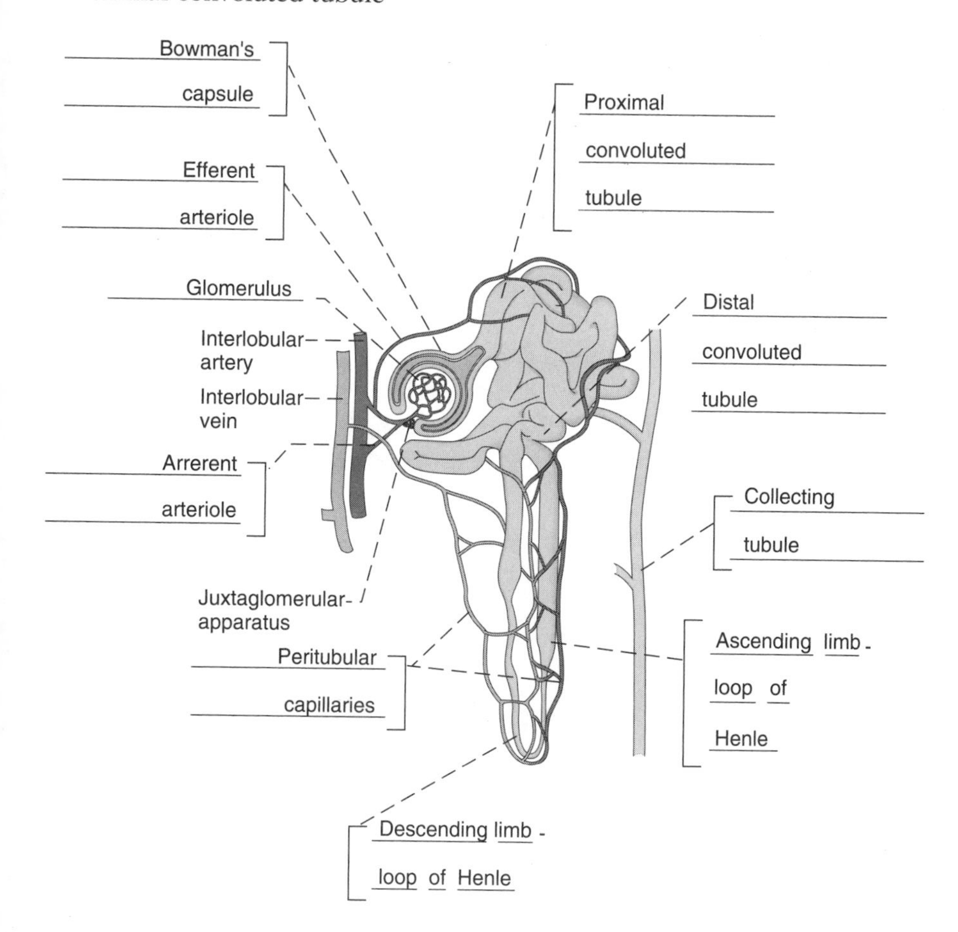


# Chapter Application

## Case Study with Critical Thinking Questions

A female patient calls to find out whether if she is experiencing a reaction to a cystoscopic examination three days ago. She has started going to the bathroom frequently, and now it is beginning to be painful. She thinks it looks like there might be a little blood in her urine. She wonders if this is common.

1. What other symptoms would you ask her if she is experiencing? Question her for other symptoms such as nausea, vomiting, and pain other than when voiding to rule out a kidney stone.

2. Why should you ask if she has done anything to treat herself? Find out if she has taken any OTC medication for urinary pain or if she has been drinking cranberry juice, both of which will give her relief fairly quickly but will not treat the cause of the infection.

CHAPTER 34

# The Endocrine System

## Words to Know Challenge

**Spelling: Each line contains three spellings of a word. Underline the correctly spelled word.**

| | | |
|---|---|---|
| 1. acromegaly | acromegally | acromegly |
| 2. adranelline | adrenelline | adrenaline |
| 3. cretanism | creatinism | cretinism |
| 4. estergen | estrogen | estragen |
| 5. goyter | goiter | goitar |
| 6. pineal | pinal | pineel |
| 7. pitutiary | pituitery | pituitary |
| 8. tetany | tettany | tateny |
| 9. thymuss | thymus | thyamus |

**Matching: Match the terms in column I with their definitions in column II.**

| | COLUMN I | COLUMN II |
|---|---|---|
| G | 1. Ovary | A. An internal secretion derived from the adrenal glands; can be commercially prepared from animal glands; acts as a stimulant |
| F | 2. Hypoglycemia | B. A metabolic disease caused by the body's inability to utilize carbohydrates |
| J | 3. Testosterone | C. A female hormone produced by the ovaries |
| H | 4. Progesterone | D. The sex organ/glands |
| I | 5. Testes | E. A chemical substance secreted by a gland or organ |
| B | 6. Diabetes mellitus | F. Deficiency of sugar in the blood |
| A | 7. Adrenaline | G. The female gonad that produces hormones causing secondary sexual characteristics to develop and be maintained |

(continues)

D 8. Gonad

E 9. Hormone

C 10. Estrogen

H. A hormone secreted by the Graafian follicle following the expulsion of the ovum

I. Male gonad that produces sperm and secretes testosterone

J. A male hormone that causes and maintains secondary sex characteristics

## Chapter Review

### Short Answer

1. Explain the difference between an exocrine gland and an endocrine gland, giving an example of each. Exocrine glands secrete substances through ducts into the body. An example is the liver excreting bile. Endocrine glands secrete substances directly into the capillaries of the circulatory system. An example is the pancreas secreting insulin.

2. What types of body functions are affected by hormones?
   a. Growth
   b. Development
   c. Metabolism
   d. Bone and blood composition
   e. Sexual maturity
   f. Endocrine gland functions

3. List the nine glands discussed in the unit, identifying the location of each gland.
   a. Pituitary—the undersurface of the brain in the sella tursica of the sphenoid bone
   b. Thyroid—the neck on each side of the larynx
   c. Parathyroid—posterior surface of the thyroid gland
   d. Adrenals—superior surface of each kidney
   e. Pancreas—behind the stomach, with its head in the curve of the duodenum
   f. Thymus—under the sternum
   g. Pineal body—roof of the third ventricle of the brain
   h. Testes—in the scrotum of the male
   i. Ovaries—in the pelvic cavity of the female, one on each side of the uterus.

4. Identify the hormones secreted by the gonads and the functions of each. Testes secrete testosterone, which causes primary and secondary male characteristics to develop. Ovaries secrete estrogen to promote primary and secondary female characteristics to develop. Progesterone affects the uterus lining and breasts.

5. What hormone secretion abnormality causes the following conditions?
   a. Giantism/Gigantism Excess pituitary growth hormone during childhood
   b. Dwarfism Insufficient pituitary growth hormone during childhood
   c. Acromegaly Excess pituitary growth hormone from the pituitary in adulthood
   d. Goiter Excess thyroid-stimulating hormone from the pituitary
   e. Tetany Lack of parathyroid
   f. Diabetes Lack of insulin production or utilization
   g. Cretinism Extreme lack of thyroxin during early development
   h. Cushing's syndrome Excess secretion of ACTH, which causes excess secretion of glucocorticords
   i. Myxedema Lack of thyroid secretions during adulthood

6. What diagnostic examinations are used to confirm the following conditions?
   a. Diabetes Blood sugar, FBS, glucose tolerance
   b. Thyroid dysfunction T3 and T4 levels, TSH
   c. Pregnancy Urine test for HCG
   d. Cushing's syndrome ACTH, cortisol levels in the blood

7. List the symptoms and characteristics in the following conditions or diseases.
   a. Cushing's syndrome Hypertensive, obese, muscle weakness, bruising, deposits of body fat between shoulders, moon face, obese trunk with slender extremities.

b. Diabetes mellitus Fatigue, hyperglycemia, polyuria, dehydration, thirst, glycosuria, weight loss, and hunger

c. Myxedema Forgetfulness, dry skin, intolerance to cold, noticeable weight gain, slowed actions, low, husky voice, carotenemia, edema, drowsy appearance, puffy eyes

8. What role does insulin play in the blood?
   a. Carries sugar into the cell for fuel
   b. Stimulates the formation of proteins and free fatty acid storage

9. Identify the six body systems that interact with diabetes and give an example of the pathology that might be present.

| | |
|---|---|
| a. Endocrine | Insulin deficiency |
| b. Urinary | Glycosuria (polyuria, UTI, kidney disease) |
| c. Circulatory | Elevated triglycerides (stroke, heart disease) |
| d. Senses | Retinopathy (lens changes) |
| e. Integumentary | Ulcers (skin infections) |
| f. Nervous | Peripheral neuropathy |

## Fill in the Blank: Use information from the chapter to fill in the blank space in the sentence.

1. Type 2 diabetes usually begins because of insulin resistance.
2. With diabetes, the body's cells resist both insulin and blood sugar.
3. Insulin resistance can also result from genetics, aging, and some medications, but being overweight and a lack of exercise are the main nongenetic factors.

## Labeling

Identify the endocrine glands on the following illustration. Refer to Figure 34–2.

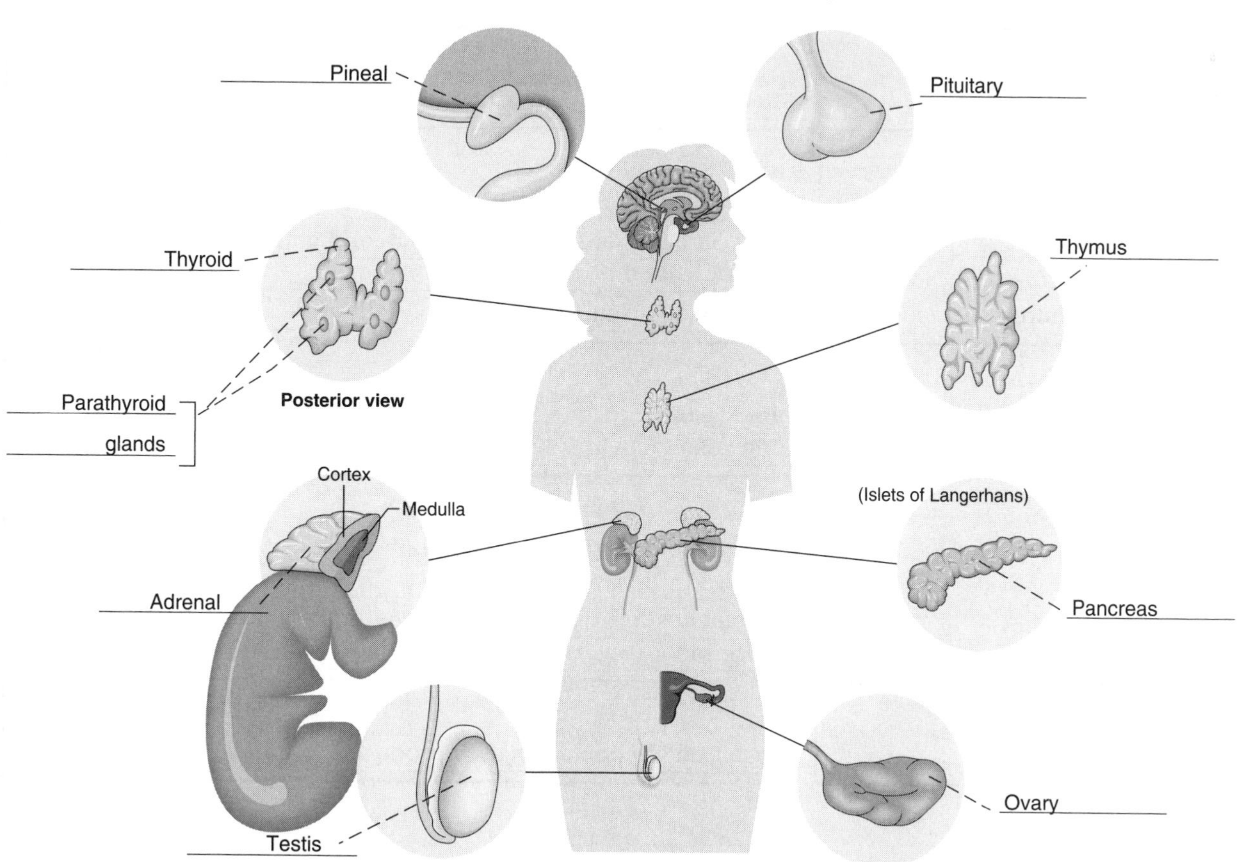

**Design a Table: Briefly identify the function(s) of the hormones from the following glands. (This will help you realize how the glands regulate the body. Many modern drugs stimulate or mimic hormones to affect body function.) Refer to Table 34–1.**

| Glands | Function |
|---|---|
| Pituitary: Anterior Lobe | |
| a. GH | a. Natural growth of tissues |
| b. TSH | b. Stimulates thyroid cells to produce and secrete thyroid hormone |
| c. ACTH | c. Stimulates adrenal gland cortex and secretion of cortisol |
| d. MSH | d. Increases skin pigmentation |
| e. FSH | e. Maturation of Graafian follicle and production of estrogen in female, as well as development of testes and production of in males |
| f. LH | f. Causes corpus luteum development and secretion of progesterone in female and causes ICSH to stimulate interstitial cells to produce testosterone in males. |
| g. PR | g. Develops breast tissue and stimulates milk secretion |
| Pituitary: Posterior Lobe | |
| a. Oxytocin | a. Contraction of uterus during childbirth and ejection of milk |
| b. ADH | b. Acts on kidney tubules to concentrate urine, conserve body fluid, and constrict blood vessels |
| Thyroid | |
| a. T4 and T3 | a. Increase metabolism; influence physical and mental activity |
| b. Throcalcitonin | b. Causes the storage of calcium in bones; reduces level of calcium in blood |
| Parathyroid | |
| a. Parathormone | a. Regulates exchange of calcium between bone and blood |
| Adrenal Cortex | |
| a. Aldosterone | a. Controls electrolyte balance of sodium and potassium |
| b. Glucocorticoids | b. Affects metabolism of protein, fat, and glucose and decreases inflammation |
| c. Sex steroids (Androgens) | c. Govern sex characteristics, especially male |
| Medulla | |
| a. Adrenaline | a. Increases heart rate, blood pressure, and blood flow; decreases intestinal activity |
| Pancreas | |
| a. Insulin | a. Essential to metabolism of carbohydrates; reduces blood sugar level |
| b. Glucagon | b. Stimulates liver to release glycogen to be converted to glucose to raise blood sugar levels |
| Thymus | |
| a. Peptides | a. React on lymphoid tissue to produce T cells |

# Chapter Application

## Case Studies with Critical Thinking Questions

### Scenario 1

A new patient calls to see when he can get an appointment. His chief complaints are that he has no energy and that he is always thirsty, which of course causes him to drink a lot, which in turn causes him to make frequent visits to the bathroom. He says it is interfering with his sleep, which is why he thinks he is so tired. He is 65 years old, so he thinks he is just having prostate problems, which could be also causing the urinary problems. He says he can wait a while for an appointment; he doesn't think it is anything serious.

1. Why do you need to determine when his symptoms began? Insidious or sudden onset helps to rule out a condition. Determine if he has other symptoms that might indicate prostate problems, such as difficulty starting a stream or a prolonged urination time.
2. Why would a family history of diabetes be important to know? Since his symptoms could indicate diabetes, determine if anyone in his family has the disease, as it tends to occur in families.
3. Why should you determine if he has ever had a problem with bleeding excessively when injured or with a dental or surgical procedure? To rule out internal bleeding, which causes thirst and weakness.

### Scenario 2

You run into an old friend whom you haven't seen in 15 years. After talking for a while, you notice she is very nervous and her eyes seem quite pronounced. She is also a lot thinner than you remember her being. When you ask her how she has been feeling, she says, "Not too great."

1. How could you question her more? You might ask her again how long she's not been feeling well to lead into more questions. You could mention her weight loss and ask if it was intentional. Tell her you are working as a medical assistant and you wonder if she has been to a doctor lately. Express concern over her eyes as a symptom of hyperthyroidism.
2. What makes you think she might have a medical problem? She appears to have symptoms of Graves' disease and may not be aware of it. It takes time to develop and, since it is gradual, she may not realize the change that has occurred. You have not seen her, so the change would be more noticeable to you.

CHAPTER 35

# The Reproductive System

## Words to Know Challenge

**Spelling: Each line contains three spellings of a word. Underline the correctly spelled word.**

| | | |
|---|---|---|
| 1. circumcision | circumsision | circumcisun |
| 2. dysmenorrhea | dismenorehea | dysmenorrea |
| 3. epididimus | epididymis | epididymus |
| 4. genetalia | genitalea | genitalia |
| 5. menapause | menopause | menoplaus |
| 6. menorrhagia | menarrhagia | menorrhagea |
| 7. prostratectomy | prostatectemy | prostatectomy |
| 8. syfhillis | syphillis | syphilis |

**Define the Terms: Define the following diseases or disorders of the female reproductive system.**

a. Abortion The spontaneous or induced loss of a pregnancy

b. Cervical erosion Ulceration of the cervical epithelium

c. Cervicitis Inflammation of the cervix by an organism

d. Cystic breast disease Presence of lumps within the breast tissue

e. Cystocele The bulging of the anterior vaginal wall and bladder into the vagina

f. Dysmenorrhea Lower abdominal and pelvic pain associated with menstruation

g. Endometriosis Presence of endometrial tissue outside the uterus

h. Fibroids Benign, smooth tumors formed by muscle cells of the uterus

i. Hysterectomy Surgical removal of the uterus

j. Malignancy of the breast Cancer of the breast

k. Ovarian cyst A sac of fluid or semisolid material on an ovary

l. PMS Prementrual syndrome; a combination of characteristics preceding menstruation

m. Polyp A growth attached by a slender stem to the membrane

n. Rectocele Bulging of the posterior vaginal wall and rectum into the vagina

## Chapter Review

### Short Answer

1. What is the difference between asexual and sexual reproduction? Asexual reproduction means the organism reproduces by simply dividing into two cells. Sexual reproduction requires a male and a female cell to unite into one single cell.
2. Explain the process of differentiation of the reproductive organs; compare the male organ to the female organ. Differentiation refers to the development of male and female sexual organs from the same embryonic tissue. The presence of androgens and a müllerian inhibitor is believed to cause male differentiation. In the embryo, the gonad tissue develops into the sexual organs. The medulla of the gonad develops into testes while the cortex becomes ovaries. The tubercle becomes the glans penis or the clitoris. The folds become the penile shaft or the labia minora. The swelling develops into the scrotum or the labia majora. The müllerian ducts become the fallopian tubes, uterus, and part of the vagina. The wolffian ducts become the epididymis, vas deferens, and ejaculatory duct.
3. How is sperm able to fertilize an egg? It attacks the corona radiata, releasing hyaluronidase, which breaks down the protection enough that one sperm can enter the ovum.
4. List the nine male sex organs or structures and describe their function.
   a. Testes—Produce sperm and testosterone
   b. Epididymis—Mature the sperm and secrete fluid as part of the ejaculant
   c. Vas deferens—Passageway for sperm
   d. Seminal vesicles—Secrete a fluid with sucrose to provide nutrition for the sperm and to add volume to the ejaculant
   e. Ejaculatory duct—Passageway for sperm
   f. Prostate—Secretes prostatic liquid to stimulate sperm motility and to preserve their life by adding alkaline to the ejaculant: also serves to empty semen into the urethra
   g. Bulbourethral glands—Secrete fluid to aid in sperm motility and make the urethra alkaline. The secretion may also aid in lubrication
   h. Urethra—Passageway for sperm and urine
   i. Penis—Organ of sexual intercourse and urinary excretion
5. How do pituitary hormones affect the function of the testes? The anterior pituitary gland releases the gonad-stimulating hormone, which causes a change in the testes. The FSH causes sperm to develop. The ICSH causes the interstitial cells to secrete testosterone.
6. List the secondary male sex characteristics.
   a. Longer, heavier bone structure
   b. Larger muscles
   c. Deep voice
   d. Growth of body hair
   e. Development of external genitalia
   f. Increased metabolism
   g. Sexual desire

7. List, in order, the structures through which sperm pass.
   a. Develop and mature in the seminiferous tubules of the testicles
   b. Epididymis
   c. Vas deferens
   d. Ejaculatory duct
   e. Urethra

8. What is the composition of semen?
   a. 5% fluids from the testes and epididymis
   b. 30% fluids from the seminal vesicles
   c. 60% fluids from the prostate
   d. 5% fluids from the bulbourethral glands

9. List the four diseases and disorders of the male reproductive system; define the condition and identify the main symptoms and/or cause of the condition.
   a. Epididymitis—Infection of the epididymis caused by strep, staph, trauma, or gonorrhea; produces severe pain, swelling in the groin and scrotum, fever, and a characteristic waddle.
   b. Hydrocele—The presence of an excessive amount of the normal fluid within the scrotum. Enlarged scrotum and discomfort. Caused by injury, inflammation, or naturally as an aging process.
   c. Erectile dysfunction—The inability to have or sustain an erection to complete sexual intercourse due to stress, organic dysfunction from chronic illness, alcohol, or drug therapies. May be caused by anxiety, fear of failure, depression, parental rejection, and previous traumatic sexual experience.
   d. Prostatic hypertrophy—Enlargement of the prostate gland caused by a change in hormonal activity. It results in reduced force and size of urine stream, dribbling, nocturia, a feeling of incomplete voiding, frequency, and eventually hematuria and retention.

10. List the eight female sexual structures and describe their function.
    a. Ovaries—Produce ova and secrete the hormones estrogen and progesterone
    b. Fallopian tubes—Serve as passageway for ova to uterus; is the usual location of fertilization
    c. Uterus—Serves as the place for the embryo to develop into an infant
    d. Vagina—Serves as passageway for menstrual flow, birth canal, and organ of sexual intercourse
    e. Vulva—No function given
    f. Clitoris—Provides heightened sexual excitement and orgasmic response
    g. Perineum—No function given
    h. Mammary glands—Provide milk for infant

11. How do hormones from the pituitary gland affect the development of the female reproductive organs? The pituitary sends out hormones that cause the ovaries to begin to release estrogen. Estrogen affects the development of the sexual organs and produces secondary sexual characteristics.

12. List the female secondary sex characteristics.
    a. Broadening of the pelvis
    b. Epiphysis becomes bone and growth ceases
    c. Soft, smooth skin develops
    d. Pubic hair
    e. Breasts develop
    f. Deposits of fat in buttocks and thighs
    g. Sexual desire
    h. Ovulation
    i. Menstruation

13. List the four phases of the menstrual cycle.
    a. Follicular
    b. Ovulation
    c. Luteal
    d. Menstruation
14. Describe the fertilization of an ovum. The sperm travel from the vagina through the uterus to the outer third of the fallopian tube, where the ovum is met. The sperm attack the protective corona radiata of the ovum, releasing an enzyme called hyaluronidase, which gradually breaks down the protection. One sperm will enter the exposed area and fertilize the ovum. The membrane of the ovum immediately seals to prevent additional sperm from entering.
15. List the usual signs and symptoms of early pregnancy.
    a. Missed menstrual period
    b. Breast tenderness
    c. Morning sickness
    d. Frequent urination
    e. Fatigue
    f. Need for additional sleep
16. List symptoms that occur later in pregnancy.
    a. Depression
    b. Fatigue
    c. Edema of hands, face, feet, and legs
    d. Constipation
    e. Urinary frequency
    f. Shortness of breath
    g. Indigestion
    h. Hemorrhoids
17. Describe the characteristics of the three stages of labor.
    First
    a. Regular uterine contractions
    b. Cervical dilation and effacement
    Second
    a. Complete dilation
    b. Head or other part enters vagina
    c. Crowning
    d. Delivery
    Third
    a. Placenta detaches
    b. Afterbirth expelled
18. List eight reasons to use contraceptives.
    a. To avoid health risks for the woman
    b. To space pregnancies
    c. To avoid babies with birth defects
    d. To delay pregnancy early in marriage
    e. To limit family size
    f. To avoid pregnancy among unmarried couples
    g. To develop career
    h. To curb population growth

19. List seven routine screening and diagnostic pregnancy tests. Blood typing, antibody screening, STD screening, urine cultures, amniocentesis, chorionic villa sampling, gestational diabetes, and group B streptococcus.

20. Name 14 methods of contraception.

a. Abstinence
b. Sterilization
c. DMPA
d. Lunelle injection
e. Birth control pills
f. IUD
g. Diaphragm
h. Male condom
i. Cervical cap
j. Female condom
k. Spermicides
l. Douching
m. Withdrawal
n. Rhythm

21. Identify the main characteristics of each of the following disease conditions.

a. Chlamydia Men experience burning while urinating and have a mucoid discharge. Women have a vaginal discharge and often dysuria. If left untreated, causes inflammation and scarring of the fallopian tubes.

b. Gonorrhea Men experience burning, itching, and pain during urination; drainage from penis or anus; swollen glands; and a sore throat. Females experience asymptomatic greenish-yellow cervical discharge, sore throat, anal discharge, and swollen glands.

c. Herpes Fluid filled vesicles on the cervix, labia, vulva, or perianal skin of the female and on the glans, foreskin, or penile shaft of the male.

d. NGU In males, urethral inflammation; in females, vaginitis and burning on urination, itching.

e. PID Pelvic inflammatory disease causes purulent vaginal discharge, fever, and malaise. There is lower abdominal pain with severe pain upon manipulation of the cervix and adjoining structures. Pelvic abscesses may develop.

f. Syphilis (four stages)
(1) Primary—Chancre lesion on female cervix or labia or on male penis or scrotum
(2) Secondary—Feneralized, painless, non-itching rash; hair loss; sore throat; headache; nausea; loss of appetite; constipation; persistent fever; pain in bones, muscles, and joints
(3) Latent—Asymptomatic but affects various internal organs
(4) Tertiary—Cardiovascular, neurological, or internal organ disease

g. Trichomoniasis Abundant, frothy, white or yellow vaginal discharge that is irritating and has a foul odor

**Matching: Match the test or procedure in column I with its description in column II.**

| | COLUMN I | COLUMN II |
|---|---|---|
| E | 1. Alpha-Fetoprotein Screening | A. Examination with an instrument connected to a monitor to view the endometrium |
| G | 2. Mammograph | B. Determines hormonal level from cells scraped from vaginal walls |
| B | 3. Maturation index | C. High-frequency sound waves that detect and aid in the diagnosis of breast irregularities |
| F | 4. Papanicolaou test | D. A urine specimen test to detect the presence of HCG |
| D | 5. Pregnancy test | E. A blood test to dectect birth defects |
| C | 6. Ultrasonography | F. Examination of cervical secretions for cancer cells |
| H | 7. Colposcopy | G. An X-ray of the breast |
| A | 8. Hysteroscopy | H. An examination of the cervix following a questionable Pap smear |

## Labeling

1. Label the male reproductive system illustration using these terms. Refer to textbook Figure 35–7.

Anal opening
Bulbourethral gland or Cowper's gland
Ejaculatory duct
Epididymis
Membranous urethra
Penis
Prepuce
Prostate gland
Rectum
Scrotum
Seminal vesicle
Spermatic cord
Symphysis pubis
Testis
Vas deferens (two times)
Urethra
Urinary bladder

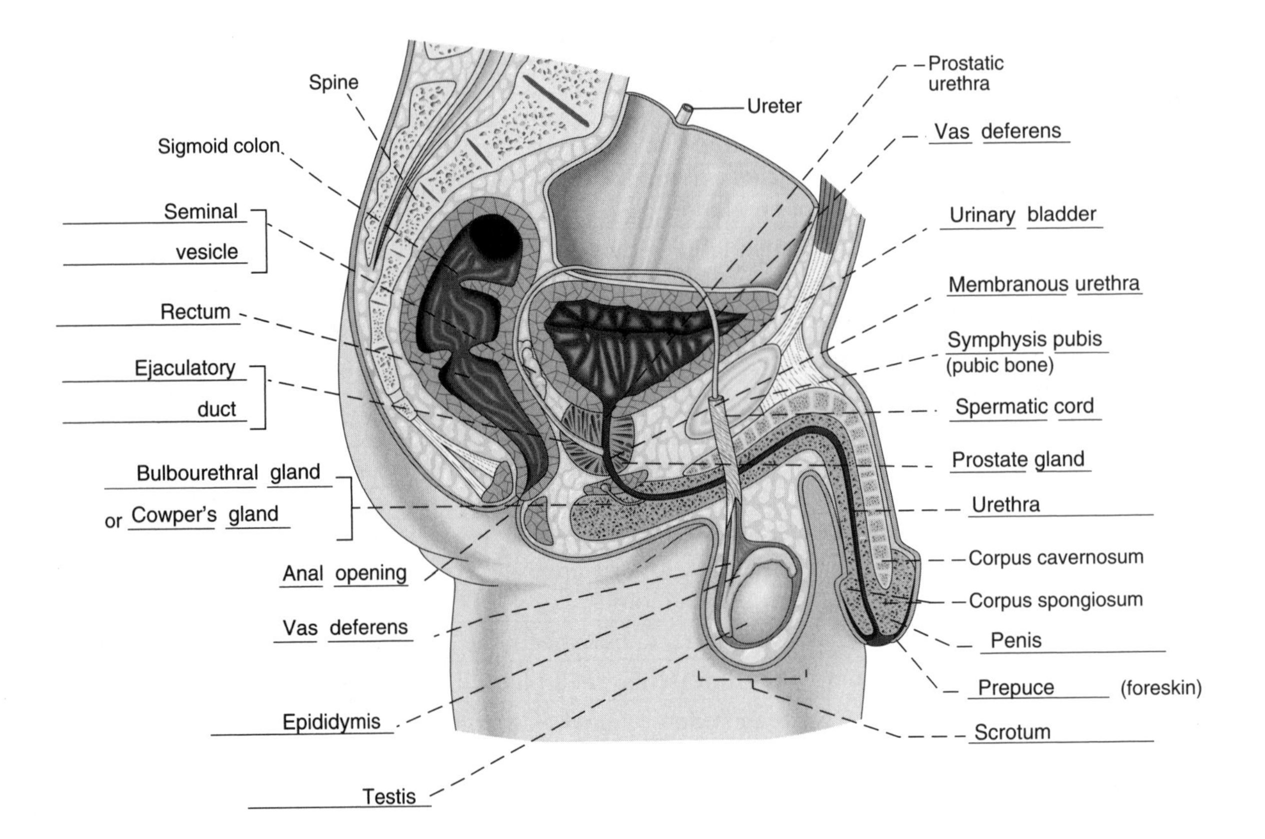

2. Label the female reproductive system illustration using the following terms. Refer to Figure 35–15 in the textbook.

Anus
Cervix
Corpus of uterus
Crus of clitoris
Fallopian tube
Fundus of uterus
Ovary
Symphysis pubis
Ureter
Urethra
Urinary bladder
Vagina

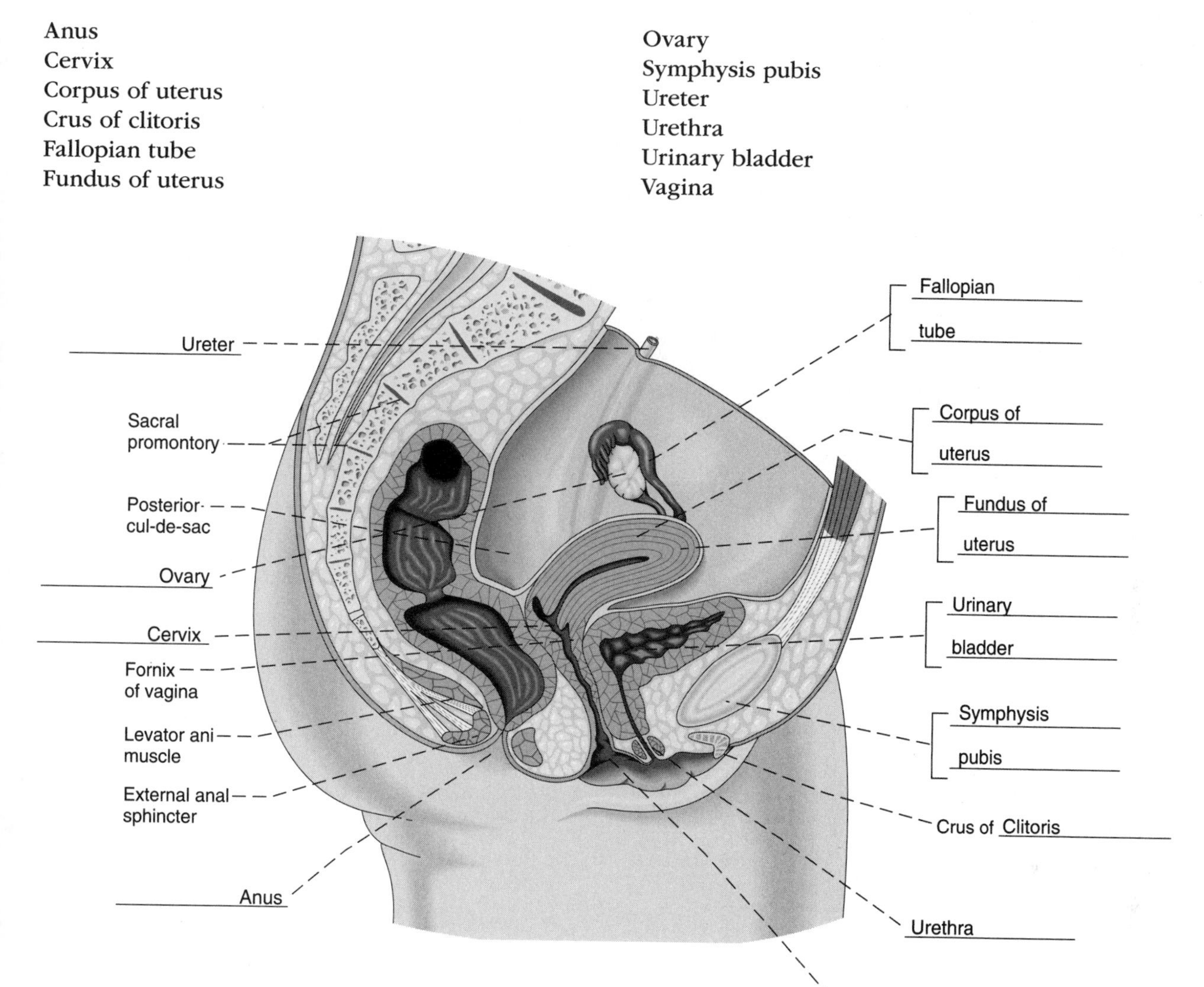

3. Label the external female structures on the illustration using the following terms. Refer to Figure 35–16 in the textbook.

Anus
Clitoris
Hymen
Labia majora
Labia minora
Mons pubis
Perineum
Urethral orifice
Vaginal orifice
Vestibule

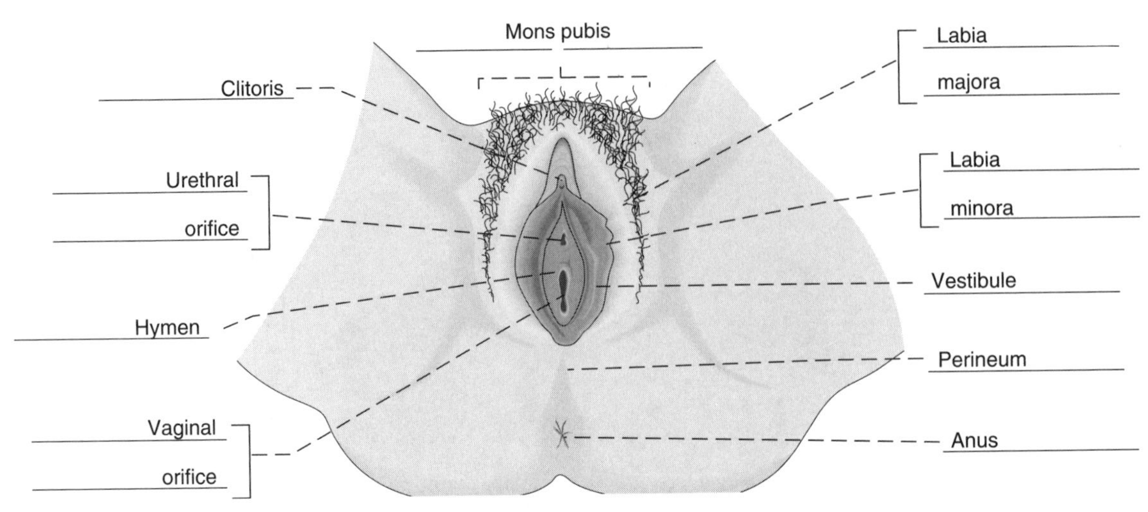


**Fill in the Blank: Use information from the chapter to fill in the blank space in the sentence.**

1. A male infant develops if the zygote contains a Y chromosome.
2. At about the seventh or eighth week, the testes begin to develop within the abdominal cavity.
3. During the eighth or ninth month, the testes move from the abdomen through the inguinal canal into the scrotum.

# Chapter Application

## Case Studies with Critical Thinking Questions

### Scenario 1

A 65-year-old male patient calls the office asking if the doctor would call in a prescription for his kidney infection. He is complaining of frequent urination, getting up at night, and even some dribbling in between. He says about a year ago his younger brother had the same problem.

1. What additional information about symptoms do you need before you talk to the doctor? What he is telling you is not adequate enough to rule out other conditions. Does he have a fever, a backache, any blood in the urine? How long has this been going on? Does he have problems starting a stream, and does it take longer to urinate? You need to explain that his brother may have had something far different than he has, and his condition cannot be diagnosed over the phone. Getting more information will help you to decide how soon he should be seen.
2. Why do you need to tell him the doctor will probably want to see him before he prescribes something? Explain to him that it is not wise to order medication without personally examining him. Often, what you think is the problem turns out to be something else. With the symptoms he is describing, it does not seem like he has an infection.

### Scenario 2

Your 16-year-old daughter tells you that some of the girls at school have been talking about having sex. One of the girls said that she didn't worry about getting any diseases or getting pregnant because she always uses a vinegar douche directly afterward. Your daughter wonders if that really works.

1. Why is it important for you to explain to your daughter the physiology of conception? Because she needs to have the correct information, explain to her that her friend is misinformed and is taking chances. Douching would be the wrong thing to do because the sperm would be assisted into the uterus. Also by the time she can perform the douche, the most mobile sperm will have already entered. Be certain she knows that vinegar will not destroy the organisms that cause sexually transmitted diseases.
2. Why would you discuss your opinions toward sexual behavior? Even if you feel you are "liberal" in your thinking and you realize controlling the desire for sex is difficult, you still may not want your daughter taking such chances. Most 16-year-old girls are not emotionally mature enough to deal with the possibility that boys may view sex as evidence of their "achievement" and often move on to another challenge, leaving the girl devastated. It is important to discuss more than just the physical act. You must especially deal with the dangers of disease transmission. Her partner may not even be aware he has an infection, since it takes time to develop. The more partners, the greater the chance of infection.

## Application Activity

This application deals with pregnancy, something many women experience and share with their friends. Suppose this is your sister's first pregnancy, and she is very excited about the development of the baby. She is constantly asking you questions. She wants to know:

1. When is the formation of the embryo complete? End of the 10th week
2. What is the baby called when it is 2 months old? Fetus
3. When can the baby's sex be determined? After 12 weeks
4. When will she feel movement? After the 20th week
5. How big is the baby at the end of 5 months? About 2 pounds
6. When can you hear its heartbeat? After 20th week

She is amazed when you tell her that at 20 weeks the fetus will open its eyes and by 24 weeks it can hear sounds inside the uterus.

SECTION 4

# The Back Office

UNIT 12

# Preparing for Clinical Procedures

CHAPTER 36

# Infection Control and Medical Asepsis

## Words to Know Challenge

**Spelling: Each line contains three spellings of a word. Underline the correctly spelled word.**

| | | |
|---|---|---|
| 1. obligate | abligate | oblegate |
| 2. susceptable | susseptible | susceptible |
| 3. rickettsiae | ricettsiae | rickettcia |
| 4. anirobes | anaerobes | anerobes |
| 5. pathagens | pathogens | pathegins |
| 6. acepcis | accepses | asepsis |
| 7. exudative | xudative | exudadiv |
| 8. malaize | malaisia | malaise |
| 9. petechial | petikial | patechial |
| 10. higene | hygiene | hyjiene |

**Matching: Match the term in column I to its definition in column II.**

| | COLUMN I | COLUMN II |
|---|---|---|
| E | 1. Bacteria | A. Pressurized device used to sterilize |
| H | 2. Communicable | B. The eggs of a louse or other parasitic insect |
| J | 3. Virus | C. Single-celled animal |
| G | 4. Pruritic | D. Organism or substance that poses a threat to human health |
| B | 5. Nits | E. Unicellular microorganism; disease-causing agent |
| I | 6. Aerobe | F. Involving entry into living tissue |
| D | 7. Biohazardous | G. Pertaining to an itching sensation |
| A | 8. Autoclave | H. Transmitted from one person to another |
| C | 9. Protozoa | I. Lives and grows only in the presence of oxygen |
| F | 10. Invasive | J. Microorganisms capable of replicating within living cells |

### Fill in the Blank

1. Sanitization is the process of washing and scrubbing to remove materials such as body tissue, blood, or other contaminants.
2. The interval between exposure to infection and the appearance of the first symptoms is called the incubation period.
3. You can use the incineration method to destroy contaminated disposable items completely by flame.
4. The Occupational Safety and Health Administration (OSHA) created the mission to prevent work-related injuries, illnesses, and deaths by issuing and enforcing rules (called standards) for workplace safety and health.
5. For an item to have all transmissible agents (such as bacteria and viruses), including their spores, eliminated, sterilization must be performed.
6. Bacterial meningitis can cause an abnormally deep stupor, known as a coma, from which a person cannot be aroused by external stimuli.
7. Sneezing or coughing can cause a droplet infection, which is a disease that results from contamination with water-based microorganisms.
8. Not all microorganisms are pathogenic. Some, known as normal flora, are helpful and necessary in humans and animals because they provide a balance in the body and destroy pathogens.
9. A pathogen is a disease-producing microorganism.
10. Hard capsules known as spores are formed by certain bacteria that enable them to resist prolonged exposure to heat.

## Chapter Review

### Short Answer

1. Name the five common infectious agents (microorganisms) known to man. Bacteria, viruses, fungi, parasites, and rickettsia.
2. What are the growth requirements for microorganisms? Oxygen, proper pH, temperature of 37°C (98.6°F), nutrients, water, and a host to inhabit.
3. Explain the preventive measures for health care professionals against the Hepatitis B virus. Hepatitis B can be prevented by obtaining the Hepatitis B vaccination series.
4. Explain the precautions to be taken when you are exposed to blood and body fluids. Blood and body fluid standard and universal precautions describe the routine wearing of appropriate protection such as gloves, gown or apron, mask, and goggles whenever the health care worker is in direct or indirect contact with blood or any body fluids, mucous membranes, or non-intact skin; is handling soiled items or surfaces; or is performing venipuncture or any other surgical procedure.
5. Why is it vitally important to follow standard and universal precautions? To avoid contamination from patients and to prevent disease transmission.
6. How are used needles, lancets, capillary tubes, glass slides, and other sharp instruments to be handled? They should be handled with extreme caution. Needles should never be recapped, broken off, or removed by hand after use from disposable syringes to prevent self-injury; all sharps products should be placed in a leak-proof, puncture-proof sharps container that is usually red in color and displays the biohazard label.
7. List the five steps in the infectious disease process and give a brief explanation of each. Incubation: period of time between exposure and appearance of first symptoms; Prodromal: appearance of first symptoms; Acute: symptoms fully developed, disease is at its peak; Declining: symptoms subside; Convalescent: body recuperates and returns to original health.

8. Explain the difference between sanitization, disinfection, and sterilization. Sanitization is the process of washing and scrubbing to remove materials such as body tissue, blood, or other body fluids; disinfection is the process by which disease-producing microorganisms or pathogens are killed, using chemical or physical means to destroy the bacteria; and sterilization is the process that destroys all forms of living organisms and their spores.

9. Define medical asepsis. Cleansing techniques, such as hand washing and disinfecting contaminated surfaces, used to destroy microorganisms found in blood or other body fluids after they leave the body.

10. Explain the purpose of using sterilization indicators for autoclaving. Sterilization indicators register proper and complete sterilization.

**Labeling: Label each link in the following chain of infection diagram and give and example of an intervention to break the chain of infection transmission.**

1. Infectious Agent: Cleansing, disinfection, sterilization

2. Reservoir or Source: Proper hygiene, clean supplies, clean equipment, clean linen

3. Portal of Exit from Reservoir or Source: Sterile dressing over wounds, isolation technique, covering mouth and nose when coughing or sneezing

4. Means of Transmission: Hand washing; proper disposal of contaminated objects; medical or surgical asepsis; wearing gloves, masks, gowns, goggles

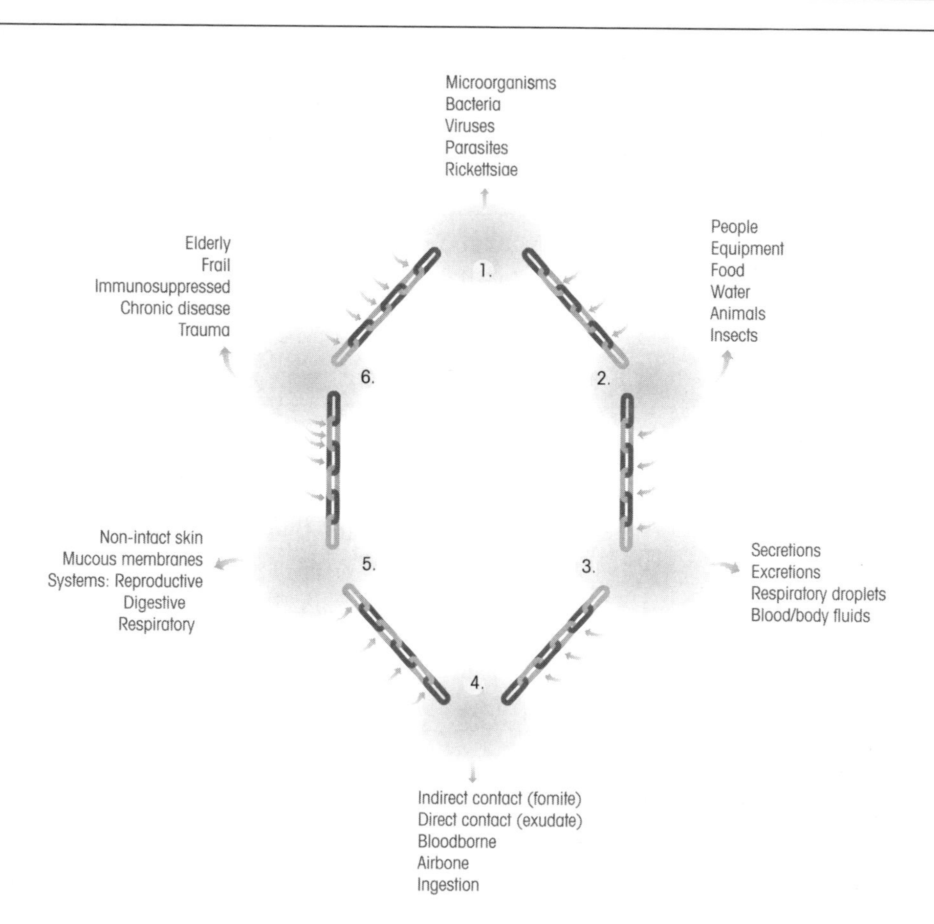


(continues)

5. Portal of Entry to Host: Proper disposal of needles or sharps, sterile technique, hand washing, PPE, skin integrity, covered wound

6. Susceptible Host: Healthy lifestyle, intact immune system, exercise, immunization, proper nutrition, stress reduction

**Matching: Match the body's defense mechanism in column I with the action it performs in column II.**

| | COLUMN I | COLUMN II |
|---|---|---|
| C | 1. Exercise | A. Gives body time to restore strength and vitality |
| E | 2. Good eating habits | B. Rids the body of invaders |
| A | 3. Getting enough rest | C. Promotes circulation, reduces stress |
| G | 4. Hair-like cilia | D. Wash pathogens from the body |
| B | 5. Coughing and sneezing | E. Keeps energy level at a maximum |
| D | 6. Tears, sweat, urine, and mucus | F. Discourages the growth |
| F | 7. Hydrochloric acid | G. Filters out invading pathogens |

# Chapter Application

## Case Studies with Critical Thinking Questions

### Scenario 1

You notice that one of your coworkers is disposing of contaminated materials in the regular trash. You have seen her throw away her gloves, blood-soaked gauze, and tubes of blood in the trash receptacle that is used for paper products and other regular waste.

1. What effect could your coworker's actions have on other employees? Other employees could become contaminated or injured if they reach into the trash.

2. What should you do about this situation? Inform your supervisor so he or she can speak with your coworker. The information will be better received coming from the supervisor rather than from you.

3. What ramifications could this have on the practice? The office could receive a fine from OSHA and have possible legal actions against it from employees if an exposure were to occur.

4. Explain how the employee should have disposed of the contaminated materials mentioned above. The gloves, depending on the amount of contamination on them, may or may not be allowed to be disposed of in the regular trash. OSHA's Bloodborne Pathogen Standard states that waste that contains liquid or semi-liquid blood or OPIM that would release blood or other OPIM when compressed must be placed in a red biohazard bag with a biohazard label. Therefore, the blood-soaked gauze must be disposed of this way. The tubes of blood, due to their sharps hazard, must be disposed of in a leak-proof, puncture-proof biohazard container displaying the biohazard warning label.

### Scenario 2

A new medical assistant is shadowing you today as part of his training. You are in a hurry because the physician is ahead of schedule and is waiting for you to get his next patient in the room. You have just finished cleaning the previous patient's room and have removed your gloves. Instead of washing your hands, you bring in the next patient, take his vitals, and begin to set up for his exam.

1. How do your actions reflect on you as a medical assistant? You failed to follow OSHA guidelines, which can result in disease transmission and/or exposures, and you are demonstrating poor work habits for the new employee.
2. What messages are you giving the new employee? Your actions say that rules and regulations don't matter and that you have to follow them only if you feel like it, not to mention that you are not respecting yourself or the patient.
3. How can you prevent a negative image in the future? Follow all the guidelines for your protection and the protection of your patients. Ask a coworker for help if you get behind or explain to the physician that you will get the patient in as fast as you can, but never compromise safety.

### Competency Practice

1. **Locate and interpret from the communicable disease chart:** Use the communicable diseases chart in your textbook to fill in the missing information in the following sentences.
   A. Antibacterial agents, antibiotics, or corticosteroids, depending on the causative agent, are the treatment for conjunctivitis.
   B. Cleansing of areas with antimicrobial soap and water and topical and/or oral antibiotics is the treatment for impetigo.
   C. Topical application of drying medications and antibiotics for secondary infections is the treatment for herpes simplex.
   D. MRSA (Methicillin-resistant *Staphylococcus aureus*) is treated with the antibiotic vancomycin to treat resistant germs.
   E. In one week, nits (eggs) hatch; in two weeks, they mature. This describes the incubation period for head lice (pediculosis).
   F. Bed rest and topical antipruritics is the treatment for chickenpox (varicella zoster virus).
   G. Blister-like lesions, which later become crusted and itchy, are symptoms of impetigo.
   H. Antibiotics, analgesics, antipyretics, increased fluid intake, and bed rest are the treatment for scarlet fever.
   I. Intense itching of small, raised areas of the skin that contain fluid or tiny burrows under the skin are symptoms of scabies.
   J. Strawberry tongue, rash on skin and inside of mouth, high fever, nausea, and vomiting are symptoms of scarlet fever.
2. **Complete an incident exposure report form:** Using the following scenario, fill out OSHA Form 301 (Incident Report form). You can download OSHA Form 301 from the Premium Website (Procedure Form 36-1).

Today's Date: Wednesday, March 3, 20XX

Lucia Lee is a medical assistant working for Dr. Roy Johnson in a busy pediatric clinic. She begins her shift at 9 a.m. At 10:15 a.m., Dr. Johnson orders a series of immunizations for his patient, Roberto Delgado, a 4-year-old boy. While Lucia is administering one of the injections, Roberto becomes agitated and pulls the needle out from his left thigh. Lucia panics and pokes herself in the right thumb while trying to activate the safety device on the syringe. She immediately washes the area with soap and water and reports the incident to the nursing supervisor, Carol Lewis. Together, they fill out the Incident Report form. Lucia is counseled by Dr. Johnson. They obtain consent from the patient's mother, and both Lucia and the patient proceed to the clinic's laboratory, where they will leave a blood sample for further testing.

**Employee Information:**

| | |
|---|---|
| Name: | Lucia Lee |
| Address: | 111 Kelly Lane<br>Wichita KS, 55119 |
| DOB: | 05/05/1982 |
| Hire date: | 01/02/2006 |

**Employer Information:**

| | |
|---|---|
| Name: | Wichita Pediatrics |
| Address: | 100 Libby Avenue<br>Wichita KS, 55119 |
| Phone: | (563)555-1234 |

**Case number from the log:** 2

3. **Perform hand washing:** Demonstrate the appropriate use of and perform hand sanitization, using antibacterial gels and foams.

4. **Select the appropriate barrier and personal protective equipment (PPE) for potentially infectious situations:** Fill in the following chart with the appropriate barrier and personal protective equipment (PPE) for each potentially infectious situation. Then demonstrate how to apply and safely remove each barrier and PPE selected.

| | Potentially Infectious Situation | Barrier/PPE Needed |
|---|---|---|
| a. | Cleaning an exam room after the patient appointment. | Gloves |
| b. | Cleaning up a blood spill. | Gloves, eyeware (goggles), and mask |
| c. | Disinfecting an endoscope. | Heavy-duty (utility) gloves, mask, eyeware (goggles), and plastic apron or gown |

5. **Prepare items for autoclaving:** Practice sanitizing, disinfecting, and wrapping or packaging instruments to be autoclaved. Properly label the package and include the necessary sterilization indicators.

6. **Perform sterilization procedures:** Divide into groups and have each person demonstrate the operation of the autoclave to the group. Stress the importance of following each manufacturer's directions because each autoclave can have slight differences. Have the group provide feedback on the performance.

CHAPTER 37

# The Medical History and Patient Screening

## Words to Know Challenge

**Spelling: Each line contains three spellings of a word. Underline the correctly spelled word.**

| | | |
|---|---|---|
| 1. emergant | emergent | emirgent |
| 2. familiel | femelial | familial |
| 3. genogram | geneogram | jeanogram |
| 4. treage | triage | treeage |
| 5. clinical diagnoses | clinical diagnosis | clinicle diagnosis |
| 6. alergies | allergys | allergies |
| 7. objective | abjective | objectiev |
| 8. sabjective | subjactive | subjective |
| 9. patronizing | patranizing | peitronizing |
| 10. remadies | remedies | remedys |

**Matching: Match the term in column I to its definition in column II.**

| | COLUMN I | COLUMN II |
|---|---|---|
| E | 1. Screening | A. Symptoms that can be observed |
| H | 2. Triage | B. Referring to accessible, nonprescription drugs |
| F | 3. Chief complaint (CC) | C. Beliefs that influence observations |
| G | 4. Interview | D. Any perceptible change in the body that indicates disease |
| B | 5. Over-the-counter | E. Process of obtaining information from patient |
| I | 6. Prioritizing | F. Main reason for office visit |
| D | 7. Symptoms | G. Talking to patients one on one and asking questions |
| A | 8. Objective | H. Sort and assess injury |
| C | 9. Biases | I. Arranging in order of importance |

### Fill in the Blank

1. Our beliefs and values tend to provide biases in how we view others.
2. An unexpected occurrence or situation demanding immediate action is considered emergent.
3. Allergies can cause an abnormal reaction by the body to substances that are normally harmless.
4. Providers who treat familial disorders and diseases may also use another type of history form called a genogram.
5. Remedies can be described as anything that relieves or cures a disease.
6. Treating a patient condescendingly is known as patronizing.
7. Subjective symptoms are felt by the individual but are not perceptible to others.
8. A provider will arrive at a clinical diagnosis from facts obtained through the medical history, physical exam, and lab testing.
9. You made need to use prioritizing skills to determine the order of importance of tasks at the medical office.

## Chapter Review

### Short Answer

1. Name five areas of knowledge that you should have to provide good patient screening. Medical terminology, anatomy and physiology, diseases and disorders, emergency procedures, and medications.
2. If a patient complains of pain, what additional questions do you need to ask? You need to identify the location, when it began, its characteristics, and its intensity; any other symptoms; things that make it better or worse; when the pain started; and what the patient was doing when it started.
3. Why might a health history form not be filled out entirely by the patient? The patient may have a language or a reading problem or may not be able to write or understand the information being asked.
4. What is the goal of patient screening? To determine why the patient is seeking health care, what the main problem is, and any other concerns. It will also seek to find out whether the patient has done anything about the problem thus far.
5. Why do some offices send out health history forms to the patient prior to the appointment? This is a provider preference. Some like the patients to have additional time to think about the questions they are answering as well as to save time when they arrive for their appointment.
6. Where should the medical assistant interview patients to obtain the health history information? In a private, confidential area where the patient is comfortable.
7. What is a genogram and why it is helpful to providers? A genogram is a diagram of medical history, including at least three generations, that can show a physician at a glance a patient's chances of developing hereditary diseases.
8. Why should you ask a patient whether he or she has any allergies, and how should you note it in the patient's medical record? A true allergy can cause severe and even life-threatening reactions. Always record the specific allergy—or write "no known allergies" ("NKA") if the patient has none—to indicate having asked the question and the patient's response.
9. After obtaining a patient's chief complaint, the medical assistant should do what next? Summarize the information with the patient for clarification and to see whether anything is missing, get the patient's approval, and sign the form.

10. Explain why health history forms vary in detail and length. This is due to the provider's preference, specialty of the practice , or both. Also, EHR programs may have a custom-built or built-in history form in their software.

**Acronym Review: Write out the following acronyms.**

1. CC Chief complaint
2. PH Past history
3. PI Present illness
4. HPI History of present illness
5. ROS Review of systems
6. UCHD Usual childhood diseases
7. NKDA No known drug allergies.

# Chapter Application

## Case Studies with Critical Thinking Questions

### Scenario 1

When obtaining a patient's chief complaint of fatigue and dizziness, you also notice that he is short of breath and is having difficulty breathing. The patient doesn't mention these symptoms in his chief complaint and talks only about the fatigue and dizziness.

1. What should you do about the apparent symptoms of shortness of breath and dyspnea? Alert the provider and let him or her handle the additional symptoms.

2. Should you chart your observed symptoms with the patient's chief complaint? No. These symptoms are not part of the patient's chief complaint, so they should not be documented as such.

3. Should you discuss this information with the provider? Because medical assistants are not permitted to perform patient assessments, the provider should definitely be informed so that he or she can decide how to handle the additional symptoms.

### Scenario 2

A patient is scheduled to see the provider today for a sore throat and a low-grade fever, which he has had for about five days. While interviewing the patient, he tells you he has also been having chest pains and difficulty breathing and would like the provider to check him for these complaints as well.

1. Will the provider be able to address all the patient's complaints in the time allotted? Probably not with so many complaints; however, chest pains and shortness of breath may be signs of a serious condition and will need to be addressed. Allotted appointments are scheduled based on the patient's chief complaint at the time the appointment is scheduled. This is why it is so important to obtain an accurate phone screening, getting as many details from the patient as possible for the reason he or she needs to be seen.

2. What should you tell the patient regarding the additional complaints? Tell the patient you will inform the provider about the additional symptoms, but let the patient know that an additional appointment may be needed to address some of the symptoms. This is a great opportunity to use patient education on why disclosing all symptoms is so important to be able to schedule the appropriate amount of time for the patient.

3. Should you document only the complaints for which the appointment time was scheduled? No, the entire chief complaint containing all the symptoms should be documented.

## Scenario 3

Amy, the medical assistant, is reviewing a completed medical history form with Mrs. Leonard. She reviews the list of medications Mrs. Leonard has listed and notices that no over-the-counter medications have been included. When Amy questions Mrs. Leonard, she says that she takes no OTC meds, even though she takes some herbal supplements and vitamins on a daily basis.

1. What should Amy have included in her questions about OTC medications? Always include vitamins and herbal supplements when questioning a patient about OTC meds.
2. Why should vitamins and herbal supplements be included in the history form? Some vitamins and herbal supplements can interfere with prescription medications.
3. What are possible implications of not including this information on the history form? Due to possible drug interactions with other substances, this information is vital to prevent adverse reaction from occurring.

## Scenario 4

Mr. Anthony is being seen by the provider for his annual physical. While screening the patient's history form, you notice that he has left the social history section blank. This is the section that includes information about alcohol and tobacco use. Mr. Anthony was told by the provider to stop smoking and drinking alcohol last year.

1. What should you do about the missing information? Give the patient the opportunity to fill in the missing information.
2. How should you approach the subject? Gently. Mr. Anthony may not want the provider to know that he has not complied with his or her orders.
3. Why is it important to obtain information concerning the patient's habits? Use of certain substances can interfere with a patient's treatment and with certain medications, not to mention affecting the patient's overall health.

## Competency Practice

1. **Perform in-person screening:** With a partner, choose an illness to portray and practice taking chief complaints. Develop the complaint, using the characteristics in the textbook to make them as complete as possible to provide the provider with the most information about what is troubling the patient. Using the mock chart below or EHR software, document the chief complaint. Refer to the textbook for charting examples. Use Procedure 37–1 as a guide.

**PROGRESS NOTE**

Patient Name: ______________________ DOB ______________

| DATE/TIME | PROGRESS NOTES | ALLERGIES |
|---|---|---|
| | | |
| | | |
| | | |
| | | |
| | | |

2. **Obtain and record a patient health history:**

   a. Select a disease condition and complete a health history form (download Procedure Form 37–2 from the Premium Website). Have another student check the form for accuracy.

   b. With a partner, have one person be the patient and the other be the medical assistant. In a private setting, practice interviewing the patient and completing the health history forms. Be as thorough as possible, using all the techniques provided in the textbook. Use Procedure 37–2 as a guide. See whether you can anticipate what type of examination and testing the physician may need to do.

CHAPTER 38

# Vital Signs and Measurements

## Words to Know Challenge

**Spelling: Each line contains three spellings of a word. Underline the correctly spelled word.**

| | | |
|---|---|---|
| 1. afibrile | afebrile | effebrial |
| 2. aral | oural | aural |
| 3. bradypnea | bradipenia | braedypenia |
| 4. fatil | fatal | fatel |
| 5. ideopathic | idiopathic | edeopathic |
| 6. menstration | menstruation | mensuration |
| 7. orthostatic | orthastatic | orthostatec |
| 8. pirogen | pyragen | pyrogen |
| 9. sphygmomanometer | spygmonometer | spygmomanometer |
| 10. sistole | systole | systoli |

**Matching: Match the term in column I to its definition in column II.**

| | COLUMN I | COLUMN II |
|---|---|---|
| C | 1. Antecubital | A. Excessively slow heart rate |
| H | 2. Apex | B. Feel by touching |
| K | 3. Arrhythmia | C. Inner elbow area |
| I | 4. Auscultate | D. A pulse site at the groin |
| J | 5. Brachial | E. Excessively rapid heart rate |
| A | 6. Bradycardia | F. A pulse site at the inner wrist |
| G | 7. Carotid | G. A pulse site near the trachea |
| D | 8. Femoral | H. Lower edge of the heart |
| B | 9. Palpate | I. To listen |
| E | 10. Tachycardia | J. A pulse site at the inner elbow |
| F | 11. Radial | K. Without a regular pattern of beats |

**Fill in the Blank: Complete the following sentences with Words to Know from this chapter.**
(*Hint*: You will use some correctly spelled words from the preceding Spelling section.)

1. Identify the four vital signs in the following sentences, indicating which body function is being measured:
   a. Blood pressure measures the force of the heart.
   b. Temperature measures the body's heat.
   c. Pulse measures the action of the heart.
   d. Respiration measures action of the lungs (breathing).
2. One respiration is the combination of one total inspiration and one total expiration. Two other terms that are frequently used and have the same meaning are inhale and exhale.
3. Patients with difficult or labored breathing are said to have dyspnea.
4. The absence of breathing is known as apnea.
5. Blood pressure is measured using a(n) stethoscope and a(n) sphygmomanometer.
6. A sphygmomanometer has a(n) aneroid dial.
7. An elevated pressure without apparent cause is said to be idiopathic or essential hypertension.
8. Excessively rapid and deep respirations are known as hyperventilation.
9. Taking a patient's temperature in the armpit is also known as the axillary method.
10. Another term for a patient running a fever is febrile.

## Chapter Review

**Short Answer: Using material from the chapter, provide a short answer in the space provided.**

1. Name five types of mensurations. Why are mensurations particularly important with infants and children?
   Height, weight, extremity length, head, chest, or abdominal circumference with infants. They are important for infants and children to determine that normal growth and development are occurring.
2. Explain why and when a patient's height and weight is measured.
   To confirm that proper growth and development are occurring. Abnormal changes could indicate the presence of a disease or disorder such as fluid retention or osteoporosis.
3. If a patient measures 70 inches, how much is that in feet and inches?
   5 feet 10 inches
4. List five types of thermometers.
   (1) Plastic disposable, (2) digital, (3) electronic, (4) tympanic infrared, (5) temporal artery
5. Name at least three situations in which oral temperature measurement is contraindicated.
   Any three of the following: Infants and small children; patients with respiratory complications or nasal obstructions; recent oral surgery or dental injuries, problems; facial paralysis; patients who are confused or disoriented.
6. Identify when a patient may be asked to monitor his or her weight at home. What suggestions could you make to a patient about measuring his or her weight?
   Patients may be asked to monitor weight at home if they have cardiac or kidney disease or if they are monitoring weight loss or gain. Patient education includes to weigh at the same time each day and with similar clothing. Suggest in the morning before breakfast while in underwear.

7. What is the normal adult rate pulse range? Discuss how pulse rate is determined and list five factors that affect the pulse rate.
   The normal adult heart rate range is 60–80. It is determined by counting the number of heartbeats per minute. Factors that affect the pulse rate include exercise or activity, age, gender, size, and the body's physical condition.

8. Name two qualities of the heartbeat that must be observed, defining the terms and listing the words to describe the characteristics.
   a. *Volume* refers to the force or strength of the pulse. Terms are *normal, full, bounding, weak,* or *thready*.
   b. *Rhythm* refers to the regularity of spacing between beats. Terms are *regular, irregular, regularly irregular,* and *intermittent*.

8. Why are respirations measured as the pulse is being measured?
   So the patient believes you are counting the pulse and does not alter his or her breathing.

9. What is the normal respiration rate for an adult?
   16–20 breaths per minute.

10. Define "blood pressure" and then name the two phases of blood pressure, describing the corresponding action that occurs and the relative amount of pressure with each phase.
    Blood pressure is the fluctuating pressure the blood exerts against the arterial walls as the heart alternately contracts and relaxes. The two phases are (1) systole (contraction phase and period of greatest pressure) and (2) diastole (relaxation phase and period of least pressure).

11. Define "auscultatory gap." It is the silent interval between systolic and diastolic pressures.

12. Explain indications for apical pulse measurements.
    Apical pulse measurement is indicated for infants and small children because of their normally rapid rate, which is easier to hear and count than to palpate. Also patients with heart conditions, especially those taking cardiac drugs, when a radial pulse is hard to feel, and if the patient has a rapid , slow, thready, or irregular beat.

13. Identify normal and abnormal blood pressure, including factors affecting blood pressure.
    An adult should have a systolic pressure less than 120 mm Hg and a diastolic pressure less than 80. Blood pressure readings persistently in the range of 140–159 and 90–99 indicate stage 1 *hypertension* (high blood pressure). Hypertension can result from factors such as stress, obesity, high salt intake, sedentary lifestyle, and aging.

**Matching: Match the routes of measuring temperature listed in column I with the corresponding normal average temperature for that route in column II.**
(*Hint*: Answers in column II may be used more than once.)

| | COLUMN I | COLUMN II |
|---|---|---|
| C | 1. Aural temperature | A. 97.6°F |
| A | 2. Axillary temperature | B. 98.6°F |
| B | 3. Oral temperature | C. 99.1°F |
| D | 4. Temporal artery temperature | D. 99.6°F |
| D | 5. Rectal temperature | |

**Labeling: Identify the labels in the following diagram, indicating the different sites where the pulse rate may be measured. Give an explanation for when or why the site is used.**

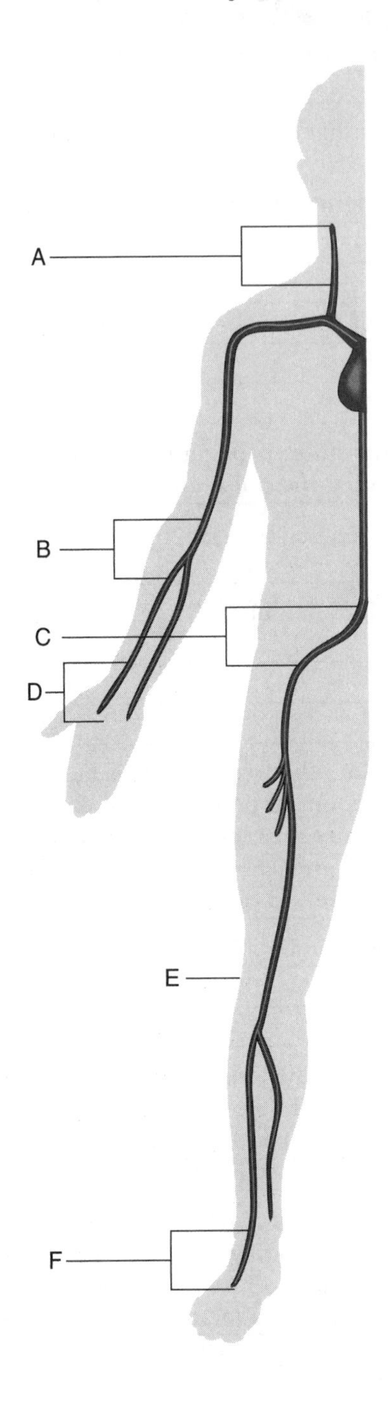


a. Carotid: Used during cardiopulmonary resuscitation (CPR)

b. Brachial: Used to palpate and auscultate blood pressure

c. Femoral: Used to evaluate circulation in the lower extremities

d. Radial: Used most frequently when measuring pulse rate

e. Popliteal: Used to evaluate circulation in the lower extremities

f. Dorsalis pedis: Used to evaluate circulation in the lower extremities

# Chapter Application

## Conversion Exercises

1. Convert the following Celsius temperatures to Fahrenheit:
   1. 36.5°C = 97.8 °F
   2. 35.7°C = 96.2 °F
   3. 39.5°C = 103.1 °F
   4. 36.8°C = 98.2 °F
   5. 38.8°C = 101.8 °F
   6. 37.4°C = 99.4 °F
2. Convert the following Fahrenheit temperatures to Celsius:
   1. 96.8°F = 36 °C
   2. 99.2°F = 37.3 °C
   3. 97.4°F = 36.3 °C
   4. 100.2°F = 37.8 °C
   5. 98.6°F = 37 °C
   6. 102.4°F = 39.1 °C
3. The National Institutes of Health has published a BMI index chart that is easy to use, and many providers prefer to have this chart posted near the scale and in the exam rooms. You can access a copy of this chart on their website at www.nih.gov. Using the chart or calculation from the textbook and the following weights and heights, calculate the BMI for each:
   1. 150 lbs/5'7 = 23.5
   2. 212 lbs/5'4 = 36.5
   3. 98 lbs/4'10 = 20.5
   4. 260 lbs/6'1 = 34.4
   5. 167 lbs/5'3 = 29.6
   6. 137 lbs/5'1 = 25.9

## Case Studies with Critical Thinking Questions

### Scenario 1

The medical assistant is having difficulty taking Mrs. Anderson's pulse and respirations. She finally locates the radial pulse and then begins to count. There are some irregularities in the pulse, so the medical assistant counts it for one full minute. Mrs. Anderson is somewhat alarmed at how long this is taking and asks the medical assistant if something is wrong. The medical assistant then takes her finger off the pulse and tells Mrs. Anderson to breathe normally while she is counting the respirations.

1. Should the medical assistant tell the patient about her irregular pulse? No. You should never tell the patient about any abnormal findings without the provider's permission.
2. How could knowing this information affect the patient? The patient may become anxious, which can affect her pulse and respirations.
3. What mistake did the medical assistant make when counting the respirations? By taking her fingers off the pulse and telling the patient to breathe normally, she alerted the patient that her respirations were being counted. If the patient is aware of the respirations being counted, she might not breathe in her normal rhythm, which would affect the results.

### Scenario 2

Carter always had trouble hearing blood pressures when he was in school, and the problem has carried over to his job. He cannot hear the blood pressure on a geriatric patient and is scared to admit this difficulty since this is only his second week on the job. Carter tries twice and gives up. He looks up the patient's last few readings and comes up with an average reading that he documents in the chart.

1. What should Carter do about his problem with hearing blood pressures? Confide his difficulty to his supervisor and ask for extra help and practice with blood pressures.
2. Was it permissible for him to document the reading he averaged? Absolutely not! An average reading may not be accurate, and this would be considered illegal documentation.

3. What possible implications might his actions have on the patient? A change in the patient's blood pressure would go undetected, which could cause the provider to misdiagnose the patient and to select the wrong treatment.

## Competency Practice

1. **Measure and record height and weight:** With a partner, practice setting the height bar and weights at different measurements and have the other partner read them. Then switch roles. When you get 10 in a row each correct, measure heights and weights on each other. In a mock patient chart or on EHR software, document the height and weight. Refer to the textbook for charting examples. Use Procedure 38–1 as a guide.
2. **Practice measuring and recording oral, axillary, tympanic (core body), and temporal artery temperatures:** Using all the types of thermometers available (disposable plastic, digital, electronic with oral probe, tympanic, and temporal artery), make a chart on a piece of paper, and obtain five of each temperature on different classmates. When finished, document two of the readings on a mock patient chart and two of the readings in an EHR (if available). Use procedures that correspond as guides.
3. **Measure and record rectal temperature with an electronic thermometer:** Using a mannequin, demonstrate the technique on obtaining a rectal temperature. Have a partner watch, critique, and provide feedback. Discuss when you should and should not use the rectal route to obtain the temperature. When finished, document on a mock patient chart or an EHR. Use Procedure 38–3 as a guide.
4. **Measure and record radial pulse rate and respirations:** With a partner, have one be the patient and the other be the medical assistant. Take turns performing the following exercises and then measure each others' pulse and respirations. Note the variations in the characteristics of your patient's pulse and respirations. Use Procedure 38–8 as a guide.

| | |
|---|---|
| Sit in a chair quietly for three minutes. | |
| Walk around the classroom for a minute. | |
| Run in place for three minutes. | |

5. **Measure and record apical pulse rate:** With a partner, locate the apex of the heart and obtain an apical pulse on each other. Document your results on a mock patient chart or an EHR. Use Procedure 38–8 as a guide.
6. **Measure and record blood pressure:** Obtain 10 blood pressures on different people and document on the following chart. Be sure to chart all the information requested. Use Procedure 38–9 as a guide.

| Gender (male or female) | Age | Position (sitting, standing, or lying down) | Blood Pressure Result | Arm Used (right or left) |
|---|---|---|---|---|
| | | | | |
| | | | | |
| | | | | |
| | | | | |
| | | | | |
| | | | | |
| | | | | |
| | | | | |
| | | | | |
| | | | | |

CHAPTER 39

# Preparing for Examinations

## Words to Know Challenge

**Spelling: Each line contains three spellings of a word. Underline the correctly spelled word.**

| | | |
|---|---|---|
| 1. anatomical | annatomical | anatonical |
| 2. dypsnea | dypnsea | dyspnea |
| 3. fenastrated | fenetrated | fenestrated |
| 4. lithotamy | lithotomy | litothomy |
| 5. recumbent | recumbant | recunbant |
| 6. supin | soopine | supine |
| 7. Trendalenburg | Trendelenburg | Trendelenberg |
| 8. aunterior | anteriour | anterior |
| 9. incompatent | incompetent | incompetant |
| 10. Fowler's | Fawler's | Foyler's |

**Fill in the Blank: Complete the following sentences with Words to Know from this chapter.**

1. Dorsal pertains to the back.
2. If someone is lying flat and even, level, and parallel to the plane of the horizon, he or she is said to be horizontal.
3. The knee-chest position is used for rectal or proctological examinations and occasionally for a sigmoidoscopy if a special table is not available.
4. The Trendelenburg position is most commonly used for a patient suffering from shock.
5. Ventral pertains to the anterior or front side of the body.
6. If a patient is lying horizontal, with his or her face down, he or she is said to be in the prone position.
7. The Sims' position is an examination position in which the patient is lying on his or her left side.

## Chapter Review

### Short Answer

1. For what purpose is each of the following examination positions used?
   A. Horizontal recumbent or supine For examination and treatment of the anterior surface of the body, breasts, and abdominal organs
   B. Dorsal recumbent Examination of the abdomen, vaginal, or rectal area
   C. Prone Examination of the back or spine
   D. Anatomical For examination of posture and movement
   E. Sims' or lateral Examination and treatment of the rectal area, rectal temperature, enemas, and sigmoidoscopy
   F. Knee-chest For rectal examination and specifically for sigmoidoscopy
   G. Fowler's For patients with respiratory or cardiovascular problems; may be used to examine the head, neck, and chest area
   H. Lithotomy For vaginal and rectal examinations; may also be used for examination of male genital area and catheterization
   I. Trendelenburg Used for patient in shock, very low blood pressure, hemorrhage, or to displace organs for some abdominal surgical procedures; may also be used to check a patient for varicose veins
   J. Jackknife or Kraske Useful for examination and instrumentation of the male urethra

2. What safety precautions must be observed for protection of both the patient and you when moving patients?
   Get help to lift a patient who is larger than you think you should try to lift. Never leave an ill patient or child alone on the table. Assist the patient on and off the table with movement on the table to prevent a fall.

3. Why is a drape used when positioning patients?
   To show respect for privacy and comfort of the patient

4. What support is used for the feet in the lithotomy position?
   Stirrups

5. What is the name of the drape that has an opening for examination?
   Fenestrated drape

6. It is routine to check for supplies when preparing an examination room. List 13 supplies you must routinely check for.
   A hand-washing product, biohazardous waste containers, face guards, gloves, gowns, drapes, paper towels, tissues, light source, tongue blades, speculums, gauze squares, and applicators

7. Explain exam room cleanup and equipment that may need to be disinfected following patient examination.
   Wash hands and put on gloves, place used supplies and disposable examination equipment in the waste or biohazard container. Check the waste container for space; replace if the bag is full. Tear the table paper near the top and roll it up with the pillow cover. Wipe the permanent examination equipment with disposable cloth or gauze squares and disinfectant. Wipe the examination room table tops with disposable cloth and disinfectant if contaminated from discarded examination supplies. Wipe any other equipment contaminated by the provider, such as a stool or exam lamp. Disinfect the examination table and dispose of cloth and gloves in the appropriate container. Prepare the exam table for the next patient. Check the hand-washing supplies and restock if needed. Check the supplies in the cabinet and exam table drawers and restock if needed. Make a final check of the room, remove gloves, and wash hands

**Labeling: Label the following illustrations, indicating the various examination positions.**

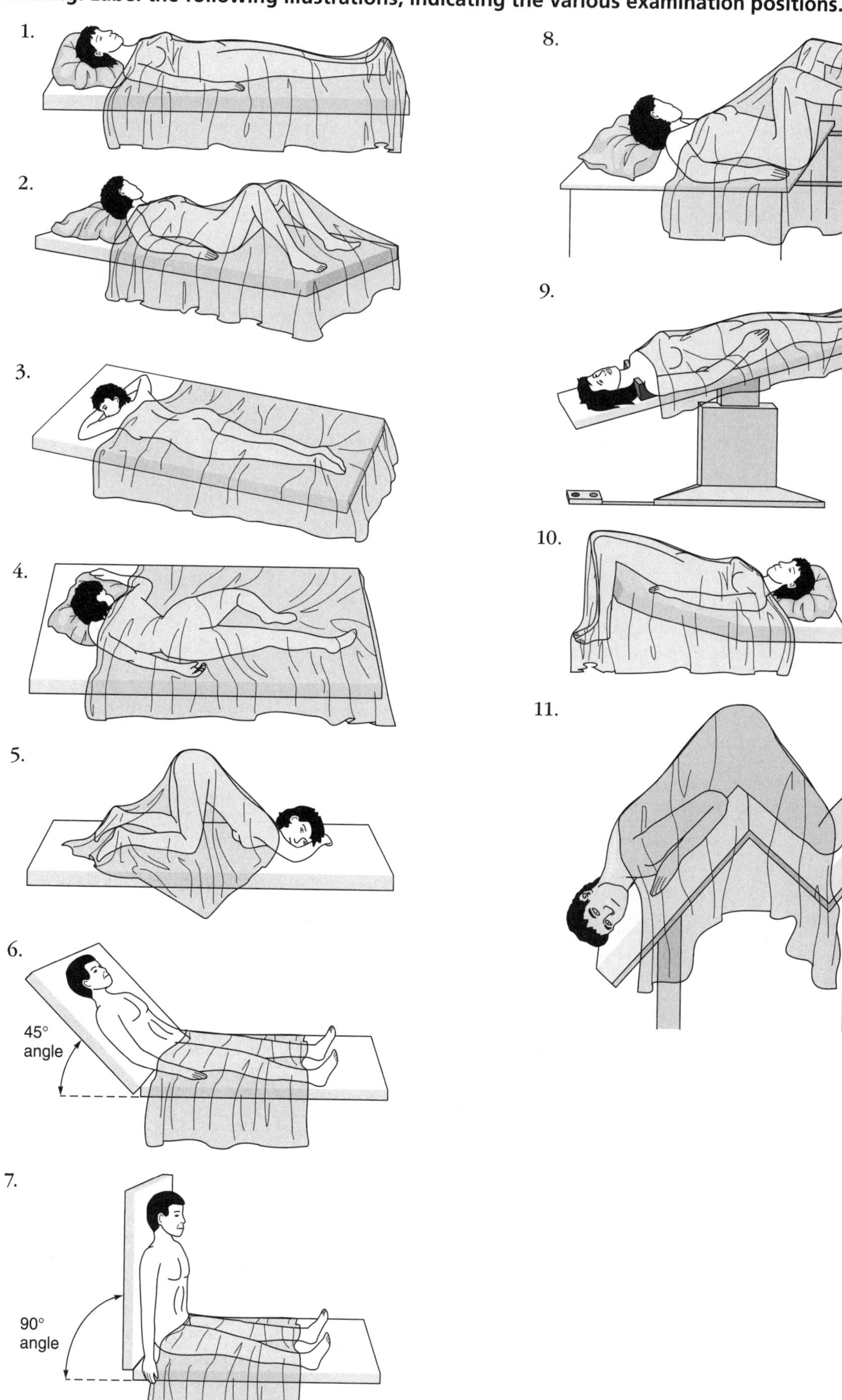

1. Horizontal recumbent or supine
2. Dorsal recumbent
3. Prone
4. Sims' or lateral
5. Knee-chest
6. Semi-Fowler's
7. Fowler's (High)
8. Lithotomy
9. Trendelenburg
10. Modified Trendelenburg
11. Jackknife or Kraske

# Chapter Application

## Case Studies with Critical Thinking Questions

### Scenario 1

Kelly escorts Mrs. Leonard into the exam room for her yearly Pap test and pelvic exam. Kelly didn't have time to clean the room before escorting Mrs. Leonard to the back office, so she asks her to have a seat on the stool while she tidies the room. She disposes the used gown and table paper and sets up all the supplies. She then asks Mrs. Leonard to disrobe and prepares her for the exam.

1. What was Kelly's first *big* mistake? She did not make sure the room was clean and ready before escorting the patient to the back office
2. What should Mrs. Leonard have been instructed to do before disrobing? Empty her bladder
3. Should equipment and supplies be set up in the presence of the patient? No. Equipment and supplies should never be set up in front of the patient because this could cause the patient to develop anxiety and not feel confident about her care

### Scenario 2

Mr. Johnson is being seen in the office for a sigmoidoscopy. The medical assistant gives Mr. Johnson disrobing instructions and leaves the room for a few minutes. When she returns, she places Mr. Johnson in the knee-chest position, and he complains about how uncomfortable it is for him. The medical assistant assures the patient that it will be only a few more minutes before the provider is ready.

1. When should the patient have been placed into the position for the exam? The patient should not be placed into the position until the provider is ready to perform the exam. The patient will need assistance from you in maintaining this position, and you must stay with the patient at all times while he or she is in the position
2. What should the medical assistant have done to make the patient more comfortable? Support and assist the patient while he is in this position
3. What is an alternative position that can be used for this procedure? A knee-elbow position can be used which is a modified version of the knee-chest position and is easier for patients to maintain

## Competency Practice

1. **Prepare and maintain examination and treatment areas.** With a partner, practice setting up an examination room for a patient coming in for a complete physical examination. Be sure to include all the supplies and equipment needed. On a blank sheet of paper, design a checklist that can be used for cleaning, maintenance, and inventory for the room. Use critical thinking skills to determine what the list should include. Use Procedure 39–1 as a guide.

2. **Transfer a patient from a wheelchair to the examination table.** Using a classmate for a partner, demonstrate the proper technique for transferring a patient from a wheelchair to the examination table. Try practicing with two people assisting the transfer. This may be needed if you are working with a large patient or with a patient who is unable to bear weight at all. Use Procedure 39–2 as a guide.

3. **Transfer a patient from the examination table to a wheelchair.** Using a classmate for a partner, demonstrate the proper technique for transferring a patient from the examination table to a wheelchair. Try practicing with two people assisting the transfer. This may be needed if you are working with a large patient or with a patient who is unable to bear weight at all. Use Procedure 39–3 as a guide.

4. **Demonstrate positioning a patient for a variety of examinations.** Using either a classmate or a mannequin, demonstrate placing the patient into a variety of positions that may be used for the provider examination. Be sure to use proper draping techniques as well. Use Procedure 39–4 as a guide.

UNIT 13

# Assisting with Examinations

CHAPTER 40

# The Physical Exam, Specialty Exams, and Procedures

## Words to Know Challenge

**Spelling: Each line contains three spellings of a word. Underline the correctly spelled word.**

| | | |
|---|---|---|
| 1. auscultation | auscutatuion | asscultation |
| 2. menipulation | manipulation | maniputation |
| 3. bimanual | bymanual | bimanule |
| 4. bruet | bruit | brute |
| 5. gate | gait | gaite |
| 6. hurnia | hernea | hernia |
| 7. laxative | laxetive | laxitive |
| 8. luman | luemen | lumen |
| 9. mucosa | mucousa | mycousa |
| 10. obtruator | obturator | abturator |
| 11. evakuant | evacuent | evacuant |
| 12. occluder | ocluder | aucluder |

**Matching: Match the term in column I to its definition in column II.**

| | COLUMN I | COLUMN II |
|---|---|---|
| F | 1. audiometer | A. means "to wash out" |
| E | 2. acuity | B. unit for measuring volume of sound |
| C | 3. cerumen | C. medical term for earwax |
| B | 4. decibel | D. another word for lavage |
| D | 5. irrigate | E. clarity/sharpness of perception |
| A | 6. lavage | F. instrument that measures hearing |
| H | 7. Snellen Chart | G. a screening tool for near vision acuity |

(continues)

| | | |
|---|---|---|
| G | 8. Jaeger Chart | H. a screening tool for distant visual acuity |
| J | 9. scribe | I. test for occult blood in stool |
| I | 10. guaiac test paper | J. documents provider's dictation during an exam |
| K | 11. enema | K. part of preparation for sigmoidoscopy |

**Fill in the Blank: Complete the following sentences with Words to Know from this chapter.**

1. Screening patients for color vision acuity is done with Ishihara color plates.
2. Pitch, quality, duration, and resonance are terms that refer to percussion.
3. Inspection is a visual exam of the body's various parts.
4. A patient told to have nothing to eat or drink for a period of time is advised to fast.
5. The heel-to-shin test and the heel-to-toe test are used to check the patient's coordination.
6. Rectal examinations may be performed by using a proctoscope or a flexible sigmoidoscope to get a better view of the colon.
7. An evacuant is used to expel fecal matter from the colon.
8. Using one finger of a gloved hand, the provider will perform a digital rectal exam to palpate the rectum to check for abnormalities.
9. When performing percussion, the provider listens to the sounds to determine the size, density, and location of underlying visceral organs.
10. Turgor of the skin is measured by pinching the back of the hand and observing the length of time for it to return to normal.
11. Side vision while looking straight forward is known as peripheral vision.
12. Lung capacity can be measured by a spirometer or a peak flow meter.

## Chapter Review

### Short Answer

1. What must the medical assistant remember to do with the ophthalmoscope and otoscope in preparing for eye and ear examinations? The medical assistant must remember to check for burned-out light bulbs, check the batteries in some handheld otoscopes and ophthalmoscopes, and check whether they are in proper working order.
2. What types of patients will require testing for visual acuity with the letter E chart? Those who have reading difficulties and non-English speaking patients.
3. Describe the role of the medical assistant in the patient examination process. The medical assistant should prepare the room, prepare the equipment, prepare the patient, provide patient teaching, and assist the provider with the examination
4. During the physical exam, what might your role entail regarding patient education?
You may be expected to provide patient education on a variety of topics. When you know about the pamphlets and other resources available in your office, you can talk with the patient and indicate that you will supply the material after the exam if the provider concurs with the necessity of it
5. What is the Ishihara screening method, and why is it administered to patients? To determine their color visual acuity and whether there are any changes

6. What is the purpose of eye irrigation? The purpose of eye irrigation is to soothe tissues, relieve inflammation, remove foreign objects, and wash out drainage.

7. What is cerumen? Why must impacted cerumen be softened and irrigated from the ear?
Cerumen is the medical term for earwax. Impacted cerumen must be softened to remove it from the ear because this hardened wax can impair hearing and cause possible injury to the ear.

8. Name the six examination techniques and provide an example of each.
   a. Inspection: visual inspection of appearance, skin, anxiety, gait, and injuries
   b. Palpation: examination of the breasts, organ size, and shape, and aortic pulsations
   c. Percussion: tapping body to locate organs, size, and density
   d. Auscultation: listening to murmurs, rhythms, and rales
   e. Mensuration: measuring height, weight, and circumferences
   f. Manipulation: passive movement of joints for ROM and flexibility

9. Describe the Rinne test for hearing. The Rinne test for hearing consists of the examiner's striking a tuning fork and then holding the shank (stem) against the patient's mastoid bone until the patient no longer hears the sound.

10. Describe the Weber test for hearing. The Weber test for hearing consists of the examiner holding the vibrating tuning fork against the patient's vertex, or crown of the head, or against an area of the skull.

11. List common behaviors that can indicate hearing loss. Inappropriately loud talking, not responding when spoken to, often asking to repeat what was said, not pronouncing words well, and responding only to very loud talking

12. List common complaints that can indicate visual disturbances. Blurriness of vision, nausea, headaches, dizziness, sensitivity to light, and feeling like something is in one's eye(s)

13. What is the purpose of the audiometer? To determine the hearing threshold of pure tones of frequencies that are normally audible to an individual

**On the following table, enter the organs in the abdominal area in which they are primarily located.**

ascending colon
descending colon
left spermatic cord
pregnant uterus
sigmoid colon
transverse colon
appendix
gallbladder
liver
right ovary
spleen
urinary bladder
cecum
left ovary
pancreas
right spermatic cord
stomach

| Abdominal Area | Organs |
|---|---|
| Right hypochondriac | Gallbladder, liver |
| Epigastric | Pancreas |
| Left hypochondriac | Stomach, spleen |
| Right lumbar | Ascending colon |
| Umbilical | Transverse colon |
| Left lumbar | Descending colon |
| Right inguinal | Cecum, appendix, right ovary, right spermatic cord |
| Hypogastric | Urinary bladder, pregnant uterus |
| Left inguinal | Left ovary, sigmoid colon, left spermatic cord |

# Chapter Application

## Case Studies with Critical Thinking Questions

### Scenario 1

The medical assistant escorts Mr. Carter into the examination room to prepare him for a complete physical exam. He tells the assistant that he hasn't been seen by a doctor for 10 years. After weighing the patient and taking his vital signs, she instructs Mr. Carter to use the rest room and collect a clean catch sample. Mr. Carter is confused and can't possibly remember all those instructions, so he just collects a specimen in a cup. She then tells Mr. Carter to disrobe and wait for the provider. Mr. Carter says he is anxious and doesn't understand why he has to do all these things. The medical assistant tells him to just relax and that the provider will be in soon.

1. List some reasons the patient might be anxious. The patient may be nervous about new procedures that have been developed since he was seen last, and he may be anxious about what the provider might find during the examination.
2. Will the specimen Mr. Carter collected be accurate for testing? Probably not because it is contaminated with surface bacteria and cells.
3. What should the medical assistant have done to calm Mr. Carter's fears? The medical assistant should have spent more time with Mr. Carter and asked if he had any questions.

### Scenario 2

Mrs. Karnes is being seen today because she found a lump in her breast. When the provider enters the room, he finds Mrs. Karnes in tears. She is still in her street clothes and the provider is quite upset that his normally efficient medical assistant did not properly prepare this patient for an exam.

1. How should the patient have been prepared for the exam? The patient should have been on the exam table and wearing a gown with the opening in the front.
2. What can this do to the provider's schedule? The fact that the provider will have to wait while the patient disrobes could push the provider's schedule behind.
3. How might the medical assistant have served the needs of the patient better? The medical assistant should have stayed with the patient and answered any questions she might have had. The medical assistant should also have given the patient proper disrobing and gowning instructions.

### Scenario 3

The provider asks the medical assistant to irrigate a patient's ear for removal of impacted cerumen. She prepares the irrigating solution but can't find the thermometer to check the temperature of the solution. She inserts the syringe straight into the ear and begins irrigation. While the medical assistant is irrigating the patient's ear, the patient complains of pain and a burning sensation in the ear. The medical assistant continues the irrigation anyway despite the patient's complaints, because the provider is in a hurry and is running behind.

1. Should the medical assistant have continued with the irrigation after the patient complained about pain and a burning sensation? No. The pain and burning sensation felt by the patient are warning signs that something is not right, and the irrigation should have been discontinued.
2. What could be the outcome of continuing with the irrigation? Injury to the tympanic membrane and other structures of the ear.
3. Did the medical assistant have the syringe properly positioned? No. The syringe should be aimed upward to irrigate the entire canal and to direct the flow away from the tympanic membrane.

## Competency Practice

1. **Prepare a Patient for and Assist with a Routine Physical Examination.** Create a table listing all the parts of a complete physical exam, along with the medical assisting duties for each part. Include a review of systems and be sure to list the medical assisting duties for each system. Use Procedure 40–1 as a guide.
2. **Irrigate the Ear.** Using a mannequin, demonstrate the technique for irrigating the ear. Have a partner watch, critique, and provide feedback. Discuss the equipment available for use to perform the procedure and what the pros and cons are for each. When finished, document in a mock patient chart or an EHR. Use Procedure 40–2 as a guide.
3. **Irrigate the Eye.** In pairs, have one student be the patient and the other be the medical assistant. The medical assistant should set up all the necessary equipment and supplies for eye irrigation and mimic the procedure without actually using any solution. Discuss the importance of irrigating from the inner canthus to the outer canthus and reasons the eye(s) might need irrigation. When finished, document in a mock patient chart or an EHR. Use Procedure 40–3 as a guide.
4. **Screen Visual Acuity with a Snellen Chart.** In pairs, have one student be the patient and the other be the medical assistant. Take turns screening visual acuity with a Snellen chart. When finished, document in a mock patient chart or an EHR. Use Procedure 40–4 as a guide.
5. **Screen Visual Acuity with the Jaeger System.** In pairs, have one student be the patient and the other be the medical assistant. Take turns screening visual acuity with a Jaeger chart. When finished, document in a mock patient chart or an EHR. Use Procedure 40–5 as a guide.
6. **Determine Color Vision Acuity by the Ishihara Method.** In pairs, have one student be the patient and the other be the medical assistant. Take turns screening color vision with the Ishihara method. Discuss the importance of color vision testing and make a list of the occupations in which color vision is critical. When finished, document in a mock patient chart or an EHR. Use Procedure 40–6 as a guide.
7. **Perform Spirometry Testing.** In pairs, have one student be the patient and the other be the medical assistant. Take turns performing spirometry testing on each other. Be sure when you are the MA to coach the patient to assist in obtaining the best results possible. When finished, document in a mock patient chart or an EHR. Use Procedure 40–7 as a guide.
8. **Perform Peak Flow Testing.** In pairs, have one student be the patient and the other be the medical assistant. Take turns educating each other on how to perform a peak flow measurement and how to obtain the patient's personal best. Discuss what the three zones are and what a patient would be advised, depending on which zone his or her result was in. When finished, document in a mock patient chart or an EHR. Use Procedure 40–8 as a guide.
9. **Perform Pulse Oximeter Testing.** In pairs, have one student be the patient and the other be the medical assistant. Take turns performing a pulse oximetry measurement on each other. Discuss what you would need to do if the patient was an infant, had dark nail polish on, or had calloused fingers. When finished, document in a mock patient chart or an EHR. Use Procedure 40–9 as a guide.
10. **Assist with a Flexible Sigmoidoscopy Procedure.** Using a mannequin and a classmate, role-play one being the provider and the other the MA. Demonstrate assisting the provider with a flexible sigmoidoscope. Use your critical thinking skills to determine what would be the next steps and what your role is. Discuss the equipment used to perform the procedure and what the cleanup process is after the procedure is complete, including chemically sterilizing the scope. Use Procedure 40–10 as a guide.

CHAPTER 41

# OB/GYN Examinations

## Words to Know Challenge

**Spelling: Each line contains three spellings of a word. Underline the correctly spelled word.**

| | | |
|---|---|---|
| 1. cervical | servical | cervacal |
| 2. fundas | fundes | fundus |
| 3. gestation | jestation | guestation |
| 4. Lamazae | Lamaze | Lemaze |
| 5. trymester | triemister | trimester |

**Matching: Match the term in column I to its definition in column II.**

| | COLUMN I | COLUMN II |
|---|---|---|
| B | 1. Atypical | A. Fetus in the uterus |
| J | 2. Cytology | B. Not the usual |
| H | 3. Douche | C. Before birth |
| G | 4. Endocervical | D. Cells shedding |
| D | 5. Exfoliated | E. Method to estimate expected date of delivery |
| E | 6. Naegele's rule | F. Doctor who developed cervical cancer test |
| F | 7. Papanicolaou | G. Within the cervix |
| A | 8. Pregnancy | H. Cleansing the vagina |
| C | 9. Prenatal | I. Inflammation of the vagina |
| I | 10. Vaginitis | J. Study of cells |

**Fill in the Blank: Complete the following sentences with Words to Know from this chapter.**

1. In place of the conventional Pap test, many providers are now using a liquid-based method known as ThinPrep.
2. Another name for a birth class is Lamaze.

3. Pap smears are sent to the cytology department to be analyzed.

4. During the prenatal examination, you assist the provider as appropriate for the trimester of the patient's gestation .

5. A flexible centimeter tape is used to measure the height of the fundus from the symphysis pubis bone to evaluate the growth of the fetus.

6. Women should be especially conscientious in scheduling Pap tests if they have a family history of uterine or cervical cancer.

7. Patient's should be advised not to douche for 48 hours prior to their Pap test because it could wash away exfoliated cells.

cervical

## Chapter Review

### Short Answer

1. List five reasons the liquid-based Pap test is preferred.
   a. Cells don't dry out
   b. Reduces mucus, bacteria, yeast, and pus cells
   c. Slightly improves cancer detection
   d. Greatly improves detection of precancers
   e. Enables additional studies from the same sample

2. When is the AutoPap used? In screening smears before a provider or technologist analyzes them. Anything identified as abnormal would still be examined by a technologist. Additionally, these computerized instruments will retest Pap samples interpreted as normal by technologists, with the intent to detect abnormal cells that are missed by humans .

3. Identify the four main guidelines regarding patient preparation for a Pap test.
   a. Do not use tampons, vaginal foams, jellies, or creams for 48 hours before the test .
   b. Do not douche for 48 hours prior .
   c. Do not have sexual intercourse for 48 hours prior .
   d. Schedule the test about five days after menstrual period .

4. Why should you have a female patient empty her bladder before a pelvic exam?
   The exam is uncomfortable with a full bladder and makes it more difficult for the provider to do. Also, it can be embarrassing to the patient to have to go after the exam has started, and it interrupts the scheduled flow of the provider's time .

5. Why is BSE necessary when a patient has an annual provider examination?
   To detect abnormalities between the provider's examinations .

6. What are the three main categories for reporting Pap results?
   a. Negative for intraepithelial lesion or malignancy
   b. Epithelial cell abnormalities
   c. Other malignant neoplasms

7. List the responsibilities of the medical assistant during a prenatal office visit.
   a. Interview patient to determine whether any new problems have been experienced; b. Request or obtain urine specimen to test; c. Measure weight and record findings; d. Check chart for lab reports of older tests; e. Measure and record vital signs; f. Prepare patient for the examination; g. Notify the provider when the patient is ready

8. How can pregnancy be confirmed?
   a. Patient interview and prenatal assessment; b. Complete physical examination; c. Lab tests; d. Diagnostic tests as indicated

**Fill in the Blank: Using material from the chapter, fill in the answers in the space provided.**

1. Initial Pap screening should begin after a female is sexually active for three years but not later than when the patient turns 21 years old.
2. A conventional or regular Pap test should be done once a year, whereas the ThinPrep test can be done every two years.
3. At 30 years old, if the woman has had three normal tests in a row, she may get screened every two to three years unless she has risk factors.
4. Women over 30 may elect to have screenings every three years if they also have the HPV DNA test.
5. If 70 or older, women who have had three normal Pap tests in a row and no abnormal findings in 10 years, and do not have any risk factors, may stop Pap screenings.
6. Women with total hysterectomy may stop screenings unless the surgery was done to treat cancer.
7. Gynecological instruments, in addition to the speculum, are used for examinations and procedures. The uterine sound measures uterine depth. The curette scrapes the lining for a specimen. A small piece of tissue may be removed with the punch biopsy forceps.

# Chapter Application

## Case Studies with Critical Thinking Questions

### Scenario 1

Lyn is being seen today for her Pap test and pelvic exam. She was given preparation instructions prior to her appointment. After the medical assistant prepares Lyn for her exam, Lyn says she is on the last day of her period and figured it would be fine to have the Pap test anyway, since her flow was light. Lyn also tells the medical assistant that she and her husband are trying to get pregnant and have been having intercourse every night for the past month.

1. Will the physician be able to collect a specimen for the Pap test? Probably not because the blood cells from her menstrual cycle and the extra cells and fluid added by intercourse could interfere with a clear specimen.
2. What should the medical assistant have done before prepping the patient for the exam? She should have questioned the patient to be sure that she had followed all preparation instructions for the exam.
3. When is the best time for the patient to have her Pap test? At least five days after the menstrual period.

### Scenario 2

Amanda calls the office to report that she is cramping and spotting. She is at 28 weeks' gestation. The first available appointment the provider has is two days from now. Amanda is very anxious and asks if she is having a miscarriage.

1. What should the office scheduling person have done about an appointment time for Amanda? This is a crucial situation, and the patient should have been worked into the schedule. Your policy may be to have the patient speak with a triage nurse or the provider first.
2. What should the medical assistant tell Amanda about her condition? Nothing. The medical assistant should not diagnose or give Amanda any information or advice without the provider's approval.
3. Who should the medical assistant consult about Amanda's problems? The provider should be consulted to see whether he or she wants the patient to go to the hospital to be evaluated or to come to the clinic.

## Competency Practice

**1. Prepare the Patient for and Assist with a Gynecological Exam and Pap Test.**
In groups of four, role play preparing the patient and assisting the provider with a gynecological exam and Pap test. Assign each person in the group to one of the following roles: narrator, provider, MA, and patient. Using Procedure 41–1 and the evaluation form below, evaluate the group's performance of the procedure (including completeness and preparedness) and communication skills (verbal and nonverbal). The final calculated grade or evaluation will be determined by your evaluation, the instructor's evaluation, and the group's evaluation. The instructor will use this same evaluation form, and a combined evaluation will be used for feedback to the group.

## Group Project Evaluation

**Prepare the Patient for and Assist with a Gynecological Exam and Pap Test**

*Based on the performance, give feedback and rate your group according to the following scale:*

**1 = poor** **2 = fair** **3 = good** **4 = exceptional**

Verbal Communication **1** **2** **3** **4**

- Communication was complete and concise with only necessary information given to the patient.
- The information given to the patient was clear (using good diction and enunciating each word distinctly). The message was audible. The MA did not use technical terms with patient.
- Patient was allowed time to process the message and verify its meaning.
- MA established rapport with the patient, acknowledging the patient by name.

**Feedback:** ______________________________

______________________________

______________________________

______________________________

Nonverbal Communication **1** **2** **3** **4**

- MA smiled when greeting patient, used appropriate facial expression according to the situation, and maintained appropriate eye contact.
- Maintained a close but comfortable position facing the patient without standing over her; respected patient's personal space.
- Used appropriate gestures to enhance communication, used appropriate touch, and displayed empathy with the patient.
- Respected patient privacy by keeping patient covered during exam.

**Feedback:** ______________________________

______________________________

______________________________

______________________________

Performance **1** **2** **3** **4**

- Group performed the procedure within 25 minutes.
- MA performed or role-played each step within Procedure 41–1. (Refer to competency assessment.)
- MA carried out each step correctly, including positioning the patient.
- Group members acted professionally.

**Feedback:** ______________________________

______________________________

______________________________

______________________________

| Preparedness | 1 | 2 | 3 | 4 |
|---|---|---|---|---|

- Equipment and supplies were gathered prior to procedure.
- Group members seemed well-prepared.
- Procedure and scenario flowed naturally.
- Each member was aware of his or her role and responsibilities.

**Feedback:** ______________________________

______________________________

______________________________

______________________________

**Final Score** _______ **/ 16 pts**

CHAPTER 42

# Pediatric Examinations

## Words to Know Challenge

**Spelling: Each line contains three spellings of a word. Underline the correctly spelled word.**

| | | |
|---|---|---|
| 1. circumfrence | circumference | circumphrence |
| 2. attachment | attachtment | atachtment |
| 3. listlessness | listlesness | lislessness |
| 4. prevantive | preventive | preventiv |
| 5. intercede | interceed | intersceed |
| 6. suscpicion | suspiscion | suspicion |
| 7. malnutrition | mallnutrition | malnutrision |
| 8. letharjic | lethargic | lethargick |

**Matching: Match the key term in column I to its definition in column II.**

| | COLUMN I | COLUMN II |
|---|---|---|
| F | 1. Pediatrics | A. Attachment of two persons |
| E | 2. Apgar | B. Inflicting emotional, physical, or sexual injury |
| C | 3. Child neglect | C. Lack of or withholding of care |
| B | 4. Child abuse | D. Advancement of abilities and knowledge |
| D | 5. Development | E. Scoring system used on infants after birth |
| A | 6. Bonding | F. Specialty medical practice that cares for infants and children |
| H | 7. Caregiver | G. Arrangement of events or dates in order of occurrence |
| G | 8. Chronologic | H. Person responsible for another's care and well-being |
| J | 9. Percentile | I. Lack of vigorous growth |
| I | 10. Failure to thrive | J. Used on a growth chart to compare a child to his or her peers. |

## Chapter Review

**Fill in the Blank: Use information from the chapter to fill in the blank space in the sentence.**

1. The American Academy of Pediatrics (AAP) has established Recommendations for Preventive Pediatric Health Care, a chart that outlines the types and frequency of examinations to provide preventive care for normally developing, healthy children.
2. Pediatric care is usually continued until age 16 or 18 or upon high school graduation.
3. An infant's growth refers to changes in height and weight.
4. An infant should be examined at 2- to 3- month intervals for the first 18 months of life.
5. Poor hygiene, inadequate clothing size, and apparent malnutrition are signs of child neglect.
6. Infants usually crawl at 8–10 months of age.
7. Most infants will walk between 12 and 15 months of age.
8. The EPSDT program, Medicaid's comprehensive and preventive child health program, is for individuals under the age of 21.
9. An infant's weight should be taken with his or her clothing and diaper removed.
10. Children older than 36 months can have their height measured on an upright scale.

### Short Answer

1. Explain the difference between child abuse and neglect. Abuse involves causing physical or mental harm, whereas neglect pertains to not providing adequate care, feeding, and hygiene to an infant or child.
2. List five signs of abuse.
   Any five of the following: (1) Discoloration or bruising of the skin; (2) Burns; (3) Suspicious story about an injury; (4) Reports by the child of sexual or physical abuse; (5) Internal abdominal pain; (6) Dislocation of joints such as the wrist or shoulder; (7) Frequent injuries requiring medical attention.
3. List five signs of neglect.
   Any five of the following: (1) Excessive length of time before seeking medical attention for an injury; (2) Apparent malnutrition; (3) Poor hygiene; (4) Inadequate clothing for season or size; unclean; (5) Developmental delay; (6) Obvious lack of dental care.
4. Explain the difference between a well-child and a sick-child visit. A well-child exam is a routine exam or visit as identified on the Recommendations for Preventive Pediatric Health Care chart. Specific well-child hours are usually set aside in each day's schedule to perform routine examinations and procedures. However, when a child is ill or has symptoms of an illness, pediatricians will attempt to see the child within a few hours of a parent's call. Parents can usually phone the pediatrician's office at all hours of the day or night, and someone who is on call will respond. Practices may also set aside early office hours to see children who have become ill overnight.
5. List five responsibilities of the medical assistant when assisting with pediatric exams. Any five of the following can be listed: Assist in gathering data, document information, perform screening tests within your skill and ability level, assist the patient, assist the provider, and provide patient education.
6. Identify immunizations given to 2- and 12-month-old children according to the Childhood and Adolescent Immunization Schedule. Refer to the annual Recommended Childhood and Adolescent Immunization Schedules for children in the United States released by the CDC to identify the immunizations given. A variety is recommended.
7. Identify two charts that assess pediatric vision acuity and explain how each is used.
   The Snellen big E chart requires the child to indicate with his or her fingers which way the E is facing. The Es become smaller and less bold as the acuity gets more difficult. Results are recorded on the last line correctly identified, the same as with adults on the regular screening chart. The kindergarten version of the chart uses various shapes and symbols in descending size to evaluate vision.

# Chapter Application

## Case Studies with Critical Thinking Questions

### Scenario 1

Jane, the medical assistant, escorts a 19-year-old single mother and her 6-month-old infant to the exam room. Jane observes that both the mother and child are wearing soiled clothing. The mother's hygiene is poor, and the infant has dried mucous around his nose and food stuck to his cheeks. While weighing and measuring the infant, Jane notices red marks on his bottom and his thigh.

1. What could Jane's observations indicate? Both neglect and abuse could be indicated ________.
2. What should Jane do about what she has observed? Alert the provider about the observations. Depending on the provider's findings, child protective services may need to be alerted ________.

### Scenario 2

Mrs. Leonard brings her son, Carter, into the office for his well-child check-up. He is very agitated today, and Amy, the medical assistant, is having a great deal of difficulty measuring and weighing him. Amy tries to measure his recumbent length with a tape measure but is not sure whether she can obtain an accurate measurement because she is unable to straighten the child's legs. Carter is squirming on the scale, and it is difficult to balance it. When Amy attempts to record the measurement on Carter's growth chart, she finds that the measurements are lower than at his last visit.

1. What should Amy do about the discrepancy in the measurements? The measurements need to be repeated because the infant is expected to have grown and gained some weight since his last checkup ________.
2. Were Amy's methods of measurement accurate? No, the recumbent length should be measured from the vertex of the head to the heel ________.
3. What could Amy have done to help remedy the situation? Amy should have asked Mrs. Leonard or a coworker to help her hold the infant ________.

## Competency Practice

1. **Measure Length, Weight, and Head and Chest Circumference of an Infant or Child.** Use infant and child mannequins and practice obtaining the length, weight, head circumference, and chest circumference. Use Procedure 42–1 as a guide. Document a mock patient chart entry in the following space or enter into an EMR and on a growth chart. You can download appropriate growth charts from the CDC's Website at www.cdc.gov.

2. **Plot Data on Growth Chart.** Use the following scenario information and a growth chart to practice plotting measurements on growth charts for both female and male patients and age groups. Be sure also to fill in the data on the bottom of the growth chart with the measurements provided. Use Procedure 42–2 as a guide. You can download appropriate growth charts from the CDC's website at www.cdc.gov.

A. Use a growth chart for **GIRLS** to plot the following measurements.

| Age | Weight | Length |
|---|---|---|
| 1 month | 8 lb. 10 oz. | 21" |
| 2 months | 11 lb. 6 oz. | 22 ½" |
| 3 months | 14 lb. 8 oz. | 24" |
| 6 months | 18 lb. | 26 ½" |
| 9 months | 23 lb. 4 oz. | 28 ¼" |
| 12 months | 24 lb. 7 oz. | 31 ½" |
| 15 months | 26 lb. 10 oz. | 32" |

B. Use a growth chart for **BOYS** to plot the following measurements.

| Age | Head Circumference Measurement |
|---|---|
| 1 month | 14 ¾" |
| 6 months | 17 ½" |
| 12 months | 18 ½' |
| 20 months | 19 ¼" |
| 32 months | 20" |

C. Calculate the percentile of WEIGHT FOR LENGTH and plot, using the example growth chart for **BOYS**. Use rounded numbers to the nearest 5% (for example, 10%, 15%, 20%; not 13%).

| Weight | Length | Percentile |
|---|---|---|
| 8# | 20 ½" | 50% |
| 12# | 24" | 25% |
| 25# | 30 ¾" | 80% |
| 28# | 32"" | 90% |
| 36# | 38" | 95% |

3. **Screen Pediatric Visual Acuity with a Modified Snellen Chart.** With a partner, have one person role play a child patient and the other person the medical assistant. Take turns screening visual acuity with one of the modified Snellen charts listed in the chapter. When finished, document a mock patient chart entry in the following space or enter into an EMR. Use Procedure 42–3 as a guide.

UNIT 14

# Laboratory Procedures

CHAPTER 43

# Blood Specimen Collection

## Words to Know Challenge

**Spelling: Each line contains three spellings of a word. Underline the correctly spelled word.**

| | | |
|---|---|---|
| 1. hemotoma | hematoma | hemitoma |
| 2. tourniquet | tournequet | tournequette |
| 3. flebotomy | phelbotomy | phlebotomy |
| 4. elasticity | elastizity | ilasticity |
| 5. plazma | palasma | plasma |

**Matching: Match the term in column I to its description in column II.**

| | COLUMN I | COLUMN II |
|---|---|---|
| G | 1. Venipuncture | A. Without any organisms |
| A | 2. Sterile | B. To scatter or spread |
| D | 3. Lancet | C. Pertaining to a vein |
| B | 4. Diffuse | D. Used for a skin puncture |
| F | 5. Puncture | E. The size of a needle bore |
| C | 6. Venous | F. A hole made by something pointed |
| E | 7. Gauge | G. The surgical puncture of a vein |

## Chapter Review

### Short Answer

1. Why is it important for the lancet to be positioned to cut across the fingerprints rather than parallel to them?
When made across the fingerprints, blood will form a bead that makes blood collection easier. When made parallel to fingerprints, the blood will most likely run down the fingerprints, making collection difficult
___________________________________________.

2. Why should the lateral sides of the infant's heel be used for capillary puncture?
   Nerve and bone damage can occur if the middle of the heel is used for collection of capillary blood in infants; there are no nerves or bony tissue in the lateral side of the infant's heel.

3. Why is the first drop of blood wiped away from the capillary puncture site?
   The first drop of blood contains tissue fluid that will dilute the specimen and jeopardize the reliability of the test results.

4. Identify the acceptable sites to perform a capillary puncture on a patient's hand.
   The ring finger and the great finger

5. During the venipuncture procedure, the tourniquet should not remain on the patient's arm for more than how long?
   1 minute (60 seconds)

6. What is the medical term for abnormal collection of blood immediately below the surface of the skin?
   Hematoma

7. The destruction of red blood cells is known as what?
   Hemolysis

**Matching: Match the item in column I with its description in column II.**

| | COLUMN I | COLUMN II |
|---|---|---|
| B | 1. EDTA | A. Sodium heparin |
| H | 2. Gray stopper | B. Hematology testing, purple stopper |
| J | 3. Syringe | C. Blood cultures |
| G | 4. Butterfly | D. Serum separator tube (SST) |
| C | 5. Yellow stopper | E. Evacuated tube holder |
| I | 6. Red stopper | F. Prevents clotting |
| D | 7. Mustard or speckled stopper | G. Multi-sample needle for small veins |
| A | 8. Green stopper | H. Sodium fluoride, blood glucose |
| E | 9. Multi-sample capability | I. No additive |
| F | 10. Anticoagulant | J. Single-use venous collection device |
| L | 11. Blue stopper | K. Anticoagulant tubes |
| K | 12. Plasma | L. Sodium citrate, coagulation studies |

# Chapter Application

## Case Studies with Critical Thinking Questions

### Scenario 1

Ben has arrived for a venous blood test to check his liver function levels and glucose. In the process of collecting the specimen, you notice a hematoma is beginning to form and you have not completed filling all the necessary tubes for the tests.

1. Why would a hematoma develop as a result of phlebotomy?
   Usually, a hematoma is a result of air getting into the site as well as blood leaking from the vessel during the venipuncture process.

2. What should you do?
   When you notice a hematoma developing, immediately stop the collection of the specimen. Remove the tourniquet FIRST and then withdraw the needle and apply pressure to the site (to help minimize the size of the hematoma and the resulting bruise)

### Scenario 2

Mrs. Johnson has a laboratory order for you to collect a capillary specimen for a random blood glucose level. You assemble your supplies in preparation of collecting and testing the specimen; when you grasp her hand, you notice her hand is exceptionally cold.

1. What do Mrs. Johnson's cold hands indicate?
   Cold hands usually indicate that the patient has poor circulation and will not be ideal for a capillary collection
2. What instructions should you give Mrs. Johnson?
   Ask her to wash her hands in warm water to help restore circulation to her fingers. You can also place a warm heating pad on the Mrs. Johnson's hands to warm her fingers; you want to make sure the patient's hands are warm so you can collect the specimen easily

### Competency Practice: Place the following steps of the capillary puncture procedure in their proper order from 1 to 10.

8 — 1. Collect the specimen.

1 — 2. Introduce yourself and identify the patient.

2 — 3. Assemble the necessary supplies.

7 — 4. Wipe away the first drop of blood.

9 — 5. Provide the patient with a clean gauze or cotton ball to apply pressure to the site.

6 — 6. Perform the puncture with the lancet, penetrating across the fingerprints.

5 — 7. Allow the selected site to dry.

4 — 8. Disinfect the site with alcohol.

3 — 9. Don gloves.

10 — 10. Dispose of lancet and contaminated materials in the appropriate biohazard containers.

### Role-Play Activities

1. Working with a partner, practice how you would explain the venipuncture procedure and capillary puncture procedure to your patient.
2. Practice palpating different classmates' veins. Try with your eyes open and eyes closed! (*Hint*: You should go by feel, *not* sight!)
3. Working with a partner, practice tying tourniquets on each other.
4. Working with a partner, pretend one of you is a patient and one is the medical assistant. Prepare the patient's arm by tying on the tourniquet and, just as you are going to perform the venipuncture, the patient (your classmate) faints! Practice removing the tourniquet quickly and ensuring that your patient is safe.

C H A P T E R **44**

# The Physician's Office Laboratory

## Words to Know Challenge

**Spelling: Each line contains three spellings of a word. Underline the correctly spelled word.**

| | | |
|---|---|---|
| 1. binnoculir | binocular | binoculare |
| 2. compensate | conpemsate | compensait |
| 3. prophicent | proficient | proficiant |
| 4. microscopie | microscopee | microscopy |
| 5. monocular | moncular | nomocular |
| 6. waved | waived | wiaved |
| 7. assurance | asurance | asurrance |

**Matching: Match each part of the microscope in column I with its description in column II.**

| | COLUMN I | COLUMN II |
|---|---|---|
| C | 1. Condenser | A. The result of combining the ocular and the lens for observation of a specimen |
| G | 2. Objectives | B. An adjective describing the size of articles examined microscopically |
| H | 3. Hpf | C. Part of the substage that regulates the amount of light directed on a specimen |
| F | 4. Ocular | D. The part of the microscope on which slides are placed for viewing |
| A | 5. Magnification | E. Part of the microscope that helps bring the specimen on the slide into sharper view |
| B | 6. Minute | F. Three or four small lenses that have different magnifying powers |
| D | 7. Stage | G. Magnifies an object about 10 times |
| G | 8. Lpf | H. Magnifies an object about 40 times |

# Chapter Review

## Short Answer

1. Explain why quality assurance (QA) and quality control (QC) are of the utmost importance in any laboratory setting.
   QA ensures that the instruments, reagents, and technician technique remain constant to ensure that patient results are reported without compromise. QC is a daily part of the QA and ensures that any results that are outside of manufacturer's range is investigated; no patient results may be reported until cause is found.

2. Identify three categories of testing within the laboratory setting.
   a. Waived
   b. Moderately complex
   c. Highly complex

3. List four forms of basic recommended personal protective equipment (PPE) that can be used when collecting specimens from patients.
   a. Gloves
   b. Face shields
   c. Fluid-resistant lab coats
   d. Respirators for airborne pathogens

4. Why is proper hand washing an important consideration when working in the laboratory and with patients?
   Prevents cross-contamination between patients, patients and workers, specimens and patients, and specimens and workers

5. List and define two of the regulatory bodies the POL falls under.
   a. CLIA – Clinical Laboratory Improvement Amendments
   b. OSHA – Occupational Safety and Health Administration

# Chapter Application

## Role-Play Activity

Pretend you are the manager of the lab. Role-play with another student how you would train him or her in proper maintenance and transport of the microscope.

## Research Activity

Go online and research the regulatory bodies that govern the POL.

a. Compare and contrast each body.

b. Next, research what types of monetary fines a laboratory might face by being noncompliant with the three regulatory bodies.

c. Present your findings in a written report.

CHAPTER 45

# Diagnostic Testing

## Words to Know Challenge

**Spelling: Each line contains three spellings of a word. Underline the correctly spelled word.**

| | | |
|---|---|---|
| 1. poloysithemia | policythemia | polycythemia |
| 2. wheel | wheal | weal |
| 3. allergie | alergy | allergy |
| 4. glycohemoglobin | glycohemaglobin | glycohemeglobin |
| 5. esinofil | esinophil | eosinophil |
| 6. imunology | immoonology | immunology |
| 7. mononuclosis | mononucleosis | mononucleusis |

**Matching: Match the term in column I with its description in column II.**

| | COLUMN I | COLUMN II |
|---|---|---|
| E | 1. Antibody | A. Released in allergic and inflammatory reactions |
| D | 2. Immune | B. Of or pertaining to the whole body |
| G | 3. Venom | C. Immunizing agent that produces antibodies |
| A | 4. Histamine | D. Protected or exempt from disease |
| B | 5. Systemic | E. A protein substance carried by cells to counteract effects of an antigen |
| C | 6. Antigen | F. A substance distilled or drawn out of another substance |
| F | 7. Extract | G. A poisonous toxin produced by several groups of animal species |

## Chapter Review

### Short Answer

1. What two tests are commonly used in screening for anemia?
   Hemoglobin and hematocrit

2. What test is used for diagnosis of diabetes mellitus?
   Glucose tolerance test (GTT)

3. Name two diseases associated with hypercholesterolemia.
   Arteriosclerosis and atherosclerosis

4. Name two tests that may be performed in the POL for immunology testing.
   Mononucleosis testing and allergy testing

5. What are the proper units of measurement for reporting hemoglobin and hematocrit results?
   Hemoglobin is reported as g/dL, and hematocrit is reported as a percent

6. Describe patient education regarding allergy injections.
   Inform patients that they should follow the schedule closely, avoid what they are allergic to, read labels on products to identify possible allergens, practice good health habits, take only prescribed medications, and if highly allergic to a particular substance, carry their kit at all times

7. What are signs and symptoms of anaphylactic shock? What can be injected to prevent anaphylactic shock?
   Intense anxiety, weakness, sweating, and shortness of breath. Adrenaline (epinephrine) can be injected to prevent anaphylactic shock

8. When performing intradermal tests, the antigen is introduced into the dermal layer of skin in what dosages?
   0.01 mL to 0.02 mL by sterile technique

9. From the following test results, place an X next to the values that would be considered a panic value.
   a. Hemoglobin (male), test result 10 g/dL: X (Panic value)
   b. Hematocrit (female), test result 40%: Normal
   c. Total cholesterol, test result 150 mg/dL: Normal
   d. Sodium (Na), test result 160 mEq/L: X (Panic value)
   e. BUN, test result 15 mg/dL: Normal
   f. Potassium (K), test result 6.0 mEq/L: X (Panic value)

**Matching I: Match the items in column I to their descriptions in column II.**

| | COLUMN I | COLUMN II |
|---|---|---|
| D | 1. Normal male hemoglobin | A. 4.0 to 5.5 million/cubic mm |
| S | 2. Normal WBC | B. Type of allergy test |
| T | 3. Normal female ESR | C. Virus that causes infectious mononucleosis |
| I | 4. PKU | D. 14–18 g/dL |
| P | 5. Normal glucose | E. ESR |
| K | 6. Normal cholesterol | F. 4.5 to 6.0 million/cubic mm |
| G | 7. Normal female hemoglobin | G. 12–16 g/dL |
| J | 8. Normal male ESR | H. Measures glycosylated hemoglobin |
| R | 9. Normal female Hct | I. Required in all states and Canada |
| F | 10. Normal male RBC | J. 0–10 mm/hr |
| M | 11. Normal male Hct | K. Below 200 mg/dL fasting |
| A | 12. Normal female RBC | L. Requires immediate attention by the health care provider |
| O | 13. Polycythemia | M. 40%–50% |
| E | 14. Test for nonspecific tissue damage | N. Glucose |
| N | 15. Screen for diabetes | O. Abnormal increase in all blood cells |
| Q | 16. Equals Hgb x 3 + 3 | P. Below 126 mg/dL fasting |
| C | 17. Epstein-Barr virus | Q. Hematocrit |
| B | 18. RAST | R. 37%–47% |
| H | 19. Hemoglobin A1C | S. 3500–11,000 |
| L | 20. panic value | T. 0–20 mm/hr |

# Chapter Application

## Research Activity

1. Go online and research types of glucometers available for patients to use. Choose three glucometers and write a brief narrative that:
   a. Compares and contrasts each glucometer.
   b. Describes which one you would prefer to use and why.

## Role-Play Activity

Pretend that you are the lead MA in the back office. You are responsible for training new employees on the allergy injection process. Practice with a classmate how you would train the employee and what you would explain and demonstrate.

## Case Studies with Critical Thinking Questions

### Scenario 1

Amy has come to the laboratory requesting that you check her hemoglobin level because she is feeling tired, is short of breath, and is sleeping more than usual. After checking with the health care provider in your office, you perform a hemoglobin test on Amy and find that her hemoglobin result is 6.0 mg/dL.

1. What does this result indicate? This value would be considered a panic value and requires immediate attention from the provider

2. What action should you take? You should ask Amy to remain in the office and report the results immediately to the health care provider. The health care provider will want to examine Amy to assess her condition for further investigative laboratory studies to determine the cause of the anemia

### Scenario 2

Mrs. Morris brings her 7-year-old son to your office to be tested for allergies. He seems to be having a lot of difficulty with congestion, sneezing, and coughing. You administer the scratch test and have been told to watch the patient closely for any severe reactions. Almost immediately, wheals begin to develop, and several swell to a +4 in a very short period of time. Mrs. Morris' son complains that his tongue feels big, and he can't breathe very well.

1. Based on the skin reactions, what could be happening to the patient? The patient appears to be having a severe allergic reaction to the allergens, possibly an anaphylactic reaction

2. What will the provider most likely do to help the patient? The physician will most likely administer epinephrine to counteract the allergens

CHAPTER 46

# Specimen Collection and Processing

## Words to Know Challenge

**Spelling: Each line contains three spellings of a word. Underline the correctly spelled word.**

| | | |
|---|---|---|
| 1. guiac | gauiac | guaiac |
| 2. bilirubin | billirubin | biliribun |
| 3. urineanalysis | urinalisys | urinalysis |
| 4. hemoturia | hematuria | hemituria |
| 5. uribilinogen | uribilinogin | urobilinogen |

**Fill in the Blank: Complete the following sentences with Words to Know from this chapter.**

. Substance used to encourage bacterial growth: agar

. The final step in the culture during which various antibiotics are tested for bacterial inhibition: sensitivity

. Bacterial staining characteristic that yields a pinkish-red color: Gram negative

. Bacterial staining characteristic that yields a bluish-purple color: Gram positive

. Drainage from a wound or affected area: exudate

. The first step in the process to isolate and identify bacterial infections: culture

. The destruction of red blood cells present in culture media: hemolysis

## Chapter Review

### Short Answer

. What is a culturette?
A sterile swab with a soft tip, protected by a plastic sleeve, used to collect cultures from various sources; an ampule is crushed to protect the integrity of the specimen after collection

2. When obtaining a throat swab for group A strep screening, what is the proper procedure for performing the swab? Do not allow the swab to touch the tongue, teeth, lips, or gums; guide the swab to the peritonsillar crypt area and collect any exudate you observe.

3. Identify three elements of a complete urinalysis. Physical, chemical, microscopic

4. Discuss the differences among random, first morning, clean-catch midstream, and 24-hour urine specimens.
   a. Random: Collected at any time of the day without special preparation
   b. First morning specimen: Collected when the patient first wakes up in the morning and is the most concentrated, yielding the most accurate results
   c. Clean-catch midstream: Requires the patient to clean external genitalia prior to collection of the specimen
   d. 24-hour specimen: Requires patient to begin timing from the first morning specimen at the onset of the 24-hour period, discard that specimen, and collect all subsequent specimens within the 24-hour time period

5. Name the three morphologic shapes and provide a description of each.
   (1) Coccus—berry-shaped or round; (2) Bacillus—rod-shaped; (3) Spirochete—spiral-shaped

6. Identify types of pathogens that can be checked for in fecal specimens.
   Ova, parasites, bacteria, and viruses

7. Which conditions might be diagnosed in a sputum specimen?
   Cancer, tuberculosis, bacterial infections, fungal infections, and viral infections

**Matching: Match the item in column I with its description in column II.**

| | COLUMN I | COLUMN II |
|---|---|---|
| H | 1. Normal fecal occult blood | A. Confirmatory test for urinary ketones |
| J | 2. Specific gravity | B. Blood in the urine |
| C | 3. pH | C. Normal urine, slightly acidic |
| I | 4. Bilirubin | D. Positive in starvation |
| D | 5. Ketones | E. Confirmatory test for urinary protein |
| E | 6. SSA | F. Confirmatory test for urinary bilirubin |
| A | 7. Acetest | G. Pregnancy |
| F | 8. Ictotest | H. Negative |
| B | 9. Hematuria | I. Might indicate liver disease when detected |
| G | 10. Human chorionic gonadotropin | J. Concentration or dilution of urine specimen |

**True or False: Place a T for true or F for false in the space provided. For false statements, explain why they are false.**

T 1. The physical testing of urine includes assessment of the color, clarity, odor, and specific gravity.

T 2. Tuberculosis is cultivated through inoculation onto a Lowenstein-Jensen slant.

F 3. It takes a minimum of four days before a culture and sensitivity report is completed.
Most culture and sensitivity results are available within a 48-hour time frame.

F 4. The majority of urine specimens will have a pH of 7.0–9.0.
The majority of urine specimens will have a pH value of 5.0–6.5.

T 5. When bacteria are present in sufficient numbers in the urine, nitrate will be reduced to nitrite by the bacterial metabolism.

F 6. Glucose is normally found in urine specimens.
Glucose is normally reabsorbed by the renal tubules and not excreted in the urine.

T 7. The four components of the Gram stain include the primary stain, mordant, decolorizer, and counterstain.

F 8. The only way to test for group A strep is a routine culture.
Several rapid tests are available on the market that yield quick results.

T 9. Special collection procedures must be used when collecting urine drug-screening specimens.

T 10. The specific gravity of most urine specimens falls in the range of 1.005–1.030

T 11. The lower respiratory tract is considered sterile.

T 12. Leukocyte esterase will be positive in pyuria.

F 13. A small amount of urobilinogen in the urine is a poor prognosis for a patient.
Urobilinogen is normally found in the urine in small amounts as a result of bacterial action in the intestinal tract.

T 14. Sputum specimens may be screened for cancer, using the same staining technique as routine gynecologic screening.

F 15. If the fecal occult blood is positive, the specimen on the slide will have a purple color.
If the fecal occult blood is positive, the specimen on the slide will have a blue color.

# Chapter Application

## Case Studies with Critical Thinking Questions

### Scenario

You are working in a multi-practice clinic that has an in-house laboratory, including a microbiology lab. Part of your duties in the laboratory includes checking and recording temperatures for all refrigerators, freezers, and incubators used in the facility. You are checking the microbiology incubators and discover that one of them is registering a temperature of 10 degrees Celsius.

1. Should you report this to anyone and, if so, who?
   This should be reported to the microbiology supervisor immediately. Cultures grow better at the same temperature as the human body (37 degrees Celsius)
   ________________________________________.

2. What is a possible result of this temperature decrease?
   This decrease in the temperature of the incubator will cause the organisms not to grow as quickly or not at all, resulting in a possible false negative report by the microbiologist reviewing the plates
   ________________________________________.

### Role-Play Activities

1. Research the health risks of untreated streptococcal infections. Write a short narrative of your findings and why these types of infections should be treated.

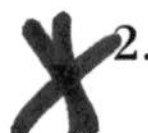

2. With a partner, role play as a medical assistant and patient and take turns explaining the various types of urine collection.

UNIT 15

# Cardiology and Radiology Procedures

CHAPTER 47

# Cardiology Procedures

## Words to Know Challenge

**Spelling: Each line contains three spellings of a word. Underline the correctly spelled word.**

1. amplyfier — amplifier — amplafyer
2. arrhythmia — arrythmia — arethmia
3. defibrillator — defibrelator — defibralader
4. eckocardiography — echocardiography — echoecardiography
5. eckoes — echoes — eckows
6. interferance — enterference — interference
7. interpretive — interpretiv — interpratif
8. meckanical — machanical — mechanical
9. multichannel — multichanel — multychannel
10. relyable — reliable — relieable
11. simaltaneous — simultanius — simultaneous
12. current — currant — curant

**Matching: Match the key term in column I to its definition in column II.**

| | COLUMN I | COLUMN II |
|---|---|---|
| D | 1. Artifacts | A. Enlarged |
| K | 2. Somatic | B. Portion of ECG between two waves |
| B | 3. Segment | C. Little activity |
| M | 4. Repolarization | D. Additional electrical activity |
| H | 5. Purkinje | E. Changes impulses into mechanical motion |
| A | 6. Augmented | F. Chest leads |
| C | 7. Sedentary | G. Difference in electrical potential |
| E | 8. Galvanometer | H. Fibers that cause muscles of the ventricle to contract |
| F | 9. Precordial | I. Momentary surge of current |
| G | 10. Voltage | J. Provides a reliable reading |
| N | 11. Interval | K. Muscle voltage artifacts |
| O | 12. Electrodes | L. Provides printed representations of ECG paper |
| J | 13. Standardization | M. Period when heart momentarily relaxes |
| I | 14. Impulse | N. Length of a wave |
| L | 15. Stylus | O. Sensors that pick up electrical impulses |

## Chapter Review

**Fill in the Blank: Using information from the chapter, fill in the blank spaces in the following sentences.**

1. All muscle movement produces electrical impulses and activity. An electrical impulse originates in the modified myocardial tissue in the SA (sinoatrial) node.
2. The current enters the electrocardiograph through the wires to reach the amplifier. Electrical impulses are transformed into mechanical motion by the galvanometer. A(n) stylus produces printed representations on ECG paper.
3. The routine ECG consists of 12 leads. The ECG is interpreted by the provider.
4. The standardization of the ECG is necessary to enable a provider to judge deviations from the standard. The usual standardization mark is 2 mm wide and 10 mm high.
5. The patient must be relaxed for a good tracing to be obtained. The tracing paper is normally run at a speed of 25 mm/second. If the ECG tracing is too large, the sensitivity should be turned down to one half.
6. Patients should keep a diary of their activities and symptoms during a 24-hour Holter monitor also known as a 24-hour ECG. Before applying the device to the patient, it is important to check the batteries and make sure it is in proper working order.
7. ECG stress tests are done by some providers on a routine basis for patients with a high risk of developing heart disease. They are more often done in a limited manner for patients interested in starting a strenuous exercise program or those who continue to have chest pain even after a routine ECG has been read as normal.
8. Echocardiography is a noninvasive diagnostic tool that tests the structure and function of the heart through the use of sound waves, or echoes reflected through the heart.
9. A defibrillator is designed to provide countershock by a trained individual to convert cardiac arrhythmias into regular sinus rhythm.

**Labeling: Label these diagrams of the ECG cycle.**

1. Place the correct letter for each wave of the ECG tracing on the line next to the number on the following diagram.

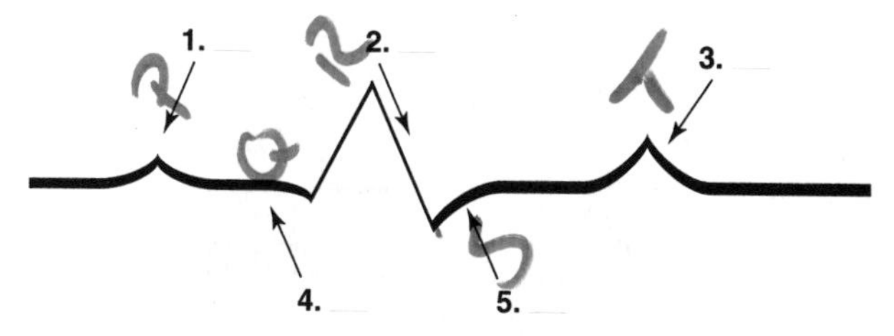

1. P
2. R
3. T
4. G
5. S

2. Label the following numbered lines with the correct name of each area of the electrical conduction through the heart.

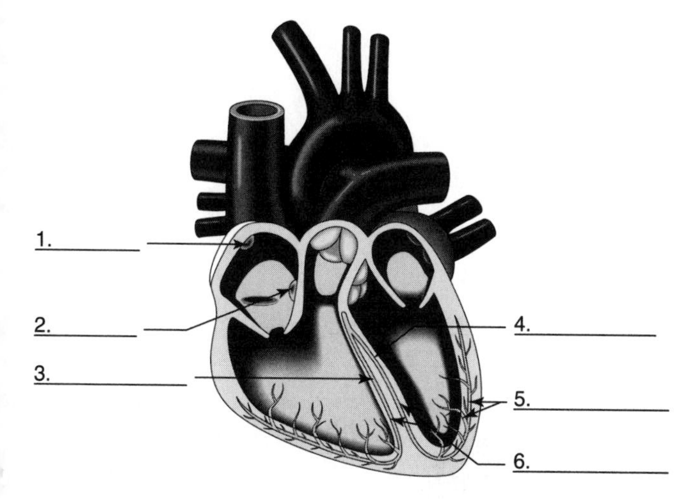

1. SA node
2. AV node
3. Right bundle branch
4. Left bundle branch
5. Bundle of HIS
6. Purkinje fibers

3. Label the following ECG tracings. State whether they are arrhythmias or interference artifacts.

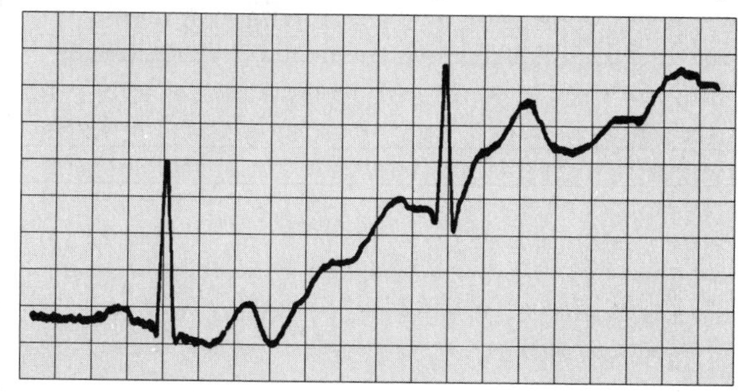

a. Wandering baseline—Interference artifact

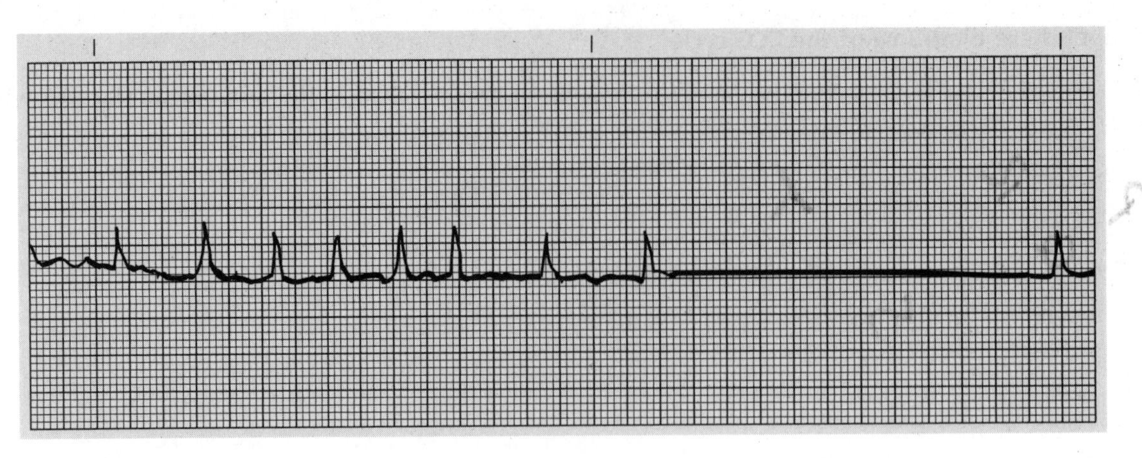

b. Atrial fibrillation with sinus pause—Arrhythmia

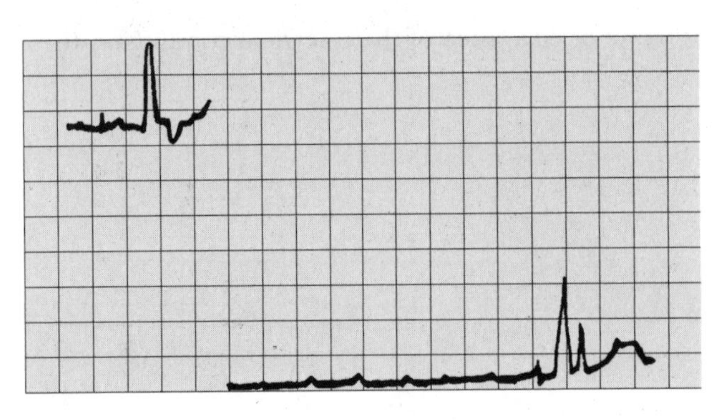

c. Interrupted baseline—Interference artifact

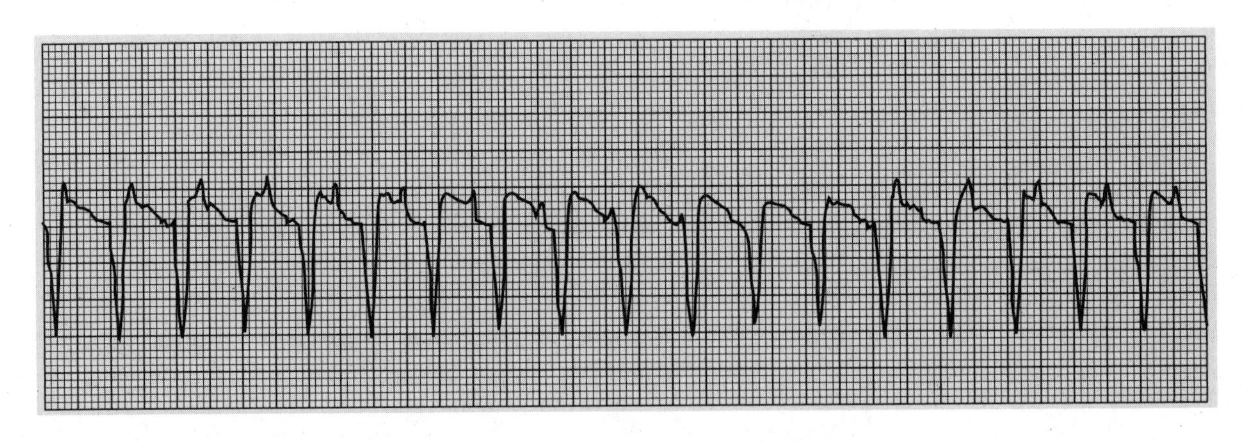

d. Ventricular tachycardia—Arrhythmia

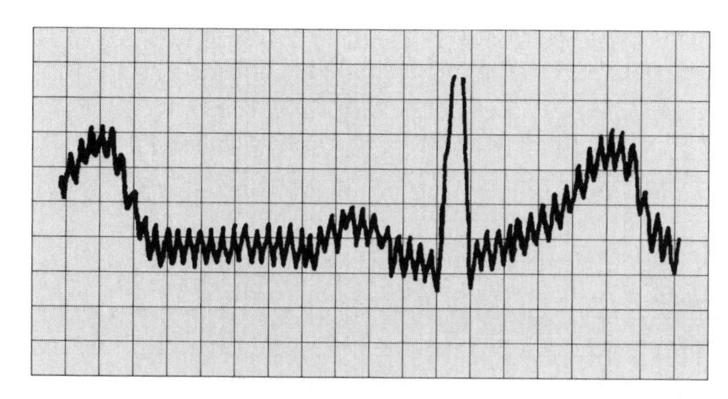

e. Alternating current—Interference artifact

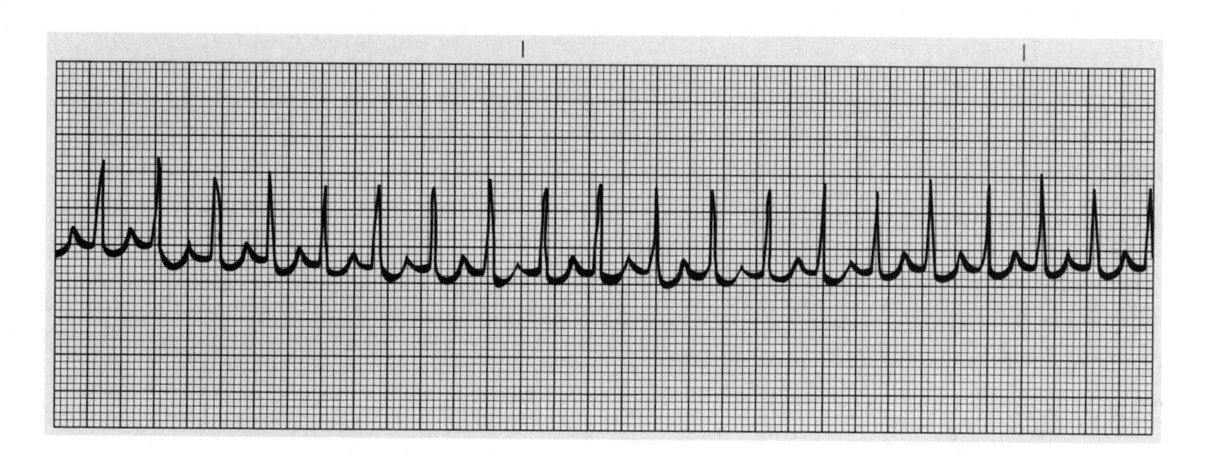

f. Paroxysmal atrial tachycardia—Arrhythmia

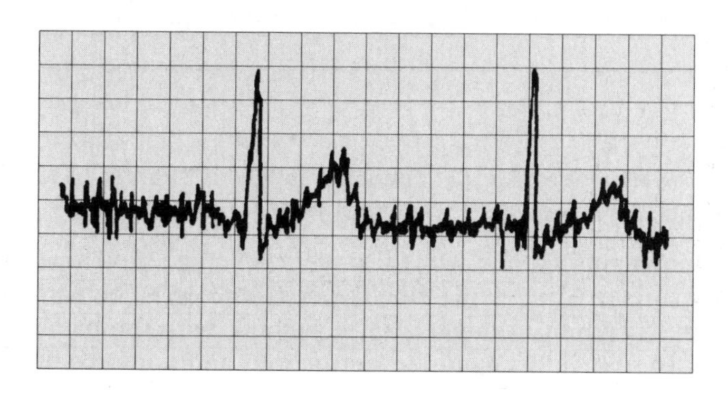

g. Somatic tremor/muscle movement—Interference artifact

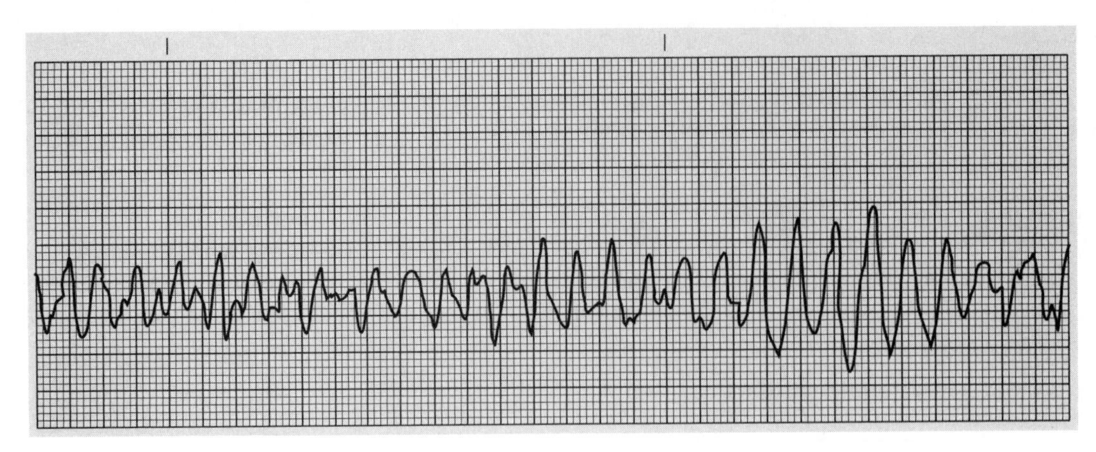

h. Ventricular fibrillation—Arrhythmia

## Chapter Application

### Case Studies with Critical Thinking Questions

#### Scenario 1

You are preparing to do an ECG on a female patient who appears to be very apprehensive about the procedure. She tells you that she has never had an ECG before; she is fearful of all the wires and afraid she will receive an electric shock.

1. What can you do to calm the patient's fears? Gently explain the procedure to the patient, stressing the fact that the machine does not discharge electricity, but rather measures the electrical impulses coming from the heart.
2. What should you do to ensure that the patient is calm and doesn't move during the procedure? Explain that the procedure will take a short time to record after all the leads are in place and that it is important for her not to talk or move because this will cause interference on the recording. Also, be sure the patient is warm enough to prevent shivering.

#### Scenario 2

You have been asked to apply a Holter monitor to a 79-year-old male patient. The patient is slightly hard of hearing and is quite confused about this machine, which he has to take home and wear.

1. What is the best way to explain the procedure to the patient? Explain why the patient is being asked to wear the monitor and go over the instructions with the patient. When explaining the dos and don'ts, be sure to have written instructions the patient can take home with him. It might also be helpful, with the patient's permission, to have a family member present who can fully understand the instructions and reinforce them after the patient returns home.
2. What must be stressed to the patient so that a proper recording is obtained? The patient must be told not to bathe or get the unit wet and not to remove any of the electrodes during the recording.
3. What can you do to ensure patient compliance? Explain to the patient how important it is to follow all directions exactly so the provider can obtain an accurate reading. If the reading is not usable, the recording will have to be repeated.

## Competency Practice

1. **Obtain a standard 12-lead ECG.** With a partner, demonstrate the proper hookup of the ECG electrodes and lead wires and run an ECG on your partner. Watch for interference and artifacts; adjust and rerun the tracing if necessary. Use Procedure 47–1 as a guide.

2. **Demonstrate the procedure for proper hookup of a Holter monitor.** With a partner, demonstrate hooking you partner up for a 24-hour Holter monitor. Provide patient education including what the patient may and may not do. Go over the patient activity diary and explain to the patient what he or she must keep track of. When completed, practice taking the Holter monitor off the patient and preparing it for storage. Use Procedure 47–2 as a guide.

CHAPTER 48

# Radiology Procedures

## Words to Know Challenge

**Spelling: Each line contains three spellings of a word. Underline the correctly spelled word.**

| | | |
|---|---|---|
| 1. distenze | distends | destends |
| 2. flatus | flates | flatis |
| 3. iodine | eyeodine | iodyne |
| 4. rentgen | roentgen | reantgen |
| 5. macherity | maturity | michrity |
| 6. systoscopy | cystascopy | cystoscopy |
| 7. electron | electran | elecktron |
| 8. ennema | enama | enema |
| 9. conjunction | congunction | cunjunction |
| 10. flexable | flexible | flecksable |
| 11. fluroscope | floroscope | fluoroscope |
| 12. thareputic | theraputic | therapeutic |
| 13. radiopaqe | radiopaiqe | radiopaque |

**Matching: Match the key term in column I to its definition in column II.**

| | COLUMN I | COLUMN II |
|---|---|---|
| J | 1. Maturity | A. Fear of being enclosed |
| A | 2. Claustrophobia | B. Used to treat cancer |
| I | 3. Sonogram | C. Laxatives and enemas |
| B | 4. Therapeutic radiation | D. Flat plate of abdomen |
| H | 5. Mammography | E. Perform with sterile catheter in conjunction with cystoscopy |
| C | 6. Evacuants | F. Barium and water mixture |
| G | 7. IVP | G. Defines structures of the urinary system |
| D | 8. KUB | H. X-ray of different angles of breast tissue |
| F | 9. Contrast media | I. High-frequency sound waves conducted through a transducer |
| E | 10. Retrograde pyelogram | J. Full development |

## Chapter Review

**Fill in the Blank: Use information from the chapter to fill in the blank space in the sentence.**

1. Diagnostic X-rays are contraindicated in pregnant women, especially during the first trimester.
2. Carbonated and alcoholic beverages should be avoided prior to X-rays of the visceral organs because they produce flatus.
3. A voiding cystogram may be ordered along with a(n) IVP.
4. Nuclear medicine uses radionuclides in the diagnosis and treatment of patients.
5. A KUB X-ray is helpful in determining the position of an intrauterine device (IUD).
6. Breast self-examination is recommended monthly for women of all ages.
7. An upper GI series is also referred to as a barium swallow.
8. To reduce the possible effects of swelling and soreness often caused by compression of the breasts during mammography, instruct the patient to omit caffeine from her diet 7 to 10 days prior to examination. Compression of the breasts during mammography allows a much clearer picture of breast tissue and requires less radiation.

### Short Answer

1. What are roentgen rays? Roentgen rays are high-energy electromagnetic radiation produced by the collision of a beam of electrons with a metal target in an X-ray tube.
2. What are therapeutic X-rays used for? Treatment of cancer.
3. What types of symptoms do patients experience if the gallbladder malfunctions? When the gallbladder malfunctions, the patient experiences abdominal discomfort, nausea, and pain.

4. What food should patients avoid if they have gallbladder trouble? Patients with gallbladder trouble should avoid fats, fatty foods, alcohol, and caffeine.

5. Why must the digestive tract be free of foods during an upper GI series? The digestive tract should be clear of all foods to avoid blockage or shadows on the anatomical structures to be observed.

6. Why is air contrast sometimes ordered with a barium enema examination? The air-contrast procedure is performed with a barium enema to distend the colon and make the structures more visible by fluoroscope.

7. What is an IVP? An IVP (intravenous pyelogram) is a study of the genitourinary system, consisting of an intravenous injection of iodine to define the structures.

8. Describe the method of radiology called a CAT (computerized axial tomography) scan. Rapid scanning of single-tissue planes performed by a process that generates images of the tissue in slices about 1 cm thick.

9. Explain why pregnant women should not have X-rays. Pregnant women should avoid X-rays because radiation from the X-ray machine is damaging to the fetus.

10. List X-ray procedures that do not require patient preparation. X-ray procedures that do not require preparation are bone studies, a chest X-ray, and a KUB.

# Chapter Application

## Case Studies with Critical Thinking Questions

### Scenario 1

Cynthia needs to be scheduled for an MRI of her head and neck. You are responsible for scheduling the test and explaining the procedure to the patient. After you have explained the procedure to Cynthia, she tells you she is extremely claustrophobic and doesn't think she can have the MRI.

1. What special preparation instructions should be given to the patient? No special instructions are needed for an MRI.

2. To whom should you relay the information regarding the patient's claustrophobia? The provider should be told about the patient's problem.

3. What could be done to help combat the claustrophobia? Often, the provider can order an open MRI for those patients with extreme claustrophobia or perhaps prescribe a sedative prior to the procedure. An open MRI does not produce as good an image as the closed MRI; therefore, some providers prefer not to use them.

### Scenario 2

A 55-year-old male calls the office to say that he had a barium enema this morning. He says that he is nauseated, bloated, and constipated and wants to know what he should do.

1. Who will determine how to treat the patient's complaint? The provider must be advised of all the patient's symptoms so that he or she can make a treatment recommendation.

2. Why can't you tell the patient what he should do about his situation? You cannot give the patient any medical advice without approval from the provider. Tell the patient that you will check with the provider and call him back.

## Scenario 3

A 35-year-old female with upper-right quadrant pain is scheduled for an ultrasound this morning. When she arrives at the facility, she is questioned about her preparation for the procedure, and it is determined that she cannot have the ultrasound because she ate a liquid, fat-free breakfast. The patient calls your office and is quite upset because she had to reschedule her appointment. She claims that the medical assistant never told her that she couldn't have anything to eat or drink after midnight. However, the medical assistant did explain all preparation instructions and gave her printed instructions to take with her.

1. How might this situation be handled in a professional manner? Try to calm the patient and ask her to locate her written instructions so you can show her where the instructions are for a morning ultrasound.

2. How might this error have been prevented? Call the patient the day before to confirm preparation instructions.

UNIT 16

# Minor Surgery Procedures

CHAPTER 49

# Preparing for Surgery

## Words to Know Challenge

**Spelling: Each line contains three spellings of a word. Underline the correctly spelled word.**

1. anticeptic    antiseptic    anticeptik
2. micorganism    mickroorganism    microorganism
3. ratchet    rachet    rachette
4. contamination    contaminition    cuntamination
5. serattions    serrations    cearations
6. asceptic    aseptic    aseptick
7. forseps    forsepts    forceps
8. microbial    microrbial    microrbital
9. skrub    sgrub    scrub

**Fill in the Blank: Complete the following sentences with correctly spelled words from the Spelling section.**

1. Because body hair encourages microbial accumulation, it is sometimes shaved.
2. The process of maintaining sterility throughout the surgical procedure is known as aseptic technique.
3. The ratchet is the locking mechanism of an instrument.
4. Serrations are etchings located on the blade of an instrument to keep it from slipping.
5. A scrub is performed prior to surgery to remove all microorganisms and aid in keeping the microbial count low.
6. Strikethrough occurs when fluid penetrates a sterile package or sterile tray and field.
7. Prepping the skin with an antiseptic solution should begin at the center of the incision site and proceed outward in one continuous circular motion as shown.
8. In compliance with Standard Precautions, proper barriers, such as gloves, gown, and face mask or shield must be worn to protect the health care staff from possible contamination while performing these procedures.

# Chapter Review

## Short Answer

1. When scheduling the patient for surgery, identify at least four items the medical assistant should advise the patient of.
   Any four of the following: (1) Appropriate length of time for the procedure, (2) appropriate clothing to wear, (3) amount of time to fast, (4) arrangement for someone to accompany the patient if necessary, (5) anticipated time off work or arranging for home care, (6) provide printed educational materials about the procedure

2. Explain how to care for surgical instruments before and following use.
   Surgical instruments should be properly sanitized and checked for flaws, autoclaved and labeled, and stored protected from moisture.

3. The three instrument classifications are: cutting and dissecting, grasping and clamping, and dilating, probing, and visualizing

4. Discuss the four sterilization techniques and identify the method most widely used.
   *Autoclave:* The autoclave renders sterility by a combination of steam and pressure. This is the most widely used. *Dry heat:* Dry heat sterilization is accomplished by raising the temperature of surgical instrumentation to the designated temperature that renders it sterile. *Gas sterilization:* Sterilization by gas occurs with ethylene oxide. *Chemical agents:* Chemicals can be used as sterilants for certain surgical instruments.

5. List three examples of when the sterile tray or field would become contaminated.
   Any three of the following: It comes in contact with an unsterile item, strikethrough occurs, an unsterile member reaches across the sterile tray or field, a sterile member turns his or her back toward the field, the field is left uncovered and unattended.

6. List the items included in the basic setup for most minor surgical procedures.
   The basic setup for most minor surgical procedures includes the following sterile items: scalpel handle and blades, hemostats, needle holder, needles and suture material, suture scissors, thumb forceps, probe, gauze squares, sponges, vial of anesthetic medication, syringes, towels, and bandages.

7. List five guidelines to follow when draping a patient.
   Always drape from the sterile to the unsterile; do not reach across a sterile area to drape; do not move drapes after they are placed; do not shake, flip, or fan drapes. Drapes should be unfolded and carefully placed in position; discard any drapes that become contaminated.

8. Describe what needs to be done when the patient arrives for the appointment.
   Provide written instructions about the procedure and care, explain the consent form and obtain signature, answer questions about the procedure, ascertain whether the patient has any allergies.

9. Select the order of procedures to prepare the skin for surgery from the following list:
   a. Drape, shave, rinse, cleanse, apply antiseptic solution
   b. Apply antiseptic solution, cleanse, rinse, shave, drape
   c. Shave, cleanse, rinse, drape, apply antiseptic solution

10. What is the purpose of the skin preparation before a surgical procedure?
    Skin preparation is performed to remove hair from the surgery site to prevent infection and to clean the skin. Antiseptic solution is applied to reduce microbial growth.

11. Why must the medical assistant be extremely careful to avoid nicking the patient's skin when performing a skin preparation?
    Microorganisms can enter the body through a break in the skin, and an infection could develop.

### Instrument Classification

Identify the classification of each instrument in the list. (*Hint*: Classifications may be used more than once.)

| | INSTRUMENT | CLASSIFICATION |
|---|---|---|
| B | 1. Forceps | A. Cutting and dissecting |
| C | 2. Retractors | B. Clamping or grasping |
| B | 3. Hemostats | C. Dilating, probing, and visualizing |
| A | 4. Scissors | |
| C | 5. Specula | |
| A | 6. Scalpels | |
| B | 7. Needle holders | |
| C | 8. Sounds | |

## Chapter Application

### Case Study with Critical Thinking Questions

Madison has not had time to sterilize the surgical instruments on the counter from an earlier procedure because she has been so busy with patient care. A coworker says that his physician needs the instruments for a procedure right away. Madison explains that the instruments have been cleaned and disinfected but not sterilized.

1. What should Madison tell her coworker? The instruments will be sterilized as soon as possible but should not be used for another procedure until then.
2. Should these instruments be used anyway? Absolutely not.

CHAPTER 50

# Assisting with Minor Surgery

## Words to Know Challenge

**Spelling: Each line contains three spellings of a word. Underline the correctly spelled word.**

| | | |
|---|---|---|
| 1. biopsy | biopsie | biopcie |
| 2. cyrosrurgery | kryosrusery | cryosurgery |
| 3. electocautery | electrocautery | elecktrocautery |
| 4. coagalate | coagulate | cogulate |
| 5. hemophilia | hemophillia | hemopilia |
| 6. anathesia | anesthesia | anathesia |
| 7. exudate | exadate | exadite |
| 8. sewture | suwture | suture |
| 9. hypoalerrgenic | hypoallergenik | hypoallergenic |
| 10. exision | excision | excison |

**Fill in the Blank: Complete the following sentences with correctly spelled words from the Spelling section.**

1. Destruction of tissue and skin lesions using extremely cold temperatures is the procedure known as cryosurgery.
2. In a needle biopsy, fluid or tissue cells are aspirated through a needle into a syringe for microscopic examination.
3. A biopsy is an excision of a small amount of tissue for microscopic examination.
4. The specimen must be preserved in a solution of 10 percent formalin until transported to the laboratory and prepared for examination.
5. Coagulate means to clot.
6. When performing a wound collection, the swab should not touch any part of the wound except the exudate.
7. A suture is a type of thread that joins skin of a wound.

8. When something is hypoallergenic, it is unlikely to cause an allergic reaction.
9. Hemophilia is a hereditary condition causing inability to clot blood.

## Chapter Review

### Short Answer

1. Discuss some of the reasons behind the upsurge in outpatient and ambulatory surgery.
   Answers will vary but can include: Significantly improved anesthesia; reduced surgery time; fewer side effects; fewer postsurgical infections
2. Identify the two most common local anesthetic agents.
   The most common local anesthetic agents are Xylocaine (lidocaine hydrochloride) and Novocain (procaine hydrochloride).
3. What is the purpose of an electrocautery device in minor surgical procedures performed in the office?
   The purpose of an electrocautery device is to control bleeding of the surgical site in removal of warts, polyps, and so on.
4. Discuss general postop instructions that should be given to a patient following a minor surgery performed in the office.
   Answers can vary but should include: Keep the site clean and dry; place no stress on the area; drink plenty of fluids; get proper rest; eat sensibly; return for a follow-up visit; report any unusual symptoms.
5. List unusual patient symptoms that should be reported to the provider following a surgical procedure.
   Unusual pain, burning, or uncomfortable sensation, bleeding or discharge, fever, nausea, and vomiting
6. List the important information that must be recorded on the patient's chart regarding a surgical procedure.
   Signed consent form, area of surgical site, type of closure of site (including number of sutures), patient education, condition of patient, immunizations noted, and return appointment date
7. Why are follow-up visits necessary in patient care? Other than the scheduled postop visit, what can the medical assistant do to follow up with patients?
   Follow-up visits are necessary to assess the patient's progress. Medical assistants can also phone the next day to see how the patient is doing and reassure him or her of the MA's (and the provider's) concern.
8. Explain how to remove sutures properly and why they should be removed.
   Suture removal should be performed by sterile technique by grasping the knot of the suture material with thumb forceps and gently but firmly pulling up, making just enough space to place the suture removal scissors to clip the suture as close to the skin as possible. Then pull the suture with the forceps back toward the healing incision so that no stress is put on it to reopen it, being careful not to pull the suture that has been on the surface of the site through the path of the suture being removed, or infection can develop.
9. Describe how to remove skin staples.
   Skin staples should be removed by sterile technique by placing the staple extractor under the staples one at a time and squeezing the handles of the extractor completely closed. Each staple is then lifted away from the skin and placed in the biohazard waste bag.

10. Describe skin closures and how they are applied.
Steri-Strips™ and butterfly closures are applied over the incision or laceration to hold the site closed and give support during healing.

**Matching: Match the procedure in column I to its description in column II.**

| | COLUMN I | COLUMN II |
|---|---|---|
| D | 1. Sebaceous cyst removal | A. Closing a wound or laceration by placing sutures or stitches or staples in the skin to hold the edges of the wound together |
| A | 2. Laceration repair | B. Fluid or tissue cells aspirated through a needle into a syringe for microscopic examination |
| E | 3. Chemical destruction | C. Incision in a localized infection, such as an abscess, to drain the exudates from the area |
| F | 4. Laser surgery | D. Excision of a small, painless sac containing a buildup of sebum, the secretion from a sebaceous gland |
| C | 5. I&D | E. Tissue destroyed by applying silver nitrate to the area |
| B | 6. Needle biopsy | F. A concentrated, intense light beam destroys a target area without harming the surrounding tissue |

# Chapter Application

## Case Studies with Critical Thinking Questions

### Scenario 1

A surgical procedure was performed at the outpatient surgery center, and the patient was instructed to return to the office for removal of the staples. When you take the bandage off, you notice that the site is infected.

1. What should you do first? Alert the provider and obtain instructions on how to proceed.
2. Describe the procedure the provider might ask you to perform. You might be asked to perform a wound collection. Use a sterile swab and insert the tip into the center of the infected area of the wound. Then transfer the swab with the specimen into the culture medium.

### Scenario 2

Joshua Leonard is having a sebaceous cyst removed from his scalp today. While you are performing the skin prep, he tells you that he is a little nervous about having the procedure because he has hemophilia.

1. What should you do with this information? Check the patient's chart to be sure this information is documented and inform the provider.
2. What are the risks while having this procedure? Bleeding might be difficult to control.

### Competency Practice

1. **Role play postop instructions:** With a partner, discuss general postop instructions that should be given to a patient following an in-office minor surgery.
2. **Removing sutures:** Practice removing sutures from an artificial arm or a suture pillow. Document the number of sutures placed and the number of sutures removed.

UNIT 17

# Medication Administration Procedures

CHAPTER 51

# Pharmacology Fundamentals

## Words to Know Challenge

**Spelling: Each line contains three spellings of a word. Underline the correctly spelled word.**

| | | |
|---|---|---|
| 1. ampeule | ampool | ampule |
| 2. generic | generic | jenerik |
| 3. prescibption | prescription | priscription |
| 4. auxillary | axillary | auxilary |
| 5. narcotic | norcatic | narcotek |
| 6. pharmocology | pharmecolagy | pharmacology |
| 7. sinergistic | synergistic | synergistic |
| 8. antigonist | antaganist | antagonist |
| 9. allergie | allergy | allurgy |

**Fill in the Blank: Complete the following sentences with Words to Know from this chapter.**

1. A synergistic drug enhances the effects of another drug, whereas a drug that prevents the action of another drug or chemical is referred to as a(n) antagonist.
2. A controlled class of drugs used to relieve pain is called a narcotic.
3. The study of medications and uses is also referred to as pharmacology.
4. A reaction to a medication that causes a immune response is called a(n) allergy, whereas a(n) intolerance to a medication can be only a symptom, such as an upset stomach, that can be controlled by taking the medication at a different time.
5. The generic name of a medication is also its official name.
6. The trade name of a medication is a label assigned by the manufacturer.
7. Drugs that have the potential for abuse or addiction are known as controlled substances.
8. Instructions written by a provider to the pharmacist for preparing, labeling, and dispensing medications that will be self-administered by a patient is called a prescription.

# Chapter Review

## Short Answer

1. Circle one: There are (1, 2, 3, (4), 5) basic categories of insulins.

2. What is meant by *generic* drug name? What is the difference between a generic name and a trade name?
   A generic drug's name is the official name assigned by the USAN (United States Adopted Names) Council. The generic name is an assigned name that remains constant, whereas the trade name is given for marketing purposes by the manufacturer

3. Explain why the correct spelling is so important when dealing with drugs.
   Many drugs have similar appearing or sounding names; incorrect spelling could lead to a drug error

4. The Drug Enforcement Administration is responsible for regulation and oversight of controlled substances; the Food and Drug Administration monitors drug safety and clinical trials and verifies that medications are safe for consumption based on available data.

5. What is a controlled substance? Describe the proper storage requirements of controlled substances in the medical office.
   A controlled substance is a drug that has the potential for abuse or addiction. It can be prescription or illegal. Controlled substances and the records of their prescribing and dispensing must be protected from misuse by storing them under double lock. Controlled substances may not be kept in the same compartments or cabinets as uncontrolled pharmaceuticals in the office setting

6. Name at least five print or online drug reference sources that are used in the medical office.
   PDR; PDR for Nonprescription Drugs; Product Inserts; Professional Drug Handbooks; USP-NF; PDR.net Downloadable applications; Online drug websites

7. Describe how refrigerated medications should be stored and handled.
   Containers should be clearly labeled with the date and time of opening or reconstitution to determine expiration. A temperature log must be maintained for all refrigerated medications and vaccinations. Medications and immunizations for patient administration should not be stored in the same refrigerator with office staff food and medications

## Matching: Drug Classifications

**Match the drug classifications in column I with its description in column II.**

| | COLUMN I | COLUMN II |
|---|---|---|
| F | 1. Anesthetic | A. thins mucous |
| I | 2. Chemotherapeutics | B. controls cardiac rhythm |
| J | 3. Antiemetic | C. relieves muscle spasms |
| H | 4. Anticonvulsant | D. produces a calming effect |
| B | 5. Antiarrhythmic | E. increases production of urine |
| D | 6. Antianxiety | F. interferes with body's ability to experience pain |
| E | 7. Diuretic | G. cures infections |
| A | 8. Expectorant | H. prevents or relieves seizures |
| G | 9. Antibiotics | I. cures cancer |
| C | 10. Muscle relaxant | J. stops or prevents nausea and vomiting |

## Matching: Controlled Substances

**Match the description items in column I with the corresponding schedule in column II.**
(*Hint*: There might be multiple answers for items in Column I.)

| | COLUMN I | COLUMN II |
|---|---|---|
| B | 1. Not able to be refilled | A. Schedule I |
| D | 2. Limited risk for physical dependence; Phenobarbital | B. Schedule II |
| A | 3. Illegal drugs | C. Schedule III |
| E | 4. Low risk of addiction, small amounts of codeine in cough syrups | D. Schedule IV |
| C, D | 5. Can be refilled up to five times in six months | E. Schedule V |
| B | 6. Requires a signed prescription to be presented with 72 hours of a phoned prescription | |
| B | 7. Legal drug but carries severe risk for psychic and physical addiction | |
| A | 8. Marijuana, heroin | |
| C | 9. Prescriptions may be written or phoned in | |

## Matching

**Recognize and describe medical, legal, and ethical concerns regarding medications and appropriate actions to be taken for each.**
*Hint*: Each can have more than one answer. Be prepared to discuss your answers and rationales in class.

| | COLUMN I | COLUMN II |
|---|---|---|
| C, B | 1. Medical assistant notices that a medication prescribed is on the list of patient's allergies. | A. Ethical concern |
| A, B | 2. Birth control pills prescribed for mentally challenged patient 14 years old. | B. Legal concern |
| B | 3. Immunizations given to a child with permission of the babysitter. | C. Medical issue |
| B | 4. Narcotics stored alongside blood pressure medications in common office cabinet. | |
| A, B | 5. Alzheimer's patient who does not have a reported injury or pain problem is prescribed a narcotic pain patch to help calm her down. | |
| B, C | 6. Prescriptions for two patients are mixed up at the time of discharge. One is for antibiotic and one is for heart rhythm control. | |
| C | 7. Prescribing antibiotics for an ear infection in a child because the parent insists rather than because it is clinically necessary. | |
| A | 8. Medical personnel's objection to participating in administration or dispensing of morning-after pill. | |

## Labeling

Drugs come in a variety of forms. Identify each of the following drug form.

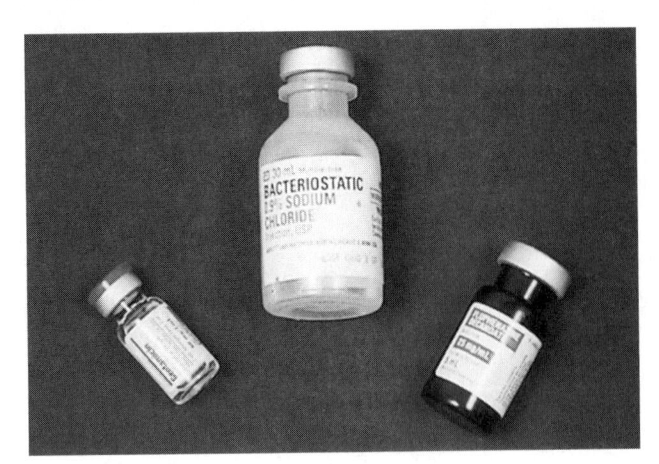


Liquids

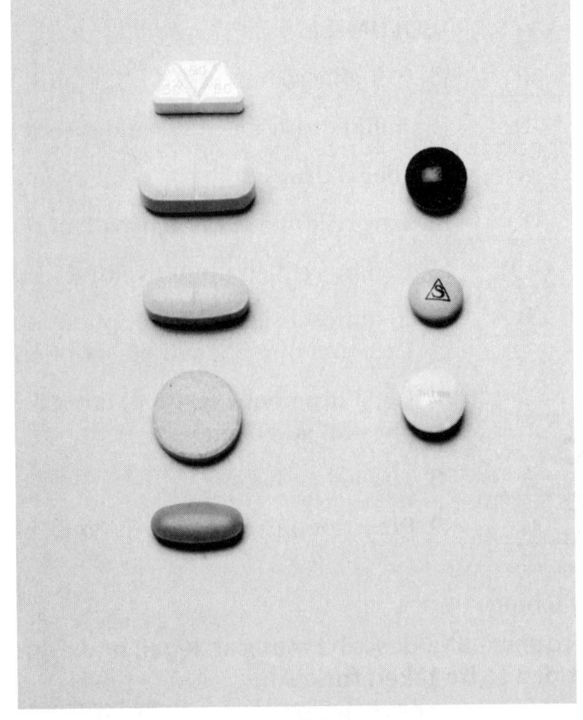

Tablets

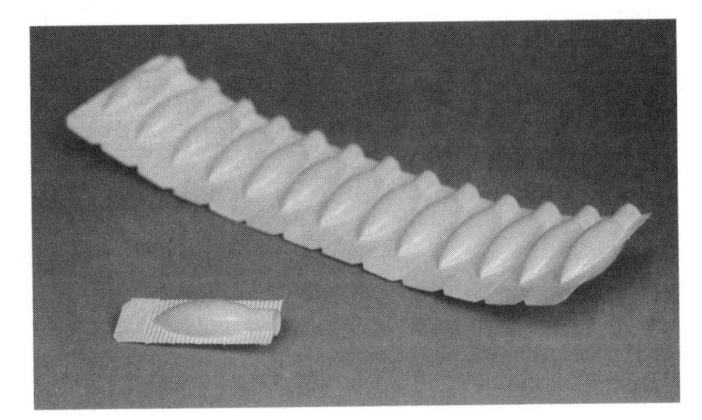

Suppositories

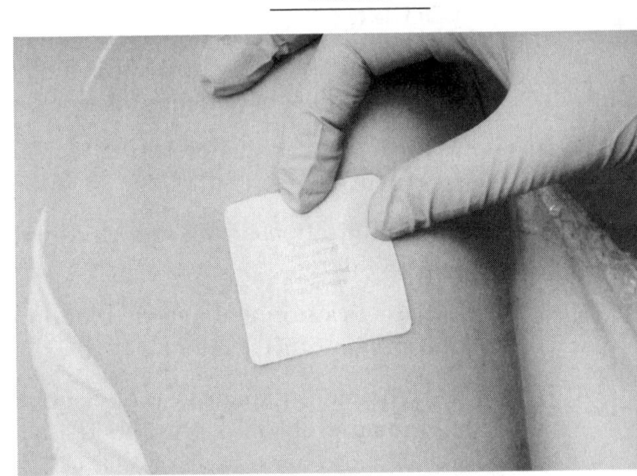

Transdermal Patch

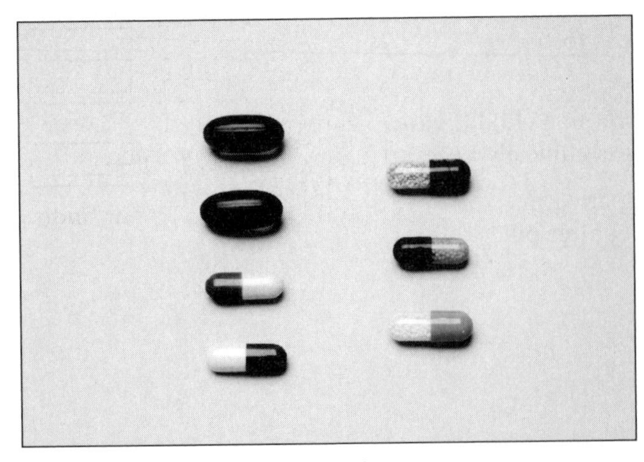

Capsules

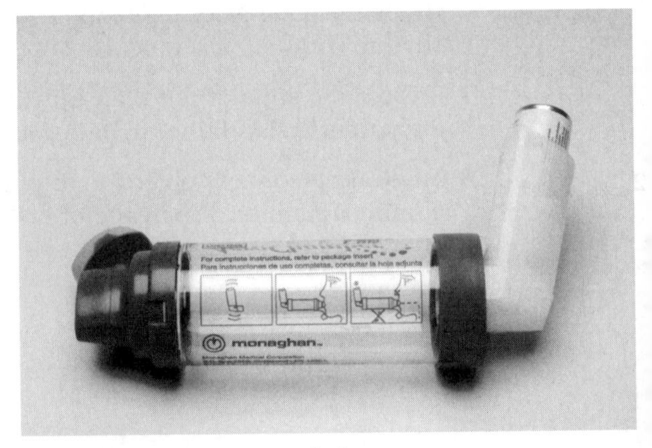


Inhalants

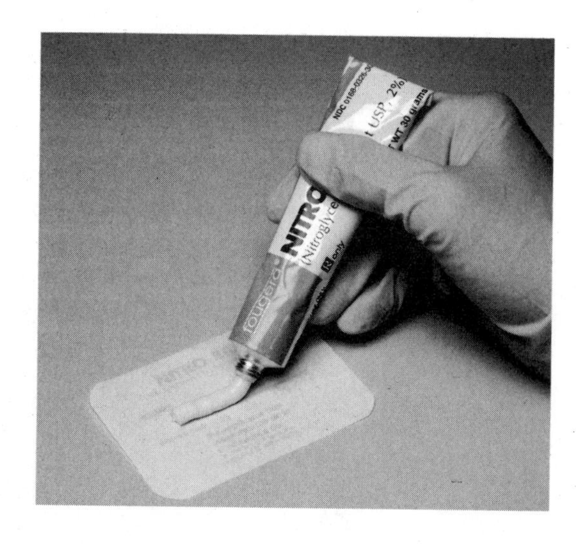


Skin Preparations

## Chapter Application

### Case Study with Critical Thinking Questions

An elderly patient presents for a new patient appointment and has brought with her a paper bag with assorted bottles: prescription, over-the-counter, and herbal remedies. Some pills are loose and unlabeled.

1. How might you help determine which medications the patient is using, and how you might identify them to arrive at an accurate medication list?
   Answers will vary but can include: determining which physicians and pharmacies prescribe and fill the prescriptions and requesting current medication lists; asking the patient whether she is able to tell you what each one does and how often she takes it, one at a time; checking loose pills against the Pillbox™ application online or the photos in a PDR or other drug reference guide.
2. What safety precautions might you discuss with the patient?
   Answers will vary but can include: discussing options for maintaining medications safely, such as requesting special caps that are easy to open; using divided pillboxes that have sections for each day of the week; or requesting the pharmacist to print labels in larger print.

### Competency Practice

1. Using the Internet or a drug reference, fill in the missing information.

| | Trade name | Generic Name | Recommended Dose and Route | Common side effects |
|---|---|---|---|---|
| a. | Captopril | capoten | Po, 12.5, 25, 50, 100 mg | Angioedema, hypotension |
| b. | Fosamax | alendronate sodium | Po, 5, 10, 35, 40, 70 mg | Abdominal pain, nausea, muscle or bone pain, headache, dizziness |
| c. | Lexapro | escitalopram oxalate | 5, 10, 20 mg po | Suicidal ideation, worsening depression |

2. Using the most current PDR available, find the following information and be prepared discuss your findings in class:
   - Determine the manufacturer for Aricept
   - Pregnancy category ratings
   - Determine what information is requested when completing a MedWatch report

CHAPTER 52

# Measurement Systems, Basic Mathematics, and Dosage Calculations

## Words to Know Challenge

**Spelling: Each line contains three spellings of a word. Underline the correctly spelled word.**

| | | |
|---|---|---|
| 1. decimal | decemul | decimol |
| 2. dividend | dividened | dividind |
| 3. devisor | diviser | divisor |
| 4. product | prodouct | prodact |
| 5. extreems | extremes | extrimes |
| 6. fraktion | fracshun | fraction |
| 7. means | miens | meens |
| 8. metric system | mitric system | metrik system |
| 9. nomerator | numerater | numerator |
| 10. purcentage | percentage | percentige |
| 11. denuminater | denominator | dinominater |
| 12. rashio | rachio | ratio |
| 13. purportion | perportion | proportion |

**Fill in the Blank: Complete the following sentences with correctly spelled words from the Spelling section.**

1. A product is the result of multiplying two numbers together.
2. The number *to be* divided is the dividend, and the divisor is the number *used to divide* another number.
3. A fraction indicates part of a whole number and is written with a numerator as the top number and a denominator as the bottom number.
4. A number expressed as part of 100 is called a percentage.
5. A ratio expresses the relationship between two components.

6. The relationship between two ratios is a proportion.
7. The metric system is based on multiples of ten; it is the most commonly used system of measurement in health care.

## Chapter Review

### Short Answer

1. Write out the formula for the basic method of calculating dosages and explain what each component of the formula means.
   The formula is: [(N) Needed/(A) Available] x Vehicle = Dose. N is the amount prescribed by the provider; A is the amount available; V is the form and amount in which the medication comes.
2. What are the three steps required for calculating dosages in the ratio and proportion method? What is the formula for this method?
   Convert, construct, calculate. dosage on hand:amount on hand = dosage desired:amount desired
3. What are the three basic units used in the metric system?
   Gram, liter, and meter
4. Why is it necessary for all health care personnel to use the same system of measurement when prescribing or administering medications?
   To avoid over- or undermedication of patients.
5. Fill in the blanks: An improper fraction has a numerator larger than the denominator, and a mixed fraction includes a whole number along with a fraction.
6. Explain why household measurement devices, such as teaspoons and tablespoons, should be avoided?
   To use a calibrated teaspoon or tablespoon would likely deliver an accurate amount. *However*, many people interpret "teaspoon" or "tablespoon" as using silverware teaspoons and tablespoons, which can vary in amounts by several milliliters, leading to potential overdose
7. What is the purpose of learning to convert medication dosages from different units?
   The order amount might not be in the same units that are on hand, so, to administer the medication safely an accurate conversion is necessary

### Abbreviations Review: Write out the following abbreviations and then tell which system of measurement it belongs to.

1. gtt Drop, household
2. g Gram, metric
3. gr Grain, apothecary
4. fl oz Fluid ounce, household and apothecary
5. lb Pound, household
6. mL Milliliter, metric
7. kg Kilogram, metric
8. pt Pint, household and apothecary

**Equivalents Review: Match the *measurement* with the appropriate *system* of measurement.** (*Hint*: The systems will be used more than once.)

| | | |
|---|---|---|
| B | 1. Cup | A. Metric |
| C | 2. Dram | B. Household |
| A | 3. Liter | C. Apothecary |
| C | 4. Grain | |
| A | 5. Gram | |
| C | 6. Drop | |
| B | 7. Pint | |
| B | 8. Quart | |
| A | 9. Meter | |
| B | 10. Teaspoon | |

# Chapter Application

## Math Review Exercises

1. How many tsp make 180 gtt? 3
   60 gtt = 1 tsp   180/60 gtt = 3 tsp
2. Convert 3 tsp into mL. 15 mL
   1 tsp = 5 mL   3 × 5 mL = 15
3. Convert 150 pounds into kg. 68.2
   2.2 lbs = 1 kg   150/2.2 = 68.18, round to 68.2
4. How many cups are in 2 quarts? 8
   1 quart = 4 cups
5. Based on the information found in the chapter, what conversions need to be performed to find the number of gtts in 20 ml?
   Convert mL into the number of tsp: 5 mL are in 1 tsp, so there are 4 tsp; then convert tsp into gtts: 1 tsp equals 60 gtts, 60 × 4 = 240 gtts
6. Add the following. Show your work.
   a. 1¼ + 68% + 0.7 = 2.63
   b. 3/8 + 0.42 + 13.5% = 1.725
7. Identify the means and extremes of the following proportions.
   a. 4:5 = 12:15 Means are 5 and 12, extremes are 4 and 15
   b. 1:3 = 3:9 Means are 3 and 3, extremes are 1 and 9

**Solving Proportions and Equations: Solve the following proportions and equations. Show your work.**

1. 1:4 = 3:$x$   $x$ = 12
2. 3:9 = $x$:12   $x$ = 4
3. 25 + $x$ = 175   $x$ = 150
4. 1.35 − 0.67 = $x$   $x$ = 0.68
5. 4.3 × 2.1 = $x$   $x$ = 9.03
6. 4 × ½ = $x$   $x$ = 2
7. 150 ÷ 3 = $x$   $x$ = 50
8. 75 × ½ = $x$   $x$ = 37.5

**Dosage Calculation Exercises: Determine the correct dosages. Use either method presented in the chapter but show your work.**

1. Order: Novolin R 10 units SubQ now
   Supplied as 100 units per 1 mL
   What is the correct volume to be administered? 0.1 mL
2. Order: Aspirin 162 mg po chew and swallow now for chest pain
   Supplied as 81 mg tablets
   What is the correct amount? 2 tablets
3. Order: Benadryl 100 mg IM now for acute allergic reaction
   Supplied as 50 mg per mL
   What is the correct amount? 2 mL
4. Order: Amoxicillin 500 mg po
   Supplied in dry powder form; when reconstituted, solution contains 200 mg per 5 mL
   What is the correct volume to be administered? 12.5 mL
5. You are asked to prepare epinephrine 0.3 mg for subcutaneous injection by the physician in an asthmatic emergency. Calculate the dose and describe the proper way to label the syringe.
   Supplied as a 1:1000 solution in a 30 mL vial containing 1 mg/mL.
   What is the correct volume? 0.3 mL
6. Order: Terbutaline 0.25 mg IM
   Supplied as 1mg/mL vial.
   What is the correct volume? 0.25 mL
7. Order: Digitek 250 mcg po as a loading dose.
   Supplied as 0.125 mg tablets
   What is the correct amount? 2 tablets
8. Order: Dexamethasone 5 mg po now
   Supplied to your office in 0.5 mg and 2 mg tablets
   What is the correct amount? Two 2 mg tablets and two 0.5 mg tablets
   *Rationale: It is preferable to use whole supplied tablets when available rather than to break tablets in half*.

CHAPTER 53

# Administering Oral and Non-Injectable Medications

## Words to Know Challenge

**Spelling: Each line contains three spellings of a word. Underline the correctly spelled word.**

| | | |
|---|---|---|
| 1. narcotic | narcotec | nercotic |
| 2. seppository | suppository | sopository |
| 3. sublingal | subblingual | sublingual |
| 4. rectul | rectal | rictal |
| 5. prescription | proscription | priscription |
| 6. topical | typical | topicul |
| 7. parental | perinteral | parenteral |
| 8. transdirmel | transdermal | trensindermal |
| 9. buccal | buckal | buckle |
| 10. mediation order | medication order | medicaton order |
| 11. dispanse | dispence | dispense |

**Fill in the Blank: Complete the following sentences with Words to Know from this chapter.**

1. A prescription ______ is a written or transmitted instruction to the pharmacist for preparing and dispensing a medication to a patient for self-administration.
2. A written instruction composed by a physician or licensed practitioner for administering medications directly to a patient is a medication order ______.
3. DAW stands for dispense as written ______.
4. Oral medications are intended for absorption through the digestive system; other methods are said to be parenteral ______, or intended for absorption from outside the digestive system.
5. Sublingual ______ medications are placed under the tongue; buccal ______ medications are placed between the cheek and gum.
6. A medication supplied as a dissolvable solid for rectal administration is called a suppository ______.

7. A(n) enema could be used to introduce contrast material rectally for imaging of the lower intestinal tract.
8. Parenteral medications are those that are given by a route outside of the digestive system.
9. Patches give medications by the transdermal route.
10. The Seven Rights are the rules that ensure safe medication administration.

## Chapter Review

### Short Answer

1. Why are different medications used to treat the same symptoms?
Medications can work through different mechanisms of action and might not produce the same side effects in different patients. Others might not be effective because the same symptom can be caused by a different underlying problem.
2. A prescription is defined as a legal document that provides instructions defined by the physician or licensed provider for preparation of a medication and authorizes its dispensing to a patient for self-administration.
3. When preparing a prescription for signature, the medical assistant should always compare all elements of the prescription with the order and verify that the information is complete and accurate.
4. What does DAW on a prescription stand for and what does it mean? Dispense as written. It is an instruction to the pharmacist not to make any substitutions or alterations in the dosing or instructions supplied to the patient.
5. What action should be taken to avoid errors when calling in prescriptions to a pharmacy? Require the pharmacist or technician to read back all the information given to verify accuracy.
6. What information is required for a complete and accurate medication order?
   a. Patient name
   b. Medication name
   c. Dosage
   d. Route of administration
   e. Frequency
   f. Date and time the order was written
   g. Specific instructions
   h. Prescriber's signature
7. What is the purpose of a medication order? Provides direct and complete instructions from a provider or other licensed practitioner for administering medications to a patient while he or she is in the facility or office
8. What must be performed before giving medications by ANY route?
Hand washing, verifying any and all the Seven Rights (Either of these answers is correct.)
9. When signing off a medication or other chart entry, how should you signify the end of the entry to prevent anyone else making an unauthorized addition to your note?
By following the signature with a straight line to the edge of the page

10. In the following chart, list the Seven Rights of medication administration and explain what each Right means.

| | **Right** | **Description** |
|---|---|---|
| 1. | Patient | Verify that you have the correct person by using two identifiers, e.g., birth date, address, social security number, etc. |
| 2. | Medication | Make sure the drug being prepared matches the order but also matches the patient's problem. |
| 3. | Dose | Check to be sure the dose prepared matches the dose ordered. It should also be within the usual range of dosing for that medication and is appropriate for the age of the patient, i.e., adult dose versus pediatric dose. |
| 4. | Route | Ensure that the correct route is to be used as ordered and that there is no contraindication for using that route. |
| 5. | Technique | Give the medication the right way by the correct route. |
| 6. | Time | Administer the medication at the appropriate time as ordered and with respect to other activities such as meals or therapy or with respect to tests that might be planned. |
| 7. | Documentation | Record accurately all the information regarding the administration of the medication and in the correct patient record as soon as possible following administration. |

11. To avoid medication errors, when should the medical assistant check the order and the medication? Before and after preparing the medication, and before and after giving the medication.

12. What steps should the medical assistant take in the event of a medication error? Ensure the patient's safety, notify the physician or ordering provider, document in the patient's record what occurred, completely and accurately, and document the patient's response.

13. List six elements required for a complete and accurate medication entry.

    **a.** Correct patient
    **b.** Medication name
    **c.** Dose
    **d.** Route
    **e.** Technique
    **f.** Time

14. When should a medication entry be completed? Immediately after the medication is given

15. Why is oral administration the most commonly used route for medications?
    It involves less risk, discomfort, and expense than other routes of administration.

16. What information is required, in addition to the standard information, when documenting immunizations?
    Manufacturer's name, lot number, serial number, and expiration date

17. What legislation requires health care providers to report adverse events following a vaccination? What is its purpose?
The National Childhood Vaccine Injury Act (NCVIA); its purpose is to detect new or unusual adverse events, monitor increases in adverse events, identify potential risk factors, identify an increase in events associated with certain lot numbers, and track safety of new vaccines.

18. Identify the routes by which a medical assistant is permitted to administer medications (unless otherwise designated by state laws).
Oral, inhaled, topical, and injectable. Additionally, it is important to be ready to provide patient education regarding medications that are generally self-administered vaginally, urethrally, and rectally.

## Matching: Routes of Administration

**Match the routes of administration in column I with their descriptions in column II.**

| | COLUMN I | COLUMN II |
|---|---|---|
| F | 1. Sublingual | A. Medication given in the ear canal |
| C | 2. Buccal | B. Applied directly to the skin |
| E | 3. Ointment | C. Placed between the cheek and gum for absorption through the mucous membranes in the mouth |
| I | 4. Inhalation | D. Medication applied into the eyelid or opening in the corner of the eye |
| A | 5. Otic | E. Emulsion of medication applied topically |
| B | 6. Topical | F. Under the tongue |
| D | 7. Ophthalmic | G. An adhesive patch containing medication worn on the skin |
| J | 8. Intraosseous | H. Into the spinal column |
| G | 9. Transdermal | I. Breathed in |
| H | 10. Intrathecal | J. How often a medication is given |

## Matching: Acceptable Abbreviations

**For each abbreviation listed, identify whether it is acceptable to use or is a Do Not Use abbreviation. Next to only the acceptable abbreviations, write what each stands for.**

| | Abbreviation | Abbreviation Written Out | Use or Do Not Use? |
|---|---|---|---|
| A | 1. kg | Kilogram | A. Use |
| B | 2. QD | | B. Do Not Use |
| A | 3. tsp | Teaspoon | |
| A | 4. tinc | Tincture | |
| B | 5. IU | | |
| A | 6. STAT | Immediately | |
| B | 7. U (unit) | | |
| A | 8. IV | Intravenous | |
| A | 9. IM | Intramuscular | |
| B | 10. MS | | |

# Chapter Application

## Identify Parts of a Prescription

In the following chart, define the purpose of each of the following parts of a prescription: "Accupril 5 mg po bid after meals. Sig #60. 3 refills. *John Smith, MD.*"

| *Part* | *Purpose* |
|---|---|
| Accupril | Drug to be dispensed |
| 5 mg | Dosage amount |
| po | Route of administration |
| bid | Frequency |
| After meals | When to take medication |
| Sig #60 | How many to be dispensed |
| 3 refills | Authorized refills |
| John Smith, MD | Authorizing practitioner's signature |

## Research Activity

1. Using the Internet, answer the following questions regarding vaccines. (*Hint*: Try the CDC website.) Instructors: Link for answers is www.cdc.gov/vaccinesafety/Vaccines/recalls.html
   a. How is a vaccine or batch recalled?
   Recalls are usually voluntary but may be requested by the FDA.
   b. How would you find out whether a vaccine has been recalled?
   The www.cdc.gov/vaccines/recs/recalls/ website has links to all recalled vaccines.
2. Make flash cards of the common abbreviations in Table 53–1 for review with a classmate.

## Case Study with Critical Thinking Questions

### Scenario 1

Kelly Anderson, 15 years old, is being seen for back pain. She strained muscles while playing volleyball at school. Her chart notes that she has an allergy to ibuprofen. The physician has seen her and left a prescription and an order for medication. You, the MA, prepare and administer Advil 600 mg, per the order. Within a few minutes, Kelly begins to complain of itching all over. When you go back to check the chart, you notice that both the chart and the prescription are for *Kevin* Anderson, another patient being seen across the hall.

1. What has occurred? This is a medication error.
2. Describe how you will handle this situation. First, ensure the patient's safety by making sure that the allergic reaction hasn't progressed to her airway. Notify the physician at once. Let the patient know what is happening. Document all actions taken, any subsequent medication orders or treatment orders received, and the patient's response. The physician likely ordered an injectable antihistamine to be given, followed by a period of observation to ensure that no additional problems developed.

3. Make a charting entry that outlines the incident and the steps taken.

   Entry may look something like this:

   2:48 p.m. 10/5/2010. Patient was given Advil 600mg po as ordered by Dr. Gibson. *Jane Adams, MA*—

   3:05 p.m. 10/5/2010. Patient complained of itching. Rash over trunk and upper extremities noted. She denied difficulty breathing or swelling of tongue. Speech is clear, no hoarseness noted. Chart reviewed, noted that order for medication was actually for another patient and that this patient has an allergy to ibuprofen. Dr. Gibson advised at once. Order for Benadryl 50 mg IM received. *Jane Adams, MA*—

   3:07 p.m. 10/5/2010. Benadryl 50 mg IM given in left gluteus max., patient identified by name and birth date. *Jane Adams, MA*—

   3:45 pm 10/5/2010. Observed patient for period of time. Rash has diminished, patient reports being drowsy but itching has stopped. Dr. Gibson discussed events with mother, who will drive patient home to rest. Dr. Gibson's discharge instructions explained. *Jane Adams, MA*—

CHAPTER 54

# Administering Injections and Immunizations

## Words to Know Challenge

**Spelling: Each line contains three spellings of a word. Underline the correctly spelled word.**

| | | |
|---|---|---|
| 1. neumonia | pnumonia | pneumonia |
| 2. meningytis | meningitis | miningitis |
| 3. wheel | weal | wheal |
| 4. intradermal | interdermal | intradurmol |
| 5. subceutaneous | subcutaneous | subcutanious |
| 6. incubation period | incubasion period | encubation period |
| 7. anaphylactic | anyphalactic | aniphylactic |
| 8. influensa | inflouinza | influenza |
| 9. hipatytis | hepatitis | hepititis |
| 10. immunization | emunization | immunozation |

**Fill in the Blank: Complete the following sentences with correctly spelled words from the Spelling section.**

Injections given at a shallow angle of injection under the dermis are referred to as intradermal; a small wheal should develop at the site of the injection to give evidence that the medication is in the dermal layer of skin.

Subcutaneous injections are given just under the skin.

Meningitis is a complication of Haemophilus influenza type B or HIB.

Measles is also known as rubeola.

The incubation period is the time in which a virus or bacterium reproduces in the host before signs and symptoms of an illness appear.

A(n) anaphylactic reaction is a serious allergic response that requires immediate treatment.

Hepatitis is another word for inflammation of the liver.

**Matching: Match the words in column I with the definitions in column II.**

| | COLUMN I | COLUMN II |
|---|---|---|
| E | 1. Hepatitis A | A. vaccine |
| G | 2. Incubation period | B. whooping cough |
| F | 3. Photosensitivity | C. period when symptoms peak |
| H | 4. Catarrhal stage | D. chickenpox |
| J | 5. Subcutaneous | E. also known as "infectious" |
| L | 6. Intramuscular | F. sensitivity to light |
| M | 7. Rubella | G. time required for a disease to develop before symptoms present |
| A | 8. Immunization | H. period when disease is highly communicable |
| D | 9. Varicella | I. flu |
| N | 10. Diphtheria | J. beneath the skin |
| C | 11. Paroxysmal stage | K. may be called "serum" |
| K | 12. Hepatitis B | L. into the muscle |
| B | 13. Pertussis | M. german measles |
| I | 14. Influenza | N. preventable disease that might require a tracheostomy and ventilatory support; highly contagious |

## Chapter Review

### Short Answer

1. List three advantages of parenteral medications.
   Any three of the following: They may administered directly to the affected organ or system [eyes, ears, etc.], bypassing the GI tract and avoiding side effects; May also be given by a route that allows for faster or more immediate effects, as in IV medications; Other routes allow for administering medications when a patient is unable to tolerate oral medications; Better predictability of absorption without interference of GI tract

2. What is the difference between a tuberculin syringe and an insulin syringe? Can they be used interchangeably?
   The tuberculin syringe is calibrated in tenths of a millimeter and has a 1.0 ml capacity. The insulin syringe is calibrated in units with a total capacity of 100 units. They are not interchangeable

3. Fill in the blanks: Medical assistants are not permitted to provide direct intravenous (IV) injections or to initiate an IV access. However, it is important to be able to recognize a problem and report it to the provider immediately.

4. Name at least one use for the intradermal route of medication administration.
   Any of the following or equivalent answer: Tuberculin testing for exposure to TB; Allergy testing for circulating antibodies to antigens

5. Fill in the following table with the correct angles of injection for each type of injection listed.

| Type of Injection | Angle of Injection |
|---|---|
| Subcutaneous | 45 degrees |
| Intradermal | 10 to 15 degrees |
| Intramuscular | 90 degrees |
| Z-Track IM | 90 degrees |

6. Why are intramuscular injections given at the angle you listed?
To allow the medication to be delivered deep into the muscle tissue for absorption and to avoid damaging more superficial subcutaneous and dermal tissues.

7. Describe the correct technique for giving a Z-track injection.
Hold the intended muscle site taut and gently displace it off to the side of the intended site. Insert the needle and begin slowly injecting the medication. Following injection of the medication, allow the tissue to return to its normal position, preventing the medication from leaking out into the more superficial tissues.

8. Name three actions that can be taken to avoid needlesticks.
Any three of the following: (1) Never recap used needles. (2) Always discard used needles and syringes into a properly labeled, hard-sided biohazard container. (3) Never allow a needle container to become overfilled. (4) The needle container should be locked before sending out for destruction. (5) Use needles and syringes that have locking shields, sheaths, or other safety devices.

9. What steps should be taken in the event of an accidental needlestick?
(1) Ensure the patient's safety and control bleeding if the needlestick caused a wound. (2) Notify the provider or other practitioner at once. (3) Might need to have blood tests performed. (4) Might need to receive or administer prophylactic medications. (5) Document carefully. (6) Abide by possible reporting requirements, based on circumstances and state laws.

### Short Essay

Discuss the following question. What comments might you offer to patients or parents who question you about why they or their children should be immunized?

Answers may include any of the following: (1) Diseases that persons are now immunized against were once potentially fatal illnesses. (2) Individuals being vaccinated protect not only themselves but an entire population from a potential catastrophic outbreak of a dangerous disease. (3) Some diseases that can be prevented with vaccinations, although not always fatal themselves, can cause lifelong health problems. For example, rubella can cause heart-valve damage, liver damage, bone malformations in children, brain damage, and blindness. Pregnant women might not suffer permanent complications, but certain preventable diseases can cause serious birth defects and death in the unborn fetus. Pertussis, which is currently a serious problem, is a disease that older children and adults can easily recover from but is deadly to babies and small children. (4) Vaccinating family animals, even those that rarely are outdoors, is still necessary to prevent introducing a fatal disease to family members.

## Chapter Application

### Labeling

1. Identify the parts of the needle pictured.

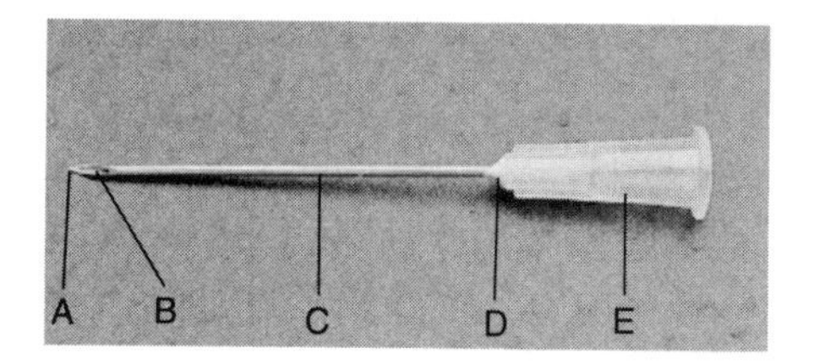


a. Point
b. Lumen
c. Shaft
d. Hilt
e. Hub

2. Identify the parts of a syringe.
   a. Luer-Lok tip
   b. Barrel
   c. Rubber stopper
   d. Plunger
   e. Flange

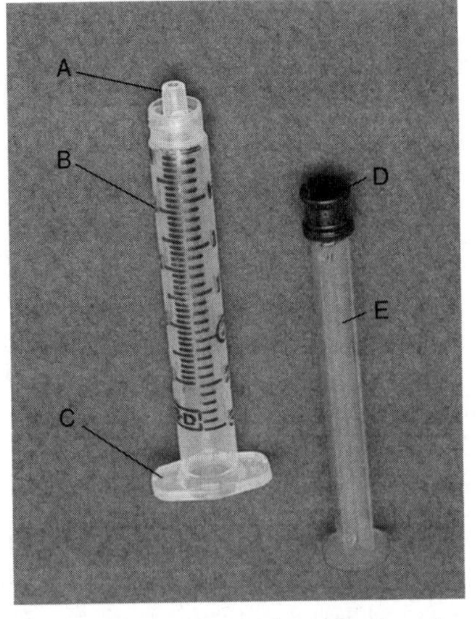


3. Next to each intramuscular injection site, identify the site name.

| Injection Site | Site Name |
|---|---|
| | Gluteus medius |
| | Ventrogluteal |
| | Vastus lateralis |
| | Deltoid |

## Case Studies with Critical Thinking Questions

### Scenario 1

A mother brings her 6-month-old in for a well-baby check. The child is playful, there is no sign of illness, and the baby's temperature is normal. Flu season is in full swing. When you ask the mother whether she is here for the baby's six-month vaccinations, she replies that she has no intention of vaccinating her baby.

1. How might you handle this conversation? (Select the best option.)
   a. Tell her that it is her legal obligation to vaccinate the baby.
   b. Give her a vaccination schedule and printed information and leave the room to hide your disapproval.
   c. Make a note in the chart and continue on with the visit.
   d. Ask her what her objections are to having vaccinations and offer to answer any questions.
2. Why did you choose this option?
   Many people fail to vaccinate children based on false beliefs or religious ideas. Very often, well-prepared education about vaccinations delivered in nonconfrontational and nonjudgmental manner can help alleviate fears. Provide only the information you know is appropriate and refer further discussion to the provider or nurse practitioner.
3. After discussion, the mother decides she would like to proceed with an immunization schedule. Where might you find information on catching up the baby's immunizations?
   www.CDC.gov. Immunizations are just not begun; rather, a catch-up schedule is often recommended. The provider will write the appropriate order, but the well-prepared MA can be very helpful in being prepared for such an order and explaining the schedule and circumstances to the parent in advance.

### Scenario 2

After preparing a vaccination for little Joey Jones, age 2, you discover that he feels warm and is just lying quietly on his mother's lap. The mother has signed the vaccination information and consent forms. The provider was about to see the baby but was called away on an emergency before seeing the child. The mother is looking at her watch and has indicated that she has another pressing appointment. Several other patients are waiting, and the provider's absence is going to put the appointment list behind schedule.

1. How will you address the situation?
   Avoid being drawn into the urgency of schedules. The baby shows signs of a temperature that might be from teething or from an illness. The reason for the temperature should be determined prior to receiving a vaccination. The provider has not yet seen the baby; therefore, a valid order has not been written or implied. The child's temperature should be taken and the provider advised. If elevated, the provider must either examine the child first or direct you to reschedule the appointment.

## Competency Practice

Look up correct amounts and routes of injection and then document, in the correct format, a note you would use to record the following injections:

a. MMR, vaccination #2 in series, pediatric
b. TB test, 0.2 mL
c. Influenza vaccination, adult

Information should be complete and contain the date, time, patient's name, age, medication name, serial number, lot number, amount delivered, route of administration, and any reaction noted along with any actions required. Instructor can build on this as a group or class exercise.

UNIT 18

# First Aid and Responding to Emergencies

CHAPTER 55

# Emergencies in the Medical Office

## Words to Know Challenge

**Spelling: Each line contains three spellings of a word. Underline the correctly spelled word.**

| | | |
|---|---|---|
| 1. asperation | aspirashun | aspiration |
| 2. diaphoresis | diephoresis | diaforesis |
| 3. profalatic | frofalytic | prophylactic |
| 4. exhaustion | eghaustion | egaustion |
| 5. ammonea | ammonia | amoania |
| 6. seezure | seazure | seizure |
| 7. cessation | sessation | cesation |
| 8. coraner | coriner | coroner |
| 9. intubation | entubation | intobacion |
| 10. poision | poison | poisen |
| 11. sincope | syncape | syncope |
| 12. resuscitation | resesutation | recessatation |

**Matching: Match the term in column I to its definition in column II.**

| | COLUMN I | COLUMN II |
|---|---|---|
| D | 1. Chronic | A. Extensive, advanced |
| K | 2. Subtle | B. Requires intervention as soon as possible |
| B | 3. Urgent | C. Can cause death |
| M | 4. Sudden | D. Long, drawn out, not acute |
| H | 5. Acute | E. Provides vital health information |
| A | 6. Severe | F. Injury |
| C | 7. Life-threatening | G. The act of reviving |

(continues)

| | |
|---|---|
| E 8. Universal emergency medical ID | H. Rapid onset, severe symptoms, short course |
| F 9. Trauma | I. Unexpected occurrence needing immediate action |
| G 10. Resuscitation | J. Another term for heart attack |
| N 11. Bandage | K. Hidden, not apparent |
| J 13. Myocardial infarction | L. Period after death |
| I 14. Medical emergency | M. Occurring quickly, without warning |
| L 15. Post mortem | N. A dressing |

**Fill in the Blank: Complete the following sentences with Words to Know from this chapter.**

1. A coma is when someone is in an abnormally deep stupor from which he or she cannot be aroused by external stimuli.
2. If you should encounter any emergency situation or if you happen to come upon an unknown person who has become ill or lost consciousness, check for a universal emergency medical identification symbol.
3. Diabetic ketoacidosis, also known as hyperglycemia, is caused by an increased amount of sugar in the blood.
4. Diabetic ketoacidosis (hyperglycemia) is caused by an increased amount of sugar in the blood. The patient might complain of confusion, dizziness, weakness, or nausea. Vomiting can occur. Respiration can be rapid and deep. The skin might be dry and flushed.
5. The patient who is exposed to high temperatures for a long period in industry or at home might suffer from heat cramps.
6. In heat exhaustion, the skin is pale, cool, and moist and the body temperature is normal. The patient becomes overheated with profuse perspiration, usually after some form of vigorous exercise.
7. Heatstroke is the most severe of the heat-related problems.
8. Hypothermia occurs when the body loses heat faster than it can produce it, resulting in a dangerously low body temperature.
9. Exposure to freezing temperatures will often result in frostbite.
10. Insulin shock, also known as hypoglycemia, can occur from an excess amount of insulin in the body.
11. One of the most common medical emergencies is an obstructed airway. The most usual cause in adults is food that is aspirated while eating.
12. Poison can be ingested, absorbed, inhaled, injected, or acquired from bites and stings.

# Chapter Review

## Short Answer

1. Identify five medical conditions for which a patient should wear an identification symbol.
   (1) Heart disease (2) Diabetes (3) Epilepsy (4) Allergies (5) Laryngectomy
2. Name the three types of visible bleeding and the characteristics of each.
   (1) Arterial: bright red bleeding produced in spurts (2) Venous: a steady flow of dark red blood (3) Capillary: a steady ooze
3. List the eight steps or stages that might occur with a major seizure.
   (1) Rigidity (2) Uncontrollable movements (3) Unconsciousness (4) Cyanosis of face and lips (5) Breathing cessation (6) Loss of bladder and bowel control (7) Confusion (8) Headache and exhaustion

4. List at least seven symptoms of a heart attack.
   Any seven of the following: (1) Severe chest pain (2) Pain radiating to one or both arms and/or left shoulder and jaw (3) Tightness of the chest (4) Weak and rapid pulse (5) Profuse perspiration (6) Cyanotic lips and fingernails (7) Nausea (8) Anxious (9) Agitated

5. What are the symptoms of internal bleeding, and how is it initially and eventually treated?
   Symptoms: (a) Rapid, weak pulse (b) Shallow breathing (c) Cold, clammy skin (d) Dilated pupils (e) Dizziness (f) Faintness (g) Thirst (h) Restlessness (i) Anxiety. Initially, the patient is kept in the recumbent position until surgery can locate and repair the site.

6. Describe the purpose of an AED and its capabilities.
   The AED is used in connection with CPR to restore cardiac function. The AED is indicated when the victim is unresponsive, is not breathing, and has no pulse. The AED can analyze the heart rhythm of a person in fibrillation or arrest; recognize a shockable rhythm; advise the operator through lights, text, and voice prompts if shock is indicated; and, with built-in diagnostic capability, permit life-saving intervention without the operator needing to evaluate the situation or interpret an ECG.

7. What are the distinguishing characteristics of arterial, venous, and capillary bleeding?
   Arterial bleeding produces bright red blood in spurts. Bleeding from a vein produces a steady flow of dark red blood. Any bleeding from capillary damage produces a steady ooze from the wound area.

8. Explain instances when obstructive airway can occur in adults and children.
   Obstructed airway most occurs in adults when food is aspirated while eating. This occurs when partially chewed food is sucked into the trachea when talking, laughing, or coughing while eating. Children, on the other hand, can get toys, toy parts, buttons, candy, or a variety of other objects, in addition to food, caught in their throat and obstruct their airway.

9. List at least 10 supplies that can be found on a crash cart.
   Any of the following may be included: gloves; alcohol wipes; stethoscope; blood pressure cuff; penlight; aromatic spirits of ammonia; oxygen tank with flow meter and wrench for opening the tank; tubing; nasal cannula and pediatric and adult masks; Ambu-bag; resuscitation masks in a variety of sizes; airways of differing sizes (nasal and oral); bandage material (sterile dressings); adhesive tape; bandage scissors; disposable syringes; tourniquets; IV supplies: tubing and needles (butterflies and angiocaths); and fluids, including D5W, NS, D10W, and lactated Ringer's

10. Compare and contrast the symptoms of hyperglycemia and hypoglycemia.
    Hyperglycemia symptoms include confusion, dizziness, weakness, or nausea. Vomiting can occur. Respiration might be rapid and deep and the skin dry and flushed. The patient's breath has a sweet or fruity odor, which might be evident some distance away. The patient can lapse into unconsciousness and die if not treated quickly. Hypoglycemia symptoms can include muscle weakness, anxiety, mental confusion, a pounding heartbeat, hunger, and diaphoresis. The skin will be cold, pale, and moist. The patient might lapse into unconsciousness and might have seizures.

**Labeling: Label the pressure points where severe arterial bleeding can be controlled.**

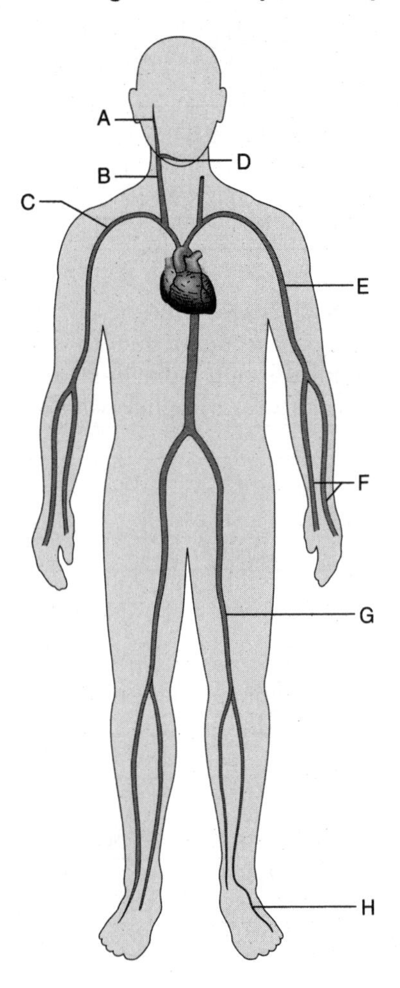


A. Temporal artery

B. Carotid artery

C. Subclavian artery

D. Facial artery

E. Brachial artery

F. Radial artery

G. Femoral artery

H. Dorsalis pedis

## Chapter Application

### Case Studies with Critical Thinking Questions

### Scenario 1

Mr. Karnes, a diabetic patient, tells the receptionist that he is not feeling very well and wants to know if he can be taken to an exam room right away. He took his insulin this morning, but didn't have time to eat before his appointment. While waiting for the medical assistant to escort him to the room, Mr. Karnes becomes unconscious and falls to the floor in the waiting room. The medical assistant summons the provider and gets the crash cart, only to find that there is no glucose in the cart.

1. What must be done immediately after the emergency has been dealt with? Any items used must be restocked immediately.

2. How can an inadequately stocked crash cart be prevented in the future? Replace items immediately after each use and routinely take inventory of the crash cart to ensure that it is fully stocked.

### Scenario 2

A frantic mother has just called your office and reports that her 3-year-old son has just ingested household cleaner. She is hysterical and is asking questions so quickly that you can hardly understand what she is saying.

1. What information should be obtained from the caller? Get the victim's name, the caller's name, and phone number immediately in case the connection is lost. Also ask when the problem occurred, what was ingested, and how much was ingested if known.
2. Who should the mother be instructed to call? Instruct the mother to call the local poison control center.

### Scenario 3

A patient in the waiting room is suffering with a hacking cough and is hurriedly trying to take a cough drop. A few seconds later, you look up and notice that the patients face is red and she is giving the universal sign for choking.

1. What is the first thing you need to do? Determine whether the patient can speak or cough by asking, "Are you choking?"
2. If the patient is indeed choking, how can you help? You should perform abdominal thrusts.
3. Should you try to dislodge the object in the patient's mouth? No. Never stick your fingers in the patient's mouth because you could force the object deeper into the throat.

### Competency Practice

**Perform an Abdominal Thrust on an Adult Victim with an Obstructed Airway.** Choose a partner and demonstrate how to perform abdominal thrusts. Explain what your next step would be if the patient loses consciousness. Use Procedure 55–1 as a guide.

CHAPTER 56

# First Aid for Accidents and Injuries

## Words to Know Challenge

**Spelling: Each line contains three spellings of a word. Underline the correctly spelled word.**

| | | |
|---|---|---|
| 1. anafalactic | anaphylactic | aniphylactic |
| 2. avulsion | evulsion | avulzion |
| 3. cravat | cravet | cravette |
| 4. moltan | molten | moltin |
| 5. superficiel | superficial | superfisual |
| 6. thermel | theremal | thermal |

**Matching: Match the term in column I to its definition in column II.**

| | COLUMN I | COLUMN II |
|---|---|---|
| I | 1. Abrasion | A. Smooth cut |
| H | 2. Chemical | B. A brisk rubbing |
| G | 3. Electrical | C. A hole |
| B | 4. Friction | D. A tear |
| F | 5. Immobilize | E. An injury |
| A | 6. Incision | F. To prevent from moving |
| D | 7. Laceration | G. Having a current |
| C | 8. Puncture | H. Acid or alkaline substance |
| K | 9. Foreign body | I. A scrape or scratch |
| L | 10. Rabies | J. State of very low blood pressure, rapid pulse, pallor |
| J | 11. Shock | K. Not normally found in the location; splinter, dirt |
| M | 12. Splinter | L. Transmitted by an animal bite |
| E | 13. Wound | M. Thin, sharp piece of wood |

## Chapter Review

**Fill in the Blank: Use information from the chapter to complete the sentence.**

1. The Rule of Nines is used to estimate the extent of a burn.
2. A third- or fourth- degree burn involves all three layers of the skin.
3. A break in the bone is also known as a fracture.
4. Injury to a muscle or muscle group is known as a strain.
5. A sprain causes a ligament injury at the joint.
6. You would place a dressing over the wound before you cover it with a bandage.
7. A scrape in the epidermis is also known as an abrasion.
8. A third- degree burn causes white, leathery tissue.
9. You should flood a chemical burn with water for 15 minutes.
10. A figure-eight bandage should be used for an injury to the palm of the hand.

## Short Answer

1. How is a bee stinger removed? By scraping the site of the sting with a sharp object
2. When is anti-rabies serum required following an animal bite? When the animal cannot be tested or observed for rabies
3. Name the three types of burns and give examples of each.
   a. Thermal—fire, electrical, firecrackers, space heaters, scalding water, curling irons, stoves, regular irons, and sunburns
   b. Chemical—acids or alkalines contact, ingestion, inhalation, or injection
   c. Electrical—faulty electrical wiring, chewing on electrical cord, high-voltage lines, lightning
4. What is the first priority in the treatment of burns? Stop the burning process
5. Compare the types of first aid treatment for the three degrees of burns.
   a. First degree—Apply cold water, antiseptic preparation, and a dressing.
   b. Second degree—Treat for shock, remove jewelry, provide ample liquids to drink, and cover area with a sterile dressing.
   c. Third degree—First aid involves only covering the area with a sterile dressing and treatment for shock. Immediate medical attention is necessary.
6. What is the benefit of adding moisture to a heat treatment? It is less likely to burn the skin and it provides deeper penetration to the tissues.
7. What action does the application of cold treatments have on the body? It decreases local circulation, bacterial growth, and body temperature. It also is a temporary anesthetic, relieves inflammation, helps control bleeding, and reduces swelling.
8. What action does the application of heat treatments have on the body? It increases tissue temperature and the rate of healing. It also decreases pain and relieves congestion in deep muscle layers, organs, and muscle spasms. It dilates blood vessels to increase circulation and reduce localized swelling.
9. Name five types of wounds.
   (1) abrasion (2) avulsion (3) incision (4) laceration (5) puncture

10. What four pieces of information are needed to determine the severity of an illness or injury?
    a. History of victim's situation
    b. Nature of injury or illness
    c. Time the accident occurred or the illness began
    d. Description of the current condition

# Chapter Application

## Case Studies with Critical Thinking Questions

### Scenario 1

Mrs. Leonard calls the office because her 3-year-old child has been stung. She thinks it was a wasp, but she isn't sure. She says he is having trouble breathing, is very restless, his head hurts very badly, and his skin is becoming mottled and blue.

1. What is happening to the child? He is suffering from a severe allergic reaction.
2. If he is going into anaphylactic shock, what medication needs to be given immediately? Epinephrine
3. What instructions should be given to Mrs. Leonard? Mrs. Leonard should be instructed to call EMS or 911.

### Scenario 2

A patient rushes into the office with a severe burn to his left hand. He says that he was deep frying some fish and spilled the hot grease on his hand. His skin is red and blistered.

1. Which class of burn is the patient suffering from? Second-degree burn
2. What is another name for this degree burn? Partial-thickness burn
3. What is the proper first aid? Remove any jewelry, have him drink lots of fluids, cover the burn with a sterile dressing, and seek medical attention.

## Competency Practice

1. **Demonstrate the proper method of cleaning a wound.** With a partner, gather the equipment and supplies and role play demonstrating the proper procedure for cleaning a wound. One is the MA and the other the patient. Be sure to provide the patient with any education regarding the wound. Use Procedure 56–1 as a guide.

2. **Demonstrate application of a tube gauze, spiral, figure-eight, and cravat bandage.** With a partner, practice these bandaging techniques. Be sure to ask the instructor to check your work for correctness. Discuss any patient education that would be needed about the bandages. Use Procedures 56–2 through 56–5 as guides.

UNIT 19

# Rehabilitation and Healthy Living

CHAPTER 57

# Rehabilitation

## Words to Know Challenge

**Spelling: Each line contains three spellings of a word. Underline the correctly spelled word.**

| | | |
|---|---|---|
| 1. angel | angle | angul |
| 2. crutches | crutzes | crutious |
| 3. sling | sleng | slinge |
| 4. suport | support | sapport |
| 5. walcher | walker | wocker |
| 6. weelchair | whealchair | wheelchair |

**Matching: Match the term in column I to its definition in column II.**

| | COLUMN I | COLUMN II |
|---|---|---|
| D | 1. Ambulate | A. Proper positioning to reduce injury |
| F | 2. Axilla | B. Manner of walking |
| H | 3. Balance | C. A type of cane |
| G | 4. Flexibility | D. To walk |
| B | 5. Gait | E. Extent of movement |
| I | 6. Mobility | F. Area under the arm |
| C | 7. Quadbase | G. The ability to twist and bend |
| E | 8. Range-of-motion | H. Equilibrium |
| J | 9. Stabilize | I. Move about freely |
| A | 10. Body mechanics | J. To hold secure |

# Chapter Review

## Short Answer

1. Identify seven situations during which the use of some form of device might be indicated to assist patients with mobility.
   Answers will vary, but some examples include: After an accident or injury; Following a stroke; After surgery; Those with a severe medical condition; Arthritis sufferers; Older adult; Physically challenged

2. Explain the importance of good body mechanics.
   Body mechanics is the practice of using certain key muscle groups together with good body alignment and proper body positioning to reduce the risk of injury to both patient and caregiver.

3. What are range-of-motion exercises?
   Any body action involving muscles, joints, and natural direction movements such as abduction, adduction, extension, flexion, pronation, and rotation

4. When are range-of-motion exercises indicated?
   They are indicated when a patient cannot perform strenuous exercise or when a patient has arthritis, bursitis, or other disabilities.

5. Identify two guidelines concerning fitting a cane.
   (1) Handle should be just below hip level.
   (2) Arm should be flexed at elbow at about 25 to 30 degrees.

6. Explain the proper height for crutches.
   They should be 2 inches below the axilla with a comfortable handhold with the arms extended.

7. List four factors that will increase safety for the patient at home.
   (1) Keep floors free of spills and clutter (2) Remove loose throw rugs or damaged floor coverings (3) Avoid using wax or other slippery products on floors (4) Use proper footwear

# Chapter Application

## Case Studies with Critical Thinking Questions

### Scenario 1

Mr. Durst has twisted his knee and cannot walk very well. He says he has no balance and is afraid of falling again.

1. Which mobility device could be helpful to the patient? A cane

2. If the provider instructs you to provide patient education regarding this mobility device, what information should be given to the patient? The patient should carry the cane on the strong or uninjured side. The cane should swing forward with the injured extremity. Part of the weight is carried by placing the cane firmly on the floor simultaneously with the injured extremity.

### Scenario 2

Sue Larson, an active 16-year-old, presented to the office with an ankle fracture. The provider has ordered you to help fit her for crutches. She states she has never had an injury like this before and that she doesn't think she needs assistance—it will be fun and easy to use the crutches.

1. What do you need to tell the patient about why you need to help with the crutch fitting? Explain that you will assist her in a proper adjustment to the crutches so they will not cause injury to her axilla area.

2. What does the patient need to know about walking with the crutches? She should be instructed that there are various crutch gaits to use depending on the type of injury she has and whether she can bear weight.

3. What can you do to ensure patient compliance? Stay with the patient and go over all the instructions for gait walking. Have the patient demonstrate the walk back to you. Reassure the patient that you are here for her if she has questions, Be sure she is totally comfortable and can ambulate well before allowing her to leave the office.

## Competency Practice

1. **Demonstrate using proper body mechanics.** With a partner or alone, practice lifting and moving various large objects, using the guidelines for proper body mechanics. For a variation, have students role play, one being the patient and the other being the MA, and apply body mechanic principles in moving the patient. Use Procedure 57–1 as a guide.

2. **Demonstrate application of an arm sling.** With a partner, demonstrate the proper application of a commercial arm sling on your partner. Be sure to choose the correctly fitting sling and go over patient education on proper use and how to watch for circulation impairment. Use Procedure 57–2 as a guide.

3. **Demonstrate fitting and instruction in use of a cane.** With a partner, demonstrate adjusting a cane to the proper height. Conduct patient education sessions on the proper use of a cane. Use Procedure 57–3 as a guide.

4. **Demonstrate fitting and instruction in use of crutches.** With a partner, practice adjusting crutches for one another. Then divide into three groups and have each group choose a crutch gait. Practice the gaits and demonstrate them to the class. Then rotate groups until each group has gotten to apply each one. Use Procedure 57–4 as a guide.

5. **Demonstrate instruction in use of a walker.** With a partner, using both walkers with wheels and those without, adjust the height of the walker and practice ambulating with it. Role play with each other instructing the patient on the proper way to walk, keeping safety in mind at all times. Discuss when a walker might be indicated for a patient. Use Procedure 57–5 as a guide.

CHAPTER 58

# Nutrition, Exercise, and Healthy Living

## Words to Know Challenge

**Spelling: Each line contains three spellings of a word. Underline the correctly spelled word.**

| | | |
|---|---|---|
| 1. anorexec | anorexic | annorhexic |
| 2. beriberi | berryberry | baribari |
| 3. scurvy | scurvey | skurvey |
| 4. tactille | tactile | tacktile |
| 5. sleep apnia | sleep apnea | sleep apniea |
| 6. protine | proteen | protein |
| 7. obesity | obeasety | obeesity |
| 8. rickettes | ricettes | rickets |
| 9. dietician | diatician | diatichian |
| 10. carbohidrate | carbohydrate | carbohydrat |

**Matching: Match the term in column I to its definition in column II.**

| | COLUMN I | COLUMN II |
|---|---|---|
| D | 1. Amenorrhea | A. A physical weakness or ailment |
| K | 2. Anorexic | B. Overeating and then initiating vomiting |
| B | 3. Bulimia nervosa | C. To rid body of food after eating |
| J | 4. Deprivation | D. Absence of menstruation |
| H | 5. Emaciation | E. To overindulge in food or drink |
| A | 6. Infirmity | F. Period of no breathing |
| C | 7. Purge | G. Non-rapid eye movement |
| F | 8. Apnea | H. Abnormal thinness |
| E | 9. Binge | I. Rapid eye movement |

(continues)

G 10. NREM — J. Having to do without or being unable to use

I 11. REM — K. No appetite, refusal to eat

## Chapter Review

### Fill in the Blank: Use information from the chapter to complete the sentence.

1. A deficiency of vitamin D can cause rickets.
2. A deficiency of vitamin C can cause scurvy.
3. People who weigh 30 percent MORE than their ideal body weight are considered obese.
4. Generally, a(n) clear liquid diet is recommended at least every two hours for patients who have diarrhea.
5. The BRAT acronym stands for bananas, rice, applesauce, and toast.
6. The BRAT diet is recommended for patients who have tolerated the 24-hour clear liquid diet.
7. Those who have been sick and are just getting over an intestinal virus might find the soft diet to be tolerable.
8. Patients who wish to reduce their weight should exercise at least three times a week and follow a(n) low-calorie diet.
9. Patients who have special dietary needs should consult with a(n) registered dietician.
10. Insomnia describes the inability to sleep.
11. Lack of sleep is termed sleep deprivation.
12. Research shows that a person needs both REM and NREM (non-rapid eye movement) stages of sleep.
13. People who sleep at least at least six hours at a time generally feel good because they benefit from the effects of the proper sequence of sleep.

### Short Answer

1. Identify three dos and three don'ts from the Guidelines for Good Health. Do (1) exercise regularly; (2) ea[t] a sensible, balanced diet; and (3) get adequate rest and recreation. (See Table 58-1 in the textbook for a ful[l] list.) Don't (1) smoke or use tobacco, (2) drink alcohol in excess, or (3) overeat or gain too much weight
2. Name the five sections in MyPlate, and list examples of foods in each section. (1) Vegetables (gree[n] section): examples include broccoli, cauliflower, carrots; beans and peas act as both vegetables an[d] proteins. (2) Fruit (red section): examples include apples, bananas, pears. (3) Grains (orange section) examples include bread, rice, pasta. (4) Protein (purple section): examples include chicken, fish, bee[f] (5) Dairy (blue section): examples include cheese, milk, yogurt

   *The purple section refers to protein.* Proteins supply nutrients such as Vitamin E, B vitamins, iron, zinc magnesium, and omega-3 fatty acids. Meat, poultry, seafood, beans and peas, eggs, processed soy products nuts, and seeds are considered proteins

   *The blue section refers to dairy.* Dairy supplies nutrients such as calcium, Vitamin D, potassium, an[d] protein. Milk, calcium-fortified soymilk, yogurt, cheese, and milk-based desserts are part of the dair[y] group; lactose-free versions of these items are also included. Foods made from milk that have little or n[o] calcium (butter, cream cheese) are not considered dairy. Choose fat-free or low-fat products in this grou[p]
3. Name the fat-soluble vitamins. Vitamins A, D, E, and K
4. Name the water-soluble vitamins. Vitamin C and B complex
5. Name two essential minerals that are most often missing from the average diet. Calcium, iron, and iodin[e]

6. List 10 diseases or conditions that can develop from poor diet and a sedentary lifestyle.
   a. Cardiovascular disease
   b. Hypertension
   c. Dyslipedemia
   d. Type II diabetes
   e. Diverticular disease
   f. Osteoporosis
   g. Obesity
   h. Iron deficiency
   i. Malnutrition
   j. Certain cancers

7. What are eight pieces of information included on food labels?
   a. Serving size
   b. Servings per container
   c. Amount per serving
   d. Listing of nutrients and gram amount
   e. Listing of fats
   f. Other items such as cholesterol, fiber, sodium, and sugar
   g. Vitamins and minerals
   h. List of ingredients

8. What two eating disorders affect primarily teenagers, and what are the underlying causes of these conditions? Anorexia nervosa and bulimia nervosa. They result from emotional stress, conflict, poor self-image, and obsessive fear of obesity.

9. Why is sleep necessary? With sleep, the body can restore itself to deal with daily activities.

10. What happens after prolonged sleep deprivation? The person becomes irritable and fatigued, has poor concentration, develops a poor memory, is clumsy, and might have visual or tactile hallucinations.

## Chapter Application

### Case Studies with Critical Thinking Questions

#### Scenario 1

Mrs. Anderson is being seen in the office to evaluate her general state of health. She is found to be malnourished and is suffering from lethargy and malaise. The provider suggests she should incorporate more protein in her diet, including some red meat, which has valuable amino acids and iron. The provider asks the medical assistant to provide Mrs. Anderson with a diet sheet listing certain meats and other foods high in protein. Mrs. Anderson tells the medical assistant she is a Seventh-Day Adventist and does not eat meat.

1. What should the medical assistant tell Mrs. Anderson about her dietary restrictions? The medical assistant should not counsel the patient about her restrictions, nor should she make any comments regarding those restrictions.

2. How can the dietary restrictions be dealt with? Should the medical assistant tell Mrs. Anderson about a dietary supplement that is very high in protein? No. The provider should always be consulted before providing the patient with any information. The provider can counsel the patient regarding other high-protein foods and dietary supplements.

### Scenario 2

Andrea, a 32-year-old in good health, calls the office to talk with the medical assistant about the diarrhea she has had for the past three days. She says she is eating only small portions of chicken noodle soup and drinking milk, but she can't seem to get over the diarrhea. She wants to know when she can expect to get better and when she can return to a normal diet.

### Critical Thinking Questions

1. With the provider's approval, what should Andrea's diet be until the diarrhea has stopped? Clear liquids
2. Which diet should Andrea follow for 24 hours after the diarrhea has stopped? The BRAT diet
3. Before resuming a normal diet, which eating plan should be followed next? The soft diet

SECTION 5

# Preparing for Employment

UNIT 20

# Workplace Readiness

CHAPTER 59

# Practicum and the Job Search

## Words to Know Challenge

**Spelling: Each line contains three spellings of a word. Underline the correctly spelled word.**

1. resame — résumé — reesume
2. transscript — transcript — transcrip
3. practicum — practical — practicam
4. chronilogical — chonological — chronological
5. targeted — targited — tarrgated
6. extirnship — externshop — externship

**Fill in the Blank: Complete the following sentences with correctly spelled words from the Spelling section.**

1. The practicum is a period of time when a student is placed in an actual health care setting to practice skills that have been learned in the classroom. Another name for this experience is externship.
2. A functional style résumé highlights your previous work experience related to the position you are seeking.
3. The goal of a résumé is to make a favorable impression so you will obtain an interview for a position.
4. This type of résumé lists education achievements followed by work experience, starting with the present or most recent job and progressing back in time. It is called a chronologic style résumé.
5. The targeted style résumé will usually include a position statement.
6. An official copy of a student's educational record is known as a transcript.

## Chapter Review

### Short Answer

1. Name three reasons participation in a practicum is beneficial to a student.
(1) Develops competency in medical assisting shills; (2) Helps decide which area of practice the student prefers; (3) Develops good work habits

2. List at least six possible areas that might be included on an externship evaluation form.
Any six of the following: (1) Appearance, (2) Attitude, (3) Maturity, (4) Dependability, (5) Initiative, (6) Administrative tasks, (7) Clinical tasks, (8) Interpersonal relationships

3. What is the goal of a résumé?
The goal of a résumé is to make a favorable impression so you will obtain an interview for a position.

4. What is the purpose of a cover letter?
To express one's desire to be interviewed for the position, to briefly describe your assets for the job.

5. List the styles of résumés and the purpose of each.
Functional—highlights previous work experience that matches job opening; Skills—emphasizes what you can do, not previous jobs; Targeted—arranges information to focus on a specific job; Chronological—lists educational achievements and work experience, starting with the most recent

6. List at least six places a medical assistant can find information about job opportunities.
Any six of the following: (1) The Internet, (2) Public or private employment agencies, (3) Public library, (4) Professional organizations, (5) Personal contacts, (6) Community service groups, (7) Newspaper and classified ads

7. Why is it important to dress professionally for an interview?
Most employers expect appropriate attire, and some require adherence to a very specific policy concerning type of dress and general appearance. Unprofessional attire and grooming (including facial piercings, unusual hair colors, and long nails) give a negative impression to employers.

8. Name six things you need to remember to be prepared for your interview.
A. Allow sufficient time to get ready.
B. Do not chew gum.
C. Do not smell of cigarettes.
D. Wear business attire.
E. Arrive 10–15 minutes early.
F. Do not bring children. Other answers are possible; see Table 59-3.

9. Why should you send a follow-up letter after an interview?
To enhance your image with the interviewer and as an indication of your interest, persistence, and follow-through ability.

10. What are six things you can do to advance in employment?
A. Show interest.
B. Show initiative.
C. Seek continuing education.
D. Acquire a new skill.
E. Be efficient.
F. Communicate well with others. Answers will vary, but should include the ideas above.

**Matching: Identify the items in the following list as desirable skills or qualities that employers seek in employees.**

A. Desirable skill
B. Desirable quality

A 1. Teamwork
B 2. Flexibility
B 3. Honesty
A 4. Critical thinking
A 5. Computer proficiency
B 6. Responsible
A 7. Time management
B 8. Positive attitude
A 9. Communication
B 10. Punctuality

# Chapter Application

## Case Studies with Critical Thinking Questions

### Scenario 1

Avery is beginning her second week at her practicum. She has been given one of the best sites, where she will gain a lot of valuable experience. She is not happy about putting in hours and not getting paid for them. Avery feels that this is just another part of her school experience and, therefore, she can skip whenever she feels like it. She has already been 10 minutes late on three occasions and has missed one whole day.

1. What does her practicum performance say about her as a medical assistant? Her behavior projects a negative image and lack of dependability.
2. What does her performance say about her school? Her performance can give the externship site a bad impression of the school. The school might appear as though it is not training the students in the importance of being dependable as well as skillful.
3. What impact could her performance have on her career? An unfavorable evaluation could affect her chances of obtaining a position in the future.

### Scenario 2

You are on your way to a job interview for a position you really want. You thought you allowed plenty of time for traffic and for any other problems that could arise. Traffic on the freeway is at a standstill because of an accident, and you realize you are going to be late for your interview.

1. What should you do? Call the site to let them know you are tied up in traffic and to give them an approximate time of arrival.
2. What impact can this situation have if you arrive late without notifying the facility? If other interviews are scheduled after yours, you might miss your interview.
3. What impression could your late arrival give to your interviewer? A late arrival could tell the interviewer you don't care about being punctual and that you are not very dependable.

## Scenario 3

You found an ad in the newspaper for a medical assisting position that you are really interested in. The ad instructed applicants to visit the clinic in person to fill out an application and drop off a résumé. You hurriedly print off a copy of your résumé and drive to the clinic, wearing clothes appropriate for the gym, since you'll be going there after. Upon arriving at the clinic, you find that there are five other people filling out applications. You hurry through your application to be the first one done, give the receptionist your résumé, and are told that they will be contacting qualified applicants for an interview next week. Three weeks later, you have not been contacted for an interview, and you are very disappointed.

1. If you could start this day over again, what would be the first thing you would do over? Review your résumé to be sure that it is current, in the style that is appropriate, and error free.

2. What are some other things that might have prevented you from receiving an interview? You may have filled out the application in cursive instead of printing, used the wrong color ink, or made mistakes on the application.

3. What could you have done to get an interview? It is often a good idea to follow up with a phone call after a suitable amount of time to let the facility know you are still interested in the position.

# Part 2

# CHAPTER GUIDES WITH LESSON OUTLINES

# SECTION 1 MEDICAL ASSISTING FOUNDATIONS

# UNIT 1 HEALTH CARE ROLES AND RESPONSIBILITIES

# CHAPTER 1 The Medical Assistant

## ABHES Curriculum

| | |
|---|---|
| MA.A.1.1.a | Comprehends the current employment outlook for the medical assistant |
| MA.A.1.1.c | Understands the medical assisting credentialing requirements and the process to obtain the credential |
| MA.A.1.1.d | Has knowledge of the general responsibilities of the medical assistant |
| MA.A.1.1.e | Defines scope of practice for the medical assistant and comprehends the conditions for practice within the state in which the medical assistant is employed |
| MA.A.1.8.aa | Is attentive, listens, and learns |
| MA.A.1.8.dd | Serves as liaison between physician and others |
| MA.A.1.11.b.1 | Exhibits dependability, punctuality, and a positive work ethic |
| MA.A.1.11.b.2 | Exhibits a positive attitude and a sense of responsibility |
| MA.A.1.11.b.3 | Maintains confidentiality at all times |
| MA.A.1.11.b.4 | Is cognizant of ethical boundaries |
| MA.A.1.11.b.5 | Exhibits initiative |
| MA.A.1.11.b.6 | Adapts to change |
| MA.A.1.11.b.7 | Expresses a responsible attitude |
| MA.A.1.11.b.8 | Is courteous and diplomatic |
| MA.A.1.11.b.9 | Conducts work within scope of education, training, and ability |

## CAAHEP Core Curriculum

| | |
|---|---|
| IV.C.13 | Identify the role of self boundaries in the health care environment |
| IV.C.14 | Recognize the role of patient advocacy in the practice of medical assisting |
| IV.A.1 | Demonstrate empathy in communicating with patients, family, and friends |
| IV.A.2 | Apply active listening skills |
| IV.A.4 | Demonstrate awareness of the territorial boundaries of the person with whom communicating |
| IV.A.5 | Demonstrate sensitivity appropriate to the message being delivered |
| IV.A.6 | Demonstrate awareness of how an individual's personal appearance affects anticipated responses |

## LESSON OUTLINE

### I. THE ROLE OF THE MEDICAL ASSISTANT

A. Most versatile allied health occupation in today's environment
B. An integral member of the health care delivery team
C. Liaison between doctor and the patient
D. To become a successful medical assistant, must acquire specific:
   1. Knowledge base (theory)
   2. Skills (procedures)
   3. Behaviors (professional characteristics or attitudes

E. Is medical assisting right for you? (Sample questions from the AAMA)
  1. Are you looking for a meaningful job?
  2. Do you like helping others?
  3. Do you have an interest in health and medicine?
  4. Are you a people person?
  5. Are you good at multi-tasking?
  6. Do you like variety in your job?
  7. Would you like to enter a career in an expanding field?

F. Skills and responsibilities of the medical assistant
  1. General skills
    a. Communication
    b. Legal and ethical
    c. Instruction
    d. Operational functions
  2. Administrative skills (two categories)
    a. Administrative procedures
    b. Practice finances
    c. Examples of skills in these categories include:
      i. Scheduling appointments
      ii. Performing inpatient and outpatient procedures
      iii. Creating and maintaining the patient's medical record
      iv. Filing medical records and other documents.
      v. Performing procedural and diagnostic coding
      vi. Performing billing and collections
      vii. Performing bookkeeping and financial procedures
      viii. Preparing submittal insurance forms
  3. Clinical Skills (three categories)
    a. Fundamental practices
    b. Diagnostic procedures
    c. Patient care
    d. Examples of skill in these categories include:
      i. Identification of the roles and responsibilities of the medical assistant as well as those of other team members in the medical office
      ii. Applying principles of aseptic technique and infection control
      iii. Performing vital signs
      iv. Performing sterilization and minor surgery procedures
      v. Collecting and processing specimens
      vi. Performing lab tests
      vii. Performing EKGs
      viii. Administering medications
      ix. Performing phlebotomy procedures
      x. Performing patient screenings

xi. Preparing patients for examinations, procedures, and treatments

xii. Responding to emergencies

(Many medical assistants work as generalists, meaning they perform both clinical and administrative duties.)

G. Boundaries of medical assistants

1. Medical assistant must be aware of the boundaries of medical assisting
2. Refer to Figure 1–4

H. Medical assisting work environment

1 Doctor's offices
2. Specialty practices
3. Urgent care centers
4. Clinics
5. Hospitals
6. Labs
7. Insurance companies
8. Billing companies
9. Government agencies

I. Types of practices

1. Solo practices
2. Partnerships
3. Multi-provider clinics
4. Urgent care centers
5. Patient-centered medical homes

J. Job outlook for medical assistants

1. According to U.S. Department of Labor, Bureau and Statistics, medical assisting expected to grow by 34% through the year 2018
2. Due to boomers retiring and the aging of the population

## II. DEMONSTRATING PROFESSIONALISM

A. Evolving into a professional doesn't just happen overnight.

B. Webster defines professionalism as "the conduct, aims, or qualities that characterize or mark a professional or professional person."

C. Altruism or selflessness is one of the most important traits of a medical professional.

D. Personal appearance

1. First impression you give to the patient and others
2. Appearance says volumes about who you are
3. Refer to Table 1–1 for how to project a professional appearance

E. Professional behaviors

1. Employers usually pursue candidates that possess professional behaviors or character traits.
2. Some characteristics seem to be almost innate or inherent.
3. Refer to Table 1–2 for a list of professional traits.

4. Be careful regarding postings you put on social networking sites.

F. Personal qualities
   1. Personality qualities affect the way character traits are perceived.
   2. An individual can demonstrate initiative, dependability, honesty, and other traits, but if he or she is not likeable, that individual will struggle in bonding or getting along with others.
   3. Positive personal qualities include:
      a. Friendly attitude
      b. Genuine smile
      c. Perception as a professional

## III. TIME MANAGEMENT

A. Refers to assortment of skills, tools, and practices to manage time during daily activities and when accomplishing specific projects

B. You must take control of your time rather than allowing time to take control of you.

C. Parento's Principle, or the 80-20 rule, states that as little as 20% of your labors result in 80% of your results. To be efficient with your time, focus on the 20% of your work that yields the greatest results.

D. List of goals that assist you in being more efficient with your time
   1. Make a daily task list and prioritize tasks in their order of importance.
   2. Learn to say no to low-priority requests
   3. Don't be a perfectionist for tasks that don't require your best efforts.
   4. Stay away from bad habits that rob you of your time, such as surfing the Internet and texting.

E. When working in an administrative capacity, patients in the office take priority over patients calling into the office except in an emergency.

F. When working in a clinical capacity, the following applies
   1. First priority: Assisting provider with emergencies and procedures
   2. Second priority: Rooming patients
   3. Third priority: Performing procedures and dismissing patients
   4. Fourth priority: Working on pending files that have tasks

G. Staying organized also assists in time management

## IV. PROFESSIONAL ORGANIZATIONS FOR MEDICAL ASSISTANTS

A. A variety of organizations, which include credentialing opportunities and continuing education opportunities, provide professional services for medical assistants.

B. Accreditation is a process by which an educational institution or program establishes credibility or legitimacy by complying with predetermined standards.

C. Accredited programs must meet or exceed established thresholds in areas such as certification pass rates, student graduation rates, and placement.

D. Two organizations specifically accredit medical assistants:
   1. Commission on Accreditation of Allied Health Education Programs (CAAHEP)
   2. Accrediting Bureau of Health Education Schools (ABHES)

E. American Association of Medical Assistants (AAMA)

1. Traces its roots to 1955
2. Has a monthly magazine referred to as *CMA Today*
3. Offers the Certified Medical Assistant credential or CMA (AAMA)
4. Must have graduated from a medical assisting program accredited by CAAHEP or ABHES
5. Must take exam at an approved Prometric Testing Center
6. Each candidate has a 90-day window to take the exam.
7. All newly and recertifying CMA (AAMA) are considered current for 60 months following the end of the calendar month of his or her initial certification or recent recertification.
8. Certified medical assistants must earn 60 CEUs every five years.
   a.) 10 administrative
   b.) 10 clinical
   c.) 10 general
   d.) 30 from any combination of categories

F. American Medical Technologists (AMT)
1. Founded in 1939
2. Certification and membership society for several allied health professionals, including:
   a. Medical assistants
   b. Medical laboratory technologists and technicians
   c. Phlebotomists
   d. Medical lab assistants
   e. Medical administrative specialists
   f. Others
   g. Publications include *AMT Events* and *Journal of CE Topics and Issues*
   h. Awards the title of Registered Medical Assistant RMA (AMT)
      i. Must have graduated from a program accredited by a recognized accrediting body if certifying via the educational route
      ii. Can take exam at any Pearson VUE Testing Center
      iii. Successful examinees must recertify every three years by receiving the appropriate number of CEUs.
   i. AMT certification also offers an administrative specialty exam for medical assistants, referred to as a Certified Medical Administrative Specialist, CMAS (AMT)

G. National Center for Competency Testing (NCCT)
1. National certification agency that has been in existence since 1989
2. Organization certifies:
   a. Medical assistants
   b. Phlebotomists
   c. Patient care technicians
   d. Medical office assistants
   e. Insurance and coding specialists
   f. ECG technicians
   g. Other healthcare specialists

3. Has special benefit, "My Professional Center (MPC)," that offers professional career development and professional and personal networking opportunities
4. Credentials for medical assistants include:
   a. National Certified Medical Assistant (NCMA)
   b. National Certified Medical Office Assistant (NCMOA)
5. Must have graduated from an NCCT-approved medical assisting program or qualified through the experience route
6. Renewal process very five years
7. Must obtain a minimum of 14 clock hours of education per year

H. National Healthcareer Association
1. Established in 1989 as a certification agency
2. Provides products and services to health care professionals in ten areas:
   a. Medical assisting certifications, including:
      i. Certified Clinical Medical Assistant (CCMA)
      ii. Certified Medical Administrative Assistant (CMAA)
   b. Must be a graduate of an NHA-approved school
   c. Exams given at NHA-approved testing sites

I. American Academy of Professional Coders (AAPC)
1. Founded in 1988
2. Promotes professionalism and encourages support education, networking, and certification in the medical billing and coding areas
3. Offers training in the billing and coding areas
4. Publishes four periodicals
5. Offers several types of certifications, including the following Certified Professional Coder specialty credentials:
   a. CPC® (Physician Practice)
   b. CPC-H® (Outpatient Hospital/Facility)
   c. CPC-P® (Payer)
6. Other certifications available as well. To remain in good standing, credentialed members required to renew membership annually and submit 36 hours of continuing education units every two years for verification and authentication of expertise.

## CHAPTER ACTIVITIES

1. Have students research three professional organizations and compare and contrast each one by writing a paper describing similarities and differences of each organization.
2. Have guest speakers come in from the different professional organizations to talk about their organizations.
3. Encourage students to attend some local, state, and national meetings of the professional organization with which your school is affiliated. Give bonus points for attending these meetings and have students share their observations from the meetings.

4. Take students on some tours of facilities in which medical assistants work. Have them write a paper about their observations.
5. Have students interview medical assistants in the field and share their findings with other classmates.

## ANSWERS TO CHECK YOUR KNOWLEDGE QUESTIONS

1. To be successful as an MA, you must learn a specific:
   a. Knowledge base
   b. Set of skills
   c. Set of behaviors
   **d. All the above**
2. All of the following are clinical skills EXCEPT:
   **a. Filing patient records**
   b. Phlebotomy
   c. Administering medications
   d. Wrapping instruments
3. Medical assistants who perform both clinical and administrative skills are referred to as:
   a. Survivalists
   b. Capitalists
   c. Generalists
   **d. Commonists**
4. Employment opportunities for medical assistants are expected to grow by what percentage through 2018?
   a. 32%
   **b. 34%**
   c. 36%
   d. 38%
5. A term that means selflessness is:
   **a. Altruism**
   b. Apathy
   c. Empathy
   d. Egocentric
6. Putting yourself in another person's shoes is:
   a. Sympathy
   b. Apathy
   **c. Empathy**
   d. None of the above
7. Which of the following would take priority over all other floor tasks?
   a. Rooming patients
   b. Performing procedures
   c. Tasking
   **d. Assisting the provider with a procedure**
8. Which of the following organizations provides the RMA credential?

a. AAMA

**b. AMT**

c. AAPC

d. NHA

9. Which of the following organizations' focus is primarily on certifying medical billers and coders?

a. NCCT

b. AMT

**c. AAPC**

d. NHA

10. Which of the following certifying organizations offers a personal Website titled "My Professional Center" that offers professional growth, career development, and professional and personal networking opportunities?

**a. NCCT**

b. AAPC

c. AMT

d. AAMA

# PROCEDURE SCENARIOS

The following scenarios, questions, and activities are provided for use with Procedure 1–1 Competency Checklist. It is optional; instructors may choose to modify the scenarios or make up their own.

## Procedure 1–1

This procedure is really not a skill, but more of a mindset. You may choose to measure different steps through a scenario, through questions and answers, or through an activity.

Sample Questions for Step 1

1. Give an example of how you can show your employer that you are dependable in regards to completing a special assignment (i.e., Designing a new brochure for the office, designing a Web page for the office, or exploring different EMR software packages.)
2. The term "Punctual" means different things to different people. Demonstrating punctuality doesn't only mean showing up for work on time, but being ready to start assigned tasks at the assigned starting time. (Not getting your first cup of coffee, checking the Internet, etc.). Explain how you can show your employer and others around you that you are punctual.

Sample Activity for Step 2

This step can be graded by simply checking the student's appearance. You should check students from head to toe and rate them accordingly. Refer to Table 1-1 for specifics.

Sample Scenario for Step 3

1. For this step, you can give the student a chief complaint and ask them to repeat back everything they can remember. Rate the student on eye contact, body language, and ability to respond appropriately. Example below:

I just don't feel good. I can't explain it but I just don't feel "normal." I feel like crying all the time. Nothing makes me happy anymore. I don't enjoy any of the activities that I use to enjoy. This all started about four months ago. It may have something to do with the death of my dog. He was such a loyal friend! I use to love to come home, but not anymore!

Have the student repeat the complaint to ascertain that he or she truly was actively listening to the patient.

Sample Question for Step 4

Ask the student to describe the difference between territorial and professional boundaries and give an example of how he or she will maintain both types of boundaries once he or she is in the industry.

Sample Activity for Step 5

Have the student list two examples of a positive work ethic.

Sample Scenario for Step 6

For this step the instructor can take on the role of the patient and talk about something that would be a sensitive topic such as being an alcoholic or the patient's battle with obesity. Observe how the student responds to the information. Was he or she sensitive to the patient's feelings and did he or she respond in a professional manner?

Sample Question for Step 7

Give the student a scenario such as the following:

You have a dinner date with a friend at 7:00 p.m.. You have been looking forward to this date for many weeks. It is 5:00 p.m. and Ashley, your co-worker, is running behind and won't be able to leave for another hour. She too had plans to go to her son's little league baseball game. What can you do to demonstrate courteousness (teamwork in this case) to Ashley, while trying to keep your dinner date with your friend?

Sample Question for Step 8

Ask the student to give an appropriate response for the following scenario:

You just wrote up the patient's complaint and left to obtain some forms for the patient to sign. When you returned, you caught the patient looking through the drawers in the examination room. How would you respond to this patient?

Sample Question for Step 9

You work for a family practice and love the team of individuals you with. Your supervisor just informed you that you are being assigned to a new team. You are not particularly fond of some of the individuals on the team. Explain how you would respond and how you can turn this into a positive experience.

Sample Question for Step 10

A patient's husband calls the office because he is concerned about his wife's diabetes. He states that she has not been compliant and has noticed some changes in her physical well-being. He asks you to disclose her latest Hgb-Alc results. The wife didn't give you permission to share any lab tests with the husband. How would you respond?

# CHAPTER 2 The Health Care Team and the Medical Environment, Past and Present

## ABHES Curriculum

| | |
|---|---|
| MA.A.1.a | Compare and contrast the allied health professions and understand their relation to medical assisting |
| MA.A.1.8.dd | Serve as liaison between physician and others |

## CAAHEP Core Curriculum

| | |
|---|---|
| IX.C.5 | Discuss licensure and certification as it applies to health care providers |
| IX.A.3 | Recognize the importance of local, state, and federal legislation and regulations in the practice setting |

## LESSON OUTLINE

### I. HEALTH CARE PROVIDERS

A. A health care provider is an individual licensed to examine, diagnose, and prescribe treatment to patients seeking assistance.

B. An organization such as a hospital or clinic may also be referred to as a health care provider.

C. Physicians are the most common health care providers.

D. A physician is trained to practice medicine. The practice of medicine includes the following components:

1. Art and science of diagnosis
2. Treatment and prevention of disease
3. Maintenance of good health

E. Physician training includes the following:

1. Four-year undergraduate degree
2. Four years of medical school
3. Three to eight years of internship and residency

F. Licensure requirements for physicians include the following:

1. Be of legal age
2. Be of good moral character
3. Have graduated from an approved medical school
4. Have completed an approved residency program or its equivalent
5. Be a resident of the state in which the physician is practicing
6. Have passed all sections of the United States Medical Licensing Examination (USMLE) prior to receiving a full medical license.

G. Reciprocity—A process in which one state recognizes another state's licensing procedures as being similar or more stringent than its own. The majority of states no longer recognize this process for physicians.

H. Revocation

1. Means suspension of a license (may be temporary or permanent)
2. State Medical Board or Special Review Committee has power to revoke a medical license
3. A physician may have a license revoked for the following:
   a. Conviction of a crime
   b. Unprofessional conduct

c. Fraud

d. Incompetence

I. Doctor of Medicine (MD) and Doctor of Osteopathic Medicine (DO)

1. Holders of either degree have similar educational requirements, are licensed physicians, and may use all accepted methods of treatment.
2. The difference in the degrees originates from different schools of thought.
3. DOs place special emphasis on the body's musculoskeletal and nervous systems, preventive medicine, and holistic patient care and education.
4. In the United States, both MDs and DOs perform the same duties, and both must pass a licensing exam by their respective boards to practice medicine.

J. General or family practitioners

1. See all types of patients.
2. Generally refer patients to specialists when the patient's symptoms are beyond the skills of the general or family practitioner.

K. Physician specialties

1. Specialty areas require additional years of study in the particular area of choice.
2. The additional study can take anywhere from two to six years.
3. Some physicians go into subspecialties.
4. Refer to Table 2–1 for complete list of physician specialties.

L. Nonphysician specialties

1. Several health specialists who are not physicians but are referred to as specialists.
2. Refer to Table 2–2 for a list of nonphysician specialists.
3. The word *doctor* is a Latin term that means to teach.
4. Someone who holds a doctorate degree or PhD has attained the highest degree awarded by a college in his or her particular discipline and may be addressed as Doctor.

a. Common disciplines in which individuals attain a PhD include:

(1) Nursing

(2) Mathematics

(3) Education

(4) Chemistry

(5) Philosophy

M. Midlevel practitioners

1. Health care providers such as nurse practitioners and physician assistants are sometimes referred to as midlevel practitioners.
2. They are able to:

a. Examine patients

b. Order diagnostic testing

c. Prescribe certain types of medication

4. Activities for a midlevel practitioner are usually directed and or dictated by a supervising physician, although in some states, nurse practitioners have more autonomy and can work independently of a physician.

N. Nurses

1. The American Nurses Association (ANA) describes nursing as the following:

   Nursing is the protection, promotion, and optimization of health and abilities, prevention of illness and injury, alleviation of suffering through the diagnosis and treatment of human response, and advocacy in the care of individuals, families, communities, and populations.

2. Several types of nurses

   a. Registered nurse (RN)

      1) Successfully completed a course of study at a state-approved school of nursing.

      2) Passed the National Council Licensure Examination (NCLEX-RN)

      3) Is licensed to practice medicine by the individual state

      4) Works in a variety of health care settings such as hospitals, convalescent centers, clinics, home health, and many other kinds of facilities

   b. Nurse anesthetist

      1) An RN certified to administer anesthesia

      2) CRNA stands for Certified Registered Nurse Anesthetist

      3) Must complete anesthesia training

      4) Works in hospitals, ambulatory surgical centers, and a host of other surgical environments

   c. Nurse midwife

      1) RN who has had extensive training and experience in labor and delivery

      2) Works in a variety of settings similar to other nurses

   d. Licensed practical nurse

      1) Has fundamentals of basic nursing

      2) Works under the supervision of a doctor or registered nurse

## I. HEALTH CARE TEAM MEMBERS

A. Many other health professionals provide services for patients.

B. Work in a variety of healthcare settings.

C. Be familiar with the role of these other team members.

D. Knowing the role of these professionals enables you to speak more intelligently with other team members and become more efficient with your role as a medical assistant.

E. Refer to Table 2–3 for a list of health care team members and their descriptions.

## II. BRIEF HISTORY OF MEDICINE

A. To understand fully the high technical level of current health care and the responsibilities of those who provide it, we must look back at its history and learn how it developed.

   1. Ancient times were filled with infectious disease and epidemics (affecting large numbers of individuals in a population).

   2. 80 percent of primitive human beings died by the age of 30 as a result of hunting accidents or violence.

   3. These individuals lived primarily alone, so there was little risk of widespread diseases or plagues.

4. When individuals began settling in communities, epidemics started, resulting in diseases such as:
    a. Tetanus
    b. Tuberculosis
    c. Tetanus
    d. Malaria
    e. Smallpox
    f. Typhus
    g. Typhoid
    h. Leprosy

B. Ancient civilizations
1. Did not understand the concept of microorganisms or the functions of the human body.
2. Disease was credited to evil spirits and demons brought on by punishment for disobedience to the gods.
3. Priests took on the role of medicine men, and treatment involved rituals to drive out demons.
4. Egypt
    a. Evidence suggests that Egyptians developed medical practice as early as 3000 BCE.
    b. Egyptian physicians were priests who studied medicine and surgery.
    c. They tried to drive out evil spirits with spells and concocted potions.
    d. In conjunction with magic, they also used about a third of the number of medicinal plants we still use today.
    e. Believed that blood flowed through canals in the body like those constructed along the Nile for irrigation.
    f. When it was thought that the body's canals were clogged, they were opened by bloodletting or the application of leeches to remove blood and disease toxins—leeches also produced hirudin, which prevents coagulation.
5. India
    a. Had the world's first nurses and hospitals.
    b. Extensive use of drugs, including those used for anesthesia—led to the main Hindu contribution: the art of healing surgery.
    c. Their knowledge of anatomy was limited but were able to perform cataract procedures and plastic surgery.
    d. Early writing indicates that they used approximately 120 surgical instruments in many kinds of surgeries.
6. China
    a. Had a highly developed center for medical learning.
    b. Belief in evil spirits as the cause of illness gradually changed as they began searching for reasons for illness.
    c. Followed a document called the Great Herbal, which contained over a thousand drugs.
    d. Used acupuncture as a means to drive out demons.
7. Greece
    a. Believed that Apollo, the sun god, taught the art of medicine to a centaur who, in turn, taught others, including Asklepios, the Greek god of healing (lived around 1250 BCE).
    b. Priests in the temples of Asklepios used massage, bathing, and exercise in treating patients.
    c. Also depended on the magical power of large, yellow, nonpoisonous snakes.
        i. Patients bathed to purify themselves, made offerings to the god, and were given tablets to read that described the cure of other patients.
        ii. They were then placed into a drug-induced sleep.
        iii. During the night, the snakes licked the wounds, and Asklepios applied salves.
        iv. This custom is thought to be where the origin of the caduceus originated (Figure 2–3).

d. Hippocrates was founder of scientific medicine
   i. Took medicine out of the realm of priests and philosophers and produced an organized method of gaining knowledge
   ii. Taught illness was the result of natural causes, not punishment for sins
   iii. Advocated examining a patient's home environment and place of work
   iv. Stressed the importance of diet and cleanliness
   v. Discovered that the course of certain diseases could be traced by listening to the chest (2000 years before the stethoscope)
   vi. Studied with the most distinguished teachers of the day
   vii. Wrote many detailed studies, among which are ones on prognostics, fractures, and surgery
   viii. Best known for his code of behavior known as the Hippocratic oath (Figure 2–4)

8. Roman Empire
   a. Romans made little contributions during early civilization other than the teachings of Claudius Galen (Table 2–4)
   b. Realized that disease was connected to filth and overcrowding, so built an elaborate sanitation system

C. Medieval history
1. From fifth to sixteenth century, learning and medicine began to decay.
2. Medicine was once again passed into the hands of the Christian church and Arab scholars—Prayer and fasting used as treatments for disease to be forgiven for sins that caused the disease.
3. Priests again became healers, and human dissection was forbidden, so anatomy and physiology died except for the erroneous teachings of Galen.
4. The second storehouse of medical knowledge was in the Muslim Arab empire.
   a. Arabs eager for knowledge; began a revival of scientific medicine.
   b. Their great knowledge of chemistry resulted in major contributions in pharmacology.
   c. They continued the Roman system of hospitals, including four major teaching centers.
      i. Had specialized wards for specific conditions
      ii. All patients admitted regardless of race, creed, or social status
      iii. Upon departure, patients given sufficient money to cover their convalescence
5. An outstanding medical school was produced in Salerno, Italy around 850.
   a. Open to men and women of all nationalities
   b. Could use a sound basis for teaching because not associated with the church
   c. By twelfth century, had a highly organized curriculum upon which students were examined and issued degrees to become the first true doctors
   d. Both anatomy and physiology taught but still based on animal dissection
   e. Other medical schools followed but again religious and scholarly factions prohibited advancement
   f. Medical teaching was predominately oral because books were scarce—medical school in Paris had only about 12 books at end of fourteenth century)
6. Barber surgeons
   a. Medieval European surgeons' practice limited to nobility, high clergy, and wealthy merchants
   b. Other patients treated by ignorant barber surgeons who cut hair, practiced bloodletting, opened abscesses, and, occasionally, performed amputations—all with the same razor

c. Trademark became white poles around which were wrapped blood-stained bandages—red and white pole still seen today outside of barbershops

7. The great diseases
    a. Two of greatest medieval diseases were leprosy and bubonic plague
    b. Leprosy was one of few diseases recognized as being contagious but was believed to be a result of sin
    c. Afflicted were herded into leper houses outside the towns, forbidden to marry, proclaimed dead citizens, and ordered to wear a black cloak with white patches
    d. In 1313, King Philip wanted to burn them all but was forbidden by the church
    e. Incidents of leprosy decreased with coming of bubonic plague (Black Death)
    f. Other plagues also surfaced such as pneumonic plague and septicemic plagues, which killed countless numbers of people because no cure at the time

D. The Renaissance
1. Beginning in Italy in fourteenth century, a revival of culture and concern for life.
2. People began gradually to escape limitations of church.
3. Classical artists—Michelangelo, Dürer, and da Vinci—began to practice dissection to depict the human body—especially bones, muscles, and internal organs—accurately.
4. Practice of medicine in beginning of seventeenth century divided among three guilds—physicians, surgeons, and apothecaries (pharmacists).
    a. Limited practice to upper classes
    b. Preferred studying, teaching, and debating theories of disease rather than working on patients
    c. Surgeons considered inferior to physicians and divided into two categories: Surgeons of the long robe and more humble barber surgeons
        i. Few surgeons held medical degrees
        ii. Trained largely in hospitals or though apprenticeships
    d. Apothecaries were tradesmen and permitted to treat people with drugs
    e. Refer to Table 2–4 for listing of medical pioneers through eighteenth century

F. Modern medicine
1. Humans practicing medicine for thousands of years, but only since development of microscope and discovery of microbes has practice of medicine progressed.
2. Emphasis on scientific inquiry changed medicine rapidly.
3. Modern pioneers provided not only technology but practices that have improved morbidity and mortality rates.
4. Refer to Table 2–5 for list of medical pioneers from nineteenth century and Table 2–6 for list of medical pioneers from twentieth and twenty-first centuries.

G. Impact of government on health care
1. Federal government provided much impetus and influence in growth of medicine through funding, grants, and regulations.
2. Refer to Table 2–7 for list of organizations and legislation affecting delivery of health care.

## IV. ALTERNATIVES TO THE TRADITIONAL MEDICAL MODEL

A. General interest has arisen in methods of health care other than traditional medical model.

B. Some authorities make distinction between various types of therapies.

C. Different types of therapies include:
   1. Complementary therapies: treatments considered to supplement or add to the conventional form of medicine. Examples include:
      a. Massage
      b. Acupuncture
      c. Acupressure
      d. Hypnosis
   2. Alternative therapy: method of treatment used instead of conventional medicine
      a. Often not validated by research
      b. No scientific evidence exists
      c. Some claims to cure but without scientific study, placebo effect cannot be ruled out
   3. National Center for Complementary and Alternative Medicine defines therapies as "medical practices that are not commonly used, accepted, or available in conventional medicine."
   4. Currently, effort being made by medical science to become more knowledgeable regarding these therapies.
   5. Refer to Table 2–8 for a listing of complementary or alternative therapies.

## CHAPTER ACTIVITIES

1. Have students pick a historical medical person from the chapter and write a research paper on the life and contributions of that person. Have them share their information with the rest of the class.
2. Invite practitioners who practice different methods of alternative medicine to speak to the class regarding their specialty.
3. Assign students a shadow day in which they have to find a practitioner who practices alternative medicine. Have them spend a day with the practitioner and write a synopsis of their experience. Have them share their findings with the class.

## ANSWERS TO CHECK YOUR KNOWLEDGE QUESTIONS

1. Which of the following would not be an example of a healthcare provider?
   **A. Medical assistant**
   B. Physician
   C. Nurse practitioner
   D. Chiropractor
2. When one state's medical board recognizes the licensing requirements of another state's medical board as being similar to or more stringent than its own.
   A. Endorsement
   B. Revocation
   **C. Reciprocity**
   D. None of the above
3. This physician specialist looks after patients admitted to the hospital.
   A. Physician partner
   **B. Hospitalist**
   C. Physiatrist
   D. Hospital physician

4. Which of the following specialists would be considered a midlevel practitioner?

   A. Podiatrist

   B. Psychologist

   **C. Nurse practitioner**

   D. None of the above

5. This health care professional administers radiopharmaceuticals to patients and then scans the body with a special camera to observe how the pharmaceuticals concentrate in specific organs.

   A. Radiological technician

   B. Radiologist

   C. Ultrasound technician

   **D. Nuclear medicine technologist**

6. Which of the following is considered one of the humors described by Galen?

   **A. Phlegm**

   B. Tears

   C. Mucus

   D. Nasal drippings

7. The legislation that was designed to make health care more accessible to those who wouldn't otherwise be able to afford health care benefits

   A. HIPAA

   B. Health Care Reform Act

   **C. PPACA**

   D. OSHA

8. These treatments are considered to supplement or add to the conventional form of medicine.

   A. Alternative therapies

   B. Supplemental therapies

   C. Addendum therapies

   **D. Complementary therapies**

9. This type of medicine identifies three types of energies that are present in all things

   **A. Ayurvedic medicine**

   B. Biofeedback

   C. Acupuncture

   D. Homeopathy

# UNIT 2 MEDICAL TERMINOLOGY
# CHAPTER 3 Introduction to Medical Terminology

## ABHES Curriculum

| | |
|---|---|
| MA.A.1.3.a | Define and use entire basic structure of medical words and be able to identify in the correct context accurately; i.e., root, prefix, suffix, combinations, spelling, and definitions |
| MA.A.1.3.b | Build and dissect medical terms from roots and suffixes to understand the word element combinations that create medical terminology |

## CAAHEP Core Curriculum

| | |
|---|---|
| IV.C.10 | Diagram medical terms, labeling the word parts |
| IV.C.11 | Define both medical terms and abbreviations related to all body systems |

## LESSON OUTLINE

### I. ORIGIN OF MEDICAL TERMINOLOGY

A. Terms as derived from Greek and Latin words.

B. Romans (Latin) developed medical procedures, diagnoses, and treatments.

C. Greeks developed medical studies.

### II. OVERVIEW

A. Prefixes modify the meaning.

B. Suffixes can change a noun to an adjective when added to word root or combining form.

C. Word roots and combining forms identify structure.

### III. WORD PARTS

A. Prefixes

1. Always in front of the words, denoted with a hyphen to the right.
2. Change or modify the word root.
3. Exceptions, for example, when a word root or combining form begins with a vowel, select the most appropriate prefix ending in a consonant.
4. Common prefixes (see Table 3–1).

B. Suffixes

1. Always at the back of the word, denoted with a hyphen to the left.
2. Can add specificity of a particular term.
3. Can be descriptive in changing a medical term to an adjective.
4. Common suffixes (see Table 3–2).

C. Word roots and combining forms (see Table 3–3).

1. Applies to part of the anatomy.
2. Can have more than one to a term.

3. Combining forms are word roots with a vowel added.
    a. Makes word easier to pronounce.
    b. Most common vowels are *o*, *a*, and *i*.

### IV. BREAKING A MEDICAL TERM APART (*VIEW MEDIA LINK: WORD PARTS WORKING TOGETHER*)

A. Identify the meaning of the suffix—always in the back of the word, denoted with a hyphen to the left.
B. Identify the meaning of the prefix—always in front of the word, denoted with a hyphen to the right.
C. Determine word roots and combining forms.
    1. Applies to part of the anatomy
    2. Can have more than one to a term

### V. BUILDING A MEDICAL TERM (*VIEW MEDIA LINK: COMBINING WORD ROOTS*)

### VI. THE IMPORTANCE OF SPELLING

A. Medical terms can sound the same or similar—for example, *ilium* and *ileum.*
B. Misspelling a term can mean the difference in a diagnosis or treatment.

### VII. FORMING PLURALS OUT OF SINGULARS

A. In English, add *s* or *es.*
B. Basic rules
    1. –a becomes –ae
    2. –is becomes –es
    3. –um becomes –a
    4. –us becomes –i
    5. –ex or –ix becomes –ices
    6. –nx becomes –nges
C. Singular to plural term examples (see Table 3–4).

## CHAPTER ACTIVITIES

1. Do a review of a medical dictionary. Guide your students to pronounce sounds appropriately. For example, the "ph" sound, which sounds like an "f"; the "ch" sound, which sounds like a "k"; etc. You could pronounce the sounds aloud for the students to repeat them aloud as a group. Select some simple and difficult terms in advance.
2. Play terms from the Audio Library in class. (The Audio Library is included within the StudyWARE™ Software, on the Premium Website.) Have students write down the words as they are pronounced and have them hand in their list to you. This could be a bonus point activity.
3. Have students make up flash cards in class and review them with their classmates in pairs.
4. Write a word part on the board and ask the students to identify it as a prefix, suffix, word root, or combining form. Also, ask the students to define the word part and provide an example term, using the word part. Write the example term on the board and ask the students how to spell this new term. You can also consider having a volunteer student write a term on the board, using the word part.

# ANSWERS TO CHECK YOUR KNOWLEDGE QUESTIONS

1. In the term "tachycardia," what part of the word is the prefix?
   a. ta-
   b. tach-
   **c. tachy-**
   d. There is no prefix in this word
2. In the term *pyromania*, what part of the word is the suffix?
   a. pyro-
   b. mani/o
   **c. mania**
   d. –ania
   e. –ia
3. The suffix in the term *rhinitis* is ____________, and it means ____________________.
   a. –is, abnormal condition
   b. –is, inflammation
   c. –itis, abnormal condition
   **d. –itis, inflammation**
4. Which of the following terms is in its singular form?
   **a. bacillus**
   b. bacteria
   c. scapulae
   d. veins
5. If a health care provider determines that more than one condition is causing a patient's illness, which of the following would be correct?
   a. diagnosis
   b. diagnosises
   **c. diagnoses**
   d. diagnoseses

# CHAPTER 4 Understanding and Building Medical Terms of Body Systems

## ABHES Curriculum

| | |
|---|---|
| MA.A.1.3.a | Define and use entire basic structure of medical words and be able to identify in the correct context accurately; i.e., root, prefix, suffix, combinations, spelling, and definitions |
| MA.A.1.3.b | Build and dissect medical terms from roots and suffixes to understand the word element combinations that create medical terminology |
| MA.A.1.3.c | Understand the various medical terminology for each specialty |
| MA.A.1.4.d | Recognize and identify acceptable medical abbreviations |

## CAAHEP Core Curriculum

| | |
|---|---|
| IV.C.10 | Diagram medical terms, labeling the word parts |
| IV.C.11 | Define both medical terms and abbreviations related to all body systems |

## LESSON OUTLINE

### I. STRUCTURE OF THE HUMAN BODY

A. Refer to Unit 11 for more in-depth knowledge of the body systems
B. The integumentary system (refer to Table 4–1)
C. The musculoskeletal system (refer to Table 4–2)
D. The cardiovascular system (refer to Table 4–3)
E. The respiratory system (refer to Table 4–4)
F. The gastrointestinal (digestive) system (refer to Table 4–5)
G. The urinary system (refer to Table 4–6)
H. The nervous system (refer to Table 4–7)
I. The endocrine system (refer to Table 4–8)
J. The special senses (refer to Table 4–9)
K. The reproductive system (refer to Table 4–10)

### II. COMMON ABBREVIATIONS (REFER TO TABLE 4–11)

### CHAPTER ACTIVITIES

1. Play terms from the Audio Library in class. (The Audio Library is included within the StudyWARE™ Software, on the Premium Website.) Have students write down the words as they are pronounced and have them hand in their lists to you. This could be a bonus point activity.
2. Have students make up flash cards in class and review them with their classmates in pairs.
3. Write a medical term on the board and ask the students to identify and define the prefix, suffix, word root, or combining form.
4. Write a word part on the board and ask the students to define the word part and use it to create a medical term.

# ANSWERS TO CHECK YOUR KNOWLEDGE QUESTIONS

1. Which of the following is the correct medical term for dry skin?
   a. xanthoderma
   **b. xeroderma**
   c. scleroderma
   d. erythemaderma
2. The term *epigastric* means:
   **a. pertaining to upon the stomach**
   b. pertaining to below the stomach
   c. pertaining to above the stomach
   d. pertaining to near the stomach
3. The combining forms *ili/o*, *lamin/o*, *mandibul/o*, and *maxill/o* pertain to which body system?
   a. lymphatic
   **b. musculoskeletal**
   c. cardiovascular
   d. integumentary
4. Aphonia means:
   a. A condition of no speech
   b. A condition of no recording
   c. A condition of painful speech
   **d. A condition of no voice**
5. The combining form in "stomatitis" means:
   a. body
   b. inflammation
   **c. mouth**
   d. stomach
6. Billie hadn't been feeling very well, so she decided to visit Dr. Burress, a ___________, a specialist in the study of the blood. Dr. Burress examined Billie and ordered some blood tests; he asked the ___________________ to draw the specimens.
   **a. hematologist, phlebotomist**
   b. hematologist, cardiologist
   c. cardiologist, phlebotomist
   d. cardiologist, venipuncturist
7. The combining form in "colposcopy" relates to the ____________ system.
   a. gastrointestinal
   b. endocrine
   **c. reproductive**
   d. nervous

# UNIT 3 MEDICAL LAW AND ETHICS
# CHAPTER 5 Legal Issues

## ABHES Curriculum

| | |
|---|---|
| MA.A.1.1.e | Define scope of practice for the medical assistant and comprehend the conditions for practice within the state where the medical assistant is employed |
| MA.A.1.4.a | Document accurately |
| MA.A.1.4.b | Institute federal and state guidelines when releasing medical records or information |
| MA.A.1.4.c | Follow established policies when initiating or terminating medical treatment |
| MA.A.1.4.f | Comply with federal, state, and local health laws and regulations |
| MA.A.1.11.b (3) | Demonstrate professionalism by maintaining confidentiality at all times |

## CAAHEP Core Curriculum

| | |
|---|---|
| IX.C.1 | Discuss legal scope of practice for medical assistants |
| IX.C.2 | Explore issue of confidentiality as it applies to the medical assistant. |
| IX.C.3 | Describe the implications of HIPAA for the medical assistant in various medical settings |
| IX.C.7 | Compare and contrast provider and medical assistant roles in terms of standard of care |
| IX.C.8 | Compare criminal and civil law as it applies to the practicing medical assistant |
| IX.C.9 | Provide an example of tort law as it would apply to a medical assistant |
| IX.C.10 | Explain how the following affect the medical assistant's practice and give examples: (a) negligence, (b). malpractice, (c) statute of limitations, (d) Good Samaritan Acts, (e) Uniform Anatomical Gift Act, (f) living will and advance directives, (g) medical durable power of attorney. |
| IX.C.11 | Identify how the Americans with Disabilities Act (ADA) applies to the medical assisting profession |
| IX.C.13 | Discuss all levels of governmental legislation and regulation as they apply to medical assisting practice, including FDA and DEA regulations |
| IX.P.4 | Practice within the standard of care for a medical assistant |
| IX.A.2 | Demonstrate awareness of the consequences of not working within the legal scope of practice |
| IX.A.3 | Recognize the importance of local, state, and federal legislation and regulations in the practice setting |

## LESSON OUTLINE

### WHAT IS LAW AND WHO MAKES IT?

A. Definition of law: system of rules, usually enforced through a collection of institutions commonly recognized as having the authority to do so

B. Sources of law
   1. U.S. Congress makes federal law
      a. Applicable to all per the Supremacy Clause of the Constitution
      b. Example: Patient Protection and Affordable Care Act ("health care reform")
   2. State legislatures make state law applicable to those living and working within the state
   3. Local governments make resolutions or ordinances applicable to those within the specific jurisdiction
   4. U.S. Supreme Court makes law, e.g., *Roe v. Wade*

5. Common law
   a. Also known as case law or law of precedent
   b. Term originated to handle situations not covered by statute

## II. CRIMINAL VERSUS CIVIL LAW

A. Criminal law
   1. Exclusively statutory
   2. Deals with one who has performed an act prohibited by law or failed to perform an act required by law
   3. Terms
      a. Defendant: the person on trial
      b. Plaintiff: the prosecution
      c. Beyond a reasonable doubt: standard of proof required to impose a penalty on the defendant
   4. Two kinds of crimes
      a. Misdemeanors
      b. Felonies

B. Civil law
   1. A collection of rules that govern the conduct and affairs of people, their rights, that are not a crime
   2. Preponderance of evidence: standard of proof required to impose a penalty on the defendant

## III. DEFINITIONS AND EXAMPLES OF CRIMES

A. Misdemeanors
   1. A crime punishable by less than one year in a jail, most commonly a county or regional jail, not a state prison
   2. Sometimes punishment can include a fine, or a fine might be imposed

B. Felony
   1. Crimes committed by people who intend to do significant harm to another, either through depriving them of their property or injuring them personally
   2. Murder
      a. The "unlawful killing of another with malice aforethought"
      b. Degrees of murder based on level of premeditation by defendant or status of victim
   3. Manslaughter
      a. The unlawful killing of a human being without malice
      b. Voluntary versus involuntary manslaughter
   4. Robbery: unlawful taking of money or goods of another from his person or in immediate presence by force or intimidation
   5. Burglary: similar to robbery but different in that burglary does not involve presence of the victim

## IV. THE LAW OF TORTS

A. Comes from the Latin *tortum*, which means "wrong"

B. Unintentional torts: accidental acts

C. Intentional torts
   1. Libel and slander (defamation of character)
   2. Trespass

3. Intentional infliction of emotional distress
4. Medical malpractice

D. Negligence

1. Unintentional tort
2. Standard of care is principle that establishes whether plaintiff can collect for damages
   a. Legal foundation for the concept of negligence: everyone owes everyone else the duty to behave reasonably
   b. When two people have a particular relationship to one another—for example, doctor and patient—the concept of an affirmative duty arises
3. Four factors that point to negligence by defendant
   a. A *duty* of care must be owed by defendant to the plaintiff
   b. Defendant must have committed a *breach* of that duty
   c. Plaintiff must have suffered harm (*injury*)
   d. Harm must be a result of the defendant's breach of duty (*causation*)
4. Simple versus gross negligence
5. The concept of *Respondeat superior*

E. Medical malpractice

1. The concept of "Standard of Care" is central to medical malpractice cases: Did the doctor render treatment—or fail to provide treatment—consistent with the standard of care expected of people with his or her training and experience in similar circumstances?
2. Six factors that point to medical malpractice
   a. A *relationship* between provider and patient
   b. That *relationship created a duty* on part of provider toward patient
   c. Duty was of a nature to be a professional *standard of care*
   d. Provider *breached* duty to patient
   e. Patient had resulting *injury*
   f. Patient would not have sustained injury but for provider's breach of duty (*causation*)
3. Defenses to medical malpractice
   a. Statute of limitations
   b. Contributory negligence
   c. Emergency

## '. DOCTOR–PATIENT CONTRACT

A. Elements of valid contract

1. Offer
2. Acceptance
3. Consideration

B. Types of contracts

1. Express
2. Implied

C. Capacity to enter into contracts: consent

D. Provider has duty of care to patient until relationship is terminated
   1. Mutual consent of the patient and the doctor
   2. Patient dismissing the doctor
   3. The changed circumstance ending care
   4. Provider withdrawal from relationship by providing patient written notice with reasonable time to find new provider
E. Patient right to privacy: patient has right to expect his or her communications with provider to be kept confidential
F. Before a doctor can treat patient, patient must provide informed consent
G. Patient Self-Determination Act
   1. Advance directives
   2. Living wills
   3. Powers of attorney
H. Medical records
   1. Providers own medical records they create
   2. Material in medical record part of privileged communication between provider and patient
   3. HIPAA and medical records
   4. Mandatory release of medical records

## VI. GOVERNMENTAL REGULATION OF THE PROVIDER OFFICE

A. Occupational Safety and Health Administration (OSHA)
   1. Ensures that employers have safe work environments for employees
   2. Employers are to maintain safe working conditions and use methods appropriate to protect workers
   3. See Chapter 36 for more information about OSHA and blood-borne pathogens
B. Clinical Laboratory Improvement Amendments (CLIA) of 1988
   1. Legislation regulating all laboratories, including relatively small ones found in provider practices
   2. See Chapter 44 for more information about CLIA and laboratory practices
C. Food and Drug Administration (FDA)
D. Drug Enforcement Agency (DEA)

## VII. FEDERAL LAWS AFFECTING THE PROVIDER OFFICE

A. Patient Protection and Affordability Act
B. Health Insurance Portability and Accessibility Act (HIPAA)
   1. Title I: continuation of health insurance coverage when workers change or lose jobs
   2. Title II
      a. Privacy Rule
      b. All personal health information protected from unauthorized disclosure
C. Good Samaritan Act
D. Americans with Disabilities Act (ADA)
E. Uniform Anatomical Gift Act

# CHAPTER ACTIVITIES

1. Discuss the standard of care in the medical office to which a medical assistant employee will be held accountable. For additional discussion on standard of care, read the following scenario and discuss: *A pregnant woman went into labor on a city bus and gave birth before help could arrive. What standard of care would the bus driver be held to? What standard of care would individuals on the bus be held to? If there was an LPN on the bus, what standard of care would that individual be held to?*
2. *Respondeat superior* is Latin for "let the master answer." It means that providers are legally responsible (liable) for their own acts of negligence *as well as* for negligent acts of employees working within the scope of their employment. *Respondeat superior* is a test to determine whether an employee was or was not acting within the scope of his or her employment when the negligent act was committed. Read the following to the class and discuss why the provider is responsible and why the patient won the case: *A patient returns after his initial visit for treatment of a leg wound. The provider had the medical assistant check the wound, change the dressings, apply antibiotic ointment, and rebind the wound over three occasions. The medical assistant did not recognize early signs of infection in the wound. Subsequently, necrosis developed, costing the patient removal of muscle tissue and a long healing process. The patient sued the provider and won the case.*
3. Have students research malpractice insurance premium rates in various states (research "provider malpractice insurance") on the Internet. Which state has the highest premiums? Why? Which state has the lowest insurance rates? Why? Do you think all health care professionals should carry malpractice insurance? Explain your answer.

# ANSWERS TO CHECK YOUR KNOWLEDGE QUESTIONS

1. In the United States, law is predominantly derived from:

   **a. legislative bodies.**

   b. executive orders.

   c. voter referendums.

   d. international courts.
2. What is the Latin phrase that means "let the master answer"?

   ***a. Respondeat superior***

   b. *Res ipsa loquitur*

   c. *Subpoena duces tucem*

   d. *Ex post facto*
3. Which of the following defines a contract?

   a. Offer, consent, acceptance

   **b. Offer, acceptance, consideration**

   c. Offer, consideration, consent

   d. Consent, consideration, acceptance
4. What is the Act that protects a provider from liability for any civil damages when he or she gives emergency care?

   a. Health Insurance Portability and Accountability Act

   b. Americans with Disabilities Act

   **c. Good Samaritan Act**

   d. Occupational Health and Safety Act

5. Which of the following is NOT considered personal health information protected from unauthorized disclosure under HIPAA?
   **a. Information included in a study that cannot be used to identify the patient**
   b. Information related to a patient's past mental health
   c. Information related to a patient's present physical health
   d. Information related to the treatment or care of a patient
6. It is the goal of which government agency to ensure that employers provide safe work environments for employees?
   a. DEA
   b. FDA
   **c. OSHA**
   d. ADA

# CHAPTER 6 Ethical Issues

## ABHES Curriculum

| | |
|---|---|
| MA.A.1.5.b | Institute federal and state guidelines when releasing medical records or information |
| MA.A.1.5.g | Analyze the effect of hereditary, cultural, and environmental influences |
| MA.A.1.11.b (3) | Demonstrate professionalism by maintaining confidentiality at all times |
| MA.A.1.11.b (4) | Demonstrate professionalism by being cognizant of ethical boundaries |
| MA.A.1.11.b (8) | Demonstrate professionalism by being courteous and diplomatic |

## CAAHEP Core Curriculum

| | |
|---|---|
| X.C.1 | Differentiate among legal, ethical, and moral issues affecting health care |
| X.C.2 | Compare personal, professional, and organizational ethics |
| X.C.3 | Discuss the role of cultural, social, and ethnic diversity in ethical performance of medical assisting practice |
| X.C.4 | Identify where to report illegal or unsafe activities and behaviors that affect health, safety, and welfare of others |
| X.C.5 | Identify the effect personal ethics might have on professional performance |
| X.P.1 | Report to proper authorities illegal and unsafe activities and behaviors that affect health, safety, and welfare of others |
| X.P.2 | Develop a plan for separation of personal and professional ethics |
| X.A.1 | Apply ethical behaviors, including honesty and integrity in performance of medical assisting practice |
| X.A.2 | Examine the impact personal ethics and morals can have on the individual's practice |
| X.A.3 | Demonstrate awareness of diversity in providing patient care |

## LESSON OUTLINE

### I. WHAT IS ETHICS?

A. We deal with ethics on a daily basis

B. Criteria for an ethical dilemma

1. There does not appear to be any justice through the legal system
2. When there is no clear-cut right or wrong answer
3. When the right behavior leads to the wrong outcome

### II. ETHICAL ISSUES IN HEALTH CARE

A. The term *bioethics* often used

B. Ethical issues considered using concepts of autonomy, beneficence, and distributive justice

1. Autonomy: patient has right to make determinations for him- or herself
2. Beneficence: requires people to do what is in best interests of others
3. Distributive justice: principle by which a society (or health care community) decides to allocate scarce resources
   a. Egalitarian approach: everyone gets equal share
   b. Earned approach: those who deserve get more
   c. Libertarian approach: each gets what he or she can legitimately get
   d. Social justice approach: allocation made to maximize number of people helped

C. Table 6–1 presents ethical issues relating to health care

D. Ethical issue: Abortion

1. Artificial termination of pregnancy
2. Consider issue of abortion from three perspectives
   a. *Autonomy:* the woman has a right to self-determination over what happens to her body
   b. *Beneficence:* because fetus cannot speak for itself, those who can should act in best interests of fetus
   c. *Distributive justice:* if procedure legally available, should be available to all, including poor

E. Ethical issue: Cryonics

1. Process to freeze body of seriously ill or deceased individual to stop decomposition of tissues
2. Consider the issue of cryonics from three perspectives
   a. *Autonomy:* person has right to decide to be frozen in time in hope of coming back to life in future
   b. *Beneficence:* may conclude that act is not in best interests of patient
   c. *Distributive justice:* may argue that procedure shouldn't be done until available to everyone

F. Ethical issue: DRGs and capitated payments

1. DRG limits amount hospital can be paid based on diagnosis, irrespective of complications that develop
2. Capitated payment to provider limits payment to set amount each month, despite how ill patient might be
3. Provider's sense of professional ethics stands between adequate care and substandard care motivated by payment structure

G. Ethics and diversity

1. Medical assistants have responsibility to care for all people equally without regard to race, creed, or color
2. To be fully respectful of all patients, must recognize and respond appropriately to ideas and elements from other ethnic and cultural backgrounds different from own
3. Consider: manner of dress, communication style, consciousness of time, values and beliefs

## III. DISTINGUISHING LEGAL, ETHICAL, AND MORAL JUDGMENTS

A. Law, ethics, and morals are types of categorizing principles

B. If situation is legal matter, always follow law

C. If situation is ethical matter, ask three questions

1. What promotes right of patient's determinations about his or her own health?
2. What is in best health interests of patient?
3. Is doing (or not doing) act in question fair to others?

D. Moral issues stem from belief system in which one makes judgment about right and wrong

E. Reporting guidelines

1. *Criminal conduct*: notify local police
2. *Patient information:* no disclosure to anyone other than patient or attending physician
3. *Physician misconduct:* notify practice administrator or office manager or even another physician in office (if others unavailable).
4. *Staff misconduct:* notify practice administrator or office manager

## IV. PROFESSIONAL ETHICS

A. Codes of ethics that prescribe behavior for professionals of a specific organization

B. Many industries, associations, and fields have ethical codes

C. AMA Code of Ethics

1. For physician conduct and behavior
2. Covers interprofessional relations, hospital relations, confidentiality, fees, records, and professional rights, among others
3. AMA Code of Ethics at www.ama-assn.org

D. Ethics for medical assistants

1. AAMA Code of Ethics for members of American Association of Medical Assistants (AAMA)
2. AMT Standards of Practice for members of American Medical Technologists
3. AAMA also has Medical Assisting Creed
4. Codes of ethics provide general framework by which to make ethical decisions but do not provide guidance for every specific question
5. Medical assistant must use best judgment regarding application of ethical considerations to given situation

## V. ORGANIZATIONAL ETHICS

A. The values the by which the organization conducts its business

B. Often, organizations have a specific Values Statement developed by leaders—two examples: Cleveland Clinic and Geisinger Health System

C. Employees in these organizations rewarded accordingly by intrinsic and extrinsic means

1. Intrinsic: reward from within such as pride in one's job
2. Extrinsic: external reward such as yearly bonus

D. Characteristics that encourage ethical behavior

1. Written code of standards
2. Ethics training for officers, managers, and employees
3. Availability of advice for employees confronting ethical issues
4. System for confidential reporting

## VI. PERSONAL ETHICS AND PROFESSIONAL PERFORMANCE

A. Professional and organizational ethics designed to inform professional performance

B. Regardless of personal perspective, adapt personal views to comply with ethical standards of profession and organization

# CHAPTER ACTIVITIES

1. Class discussion topics: The following topics provide opportunities for students to think critically about relevant issues. Question prompts follow each topic.

   a. The Terry Schiavo case made national headlines a few years ago. Orders came down from physicians, lawyers, and her husband that the feeding tube was to be removed, and a do-not-feed order was given.

   - Discuss this case in terms of the concepts of autonomy, beneficence, and distributive justice.
   - If you were a medical assistant taking care of a patient in a vegetative state, such as Terry Schiavo, how would you feel?

   b. The U.S. recession of 2007–2009 has caused a new group of people to become poor. Many people lost jobs, homes, and health care, and Wall Street behavior caused some people to lose lifetime savings. These people are being called the new poor. In contrast, babies were born to a welfare mom up to 40 years ago who were raised on welfare, then had children of their own they raised on welfare, and now have grandchildren growing up on welfare. This group of people have always received a helping hand from the government for health care (Medicaid) and living arrangements (low-income housing or housing assistance), and many have even received job training. As more people request help and assistance from the government, resources are becoming even scarcer.

- Who then should be allocated the limited resources?
- Should those who still have jobs be expected to carry the burden of those who never worked?
- Should those who can afford to pay get medical preference over those who cannot pay?
- Should funds be channeled to the young and taken away from the elderly?

c. Many issues have surfaced due to advances in technology. One issue of much controversy relates to the *right* to have a child. Part of discussion on this issue relates to financial responsibilities for genetic testing.

- Should insurance companies or Medicare be covering the costs for artificial insemination?
- Should this be a national or state issue?

d. By the year 2014, the majority of Americans should have an online electronic medical record (EMR). Many issues have surfaced regarding who should be allowed to access this information, when should they have access, and where they should be able to access this information (e.g., home, office, medical facility).

- Discuss how long some information needs to stay on an EMR.
- Does every physician need access to *all* of the EMR? (e.g., Does the podiatrist need to know a patient had a mastectomy, or does a dentist need to know you go to a chiropractor?)

## ANSWERS TO CHECK YOUR KNOWLEDGE QUESTIONS

1. Recognizing that the patient has the right to make decisions about his or her life, death, and health describes the concept of:

   **a. autonomy.**

   b. beneficence.

   c. distributive justice.

   d. bioethics.

2. The principle by which we as a society (or health care community) decide to allocate resources that are in scarce supply is:

   a. autonomy.

   b. beneficence.

   **c. distributive justice.**

   d. bioethics.

3. The organization that has a comprehensive Code of Ethics that speaks to a wide range of matters arising in the professional conduct of a doctor is the:

   a. AAMA.

   **b. AMA.**

   c. AMT.

   d. Cleveland Clinic.

4. The organization that publishes a Standards of Practice for the medical assistant is the:
   a. AAMA.
   b. AMA.
   **c. AMT.**
   d. Cleveland Clinic.
5. Studying hard for an exam to achieve a good grade is an example of this type of motivation.
   **a. Extrinsic**
   b. Intrinsic
   c. Beneficent
   d. Autonomous

# UNIT 4 PROFESSIONAL COMMUNICATIONS
# CHAPTER 7 Verbal and Nonverbal Communications

## ABHES Curriculum

| | |
|---|---|
| MA.A.1.8.aa | Are attentive, listen, and learn |
| MA.A.1.8.bb | Are impartial and show empathy when dealing with patients |
| MA.A.1.8.cc | Communicate on the recipient's level of comprehension |
| MA.A.1.8.dd | Serve as liaison between physician and others |
| MA.A.1.8.ii | Recognize and respond to verbal and nonverbal communication |
| MA.A.1.8.kk | Adapt to individualized needs |

## CAAHEP Core Curriculum

| | |
|---|---|
| IV.C 1 | Identify styles and types of verbal communication |
| IV.C.2 | Identify nonverbal communication |
| IV.C.3 | Recognize communication barriers |
| IV.C.4 | Recognize techniques for overcoming communication barriers |
| IV.C.5 | Recognize the elements of oral communication, using a sender–receiver process |
| IV.C.13 | Identify the role of self boundaries in the health care environment |
| IV.C.16 | Differentiate between adaptive and nonadaptive coping mechanisms |
| IV.P.11 | Respond to nonverbal communication |
| IV.A.1 | Demonstrate empathy in communicating with patients, family, and staff |
| IV.A.2 | Apply active listening skills |
| IV.A.3 | Use appropriate body language and other nonverbal skills in communicating with patients, family, and staff |
| IV.A.4 | Demonstrate awareness of the territorial boundaries of the person with whom communicating |
| IV.A.6 | Demonstrate awareness of how an individual's personal appearance affects anticipated responses |
| IV.A.10 | Demonstrate respect for individual diversity, incorporating awareness of one's own biases in areas including gender, race, religion, age, and economic status |

# LESSON OUTLINE

## I. THE COMMUNICATION PROCESS

A. Review Figure 7–1 to conceptualize the communication process

B. Communication styles

   1. Visual people need to see pictures or see it in writing
   2. Auditory people learn by hearing
   3. Kinesthetic people think in terms of sensations or feeling, often move their hands when talking, and respond physically as well as verbally
   4. Important to identify and adapt to the communication styles of others

C. Communication barriers

   1. Anything that gets in the way of clear communication.
   2. Three common barriers

a. Physical disabilities
b. Psychological attitudes and prejudice
c. Cultural diversity

D. Active listening
1. Giving attention to the persons trying to communicate with you and taking an active interest
2. Examples include repeating words and phrases or giving approving or disapproving nods
3. Signals to the sender that you are hearing and following what is being said

E. Perception
1. Being aware of one's own feelings and the feelings of others
2. A skill acquired with experience and practice
3. Being attentive to the needs of others and your surroundings improves your perception skills
4. Anticipating the needs of others is a part of perception that enhances your effectiveness

## II. NONVERBAL COMMUNICATION (PROCEDURE 7–1)

A. Communicating without using any form of speech
B. Possible to contradict a verbal message by using incongruous nonverbal communication
C. Body language
1. A complex communication process
2. Involves unconscious use of posture, gestures, and other forms of nonverbal communication

D. Types of nonverbal communication
1. Appearance
2. Facial expression
3. Eye contact
4. Gestures
5. Distance
a. If you are engaged in a personal conversation, the generally accepted space between two people is from 1.5 to 4 feet.
b. For social conversation among people, the distance between people is from 4 to 12 feet.
c. In a public setting, the space can be 12 to 25 feet.
6. Silence

## III. THERAPEUTIC TOUCH AND RELATIONSHIPS

A. A comforting touch helps patients feel that you care and gives them a sense of security and acceptance.
B. A handshake is a sign of friendship.
C. A hug can convey feelings of warmth and affection (only if you are certain of the acceptable boundaries expressed by the patient or by office protocol)
D. Be sensitive to the patient's reaction when touching is involved.

## IV. COMMUNICATING EMOTIONAL STATES

A. Common questions used to find out the emotional states of patients:
1. "What seems to be the problem today?"

2. "What brings you here to see the doctor today?"
3. "Can you tell me about the problem you seem to be having?"
4. "Can we talk about what has been giving you concern that brings you in to see the doctor?"

## V. FUNDAMENTALS OF PSYCHOLOGY

A. Maslow's model consists of five stages of needs.
   1. The first four are grouped together as deficit needs, meaning that if you have a deficit in any of the first four categories, you experience that as a need. These four stages are:
      a. Physiological – *Basic survival needs*
      b. Safety – *Stability*
      c. Belongingness and Love – *Being with someone or a group*
      d. Esteem – *Respect, self-respect, confidence, and independence*
   2. The fifth and highest level: Self-actualization—*You tend to be a problem solver and place a great deal of emphasis on family and long-term relationships* (Figure 7–8).

B. Kubler-Ross's stages of grief
   1. Denial
   2. Depression
   3. Bribery
   4. Anger
   5. Resolution

## VI. DEFENSE MECHANISMS

A. Used to help deal with unpleasant and socially unacceptable circumstances or behaviors
B. Used to help make an emotional adjustment in everyday situations
C. Everyone uses various defense mechanisms from time to time, but habitual use can result in negative feelings or outcomes.
D. Types of defense mechanisms
   1. Repression—The most commonly used defense mechanism
   2. Suppression
   3. Displacement
   4. Projection
   5. Rationalization
   6. Intellectualization
   7. Sublimation
   8. Compensation
   9. Temporary withdrawal
   10. Daydreaming
   11. Malingering
   12. Denial
   13. Regression
   14. Procrastination

## VII. COPING SKILLS

A. Can be positive or negative
B. Used to offset disadvantages in day-to-day life
C. Positive coping helps you through situations at nearly the same level of effectiveness as those who do not have the disadvantage.
D. Use of negative coping skills can provide short-term relief or distraction but can ultimately worsen the circumstance. Common example of negative coping skill: abuse of alcohol or drugs.
E. Adaptive and nonadaptive coping skills; refer to Tables 7–3 (adaptive) and 7–4 (nonadaptive).
F. Self awareness
   1. Medical assistants, in both administrative and clinical capacities, have many opportunities daily to observe patients' mental and emotional states.
   2. These observations have a direct influence on the medical assistants' behaviors, which in turn directly influence their overall health.

# CHAPTER ACTIVITIES

1. Set up the classroom as a medical office and role-play, taking the roles of the MA and the patient for a class period. Half participates while the other half critiques, then reverse the groups.
2. Have a motivational speaker relate to the students how important attitude and communication are in the workplace and elsewhere.
3. Arrange for a speaker from the senior services to explain the organization and distribute information pamphlets to students. These speakers often bring a video to enhance their purpose.
4. Choose two of the defense mechanisms discussed in this chapter and write a short scenario for each mechanism about a real-life situation in with the mechanism was used. Present the scenarios to the class and ask the class to identify which of the mechanisms you are describing.
5. Search the Internet to see whether you can find other problem-solving skills that were not discussed in this chapter.

# ANSWERS TO CHECK YOUR KNOWLEDGE QUESTIONS

1. A patient who is grimacing and wincing would be communicating:
   **a. nonverbally.**
   b. verbally.
   c. affectively.
   d. intellectually.
2. Which of the following terms describes being aware of one's own feelings and the feelings of others?
   a. Body language
   b. Gestures
   c. Empathy
   **d. Perception**

3. All the following are examples of body language except:
   a. appearance.
   b. facial expressions.
   **c. tone of voice.**
   d. gestures.
4. Which of the following would convey a positive attitude?
   a. Frown
   **b. Smile**
   c. Clenched teeth
   d. Fist
5. Which of the following would be part of active listening?
   a. Handshake
   b. Eye contact
   c. Repeating information given by the patient
   **d. Both b and c**
6. Which of the following describes an unconscious act that helps one deal with an unpleasant situation?
   a. Coping skills
   **b. Defense mechanism**
   c. Excuse
   d. Problem-solving
7. The ongoing method inside each of us that deals with changes and adjustments in our lives is our:
   a. ideal self.
   b. social self.
   **c. self-as-process.**
   d. self-image.

# PROCEDURE SCENARIO

The following scenario is provided for use with the Competency Checklists. They are optional; instructors may modify the scenarios or make up their own.

## Procedure 7–1 Scenario

An elderly female patient of Korean descent is being seen by the physician at the request of family members for signs of dementia. You have brought the patient to the exam room, confirmed the correct patient with two identifiers, and taken the patient's vital signs. You must now elicit information about the patient's chief complaint for the physician. Additionally, you notice in the chart that today is the patient's birthday. You perform the patient intake, responding to nonverbal communication. Students can download the following forms from the Premium Website to complete this activity and use as Work Product for this procedure:

- Procedure Form 7–1: Progress note

# CHAPTER 8 Applying Communication Skills

## ABHES Curriculum

| | |
|---|---|
| MA.A.1.8.aa | Are attentive, listens, and learns |
| MA.A.1.8.bb | Are impartial and show empathy when dealing with patients |
| MA.A.1.8.cc | Communicate on the recipient's level of comprehension |
| MA.A.1.8.dd | Serve as liaison between physician and others |
| MA.A.1.8.kk | Adapt to individualized needs |
| MA.A.1.8.ll | Apply electronic technology |
| MA.A.1.9.q | Instruct patients with special needs |

## CAAHEP Core Curriculum

| | |
|---|---|
| IV.C.7 | Identify resources and adaptations that are required based on individual needs, i.e., culture and environment, developmental life stage, language, and physical threats to communication |
| IV.C.13 | Recognize the role of self-boundaries in the health care environment |
| IV.C.14 | Recognize the role of patient advocacy in the practice of medical assisting |
| IV.C.15 | Discuss the role of assertiveness in effective professional communication |
| IV.P.5 | Instruct patients according to their needs to promote health maintenance and disease prevention |
| IV.P.9 | Document patient education |
| IV.P.11 | Respond to nonverbal communication |
| IV.P.13 | Advocate on behalf of patients |
| IV.A.1 | Demonstrate empathy in communicating with patients, family, and staff |
| IV.A.2 | Apply active listening skills |
| IV.A.3 | Use appropriate body language and other nonverbal skills in communicating with patients, family, and staff |
| IV.A.4. | Demonstrate awareness of the territorial boundaries of the person with whom communicating |
| IV.A.7. | Demonstrate recognition of the patient's level of understanding in communications |
| IV.A.8. | Analyze communications in providing appropriate responses and feedback |
| IV.A.9. | Recognize and protect personal boundaries in communicating with others |
| IV.A.10. | Demonstrate respect for individual diversity, incorporating awareness of one's own biases in areas, including gender, race, religion, age, and economic status |
| V.P.7 | Use the Internet to access information related to the medical office |

## LESSON OUTLINE

### I. CRITICAL THINKING SKILLS

A. Also referred to as problem-solving skills or analytical skills

B. Critical thinking process

1. Decide what you think and why you think it.
2. Seek other views and evidence (develop arguments by using supportive evidence).
3. Decide which view is most reasonable.

C. Students should use these basic steps when problem solving:
   1. Determine just what the problem is and write it down.
   2. Ask whether there is a contributing problem chain or a series of events.
   3. Gather facts and ideas to help you decide what to do about it.
   4. Use analytical and creative thinking. List your decisions and what you think their outcome will be.
   5. Prioritize your decisions and begin testing them one by one until results are satisfactory to you and others concerned.

## II. COMMUNICATING WITH PATIENTS

A. Communication is a skill that will set you apart from others
B. Communication tips are provided in Table 8–1 (dos and don'ts)
C. Communication skills take time to develop
D. Communicating with special needs patients
   1. Patients with special needs (deaf, blind, and so on) require unique and individually tailored methods to communicate instructions.
   2. Reflective communication (acting as a verbal mirror) can be especially helpful for any patient requiring special attention.
E. Communicating with culturally diverse patients
   1. It is important to understand and respond with sensitivity to the needs and preferences of diverse patients.
   2. Incorporate cultural diversity awareness into your routine when performing your medical assistant duties.
F. Communicating with pediatric patients
   1. Children are not just small adults and require a much different approach than do adult patients.
   2. Use the four Es (*encouragement*, *empathy*, *enlistment*, and *education*) to engage the child in health care matters.
   3. Use appropriate terminology. Refer to examples in Table 8-3.
G. Communicating with geriatric patients
   1. A number of factors affect the geriatric patient's ability to communicate effectively with health care providers and willingness to comply with medical regimens.
   2. The normal aging process involving sensory loss, decline in hearing or memory, retirement from work, and separation from family and friends affect communication functionality.
H. Communicating with families
   1. Be careful to respect the patient's privacy when discussing health care issues with family members.
   2. Do not relay information to the patient or family that the physician has not directed you to do so.
   3. Refer to the Comprehensive Communication Preference (CCP), a legal document enumerating the patient's communication wishes.
I. Communicating with difficult or uncooperative patients
   1. The best approach is to hold off any negative judgments and try your best to accommodate the requests.
   2. Follow these steps to defuse and resolve the matter:
      a. Let the patient vent.
      b. Avoid getting trapped in negative feelings.
      c. Express empathy to the patient.
      d. Begin problem solving.

e. Mutually agree on the solution.

f. Follow up.

## III. PATIENT EDUCATION (PROCEDURE 8–1)

A. Can include verbal instructions, printed materials, or electronic formats

B. Steps in providing patient education

1. Assess the patient's ability to comprehend the instructions.
2. Use reflective (mirror) communication skills, repeating the clear, concise instructions to patient.
3. Provide a written copy of the educational materials for the patient to take with him or her.

C. The importance of documenting patient education

## IV. PATIENT ADVOCACY (PROCEDURE 8–2)

A. Advocates promote and protect the rights of patients, frequently through a legal process.

B. Patients are also represented in response to health care, insurance matters, prescription drug coverage, DMV, and matters with large health care institutions.

C. Counseling and information is also provided to patients about their rights as well as intervention with health care providers as needed.

D. An advocate can assist patients on any matter affecting their health, legal, or financial status such as medical bills and job discrimination related to the patient's medical condition.

## V. COMMUNICATING WITH THE HEALTH CARE TEAM

A. Will be in a variety of methods: verbal, written, and electronic

B. All communications should be respectful and professional

C. The medical assistant is part of a team, which includes the office staff, doctor(s), office manager, and patients

D. It is essential for medical assistants to commit themselves to the common goal of quality patient care

E. Communicating effectively with all members of the team is fundamental to job performance

G. Effective professional communication—The difference between assertive and aggressive communication

H. Roles and responsibilities in the medical office

1. For a medical office to run efficiently, employees should know and understand the roles and responsibilities of all parties.
2. Coordinating a medical office requires great skill. There are multiple layers of policy, regulation, and personalities that affect the day-to-day operations.
3. Each member of the staff has a unique set of values, principles, and standards to offer. Mutual respect and trust enhance the teamwork and efficiency.

I. Methods of communication in the medical office

1. Intra-office communication

a. Electronic (email or instant messaging)

b. Written document (a memo) provided, requiring each employee to read and sign

c. Bulletin board, often used for notices, educational programs, seminars, or meetings

2. Participating in staff meetings
   a. Most medical offices hold regular staff meetings that all employees are expected to attend.
   b. They are usually set and chaired by the office manager or the physician.
   c. The meetings are usually held in the medical office either before or after patient care hours and are announced far enough in advance so that arrangements can be made for staff to attend.
   d. At these meetings, decisions concerning office policy changes are reached, problems are discussed, new ideas can be expressed, and staff members can get more acquainted with each other.
3. Performance reviews as an avenue for communication
   a. In most employment situations, an evaluation of work performance is made on an annual basis.
   b. It is filed in the employee's permanent employment record.
   c. An initial employment review is usually held after a probationary period of 30, 60, or 90 days.
   d. Evaluation forms outline the most important qualities and abilities needed for the job and include a section for strengths and weaknesses to be listed.
   e. Employers are always aware of an employee's behavior. A person's attitude shows at all times.

## CHAPTER ACTIVITIES

1. Make a list of interferences that can block communications between staff members in the medical office and then list ways to eliminate the blocks.
2. Write an office memo concerning a new policy about clocking in. Have each student read your memo and then initial it.
3. Contact a local medical office and ask whether a student can sit in on one of the staff meetings. Have the student take notes and then share some of the things discussed with the class. Be sure that the identity of those in the staff meeting is protected when student is presenting his or her comments.
4. Set up the classroom as a medical office and role-play for a class period. Half participate while the other half critiques; then reverse the groups.
5. Have a motivational speaker relate to the students how important attitude and communication are in the workplace and elsewhere.
6. Invite a funeral director to speak to the class about bereavement and what the medical assistant can do to help. Funeral directors are often most willing to share their experiences in this area. They are empathic and insightful and will be helpful to students in realizing how important their influence may be with patients and families.
7. Arrange for a speaker from the hospice movement to explain the organization and distribute information pamphlets to students. These speakers often bring a video to enhance their purpose.
8. Rotate students weekly to be in charge of a bulletin board and post information about related activities, school and community events, and seminars. Include information from the bulletin board in quizzes to check the students' awareness of what is posted. This helps them get used to interoffice communications and encourages better communication skills.
9. Have students share in discussing their hobbies or favorite leisure activities and the importance of time for self.

# ANSWERS TO CHECK YOUR KNOWLEDGE QUESTIONS

1. All the following are steps to problem solving except:
   a. determining what the problem is and writing it down.
   b. using creative thinking.
   c. gathering facts and ideas to help you decide what to do.
   **d. putting off dealing with the problem until you are able to solve it.**
2. Which of the following is key to patient compliance when providing patient education?
   a. Information
   **b. Motivation**
   c. Criticism
   d. Nonchalance
3. The medical assistant must learn to relate to which of the following people?
   a. Patient
   b. Provider
   c. Coworkers
   d. a and b only
   **e. All of the above**
4. All the following are necessary for an enjoyable work atmosphere except:
   a. cooperation.
   b. respect.
   **c. liking your coworkers.**
   d. honesty.
5. All the following qualities of an efficient medical assistant except:
   a. versatility.
   **b. beauty.**
   c. initiative.
   d. self-starting.
6. Which of the following could be part of a staff meeting?
   a. In-service program
   b. Policy changes
   c. Discussing a personality conflict
   d. None of the above
   **e. Both a and b**
7. Which of the following can be used as a means of intra-office communication?
   a. Bulletin board
   b. Email
   c. Intra-office memo
   **d. All of the above**

# PROCEDURE SCENARIOS

The following scenarios are provided for use with the Competency Checklists. They are optional; instructors may modify the scenarios or make up their own. The forms referenced in the following scenarios can be downloaded from the student's Premium Website.

## Procedure 8–1

The patient and his son are at the office to discuss the upcoming hip replacement surgery. The patient is blind and of Japanese descent. You will perform the patient intake and instruct the patient and family according to their needs. You brought the patient and son to the exam room, confirmed the correct patient with two identifiers, checked the patient's Comprehensive Communication Preference (CCP) form, and took the patient's vital signs and chief complaint. After the physician has completed the patient's exam and review of tests and consultation report, he asks you to give the patient presurgical and postsurgical instructions.

Students can download the following forms from the Premium Website to complete this activity and use them as work product for this procedure:

- Procedure Form 8–1: Progress Note

## Procedure 8–2

You are a medical assistant at Douglasville Medicine Associates, 5076 Brand Blvd, Suite 401, Douglasville, NY 01234. The office phone number is (123) 456-7890, and fax number is (123) 456-7891. Jane Patient (SS#999-99-1234) is a patient of Dr. L.D. Heath (DEA# B2177EXAMPLE).

Jane Patient lives with her husband at 1234 Main Street, Douglasville, NY 01234. She is currently taking the following medications: Nexium (40 mg), Micardis (20 mg), and Lasix (10 mg). She is allergic to lidocaine. Her total monthly income is $2000.

*Instructor Notes:* The instructor may choose to have students go online and fill out a "live" form downloaded from the RxAssist Website (www.rxassist.org), following the instructions on the site for any one of the listed medications. Students may also complete Procedure Form 8–2, which is a mock form. Students can download the following forms from the Premium Website to complete this activity and use them as work product for this procedure:

- Procedure Form 8–2: Mock Drug Application Form

# SECTION 2 THE FRONT OFFICE

# UNIT 5 BUSINESS COMMUNICATIONS
# CHAPTER 9 Telephone Communication

## ABHES Curriculum

| | |
|---|---|
| MA.A.1.4.a | Document accurately |
| MA.A.1.8.ee | Use proper telephone techniques |
| MA.A.1.8.aa. | Are attentive, listen, and learn |
| MA.A.1.8.bb | Are impartial and show empathy when dealing with patients |
| MA.A.1.8.dd | Serve as liaison between physician and others |
| MA.A.1.8.hh | Receive, organize, prioritize, and transmit information expediently |
| MA.A.1.11.b(3) | Maintain confidentiality at all times |

## CAAHEP Core Curriculum

| | |
|---|---|
| IV.C.4 | Identify techniques for overcoming communication barriers |
| IV.C.9 | Discuss applications of electronic technology in effective communication |
| IV.P.2 | Report relevant information to others succinctly and accurately |
| IV.P.7 | Demonstrate telephone techniques |
| IV.P.8 | Document patient care |
| IV.P.12 | Develop and maintain a current list of community resources related to patients' health care needs |
| IV.A.2 | Implement time management principles to maintain effective office function |
| V.P.7 | Use Internet to access information related to the medical office |
| XI.P.12 | Maintain a current list of community resources for emergency preparedness |
| IV.A.1 | Demonstrate empathy in communicating with patients, family, and staff |
| IV.A.2 | Apply active listening skills |
| IV.A.5 | Demonstrate sensitivity appropriate to the message being delivered |
| IV.A.8 | Analyze communications in providing appropriate responses and feedback |

## LESSION OUTLINE

### I. THE "DIRECTOR OF FIRST IMPRESSIONS"

A. The telephone is the center of all activity in the medical office. The professional attitude conveyed is critical to the success of the business of practicing medicine.

B. You are the "Director of First Impressions."

C. Developing excellent telephone customer service (in both tone and words) is one of the most valuable business skills you can acquire.

### II. ANSWERING THE TELEPHONE

A. The phone call is often the first contact a patient has with the office.

B. Your manner of speaking and the empathy you convey are part of establishing an appropriate image of the practice (review Table 9–1).

C. Answer each call as soon as possible—at least by third ring
   1. Make sure you get all the information needed, repeating back the information to the caller to make sure you have recorded his or her request accurately.
   2. Let the caller know when he or she may expect a response (giving a reasonable time frame and one you can keep).

## III. HANDLING MULTIPLE RINGING LINES

A. Excuse yourself and ask the patient you are speaking with whether you may place him or her on hold.

B. Answer the second call, determine the nature of the call (be sure it is not an emergency), and ask whether the caller can hold. (Exception: If a doctor or hospital is calling asking to speak with the doctor in your office, the caller should be put through immediately and not placed on hold, or into a queue.)

C. Return to the first call and thank him or her for holding.

D. Resolve the first call and return to the second call.

## IV. TELEPHONE SCREENING (SEE PROCEDURE 9–1)

A. An established phone screening manual should be kept near each phone for reference.

B. If you do not know how to handle a patient or if the questions have not been addressed in the manual, referring the problem to one who is more experienced is necessary and appropriate.

C. Never guess in response to a patient's question and do not treat any question lightly.

D. Document, in detail, all the information obtained from the patient and relay or attach to the message for the doctor to review.

E. Anticipate what the doctor will need, such as relevant patient information and symptoms, lab results, consult results, date of last appointment, next appointment (if scheduled), blood pressure, and temperature and mark the message urgent if determined so or advised so by patient.

F. Routing calls in the medical office
   1. Table 9–3 lists examples of calls received in the medical office and where they should be routed.
   2. Knowing where to send a call when it comes in will save time, avoid frustration, and score service points.

G. Nonemergency calls
   1. If the person on the phone needs additional information, or the call is going to take a while, excuse yourself from the phone call by saying, "May I put you on hold for a moment?"
   2. If it will be more than one minute, the caller should not be put on hold; in this case, say "May I call you back with that information?"
   3. Be sure to confirm the patient's phone number before hanging up.
   4. Find out a good time to call back, including later times in case the provider wants to talk with the patient.
   5. When a caller is on hold, be mindful of the length of the hold time.

H. Transferring telephone calls
   1. If you need to transfer a patient's call to another department or office, first give the caller the phone number, extension, and the person's name to whom you are transferring him or her in case there is a disconnection.
   2. Signal (or page) the person for whom the patient is calling, explain who is waiting to speak to him or her, and give a brief summary of the issue.

3. Pull the chart for the provider if the patient is calling for information and have the pertinent data readily available (e.g., labs, test results, consults, chart notes).
4. If using a public address system, be very careful with confidentiality, stating only the person's name and that he or she has a call on a particular line.

I. Interpreter services

1. Offices should have policies in place regarding the provision of language services and should not rely on patients' friends, family, or other ad hoc interpreters.
2. It is your responsibility to become familiar with your office policies regarding interpreter services, how to access language services, and how to work with an interpreter.

## V. DOCUMENTING TELEPHONE CALLS

A. It is critical to record the date, time, name, date of birth, M/F, phone number(s), and detailed and accurate message along with your name or initials. All calls should be documented in the same manner; see Figure 9–3.

B. Urgent messages should be marked urgent and given to the doctor immediately.

C. Pull the chart and have all information relevant to the call attached to the message (e.g., lab reports, test results, consults, prescription requests, and so on).

D. If electronic messaging with EMR, attach the relevant information to the message to expedite care (Figure 9–4).

E. All messages must be signed off (both paper and electronic) to confirm final action has been taken. Usually, the last person to contact the patient shall sign off and file or save to chart and notify patient of action.

F. Confidentiality and returning patient messages

1. Data regarding patients may not be given out over the telephone to anyone unless the patient has given written permission with a signature for the release of specific information.
2. This authorization is often given with a Confidential Communication Preference (CCP) (refer to Figure 9–7).

G. Recording messages from messaging devices (see Procedure 9–2)

1. Internal EMR messaging, lab portals, and prescription refills can be available to doctors 24/7, although replies to patients are not to be expected outside normal business hours.
2. Answering machines are useful for short periods such as during lunch time; however, answering services are more likely used outside office hours.
3. The answering service can relay a message to the office by email, fax, or phone or contact the doctor by cell phone or pager if the call is determined to be an emergency or the doctor is on call.
4. Messages from the answering service need to be returned in the order of importance within an appropriate and reasonable time period. Remember to check the fax machine and patient portal for other patient-related messages.

## VI. COMMON TYPES OF PHONE CALLS

A. Appointments

1. When scheduling appointments, positively identify the patient and confirm the last appointment date.
   a. Use at least two identifiers of the patient, including date of birth and last and first names.
   b. If you are working for a doctor with a closed practice (no longer accepting new patients), it is important to confirm that you are booking only current patients.

2. Assess the type of appointment needed and note so in the schedule because each type of appointment can carry a different CPT billing code, require a different amount of time for the visit, and have different eligibility for insurance reimbursement.
3. Use time slots held for same-day or urgent visits to book first from your phone calls of the day for patients requiring more immediate attention—use screening methods to determine which patients need to be seen the same day or need urgent time slots.
4. Book any open appointment slots in order during the day. (For example, if you have three morning and two afternoon appointments open at the beginning of the day, fill your morning appointments first.)
5. The appointment should be confirmed by reading the scheduled time back to the patient after it has been recorded in the appointment book or scheduling system.
6. Frequently, medical offices place reminder calls to patients 24 to 48 hours in advance of appointments. Refer to Table 9–4 for some helpful telephone scheduling tips.

B. Prescription refills
   1. Verify office rules for prescription refills and follow them without exception.
   2. The general rule is that a medical assistant does not give out information or call in a prescription without the express direction of the provider.
   3. Write a message of the request for prescriptions in legible handwriting with detailed accuracy or document in the EMR.
   4. For a patient request of a prescription refill, document the name and phone number of the pharmacy as well as the name of the medication, strength, and prescription number, and when the prescription was last filled.
   5. Record the telephone number where the patient can be reached in case the provider needs to talk with the patient before prescribing the medication or if the provider determines the patient might need an examination first.
   6. Many prescriptions are currently sent to the office by electronic messaging, known as easyscripts or surescripts (often referred to as e-scripts) directly from the pharmacy.
   7. Additionally, patients might request prescription refills through patient portals (Figure 9–9).

C. Test results (see Procedure 9–3)
   1. Always observe office policy for releasing results.
   2. Most providers will want to speak with the patient if the test results are abnormal, although some allow the medical assistant to give normal results over the telephone.
   3. Attach result of the test, lab, or consult report for the provider to review along with the message for the provider to call the patient.
   4. Review the patient's CCP prior to calling with any results. Confirm which number to call and authorization to leave messages or speak with other parties.
      a. It is generally best not to leave a message with abnormal results.
      b. You should leave a message for the patient to return your call, without revealing a sense of urgency in your voice.

D. Follow-up calls
   1. Providers often advise patients to call the next day to report their progress.
   2. The medical assistant should determine whether to take the call and relay the message to the doctor (always attach the patient's report on the chart) or whether the provider wishes to speak directly to the patient.

3. Make sure you have the patient's current home and cell phone, pager, or work number(s) before the patient leaves your office so you will be able to call if necessary.
4. Verify that the patient's chart has a current phone number of a relative or friend if the patient cannot be contacted (and contact is authorized per the CCP).

E. Professional calls
   1. When another provider telephones to speak to your provider, politely ask the caller for his or her name and inform the provider.
   2. Professional etiquette dictates that the provider does not keep a colleague waiting unless the provider is involved with an emergency or surgical procedure.
   3. Be sure to ask whether the call is regarding a patient and whether you should pull the chart.
   4. It is wise to obtain the name and phone number of the caller in case the call is disconnected.
   5. Calls received regarding X-ray or laboratory results need to be recorded with precise accuracy:
      a. Always record the name of the person giving the report and phone number in case your doctor wants to call back for further information.
      b. Read back everything you have written down to be sure it is correct and complete before allowing the caller to leave the line.
      c. Attach the message along with the patient's chart for review by the doctor.

F. Business, personal, and legal calls
   1. Office policy will dictate protocol for business, personal, and legal calls.
   2. Calls from attorneys requesting information about a patient must be handled with great caution.
      a. Attorneys know that patients must give written permission to divulge information to anyone regarding their health, yet lawyers still call.
      b. Pull the patient chart and look for authorization listing the name of the attorney and the signature of the patient.
      c. If you find the authorization, you may answer questions about the patient. Some providers might still want you to check with them before releasing information.
      d. You must confirm information written on the patient's CCP. If you do not find authorization listing the name of the attorney, you must tell the caller an authorization signed by the patient is required prior to releasing information.
      e. It is advisable to return a call from an attorney even if you have authorization so you can ensure to whom you are talking.
      f. Most doctors prefer to be advised of requests from attorneys.
      g. Additionally, a quality department review might be required prior to release of patient information.
      h. Only information that has been authorized by the patient in writing, with the patient signature, may be given to another party.
      i. Record the call and information released by telephone or copied for attorneys or other parties from patient charts. Patients have the right to know who has accessed their medical information, and their charts should reflect each and every release of information.
      j. Common practice is to refer business or legal calls to the office manager. Check with the doctor or employer regarding the policy.

G. Long-distance calls

1. If you are calling an area outside of your time zone, consult the telephone directory for the map of time zones (refer to Figure 9–11) so you can establish the appropriate time to call.
2. Take into consideration when it is lunch break in a different time zone so that you will not waste time trying to phone an office when the staff is not available to take your call.
3. Be sure you know the code needed to dial for your long-distance service in addition to the telephone numbers of the persons you need to call.
4. A record book should be kept on all long-distance calls.

H. Difficult calls:

1. You will encounter difficult callers.
    1. When patients make demands by asking for something that is unreasonable and difficult to provide, the best approach is to hold off any negative judgments and try your best to accommodate the requests.
    2. If the caller is cursing, give the caller the benefit of the doubt and politely say, "I really want to help you, but I'm having trouble with the kind of language you are using. Can you please refrain from using that kind of language?" Give the caller a second chance and another warning if the language persists.
    3. If this does not work, let the caller know that you are no longer the person who can help and inform your supervisor of the problem.
    4. If a caller makes any threats, document the identity of the caller and the nature of the threat; advise that you are no longer the person who can help and inform your supervisor (Figure 9–12).
    5. End the call in a professional manner.

## VII. TELEPHONE SERVICES

A. Phone menus

1. Most business phone systems have a menu for the caller to be connected to the proper person or department (e.g., "Press one to reach the billing department, press two to speak to the scheduling department, press three for prescription refills").
2. This system is designed to be more efficient, route to the proper person or department, and prevent the caller from being disconnected or kept on hold too long.
3. The caller should be instructed at the beginning of the recording to hang up immediately and call 911 or EMS (as applicable to caller's geographical area) if the call is for a medical emergency.

B. Conference calls

1. The telephone can be used to conduct conversations simultaneously with several people in various locations to conduct meetings and professional or personal communications.
2. Conference calling saves time, travel, and money.
3. If your phone system is not equipped to allow multiple connections, conference calls can be arranged with your local phone service provider.

C. Teleconferencing

1. Teleconferencing means exchanging information like a conference call, except everyone can see and hear each other at the same time, linked through telecommunications equipment.
2. Cameras, speaker phones, connection devices, and television or computer monitors are in each location.
3. The phone company or the meeting originator contacts all other sites and networks the phones.

## VIII. COMMUNITY RESOURCES

A. Patient health care needs (see Procedure 9–4)

1. Keep an up-to-date index of your most frequently called numbers, as well as resources for patients and emergency preparedness, by the telephone (see Procedures 9–4 and 9–5). Review Table 9–5 for a list of frequently called numbers in a medical office.
2. Locate these resources through such means as office materials and directories, the Internet, intranet, and telephone book.
3. Use Internet portals for access to telephone numbers and addresses to research available additional community resources, both for patient health services and emergency preparedness (see Tables 9–6 and 9–7).
4. Have a copy of the most current telephone book, as well as the current directory for the local emergency clinics, hospitals, and physicians (in network) and specialists, on hand in the office. Be sure to verify that the information is current.

B. Emergency preparedness (see Procedure 9–5)—Keep an up-to-date list of emergency contact information and resources, including, for example:

1. Medical Reserve Corps
2. American Medical Association
3. OSHA
4. CDC
5. Fire department
6. Police department
7. Ambulance and patient transport companies
8. Local hospital directory of contact information
9. United States Department of Homeland Security (www.ready.gov)

## CHAPTER ACTIVITITES

1. Role play: Assign students specific types of telephone calls to answer. (The student should record the situation briefly and how it was handled and review the answers with the instructor if not observed by the instructor during the actual practice.)
   a. Show how to be the Director of First Impressions (patient calling for new patient appointment).
   b. Screen (triage) a patient call with chest pain.
2. Prepare a proper message for the physician based on one or more of the preceding scenarios.
3. Ask a local physician to address the class on the importance of telephone screening and proper messaging techniques to enhance provider efficiency and patient safety.
4. Using the United States Department of Homeland Security Website (www.ready.gov), create a list of community resources and emergency response, using the example templates provided.

## ANSWERS TO CHECK YOUR KNOWLEDGE QUESTIONS

1. Which of the following is NOT considered a guideline (protocol) for answering the telephone in the medical office?

   a. Answer the telephone as promptly as possible, with a smile.

   b. Put the caller on hold as quickly as possible.

   c. Handle as many telephone calls as you possibly can without disturbing the provider. Provide message and documentation, including attaching the call-back number and chart when needed by the provider for review.

   d. Document only the important calls.

   e. None of the above

   **f. b and d**

2. Identify methods of screening and routing incoming calls.

   a. Determine nature of call.

   b. Accurately describe patient symptoms.

   c. Determine level of urgency.

   d. Use standard questions and respond in a template form pre-authorized by the provider.

   **e. All of the above**

   f. b and c only

3. Which of the following is incorrect when documenting a telephone message?

   **a. Record nature of call only if urgent message**

   b. Caller's full name

   c. Date of birth

   d. M/F (sex)

   e. Date and time of call

4. Which types of telephone calls will a medical assistant have to answer in the medical office?

   a. Appointments

   b. Prescription refills

   c. Follow-up calls

   d. Difficult calls

   **e. All of the above**

   f. a, b, and d

5. Which of the following describe the types of community resources for patients' health care needs?

   a. Senior services

   b. Lab services and locations

   c. Occupational Health and Safety Administration

   d. Police department

   e. All of the above

   **f. a and b only**

## PROCEDURE SCENARIOS

The following scenarios are provided for use with the Competency Checklists. They are optional; instructors may modify the scenarios or make up their own. The following forms can be downloaded from the students' Premium Website.

## PROCEDURE 9–1 SCENARIO

Joan Anthony calls the office at 8:00 a.m. on Tuesday, January 6 (current year): "This is Mrs. Anthony. I am having trouble breathing and I need the doctor to call me back immediately! I am very anxious and have used my inhaler three times, but it doesn't seem to help. Please call me soon."

Students can download the Procedure Form 9–1: Progress Note form from the Premium Website to complete this activity and use as work product for this procedure.

## PROCEDURE 9–2 SCENARIO

Upon returning from lunch, there is a telephone message from the office's answering service. Record the following information on the telephone message form (Procedure Form 9–2): Ms. Jamison telephoned complaining of a high fever, tight chest, and deep cough. She has been sick for about three days and has been taking OTC medication with no relief. She is at work now, 272-2222, but will be leaving to go home at 2:00 p.m. and can be reached there at 888-8888.

Students can download Procedure Form 9–2: Telephone Message Form from the Premium Website to complete this activity and use as work product for this procedure.

# CHAPTER 10 Written Communications

## ABHES Curriculum

| | |
|---|---|
| MA.A.1.7.a (1) | Locate the keys of a keyboard |
| MA.A.1.7.a (2) | Type medical correspondence and basic reports |
| MA.A.1.7.b (1) | Efficiently maintain and understand different types of medical correspondence and medical reports |
| MA.A.1.7.b (2) | Apply computer application skills, using a variety of electronic programs, including both practice management software and EHR applications |
| MA.A.1.8.a | Perform basic clerical functions |
| MA.A.1.8.dd | Serve as liaison between provider and others |
| MA.A.1.8.gg | Use pertinent medical terminology |
| MA.A.1.8.jj | Perform fundamental writing skills, including correct grammar, spelling, and formatting techniques when writing prescriptions, documenting medical records, etc. |
| MA.A.1.8.ll | Apply electronic technology |

## CAAHEP Core Curriculum

| | |
|---|---|
| IV.C.8 | Recognize elements of fundamental writing skills |
| IV.C.9 | Discuss applications of electronic technology in effective communication |
| IV.C.10 | Organize technical information and summaries |
| IV.P.3 | Use medical terminology, pronouncing medical terms correctly, to communicate information, patient history, data, and observations |
| IV.P.10 | Compose professional and business letters |

# LESSON OUTLINE

## CORRESPONDENCE IN THE MEDICAL OFFICE

A. Interoffice communication

1. An informal, memo-style communication that is usually specific to one concern.
2. An effective way of being certain that everyone is aware of some event, policy, concern, and other internal communication, circulated electronically (email) or by copy of a memo.

B. Informal notes

1. Indicated for times when thanks, congratulations, or similar expressions are desired.
2. Usually personal and informal in nature, written on a first-name basis.

C. Personal letters

D. Professional letters

1. Providers might need to write to their professional associations, licensing boards, and other providers regarding some issue or concern affecting personal medical activities or their professional practice.
2. These specific writings require detailed dictating and perfect transcription.

E. Form letters and templates

1. Form letters are used for referrals, consults, annual examination reminders, collection letters, school and work releases, suppliers of equipment and materials, and other correspondence necessary to the office operation.

2. A template is an electronic file (or preprinted document) with a predesigned, customized, format.
    a. Examples of templates are fax cover sheets or patient information letters, ready to be filled in.
    b. Your PC word processing program (Word, for example) has numerous built-in templates.
    c. Explore these to create documents you will use frequently.
    d. Use the mail merge feature to send the same letter to multiple recipients..

F. Information sheets
1. Provide specific written instructions regarding the examinations and diagnostic tests performed in your office.
2. Reinforce what you have explained and serve as reminders after patients leave the office.
3. Can be prepared and stored in the files to be used as needed and are an excellent example of patient education material.

G. Clinical email
1. Allows for the almost instant exchange of information without the costs associated with long-distance phone calls.
2. Offers the advantage of transmitting written material, making it appropriate for transferring reports, documents, correspondence, and most forms of written communication.
3. To comply with patient privacy and HIPAA guidelines, all electronic communications, including email, must provide security measures such as restricted user access, encryption, and passwords.
4. Some pros and cons of using email must be considered.
5. Email and computer viruses—Standard methods of protection are available, such as employing firewalls and antivirus software (with the virus database kept up to date) to protect your computer while browsing and downloading files.

## II. COMMUNICATION AND HIPAA REGULATIONS

A. Communications that include personal information about patients require specific handling.

B. You must adhere strictly to ethics and laws of confidentiality.

C. With the enactment of HIPAA, rules about the security of patients' personal health information (PHI) as contained in medical records were identified.

D. Most providers have developed specific Release of Information forms that follow the HIPAA guidelines.

E. Patients are requested to sign these forms, giving permission for providers to communicate personal information. Some instances would be:
1. Patient personal use
2. Life insurance questionnaire
3. Disability insurance questionnaire

F. A release is not required when releasing information pertaining to the patient's care. Some examples of instances would be:
1. To request a consultation from a specialist.
2. To provide results to the referring physician from a specialist.
3. To provide information to a hospital or nursing care facility.
4. To an insurance company for payment of services.

G. The patient is provided with a written statement from the provider's practice that explains its adherence to the HIPAA regulations regarding his or her personal information.

H. Patients are asked to sign a form indicating they have received a copy of this document. This is often referred to a Notice of Privacy Practices (NOPP).

I. Procedures must be in place to comply with HIPAA and protect the privacy of patient information with electronic applications (email and EHR).
   1. Security measures must include encryption, firewall software and hardware, personnel passwords, access restrictions, and activity logs.
   2. Access to the patient's record may be limited within an office to only those people who need to view the chart.
   3. Preparing written (or electronic) communication may be limited to those approved individuals.
   4. Some employees would be prohibited from access to patient information by the security officer as directed by HIPAA regulations.

## III. WRITING GUIDELINES

A. Spelling
   1. You must check any word if you are not sure of its accuracy.
   2. You might find that when using a word processing program, the spell check feature will be a great assistance; however, do not rely solely on spell check because it is possible that the word is spelled correctly but you have entered the wrong word or a word out of context.
   3. Examples of this are "their" for "there," "cite" for "sight," and others.
   4. There are 14 rules about spelling that are very helpful (refer to Figure 10–1)
      a. If you cannot seem to spell certain words correctly, try making an alphabetical list of them to use as a quick reference.
      b. Make a mental picture of the word correctly spelled.
      c. Pronounce the word correctly several times.
      d. Write the word, dividing it into syllables and inserting accent marks.
      e. Write or type the word several times.
      f. Learn to use a general dictionary and a medical dictionary when you are in doubt.

B. Parts of speech—To compose effective, well-written communications, you need to be aware of the eight parts of speech and how they are used (refer to Table 10–3)
   1. Noun
   2. Pronoun
   3. Verb
   4. Adjective
   5. Adverb
   6. Preposition
   7. Conjunction
   8. Interjection

C. Sentence structure
   1. Write in complete thoughts.
   2. A *simple sentence* consists of only one complete thought, that is, one independent clause with a subject and a verb.

D. Punctuation

1. To make sentences easier to read and to tell a reader when you come to the end of a thought, a variety of markings called punctuation are used (refer to Table 10–4).
2. The most common are the comma, period, apostrophe, hyphen, and ellipses.

E. Capitalization

1. Capitalize names of persons and places, the first word in a sentence, names of holidays, principal words in titles of major works, and any product or title that might be trademarked.
2. Many medical terms begin with a capital letter because they are names of the physicians who named them.
3. Medications are usually trademarked.
4. Use your dictionary when in doubt.

F. Numbers

1. In the absence of other references and if the provider's preference is unknown, usually any number under 10 is spelled out, whereas those above are expressed in numeric form.
2. A partially contradicting general rule says to spell out the number if it can be done in one or two words.
3. A number at the beginning of a sentence must be spelled out.
4. A person's age and the time of day are usually written in numeric form.
5. Dates, street numbers, and page numbers are written in figures.
6. When several numbers are mentioned within a short space, figures should be used for all of them.

G. Proofreading

1. All written communication must be proofread before it is sent.
2. Spell check and immediate feedback of composition errors from word processing software can identify most common errors.
3. Do not rely on spell check; it will still miss the correctly spelled wrong word and out-of-context words.

## IV. PREPARING BUSINESS LETTERS

A. Components of a business letter

1. Letterhead: Preprinted name, complete address, and phone number (optional)
2. Date line: Date letter is dictated or composed
3. Inside address: Address of person to whom the letter is being sent
4. Salutation: The greeting to the recipient
5. Reference: To identify what or about whom the letter is concerning
6. Body: The content of the letter
7. Complimentary closing: Expressing the closing of the letter
8. Sender's signature: Signature of the writer
9. Title: Writer's title if appropriate (e.g., Vice President, Director)
10. Reference initials: Initials of the letter typist
11. Enclosures: Any identified materials to be sent with the letter
12. Copies: "cc," meaning "carbon copy," identifies another person or persons to whom a copy of the letter is sent.

B. Letter styles

1. See Figures 10–3 A, B, and C, which are samples of the full block letter, the modified block letter, and the modified block letter with indented paragraphs.

2. Full block style: The dateline, address, salutation, body of letter, complimentary close, typed signature, and the initials of the typist are flush with the left margin.
3. Modified block: The dateline, complimentary close, and typed signature begin a bit right of center.

C. Stationery—Letterhead stationery and matching envelopes are usually 16-, 20-, or 24-pound weight.

D. Composing the letter (see Procedure 10–1)

1. Determine what information needs to be included (a) to answer a letter, (b) to respond to a verbal request, (c) to request information, and (d) to obtain a specific response.
2. Determine the style for the letter and set margins for appropriate placement on the page.
3. Select the typeface and font size.
4. Compose a rough draft, using concise, clear sentences.
5. Proofread the draft and edit the content. Eliminate redundant (extra, unnecessary) phrases.
6. Compose the final copy and prepare the envelope.
7. Sign it or give it to the sender to sign.

E. Consultation letters

1. In a specialist's office, one of the most common letters received is a request from another provider for a consultation of a patient (Figure 10–4).
2. The content of the correspondence usually covers:
   a. The reason for the appointment.
   b. The date and time of the appointment.
   c. A statement that if there are any questions, please feel free to call the office.
   d. The office's phone number.
   e. *Note: If a prior authorization is required by the patient's insurance company, it should be so stated in an appointment or referral correspondence.*
   f. The office visit will require a follow-up letter from the specialist to the referring provider, identifying the findings, diagnosis, and recommended course of treatment.

## V. HANDLING INCOMING MAIL

A. Incoming mail

1. The amount of mail coming into providers' offices depends on the number of providers.
2. Many types of mail come into a provider's office.
3. Office policy determines whether it is sorted and placed on the provider's desk, the office manager's desk, or a combination of both according to the type of mail received.

B. Sorting mail

1. Incoming mail should first be sorted.
2. Any mail marked *personal* should be placed on the provider's or office manager's desk unopened.

C. Opening mail

1. Supplies: letter opener, paper clips, stapler, and date stamp
2. Stack all envelopes so that they are facing in the same direction.
3. Open each letter along the flap edge, being careful to remove all contents from each envelope.
4. As the mail is removed, be sure the contents contain the same name and return address shown on the envelope.

5. Date-stamp the correspondence and attach any enclosures.
6. If an enclosure is indicated on the letter but is missing, write "None" after the "Encl." notation and circle it to indicate need for follow-up.

D. Processing incoming mail
   1. Follow office policy and physician preference when processing incoming mail, including routine office expense bills, insurance forms, and checks for deposit.
   2. Immediately endorse stamp with the practice stamp any checks received.
   3. If cash is received in the mail, seek a witness to verify the amount of money and have that person sign a receipt along with you to be sent to the patient.

E. Mail received during vacation
   1. Discuss, before the physician leaves, what to do with urgent mail.
   2. Never send an original document by mail; send only copies and comply with HIPAA regulations.
   3. If the physician will be away for a long time, you might need to send mail more than once.
   4. If so, be sure to number the envelopes consecutively and keep track of what you send so that you can be sure all the mail is received.

F. Preparing mailings

G. Addressing the envelope
   1. Addresses can now be read by computers and optical character readers (OCRs) if handwritten or typed.
   2. Use a standard type font; script or executive type letters run together.

H. Preparing the envelope
   1. When the mail has been signed, fold it and place it in the envelope (see Figure 10–7 A–C).
   2. Ensure that the envelope is a proper size.

I. Stamp or meter mail
   1. Stamps may be purchased at a post office or purchased online and printed.
   2. If you have a large volume of mail, it is preferable to use a postage meter.

J. Mail classifications
   1. Express mail
   2. Priority mail
   3. First class mail
   4. Periodicals
   5. Standard mail (A)
   6. Standard mail (B)

K. Special mailing services
   1. Certificate of mailing
   2. Certified mail
   3. Collection on delivery (COD)
   4. Insurance
   5. Registered mail
   6. Return receipt
   7. Restricted delivery

## CHAPTER ACTIVITIES

1. Prepare sample forms of written communication using examples in text.
2. Use a word processing application to prepare a letter, envelope, and interoffice memo.
3. Assign students a list of names, places, ZIP codes, and organizations they must find in your telephone directory.
4. Quiz students on state abbreviations.
5. Assign spelling rules each week for study and quiz weekly until the terms are mastered.
6. Explore templates available in Microsoft Excel and Word and prepare samples of written communication.
7. Encourage practice in the area of written communications with extra assignments in composing and transcribing letters, always being sure to inform students of the standards required for the assignments.

## ANSWERS TO CHECK YOUR KNOWLEDGE QUESTIONS

1. Of the following items, which are advantages of using email?
   a. Can be used in a court of law as evidence
   b. Provides easy reference to past communications
   c. Saves time and paper
   d. a and c
   **e. b and c**
2. Identify which is NOT a type of form letter or information sheet.
   **a. Reply to AMA regarding provider speaking engagement**
   b. Work status note
   c. Athletic participation approvals
   d. Annual diagnostic test or examination notice
3. Name the parts of speech.
   a. Noun
   b. Verb
   c. Adjective
   d. Pronoun
   **e. All of the above**
   f. a and d
4. Describe how mail received during vacation might be handled.
   a. Hold all mail until the provider returns.
   b. Read all mail and decide how each piece will be handled.
   c. Call the physician to discuss daily mail.
   d. Call the physician to discuss urgent mail.
   **e. b and d**
   f. a and c
5. Which is not a classification of mail?
   a. Certified
   **b. Internet address**
   c. Registered
   d. Express

## PROCEDURE SCENARIO

The following scenario is provided for use with Procedure 10–1 Competency Checklist. It is optional; instructors may modify the scenario or make up their own. The following forms can be downloaded from the students' Premium Website.

*Hint*: Some words may be misspelled. Use your proofreading skills carefully.

### Procedure 10–1 Scenario

Type a letter, using modified block style (as shown in Figure 10–3 B in the text). Address the letter to John Jones, MD, 3530 Main Street, Cold Springs, KY 41076. The name of the patient is Ms. Patty Segal. The dictating provider is Samuel E. Matthews, MD. For the date, use two working days before today's date. The letter content follows:

*Hint*: Some words are misspelled, so students will need to use proofreading skills additionally.

I saw _________ on ____________ for X-ray examination.

AP and lateral roentgenograms of the cervical spine show an aberration of the normal cervical curve. The curve is slightly convexed posteriorly at the level of the fith, sixth, and seventh cervical vertebrae. Normally, the posterior curve should be concave. There are no significant hypertrophic changes, but there are minimal true arthritic changes involving the articular facets in the lower cervical region.

A roentgenogram of the right shoulder shows no evidence of intrinsic done disease. There is no periarticular soft tissue calcification in the region of the bruise.

Thank you for your referal

Very truly yours,

Students can download the following forms from the Premium Website to complete this activity and use as work product for this procedure:

- Procedure Form 10–1: Letterhead

## PROCEDURE 10–1 ANSWER KEY

**SAMUEL E. MATTHEWS, MD**
**100 EAST MAIN STREET, SUITE 120**
**YOURTOWN, US 43200-4321**

Date [as instructed]

John Jones, MD
3530 Main Street
Cold Springs, KY 41076

RE: Ms. Patty Segal / DOB 01-29-19XX

Dear Dr. Jones:

I saw Ms. Segal on [date as instructed] for X-ray examination. AP and lateral roentgenograms of the cervical spine show an aberration of the normal cervical curve. The curve is slightly convexed posteriorly at the level of the fifth, sixth, and seventh cervical vertebrae. Normally, the posterior curve should be concave. There are no significant hypertrophic changes, but there are minimal true arthritic changes involving the articular facets in the lower cervical region.

A roentgenogram of the right shoulder shows no evidence of intrinsic bone disease. There is no periarticular soft tissue calcification in the region of the bruise.

Thank you for your referral.

Very truly yours,

Samuel E. Matthews, MD

SEM:bw

# CHAPTER 11 Operating Computers and Office Equipment

## ABHES Curriculum

| | |
|---|---|
| MA.A.7.b | Identify and use office machines, computerized systems, and medical software properly |
| MA.A.8.y | Perform routine maintenance of administrative and clinical equipment |
| MA.A.8.ll | Apply electronic technology |

## CAAHEP Core Curriculum

| | |
|---|---|
| IV.C.9 | Discuss applications of electronic technology in effective communication |
| V.C.11 | Discuss principles of using electronic medical records (EMR) |
| V.C.14 | Discuss the importance of routine maintenance of office equipment |
| V.P.6 | Use office hardware and software to maintain office systems |
| V.P.9 | Perform routine maintenance of office equipment with documentation |
| XI.P.10 | Identify principles of body mechanics and ergonomics |

## LESSON OUTLINE

### I. THE COMPUTER

A. Computer terms (Table 11–1)

B. Hardware and software

1. *Hardware* refers to the hard disk drive, the CPU, the monitor, and the keyboard.
2. *Software* refers to the programs containing instructions to the computer that enable it to perform tasks.

### II. ERGONOMICS AND COMPUTER USE

A. When using the computer, evaluate the workstation for health and safety considerations. Proper lighting, height, keyboard, mouse, and headset are items that should be addressed. (Refer to Figure 11–4 and Table 11–3.)

B. Ergonomics programs provide a work environment that promotes wellness and minimizes musculoskeletal disorders.

C. Improper setup of workstations or repeated use of computer equipment can result in injury.

### III. COMPUTER APPLICATIONS SOFTWARE

A. These enable computers to perform specific tasks. Examples include word processing, managing databases, preparing spreadsheets, practice management, and more.

B. Practice management software

1. A type of applications software that manages the operations of a medical practice.
2. Available from a variety of companies.
3. Functionality of practice management software varies, depending on the program but typically enables a medical office to schedule appointments, record patient demographics and insurance information, process claims, perform insurance and billing routines, and generate financial reports.

C. Electronic health records (EHR) software
   1. Captures all patient health information harvested from one or more encounters in any health care delivery system (such as a medical office, hospital, urgent care center, and so on).
      a. Includes demographics, progress notes, vital signs, current medications, allergies, immunizations, lab orders, and more.
      b. Enables providers to document all care received by the patient—tests performed, treatments prescribed, patient education given, and so on.
      c. Use of EHR software significantly enhances efficiency in the medical office by improving workflows, reducing paper usage, and shrinking costs.
      d. As you document in an EHR, it is your responsibility to ensure data integrity.
   2. EHR software and downtime
      a. Inevitably, the practice will experience times when the computer systems are not operating.
      b. Preparations must be made to convert to paper, using manual scheduling and messaging, billing, and a downtime form for the patient encounter.

D. Encoder software
   1. Available for all CPT®, HCPCS, and ICD-9-CM code sets and Medicare coding guidelines.
   2. Improves coding accuracy and billing performance and reduces rejected claims.
   3. With optional functionality features, other advantages of using encoder software include:
      a. Compliance editing
      b. Robust code checking
      c. Increase in the rules set
      d. Improved compliance and accuracy for accelerated claims payments
      e. Fee calculator
      f. Color code edits
      g. Modifier crosswalk
      h. Cross-coder relationships
      i. Medicare CCI edits
      j. LMPR/LCD and NCD policies

E. The Internet
   1. The Internet is a system of interconnected computer networks by which to access information from all over the world.
   2. It is possible to enter, obtain, and exchange information as well as conduct business transactions such as banking, all electronically.
   3. However, be cautious. The Internet contains a wealth of information, but not all of it is good information.
   4. Guidelines for evaluating Websites:
      a. Check the source. Are there links to professional affiliations or are there professional credentials?
      b. Be cautious about personal testimonies from users; they often are receiving monetary compensation for making statements.
      c. Watch for dates of the information; the information might be very old and no longer valid.
      d. Use your analytic and critical thinking skills to interpret scientific studies or reports. Who did the research? How many people were included in the study? Is the amount of time spent appropriate to arrive at the stated conclusions? Is there more than one study on the subject to give its results credibility?

## IV. COMPUTER SECURITY

A. Physical access (computers, screens, printers, fax, copier)
   1. Use screen privacy shields and automatic screen savers.
   2. Place equipment out of high traffic and visual sight areas.

B. Use passwords for each computer and software application and set applications to log off automatically if inactive for a specified period of time.

C. Catalog all information system components
   1. Hardware: computer workstation and tablets, printers, PDAs, scanners, and modems.
   2. Software: Operating system, billing software, practice management, email, EHR, database.
   3. Network: Routers, hubs, phone and cable lines, wireless, firewall software and hardware.

D. Ensure integrity from loss, disaster, human error, hard drive error, virus, or equipment damage by backing up data
   1. Use appropriate level of secure backup for the practice.
      a. Tapes
      b. CDs
      c. Offsite storage
   2. Keep network and communication safeguards intact.
   3. Defend against attacks and viruses: Install firewalls (hardware and software devices that protect an organization's network from intruders).
   4. Understand encryption
      a. HIPAA security standards require you to assess whether unencrypted transmissions of health information are at risk of being viewed by unauthorized entities.
      b. If they are, some form of encryption should be considered for:
         i. Patient billing and information exchanged with payers and health plans
         ii. Usage, case management, authorization, and referrals
         iii. Patient health information gathered from or displayed on a Website or portal
         iv. Lab and other clinical data electronically sent to and received from outside labs
         v. Word processing files used in transcription and transferred electronically
         vi. Emails between providers and patients and between attending and referring providers and their offices
   5. Vendor and business relationships chain of trust: Demand that all vendors and business partners fully understand the HIPAA security standards.
   6. Access and security levels to EHR should be monitored and tracked.

## V. OFFICE EQUIPMENT

A. Copy machines (see Procedure 11–1)
   1. A photocopy of correspondence, an insurance form, a patient's record, laboratory reports, or account information is often needed.
   2. Most machines can be set to use either letter- or legal-sized paper.

B. Fax machines
   1. The machine can send and receive letters, medical reports, laboratory reports, and insurance claims.
   2. Providers can use the fax machine to receive and send prescription orders to pharmacies.

C. Dictation-transcription machine (see Procedure 11–2)

1. Several kinds of machines are available: a unit for **dictation** only, a unit for **transcription** only, or a combination unit that can be used for both purposes.
2. Many providers use portable dictation equipment.
3. Keep up to date with the changes in technology for efficiency in dictation and transcription and the integration and interoperability with other software programs.

D. Printers

1. To produce hard copy from computer files, you must have a printer.
2. Two types of printers are appropriate for a medical office: inkjet or laser. An inkjet printer might print in three modes.

E. Smart phones and pagers

1. Providers commonly use smart phones or pagers so they can be contacted regardless of where they are or what they are involved in.
2. Providers commonly use cell phones with data features (smart phones) in lieu of or in addition to pagers.
3. A pager is a small electronic device that is activated by a telephone signal.

### VI. EQUIPMENT MAINTENANCE (SEE PROCEDURE 11–3)

A. The medical assistant may be asked to keep track of equipment maintenance because the office has a number of clinical equipment pieces that must remain operational.

B. Most machines come with a manual for routine maintenance.

C. Daily maintenance includes cleaning various parts (with appropriate materials), checking and resetting consumables, replacing parts, and troubleshooting.

## CHAPTER ACTIVITIES

1. Demonstrate the copy machine and have each student operate it at least once.
2. Arrange a field trip to an office in which all office equipment items are used (if they are not available in the class laboratory).
3. Assign computer lessons for students to complete after demonstration of the equipment. Check to be sure students operate it properly.
4. Have students type lecture notes on a computer for a week.

## ANSWERS TO CHECK YOUR KNOWLEDGE QUESTIONS

1. Which types of material are often photocopied?
   a. Patients' insurance card(s)
   b. Patients' drivers license
   c. Patients' Social Security card
   d. Lab reports
   e. a, b, and c
   **f. a and d**

2. Identify when dictation is NOT used.
   a. Patient notes
   **b. Patient appointment time**
   c. Patient observations
   d. Patient findings
3. Which is NOT a computer term listed in the unit?
   **a. IOC**
   b. Virus
   c. Bug
   d. Attachment
   e. Interface
4. Which is NOT a computer program listed in this unit?
   **a. Digital voice recorder**
   b. Medical practice management software
   c. Electronic health record software
   d. Encoder software
5. Which is NOT referred to as computer hardware?
   a. PDA
   **b. Router**
   c. Printer
   d. Scanner
   e. Modem
6. Explain why backing up computer data is necessary.
   a. Deletes unwanted information
   b. Human error
   c. Virus
   d. Hard drive error
   e. All of the above
   **f. b, c, and d**

# UNIT 6 BEGINNING THE PATIENT'S RECORD
# CHAPTER 12 Scheduling Appointments and Receiving Patients

## ABHES Curriculum

| | |
|---|---|
| MA.A.8.c | Schedule and manage appointments |
| MA.A.8.d | Apply concepts for office procedures |
| MA.A.8.f | Schedule inpatient and outpatient admissions |

## CAAHEP Core Curriculum

| | |
|---|---|
| I.A.2 | Use language and verbal skills that enable patients' understanding |
| IV.A | Concepts of effective communication |
| V.C.1 | Discuss pros and cons of various types of appointment management systems |
| V.C.2 | Describe scheduling guidelines |
| V.C.3 | Recognize office policies and protocols for handling appointments |
| V.C.4 | Identify critical information required for scheduling patient admissions and procedures |
| V.C.11 | Discuss principles of EMR |
| V.P.1 | Manage appointment schedule, using established priorities |
| V.P.2 | Schedule patient admission and procedures |
| V.P.4 | Explain general office policies |
| V.P.3 | Organize a patient's medical record |
| V.A.2 | Implement time management principles to maintain effective office function |
| IX.C.4 | Summarize the Patient Bill of Rights |
| IX.P.3 | Apply HIPAA rules regarding privacy and release of information |
| IX.P.5 | Incorporate the Patient's Bill of Rights into personal practice and medical office policies and procedures |

# LESSON OUTLINE

## I. ESTABLISHING A MATRIX

A. Definition of matrix

B. How the matrix organizes the schedule and promotes a predictable, smooth course to the day

C. Orally review or quiz students regarding what types of time blocks or appointments would be best scheduled as:

1. Cluster
2. Double-booking
3. Flex time
4. Modified wave
5. Single-booking
6. Streaming
7. Unstructured
8. Wave

D. Discuss what different types of medical practices might benefit most from different types of scheduling practices.

## II. APPOINTMENT DOCUMENTATION

A. Describe how to enter information correctly in the appointment schedule.

B. What are the ethical and legal considerations of making corrections?

## III. CREATING NEW APPOINTMENTS (PROCEDURE 12–1)

A. Required information

1. Correctly spelled name
2. Next available appointment or based on prescribed time
3. Date and time understood by patient
4. Appropriate amount of time to be reserved
5. Preference for time of day
6. Consistent times and days for multiple appointments
7. Alternate time to first offered appointment
8. Accurate entry made in book or computer
9. Appointment card containing necessary information

B. Telephone appointments

1. Discuss communication methods over phone, lacking benefit of facial expressions and body language.
2. Stress importance of obtaining all necessary information and contact information before patient hangs up.
3. Read back information to verify.
4. Have students simulate process of scheduling and appointment over the phone.

C. Follow-up appointments

1. Discuss obtaining information about type of appointment and specific information necessary to schedule follow-up appointment.
2. Have students practice as patient and MA.

D. Referral appointments (Procedure 12–2)

## IV. MAINTAINING THE SCHEDULE

A. Walk-in or chronically late patients

1. Describe the conflict that a patient without an appointment or one who is habitually late can introduce into the schedule.
2. Have students practice as both patient and scheduler.

B. Missed appointments

C. Business appointments

1. Review different methods of handling business associates or colleagues during the schedule day.
2. Explore options for scheduling and ways to work them in while maintaining an on-time office schedule.

## V. GREETING PATIENTS

A. Ask students to identify appropriate greetings and titles: Mr., Mrs., Ms. Discuss not addressing elderly patients as "honey" or "dear" and how this is unprofessional and demeaning to an older person.

B. Active listening

C. Eye contact

D. Clear and complete explanations

E. Confidentiality

## VI. SIGN-IN

A. Helps maintain scheduling

B. Important to protect confidentiality

C. Ask for ways in which this confidentiality might be preserved when signing in.

## VII. OBTAINING NEW PATIENT INFORMATION (PROCEDURE 12–3)—DISCUSS HOW EACH OF THE FOLLOWING IS USEFUL

A. Patient's complete, correctly spelled name

B. Date of birth (DOB)

C. Social Security number (SSN)

D. Marital status

E. Current address and length of time at that address

F. Telephone numbers: home, work or pager, cell phone, email, and fax numbers

G. Name and relationship of person legally responsible for charges

H. Occupation: name, address, and phone number of employer; spouse's work information if available

I. Health insurance information

J. A copy of the patient's driver's license or the driver's license number and expiration date

K. If referred, write down the referral source.

## VIII. EXPLAINING OFFICE POLICIES (PROCEDURE 12–4)

A. Discuss importance of communicating policies to patients to avoid misunderstandings.

B. Have students simulate process.

# CHAPTER ACTIVITIES

1. Have students make up flash cards in class and review them with their classmates in pairs.
2. Prepare a blank schedule; have students apply a matrix and schedule different types of appointments appropriately.

# ANSWERS TO CHECK YOUR KNOWLEDGE QUESTIONS

1. A *matrix* refers to what?

   **a. Establishing blocks of time in a schedule for different types of appointments and scheduled breaks**

   b. The material that holds printed or copied material together

   c. A method to connect different computers in the office

   d. Tangle of ethical and legal dilemmas faced by an office practice

2. Which type of scheduling might be most helpful in a general surgeon's office?

   a. Double-booking

   b. Wave

   c. Streaming

**d. Cluster (Rationale: General surgeons perform a number of types of procedures, both in the office and in the hospital, as well as follow-ups and rounding on hospital patients. Clustering appointments is the most efficient method for this type of practice.)**

3. When explaining office policies to patients, all the following should be included EXCEPT:
   a. What the patient can expect from the office staff
   **b. How the provider allocates the earnings made through the business management of the practice (Rationale: The patient has no right to this type of information because it does not affect his or her care.)**
   c. What types of confidentiality protections are in place
   d. How the patient is expected to behave while receiving services from the office
4. Which of the following types of information will not be required when prearranging a hospital admission?
   a. Insurance numbers
   b. Patient's demographic data
   c. Types of services expected during the admission
   **d. Diagnosis chosen by the medical assistant (Rationale: The admitting diagnosis should not be made based on the medical assistant's determination but only on a diagnosis specifically indicated by the provider.)**
5. Which is the most appropriate action for greeting patients when they arrive in the office?
   a. They should be taken immediately to an exam room to protect their confidentiality.
   b. Have them sign in on the sign-in sheet with their full name, specific reason for visit, and social security number to avoid confusing them with other patients who might have similar names.
   **c. Greet the patient by his or her full name and make eye contact. (Rationale: A is unnecessary, and B reveals far too much information, violating the patient's right to confidentiality.)**
   d. None of these is appropriate

## PROCEDURE SCENARIOS

The following scenarios are provided for use with the competency checklists. They are optional; instructors may modify the scenarios or make up their own. The following forms can be downloaded from the students' Premium Website.

### PROCEDURE 12–1

Schedule patients, using the information below and the established appointment scheduling guidelines. Students can download the following forms from the Premium Website to complete this activity and use as work product for this procedure:

- Procedure Form 12–1 A: Appointment schedule (blank)
- Procedure Form 12–1 B: Appointment card (blank)

1. Using the procedure form, prepare an appointment matrix, using the following criteria:
   a. Office hours are from 8:00 a.m. to 5:30 p.m.
   b. Lunch for staff and personal appointments at noon for 1½ hours
   c. Mornings: Schedule Monday, Wednesday, and Friday mornings for 20-minute appointments to see follow-ups and well-person physicals.
   d. Tuesday afternoons: Childhood immunizations in 20-minute visits
   e. Thursday afternoons: 40-minute new-patient appointments
   f. Tuesday and Thursday mornings: Surgeries or special procedures

2. Using the appointment matrix you created, schedule the following appointments for:
   a. Andrew Wu for a follow-up appointment. He can come in only on Thursday or Friday.
   b. John Anderson, a new patient to the practice, for a physical.
   c. Sofia Vasilakos calls to make an appointment for her son Nicholas for an immunization.
   d. Angela Rodriguez, for a colposcopy. She prefers an appointment early in the week if possible.
   e. Amy Bartlett has a 3-month-old baby, Molly, who has a temp of 101 and needs to be seen today.

## PROCEDURE 12–2

Scenarios 1 and 2 are provided to complete this competency.

*Scenario 1: Outpatient Procedure*

Kenneth Jones, age 50, has had a positive treadmill test that suggests an underlying cardiac condition. The cardiologist has asked you to schedule him for a cardiac catheterization with planned stent placement, which will require an overnight stay. He also needs a CBC, electrolyte panel, and an echocardiogram done prior to the catheterization. What information will you need to make sure all required preoperative testing is done in advance and that the catheterization is scheduled?

*Scenario 2: Inpatient Admission*

Katherine Jameson is 45 years old and has a history of endometriosis. Her OB/GYN physician has determined that she needs to have a total abdominal hysterectomy. Ms. Jameson needs her laboratory work and a KUB done prior to admission. She will need to be in the hospital approximately five days following her procedure. A medical-surgical unit will be appropriate following surgery unless complications arise. Postoperative laboratory, abdominal X-ray, and pain medications should be anticipated. What kind of paperwork must be completed, and what information will the hospital require prior to admission?

## PROCEDURE 12–3

Students can download the following forms from the Premium Website to complete this activity and use as work product for this procedure:

- Procedure Form 12–3a: Patient information form (blank)
- Procedure Form 12–3b: Encounter form (blank)

# CHAPTER 13 The Medical Record, Documentation, and Filing

## ABHES Curriculum

| | |
|---|---|
| MA.A.4.a | Document accurately |
| MA.A.4.b | Institute federal and state guidelines when releasing medical records or information |
| MA.A.8.b | Prepare and maintain medical records |
| MA.A.8.d | Apply concepts for office procedures |

## CAAHEP Core Curriculum

| | |
|---|---|
| V.C.5 | Identify systems for organizing medical records |
| V.C.6 | Describe various types of content maintained in a patient's medical record |
| V.C.7 | Discuss pros and cons of various filing methods |
| V.C.8 | Identify both equipment and supplies needed for filing medical records |
| V.C.9 | Describe indexing rules |
| V.C.10 | Discuss filing procedures |
| V.C.11 | Discuss principles of using electronic medical record [EMR] |
| V.C.12 | Identify types of records common to the health care setting |
| V.P.3 | Organize a patient's medical record |
| V.P.4 | File medical records |
| V.P.8 | Maintain organization by filing |
| V.A.1 | Consider staff needs and limitations in establishment of a filing system |

## LESSON OUTLINE

### I. PURPOSE OF RECORDS

A. Define

B. Identify types of information contained in demographics

C. Identify pertinent legal information

D. Discuss how data mining using EMRs can help in insurance audits and identifying patients for clinical trials or new treatments

### II. HIPAA AND THE MEDICAL RECORD

A. Maintaining the privacy of health information

B. Establishing standards for any electronic transmission of health information and related claims

C. Ensure the security of all electronic health information

D. Ensure compliance with federal and state privacy laws

### III. ELECTRONIC HEALTH RECORDS

A. Definition

B. Show students information from the www.nih.gov Website

C. Advantages

D. Disadvantages

## IV. PARTS OF THE MEDICAL RECORD (PROCEDURE 13–1)

A. Discuss subjective versus objective data (Table 13–1)

B. Administrative data

C. Financial and insurance information

D. Correspondence

E. Referral

F. Past medical records

G. Clinical data

H. Progress notes

I. Diagnostic information

J. Lab information

K. Medications

## V. CHARTING IN THE PATIENT RECORD

A. Problem Oriented Medical Record (POMR)

B. Methods of charting patient medical information
   1. SOAP
   2. HPIP
   3. CHEDDAR

C. Dating, correcting, and maintaining the chart
   1. Dates; military or 12-hour time
   2. Proper method for making corrections
   3. Legal implications

D. Tracking medical records
   1. Charts to be filed
   2. Prescription refills
   3. Lab results
   4. Coding/financial corrections
   5. Charts awaiting dictation
   6. Referrals

## VI. FILING MEDICAL RECORDS

A. Steps in filing
   1. Inspecting
   2. Indexing
   3. Coding
   4. Sorting
   5. Storing
   6. Supplies

B. Filing supplies
   1. OUTguides or OUTfolders
   2. Vertical pockets
   3. Index tabs
   4. Colored alphanumeric labels
   5. Standard office equipment
   6. Storage units

**VII. FILING SYSTEMS**

A. Chronologic
B. Alphabetic (Procedure 13–2)
C. Numeric (Procedure 13–3)
D. Subject
E. Tickler files
F. Locating a missing chart
G. Storing and purging files

## CHAPTER ACTIVITIES

1. Provide examples of different types of reports contained within a medical record. Have student sort and file report accordingly.
2. Have student identify different types of medical records and their uses.
3. Scramble dummy patient records; have student use different types of indexing methods to organize records in a timed game between teams of students.

## ANSWERS TO CHECK YOUR KNOWLEDGE QUESTIONS

1. Which of the following items are NOT part of a patient's demographic information?
   a. Gender
   b. Ethnicity
   c. Religion
   **d. Lab values**
   e. Marital status
2. The medical record:
   a. Documents patient progress.
   b. Verifies necessity of services to insurance billing.
   c. Serves as a means of communication between providers.
   **d. All the above**
3. The S in SOAP stands for:
   **a. Subjective.**
   b. Subordinate.
   C. Symptomatic.
   d. Standard.

4. CHEDDAR is an acronym used for:
   a. Determining which accounting method is to be used in the practice.
   **b. Conducting a patient encounter.**
   c. Retrieving patient billing information.
   d. Evaluating laboratory results.
5. "Meaningful use" refers to:
   a. How a prescription is taken.
   b. What type of labs are ordered.
   c. Billing practices.
   **d. The manner in which electronic health records are used.**
6. Advantages of electronic health records include:
   a. Eliminating the need for transcription.
   b. Decreasing or eliminating errors related to poor or illegible handwriting.
   c. Abolishing the need to secure patient files.
   d. Providing a means for patients to diagnose themselves and decrease medical costs.
   e. **a and b only.**
   f. All the above.
7. Regarding storing medical records, which is TRUE?
   a. Patient records must stored indefinitely.
   b. Records must be maintained for 15 years.
   c. **Records may be purged on a regular basis to make room for new charts.**
   d. Records of deceased patients may be destroyed after a death certificate is received.

# UNIT 7 HEALTH INSURANCE AND CODING
# CHAPTER 14 Health Insurance

## ABHES Curriculum

| | |
|---|---|
| MA.A.1.8.r | Apply third-party guidelines |
| MA.A.1.8.s | Obtain managed care referrals and precertification |
| MA.A.1.8.v | Use physician fee schedule |

## CAAHEP Core Curriculum

| | |
|---|---|
| VII.C. 1 | Identify types of insurance plans |
| VII.C.2 | Identify models of managed care |
| VII.C.3 | Discuss workers' compensation as it applies to patients |
| VII.C.4 | Describe procedures for implementing both managed care and insurance plans |
| VII.C.5 | Discuss utilization review principles |
| VII.C.6 | Discuss referral process for patients in a managed-care program |
| VII.C.10 | Discuss types of physician fee schedules |
| VII.C.11 | Describe the concept of RBRVS |
| VII.C.12 | Define diagnosis-related groups (DRGs) |
| VII.P.2 | Apply third-party guidelines |
| VII.P.4 | Obtain precertification, including documentation |
| VII.P.5 | Obtain preauthorization, including documentation |
| VII.P.6 | Verify eligibility for managed care services |
| VII.A.2 | Demonstrate sensitivity in communicating with both providers and patients |
| VII.A.3 | Communicate in language the patient can understand regarding managed care and insurance plans |

## LESSON OUTLINE

### I. THE PURPOSE OF HEALTH INSURANCE—TERMS USED IN HEALTH INSURANCE (SEE TABLE 14-1)

### II. MANAGED CARE DELIVERY SYSTEMS

### III. TYPES OF INSURANCE PLANS

A. Commercial health insurance plans

B. Indemnity-type insurance

C. Health maintenance organizations (HMOs)

1. Staff-model HMO
2. Group-model HMO
3. Preferred provider organization (PPO)
4. Point-of-service (POS) plans
5. Independent practice associations (IPAs)

## IV. CONSUMER-DRIVEN HEALTH PLANS (CDHPS)

A. Health savings account (HSA)

B. Health reimbursement account (HRA)

C. Flexible spending account (FSA)

## V. GOVERNMENT HEALTH PLANS

A. Medicare

1. Medicare administration and processing
2. Medical necessity and non-covered services
3. Medicare reimbursement

B. Medicaid

C. Workers' compensation

D. TRICARE and CHAMPVA

## VI. PATIENTS WITH NO INSURANCE

## VII. PRIMARY AND SECONDARY INSURANCE COVERAGE

A. Coordination of benefits and birthday rule

B. Medicare and supplemental insurance

## VIII. VERIFYING INSURANCE COVERAGE (SEE PROCEDURE 14–1)—PREAUTHORIZATION AND PRECERTIFICATION

A. Procedure 14–2: Obtain Managed Care Referral and Precertification

B. Procedure 14–3: Obtain a Preauthorization for a Procedure

## IX. ACCEPTING ASSIGNMENT AND FEE SCHEDULES

A. Usual, customary, and reasonable (UCR)

B. Resource-based relative value scale (RBRVS)

C. Diagnostic-related groups (DRGs)

## X. MAINTAINING CURRENCY

# CHAPTER ACTIVITIES

1. Have a guest speaker from a major insurance group speak to the class.
2. Contact a local medical assistant to speak to the class on the completion of insurance forms.
3. Contact the local Medicare office; in many cases, it will give instruction in the completion of its forms and provide exercises for students to complete.

# ANSWERS TO CHECK YOUR KNOWLEDGE QUESTIONS

1. If a Medicare patient is being provided with a service that might not be covered, the office should:
   a. not provide the service.
   b. have the patient sign a waiver.
   c. have the patient call Medicare.
   **d. have the patient sign an ABN.**
2. The components used to calculate the Medicare physician fee schedule are:
   **a. practice expense, malpractice expense, and work experience.**
   b. time spent to perform a service.
   c. rent, utilities, staff salaries.
   d. none of the above.
3. A consumer-driven health plan in which only the employer contributes and the money is not lost at the end of the year is called a:
   a. health savings account.
   b. flexible savings account.
   **c. health reimbursement account.**
   d. medical savings account.
4. The government health plan that covers individuals who have a limited or low income is:
   a. medicare.
   b. TRICARE.
   **c. medicaid.**
   d. social Security.
5. The percentage that a patient pays for services after the deductible has been met is called:
   a. copayment.
   b. deductible.
   c. fee for service.
   **d. coinsurance.**
6. Commercial insurance that provides coverage only for catastrophic illnesses and injuries is referred to as:
   a. self-pay.
   b. workers' compensation.
   **c. indemnity.**
   d. managed care.
7. Methods used to verify patient coverage include:
   a. telephone.
   b. point-of-service device.
   c. plan Website.
   **d. all of the above.**
8. The maximum amount a nonparticipating provider can charge for a Medicare patient service is called the:
   **a. limiting charge.**
   b. maximum reimbursement.

c. fee schedule.

d. capitation.

9. What do managed-care delivery systems emphasize to help control costs?

a. Quality assurance

b. Preventive care

c. Utilization review

d. a and b

**e. a and c**

10. The amount that a patient must pay before his or her insurance will begin to pay is known as:

a. coinsurance.

b. copayment.

**c. deductible.**

d. fee for service.

# HAPTER 15 Procedural and Diagnostic Coding

## 3HES Curriculum

MA.A.1.8.t Perform diagnostic and procedural coding

MA.A.1.8.dd Serve as liaison between provider and others

MA.A.1.8. u Prepare and submit insurance claims

MA.A.1.11.b (5) Demonstrating professionalism: Exhibiting initiative

## AAHEP Core Curriculum

VII.P.3 Complete insurance claim forms

VIII.C. 1 Describe how to use the most current procedural coding system

VIII.C. 2 Define upcoding and why it should be avoided

VIII.C. 3 Describe how to use the most current diagnostic coding classification system

VIII.C. 4 Describe how to use the most current HCPCS coding

VIII.P. 1 Perform procedural coding

VIII.P. 2 Perform diagnostic coding

VIII.A. 1 Work with provider to achieve the maximum reimbursement

## ESSON OUTLINE

### INTRODUCTION TO CODING

A. Converting descriptions of disease, injury, procedures, and services into numeric or alphanumeric designations

B. Accurate coding optimizes reimbursement

### THE HISTORY OF CODING

A. International Classification of Diseases (ICD)
   1. As early as the 1890s, a physician developed a classification of causes of death.
   2. The American Public Health Association recommended this classification system to be adopted by those recording deaths in Canada, Mexico, and the United States
   3. 1938: ICD-5
   4. 1978: ICD-9
   5. 2013: ICD-10 (adopted in the United States)

B. Current Procedural Terminology (CPT)
   1. First published in 1966 by the American Medical Association
   2. 1970: Five-digit codes introduced
   3. 1983: CPT was adopted as part of the Healthcare Common Proceduel Coding System (HCPCS)
   4. 2004: Per the Medicare Modernization Act, new, revised, and deleted codes must be implemented every January 1.

### . HCPCS

A. Level I: CPT codes

B. Level II: National codes

1. Level II codes developed to identify products and services not covered by CPT
2. One alpha and four numeric characters
3. Two sections
   a. Index
   b. Tabular list of codes
4. When appropriate, the correct HCPCS modification should be appended to provide additional information about the service.

C. Possible to report both CPT and HCPCS codes on the same claim

D. HCPCS codes are published annually.

## IV. CPT (SEE PROCEDURE 15–1)

A. Codes for procedures or services

B. Sections of the CPT Manual
1. Evaluation & Management
2. Anesthesiology
3. Surgery
4. Radiology
5. Pathology and Laboratory
6. Medicine

C. Modifiers
1. Covered in Appendix A of the manual
2. Used when a procedure or service needs to be slightly altered
3. Examples when one would use modifiers
   a. If an unusual event occurred
   b. If more than one provider performed the procedure

D. Unlisted codes

E. CPT manuals are updated annually.

F. CPT symbols (see Figure 15–1)

G. E/M services guidelines (see Table 15–2)
1. Key components
2. Contributory factors

H. CPT coding rules
1. Select the name of the procedure or service that most accurately identifies the service performed.
2. This is typically marked on an encounter form.
3. If clarification is needed to determine the correct code, seek the provider to clarify.

## V. ICD-9 (SEE PROCEDURE 15–2)

A. Codes for diseases or conditions

B. Establishes medical necessity

C. Using the ICD-9-CM manual

1. Volume I: Tabular List
2. Volume II: Alphabetic Index
3. Volume III: Used by hospital coders

D. ICD-9 coding rules
1. Follow the reason rule
2. Code each problem to the highest level of specificity

### I. ICD-10-CM

A. Coding system that has been in place since 1990
B. Used by most other industrialized countries in the world
C. ICD-9-CM is inadequate to meet the needs of the twenty-first century
D. Contains over 68,000 codes
E. Allows for greater specificity in reporting diseases

### II. ICD-10-PCS—INPATIENT HOSPITAL PROCEDURAL CODING SYSTEM

### III. ELECTRONIC CODING

### . CODING ACCURACY

A. Unbundling
B. Upcoding
C. Bundling codes
D. Downcoding
E. Medicare audit

## HAPTER ACTIVITIES

1. Have a guest speaker from a major insurance group speak to the class.
2. Assign lists of diseases and disorders you find in the anatomy section of the text for students to find code numbers for.
3. Prepare lists of surgical procedures to which students can apply code numbers.
4. Supply students with a folder of chart notes for several patients. The students should locate the diagnosis and complete the standard insurance form for each with the appropriate code numbers.

## NSWERS TO CHECK YOUR KNOWLEDGE QUESTIONS

1. There are ______ coding systems for providers to use in reporting their services for reimbursement.
   **a. 2**
   b. 3
   c. 6
   d. 4
2. HCPCS stands for:
   a. Health Codes and Procedure Coding System.
   **b. Healthcare Common Procedure Coding System.**

c. Health & Common Procedure Caring System.

d. Healthcare Current Procedural Coding System.

3. How many sections can be found in the CPT manual?

a. 4

**b. 6**

c. 5

d. 7

4. Which section of CPT is used by almost every provider specialty?

a. Surgery

b. Anesthesia

c. Radiology

**d. Evaluation & Management**

5. Which form do providers use to indicate services they have provided?

a. Superbill

b. Invoice

c. Encounter form

d. a and b

**e. a and c**

6. Which key components must be considered when a provider is selecting a visit level?

a. History, exam, patient condition

b. Exam, medical decision making, number of tests performed

**c. History, exam, medical decision making**

d. Medical decision making, number of diagnoses, time spent

7. ICD-10/PCS will be implemented in the United States on:

a. October 31, 2011.

b. January 1, 2012.

c. January 1, 2013.

**d. October 1, 2013.**

8. What can a coder use to ensure correct coding?

a. CPT manual

**b. Coding guidelines**

c. Provider directives

d. State government regulations

9. Using ICD-9 to report diagnoses is required to establish:

**a. medical necessity.**

b. reimbursement.

c. history of the patient.

d. none of the above.

10. Coding correctly helps providers avoid:

a. being accused of inflating their fees.

**b. being accused of fraud.**

c. being sued.

d. having to send in appeals.

# PROCEDURE SCENARIOS

The following encounter form is provided for use with the Competency Checklists for Procedures 15–1 and 15–2. It is optional; instructors may modify the scenario or make up their own.

# PLEASE RETURN THIS FORM TO RECEPTIONIST

NAME ____________________

Receipt No: ____________________

PLACE OF SERVICE:
( ) OFFICE
( ) NEW YORK COUNTY HOSPITAL
( ) COMMUNITY GENERAL HOSPITAL
( ) RETIREMENT INN NURSING HOME
( ) ____________________

DATE OF SERVICE ____________________

**A. OFFICE VISITS - New Patient**

| Code | History | Exam | Dec. | Time | |
|---|---|---|---|---|---|
| ___99201 | Prob. Foc. | Prob. Foc. | Straight | 10 min. | ______ |
| ___99202 | Ex. Prob. Foc. | Ex. Prob. Foc. | Straight | 20 min. | ______ |
| ___99203 | Detail | Detail | Low | 30 min. | ______ |
| ___99204 | Comp. | Comp. | Mod. | 45 min. | ______ |
| ___99205 | Comp. | Comp. | High | 60 min. | ______ |

**B. OFFICE VISIT - Established Patient**

| Code | History | Exam | Dec. | Time | |
|---|---|---|---|---|---|
| ___99211 | Minimal | Minimal | Minimal | 5 min. | ______ |
| ___99212 | Prob. Foc. | Prob. Foc. | Straight | 10min. | ______ |
| ___99213 | Ex. Prob. Foc. | Ex. Prob. Foc. | Low | 15 min. | ______ |
| ___99214 | Detail | Detail | Mod. | 25 min. | ______ |
| ___99215 | Comp. | Comp. | High | 40 min. | ______ |

**C. HOSPITAL CARE**

| | Dx | Units | Code | |
|---|---|---|---|---|
| 1. Initial Hospital Care (30 min) | ___ | ___ | 99221 | ______ |
| 2. Subsequent Care | ___ | ___ | 99231 | ______ |
| 3. Critical Care (30-74 min) | ___ | ___ | 99291 | ______ |
| 4. each additional 30 min. | ___ | ___ | 99292 | ______ |
| 5. Discharge Services | ___ | ___ | 99238 | ______ |
| 6. Emergency Room | ___ | ___ | 99282 | ______ |

**D. NURSING HOME CARE**

| | Dx | Units | Code | |
|---|---|---|---|---|
| Initial Care - New Pt. | | | | |
| 1. Expanded | ___ | ___ | 99322 | ______ |
| 2. Detailed | ___ | ___ | 99323 | ______ |
| Subsequent Care - Estab. Pt. | | | | |
| 3. Problem Focused | ___ | ___ | 99307 | ______ |
| 4. Expanded | ___ | ___ | 99308 | ______ |
| 5. Detailed | ___ | ___ | 99309 | ______ |
| 5. Comprehensive | ___ | ___ | 99310 | ______ |

**E. PROCEDURES**

| | Dx | Code | |
|---|---|---|---|
| 1. Arthrocentesis, Small Jt. | ___ | 20600 | ______ |
| 2. Colonoscopy | ___ | 45378 | ______ |
| 3. EKG w/interpretation | ___ | 93000 | ______ |
| 4. X-Ray Chest, PA/LAT | ___ | 71020 | ______ |

**F. LAB**

| | Dx | Code | Units |
|---|---|---|---|
| 1. Blood Sugar | ___ | 82947 | ______ |
| 2. CBC w/differential | ___ | 85031 | ______ |
| 3. Cholesterol | ___ | 82465 | ______ |
| 4. Comprehensive Metabolic Panel | ___ | 80053 | ______ |
| 5. ESR | ___ | 85651 | ______ |
| 6. Hematocrit | ___ | 85014 | ______ |
| 7. Mono Screen | ___ | 86308 | ______ |
| 8. Pap Smear | ___ | 88150 | ______ |
| 9. Potassium | ___ | 84132 | ______ |
| 10. Preg. Test, Quantitative | ___ | 84702 | ______ |
| 11. Routine Venipuncture | ___ | 36415 | ______ |

**F. Cont'd**

| | Dx | Units | |
|---|---|---|---|
| 12. Strep Screen | ___ | 87081 | ______ |
| 13. UA, Routine w/Micro | ___ | 81000 | ______ |
| 14. UA, Routine w/o Micro | ___ | 81002 | ______ |
| 15. Uric Acid | ___ | 84550 | ______ |
| 16. VDRL | ___ | 86592 | ______ |
| 17. Wet Prep | ___ | 82710 | ______ |
| 18. ____________ | ___ | ___ | ______ |

**G. INJECTIONS**

| | Dx | Code | |
|---|---|---|---|
| 1. Influenza Virus Vaccine | ___ | 90658 | ______ |
| 2. Pneumoccocal Vaccine | ___ | 90772 | ______ |
| 3. Tetanus Toxoids | ___ | 90703 | ______ |
| 4. Therapeutic Subcut/IM | ___ | 90732 | ______ |
| 5. Vaccine Administration | ___ | 90471 | ______ |
| 6. Vaccine - each additional | ___ | 90472 | ______ |

**H. MISCELLANEOUS**

1. ____________ ___ ______
2. ____________ ___ ______

**AMOUNT PAID $** ____________

**Mark diagnosis with (1=Primary, 2=Secondary, 3=Tertiary)**

DIAGNOSIS NOT LISTED BELOW ____________________

| DIAGNOSIS | ICD-9-CM 1, 2, 3 | |
|---|---|---|
| Abdominal Pain | 789.0_ | ______ |
| Allergic Rhinitis, Unspec. | 477.9 | ______ |
| Angina Pectoris, Unspec. | 413.9 | ______ |
| Anemia, Iron Deficiency, Unspec. | 280.9 | ______ |
| Anemia, NOS | 285.9 | ______ |
| Anemia, Pernicious | 281.0 | ______ |
| Asthma w/ Exacerbation | 493.92 | ______ |
| Asthmatic Bronchitis, Unspec. | 493.90 | ______ |
| Atrial Fibrillation | 427.31 | ______ |
| Atypical Chest Pain, Unspec. | 786.59 | ______ |
| Bronchiolitis, due to RSV | 466.11 | ______ |
| Bronchitis, Acute | 466.0 | ______ |
| Bronchitis, NOS | 490 | ______ |
| Cardiac Arrest | 427.5 | ______ |
| Cardiopulmonary Disease, Chronic, Unspec. | 416.9 | ______ |
| Cellulitis, NOS | 682.9 | ______ |
| Congestive Heart Failure, Unspec. | 428.0 | ______ |
| Contact Dermatitis NOS | 692.9 | ______ |
| COPD NOS | 496 | ______ |
| CVA, Acute, NOS | 434.91 | ______ |
| CVA, Old or Healed | 438.9 | ______ |
| Degenerative Arthritis (Specify Site) ______ | 715.9 | ______ |
| Dehydration | 276.51 | ______ |
| Depression, NOS | 311 | ______ |
| Diabetes Mellitus, Type II Controlled | 250.00 | ______ |
| Diabetes Mellitus, Type II Controlled | 250.02 | ______ |
| Drug Reaction, NOS | 995.29 | ______ |
| Dysuria | 788.1 | ______ |
| Eczema, NOS | 692.2 | ______ |
| Edema | 782.3 | ______ |
| Fever, Unknown Origin | 780.6 | ______ |
| Gastritis, Acute w/o Hemorrhage | 535.00 | ______ |
| Gastroenteritis, NOS | 558.9 | ______ |
| Gastroesophageal Reflux | 530.81 | ______ |
| Hepatitis A, Infectious | 070.1 | ______ |
| Hypercholesterolemia, Pure | 272.0 | ______ |
| Hypertension, Unspec. | 401.9 | ______ |
| Hypoglycemia NOS | 251.2 | ______ |
| Hypokalemia | 276.8 | ______ |
| Impetigo | 684 | ______ |
| Lymphadenitis, Unspec. | 289.3 | ______ |
| Mononucleosis | 075 | ______ |
| Myocardial Infarction, Acute, NOS | 410.9 | ______ |
| Organic Brain Syndrome | 310.9 | ______ |
| Otitis Externa, Acute NOS | 380.10 | ______ |
| Otitis Media, Acute NOS | 382.9 | ______ |
| Peptic Ulcer Disease | 536.9 | ______ |
| Peripheral Vascular Disease NOS | 443.9 | ______ |
| Pharyngitis, Acute | 462 | ______ |
| Pneumonia, Organism Unspec. | 486 | ______ |
| Prostatitis, NOS | 601.9 | ______ |
| PVC | 427.69 | ______ |
| Rash, Non Specific | 782.1 | ______ |
| Seizure Disorder NOS | 780.39 | ______ |
| Serous Otitis Media, Chronic, Unspec. | 381.10 | ______ |
| Sinusitis, Acute NOS | 461.9 | ______ |
| Tonsillitis, Acute | 463. | ______ |
| Upper Respiratory Infection, Acute NOS | 465.9 | ______ |
| Urinary Tract Infection, Unspec. | 599.0 | ______ |
| Urticaria, Unspec. | 708.9 | ______ |
| Vertigo, NOS | 780.4 | ______ |
| Viral Infection NOS | 079.99 | ______ |
| Weakness, Generalized | 780.79 | ______ |
| Weight Loss, Abnormal | 783.21 | ______ |

**ABN: I UNDERSTAND THAT MEDICARE PROBABLY WILL NOT COVER THE SERVICES LISTED BELOW**

A. ____________ B. ____________ C. ____________

Date ____________ Patient Signature ____________

Doctor's Signature ____________________

RETURN: ____________ Days ____________ Weeks ____________ Months

**DOUGLASVILLE MEDICINE ASSOCIATES**
5076 BRAND BLVD., SUITE 401
DOUGLASVILLE, NY 01234
PHONE No. (123) 456-7890
EIN# 00-1234560

❑ L.D. HEATH, M.D. NPI# 9995010111
❑ D.J. SCHWARTZ, M.D. NPI# 9995020212
❑ SARA O. MENDENHALL, M.D. NPI #9995030313

# UNIT 8 BILLING AND PAYMENT FOR MEDICAL SERVICES
# CHAPTER 16 Patient Accounts

## ABHES Curriculum

| | |
|---|---|
| MA.A.1.7.b | Apply computer application skills using a variety of different electronic programs including both practice management and EMR software |
| MA.A.1.8.h | Post entries on a daysheet |
| MA.A.1.8.k | Perform accounts receivable procedures |
| MA.A.1.8.m | Post adjustments |
| MA.A.1.8.w | Use manual or computerized bookkeeping systems |
| MA.A.1.8.y | Effective communication (aa, bb, cc, dd, ii, kk, ll) |

## CAAHEP Core Curriculum

| | |
|---|---|
| VI.C.1 | Explain basic bookkeeping computations |
| VI.C.2 | Differentiate between bookkeeping and accounting |
| VI.C.7 | Compare manual and computerized bookkeeping systems used in ambulatory health care |
| VI.C.10 | Identify procedure for preparing patient accounts |
| VI.C.13 | Discuss types of adjustments that may be made to a patient's account |
| VI.P.2 (a) | Perform accounts receivable procedures, including: post entries on a daysheet |
| VI.P.2 (d) | Perform accounts receivable procedures, including: post adjustments |
| VI.P.3 | Us;e computerized office billing systems |

## LESSON OUTLINE

### I. BOOKKEEPING PROCESS

A. Recording the financial transactions of a business
B. Bookkeeper versus accountant
C. Basic terminology used in bookkeeping
   1. Account or ledger
   2. Daysheet
   3. Posting
   4. Accounts receivable
   5. Accounts payable
   6. Debit
   7. Credit
   8. Balance
   9. Adjustment
   10. Debit balance
   11. Credit balance
D. Business Associate Agreement used when outside company provides bookkeeping for a business
E. Accuracy in bookkeeping is critical

## II. POSTING PROCEDURES TO PATIENT ACCOUNTS

A. Several methods to post procedures: manual and computerized

B. Encounter forms

1. Also called charge slip or superbill
2. Charges entered on an encounter form by provider
3. Contains list of procedures performed in that medical office
4. May be preprinted and coordinated with computerized practice management software

C. Patient ledger: record of all charges (services rendered), payments, and adjustments made

D. Computerized systems

1. Practice management software most commonly used in clinics and medical offices
2. Provides up-to-date financial information about office
3. Some electronic health records software can link with practice management software, eliminating need for printed encounter forms
4. Printed encounter forms used with practice management software
   a. Charges selected on the form
   b. Form given to front office medical assistant
   c. Charges entered in practice management software, either by front office personnel or billing department

E. Pegboard system

1. Uses base with pegs, daysheet, ledger, and encounter forms
2. Daysheet
   a. Captures all daily entries
   b. Patient ledger card overlaid and entries recorded on both ledger and daysheet at same time
   c. At end of day, charges totaled

## III. BOOKKEEPING SYSTEMS

A. Single-entry bookkeeping system

1. In its basic form, similar to checkbook register
2. Journal for each transaction recorded in one column
3. Only revenue and expenses totaled
4. Disadvantages
   a. No tracking of asset and liability accounts
   b. No direct linkage between income and the balance sheet
   c. Undetected errors can occur

B. Double-entry bookkeeping system

1. More sophisticated method
2. Each transaction recorded in two columns; each account has two columns
3. For each debit, an equal and opposite credit
4. Total of all debits must equal total of all credits
5. Advantages
   a. Accurate calculation of profit and loss
   b. Inclusion of assets and liabilities

c. Ability to prepare financial statements directly from accounts

d. Detection of errors and fraud more visible

e. Allows for balance in the accounting equation (assets = liabilities + owner's equity)

C. Computerized systems

1. Advantages

a. Speed

b. Efficiency

c. Automation

d. Calculations

e. Accuracy

f. System integration

g. Concurrent information

h. Availability of information

i. Management information

j. Legibility

k. Staff motivation

l. Reduction of frustration

m. Cost savings

2. Disadvantages

a. Computer system problems

b. Garbage in, garbage out

c. Must be properly programmed

d. Computer fraud

## IV. COMMUNICATING FEES TO PATIENTS

A. Common for MA to answer questions about patient accounts

B. When known in advance fees will be costly, cost estimate sheet is given

C. Assist patient in planning a reasonable payment schedule following office policy

D. Discounts sometimes given for professional or hardship reasons

1. Physician authorizes discount

2. No discount without authorization

# CHAPTER ACTIVITIES

1. Go on a field trip to a physician's office to watch how accounts are handled.
2. Have students first post patient charges in a manual system (using the activities in the Workbook). Then, have them post the same charges using practice management software. Discuss their experiences using each system.

## ANSWERS TO CHECK YOUR KNOWLEDGE QUESTIONS

1. A(n) _________ records the financial transitions of a business; a(n) ______________ analyzes these transactions and prepares current reports and comparison reports with other periods of time.
   a. daysheet; accountant
   b. daysheet; bookkeeper
   c. accountant; bookkeeper
   **d. bookkeeper; accountant**
2. In which of the following bookkeeping systems are all necessary forms generated with one posting?
   a. Single-entry
   b. Double-entry
   **c. Pegboard**
   d. Standard
3. This is a record of all charges or services rendered, any payments made by the patient or the insurance carrier, and any adjustments; it is:
   a. a daysheet.
   **b. a patient ledger.**
   c. accounts receivable.
   d. a credit balance.
4. When an entry is made on the daysheet, it is called:
   **a. journalizing.**
   b. journaling.
   c. posting.
   d. accounting.
5. An encounter form is also known as a:
   a. cost estimate sheet.
   b. patient ledger.
   c. business associate agreement.
   **d. charge slip.**
6. For each debit, there is an equal and opposite credit, and the total of all debits must equal the total of all credits. This describes which bookkeeping system?
   a. Single-entry bookkeeping
   **b. Double-entry bookkeeping**
   c. Computerized bookkeeping
   d. Trial balance bookkeeping

## PROCEDURE SCENARIOS

The following scenarios are provided for use with the Competency Checklists. They are optional; instructors may modify the scenarios or make up their own. Forms referenced can be downloaded from the students' Premium Website.

**Procedure 16–1**

Students can download the following form from the Premium Website to complete this activity and use as work product for this procedure.

- Procedure Form 16–1: Patient Ledger (Note that there are existing entries; the student will need to add to these entries and calculate totals.)

Provide the following information to the student for completion of the Patient Ledger for scoring of the Competency Checklist:

- Use yourself as the patient and your provider's name as the doctor. Use today's date.
- Insurance information: Insurance Company – Health Care One; Insurance ID – 123-45-6789-A; Coverage Code A – Group II; office visit copayment ($30); this is your own health insurance through your job. You pay with a personal check (#1600).
- Description: You are an established patient requiring an intermediate exam (99213, $100), urinalysis (81000, $30), therapeutic injection of pain medication (90782, $100), venipuncture (36415, $120), injection of B12 (90782, $40), renal and pelvic X-rays review (76140-26, $45).
- Diagnosis: hematuria (599.7), pyelonephritis (590.10). The doctor wants to see you in two weeks.
- Insurance payments: On 08/01/20XX, your insurance company made a $75 payment for the intermediate exam and, on 09/01/20XX, your insurance company made a $150 payment for the office procedures performed on the intermediate exam date. On 09/15/20XX, the insurance company made a $25 adjustment for underpaying on the office procedures performed on the intermediate exam date.

Procedure 16–1 Answer Key

# PATIENT LEDGER

**Date:**

**MR#:** **Address:** **Provider:**

**Name:** **City/State/Zip:** **Date of Birth:** **Sex:**

## Charges

| *Date of Service:* | *Procedure:* | *Description:* | *Diagnosis Codes* | *Amount* |
|---|---|---|---|---|
| 2/1/20XX | 70373 | X-Ray | 052.9 354.0 503 847.2 | $75.00 |
| 2/1/20XX | 29130 | App. of Finger Splint | 052.9 354.0 503 847.2 | $30.00 |
| 2/1/20XX | 99204 | Office Visit New | 052.9 354.0 503 847.2 | $75.00 |
| 3/1/20XX | J1820 | Inj, Insulin, Up to 100 Units | 052.9 354.0 503 847.2 | $20.00 |
| **X/X/20XX** | **99213** | **Intermediate exam** | **599.7 590.10** | **$100.00** |
| **X/X/20XX** | **81000** | **Urinalysis** | **599.7 590.10** | **$30.00** |
| **X/X/20XX** | **90782** | **Inj, therapeutic** | **599.7 590.10** | **$100.00** |
| **X/X/20XX** | **36415** | **Venipuncture** | **599.7 590.10** | **$120.00** |
| **X/X/20XX** | **90782** | **Inj, B12** | **599.7 590.10** | **$40.00** |
| **X/X/20XX** | **76140-26** | **Review x-ray** | **599.7 590.10** | **$45.00** |
| | | | **Total:** | **$635.00** |

## Insurance Payments

| *Date of Payment:* | *Payment Code:* | *Line Description:* | *Transaction Description:* | *Amount* |
|---|---|---|---|---|
| 2/1/20XX | XP | XYZ Insurance Payment | XYZ | ($40.00) |
| 2/1/20XX | XP | XYZ Insurance Payment | XYZ | ($20.00) |
| **8/1/20XX** | | **Health Care One Payment** | **Exam** | **($75.00)** |
| **9/1/20XX** | | **Health Care One Payment** | **Procedures** | **($150.00)** |
| | | | **Total:** | **($285.00)** |

## Insurance Adjustments/Other Credits & Adjustments

| *Date of Payment:* | *Payment Code:* | *Line Description:* | *Transaction Description:* | *Amount* |
|---|---|---|---|---|
| 5/1/20XX | MED ADJ | Medicare Writeoff | Adjustment | ($10.00) |
| 5/1/20XX | MED ADJ | Medicare Writeoff | Adjustment | ($10.00) |
| **9/15/20XX** | | **Health Care One** | **Adjustment (Proc)** | **($25.00)** |
| | | | **Total:** | **($45.00)** |

## Patient Payments

| *Date of Payment:* | *Payment Code:* | *Payment Description:* | *Transaction Description:* | *Amount* |
|---|---|---|---|---|
| 2/1/20XX | COCHECK | Copay Check Payment | | ($20.00) |
| 3/1/20XX | CCARDCOP | Credit Card Copay | | ($20.00) |
| **X/X/20XX (exam date)** | **COCHECK** | **Copay Check** | **#1600** | **($30.00)** |
| | | | **Total:** | **($70.00)** |
| | | | **Total Payments** | **($400.00)** |
| | | | **Amount Due:** | **$235.00** |

# CHAPTER 17 Preparing Insurance Claims and Posting Insurance Payments

## ABHES Curriculum

| | |
|---|---|
| MA.A.1.8.i | Perform billing and collection procedures |
| MA.A.1.8.k | Perform accounts receivable procedures |
| MA.A.1.8.m | Post adjustments |
| MA.A.1.8.r | Apply third party guidelines |
| MA.A.1.8.u | Prepare and submit insurance claims |
| MA.A.1.8.w | Use manual or computerized bookkeeping systems |
| MA.A.1.8.y | Effective communication (hh) |

## CAAHEP Core Curriculum

| | |
|---|---|
| VI.P.13 | Discuss types of adjustments that may be made to a patient's account |
| VI.P.2.d | Post adjustments |
| VI.3 | Use computerized office billing systems |
| VII.C.7 | Describe how guidelines are used in processing an insurance claim |
| VII.C.8 | Compare processes for filing insurance claims both manually and electronically |
| VII.C.9 | Describe guidelines for third-party claims |
| VII.P.1 | Apply both managed care policies and procedures |
| VII.P.2 | Apply third party guidelines |
| VII.P.3 | Complete insurance claim forms |
| IX.C.3 | Describe the implications of HIPAA for the medical assistant in various medical settings |

# LESSON PLANS

## I. THE HISTORY OF CLAIMS

A. History of third-party reimbursement

B. HIPAA and electronic claims submission

## II. COMPLETING THE CLAIM FORM (PROCEDURE 17–1)

A. Standard form used in medical offices

B. Must obtain patient's insurance card and assignment of benefits

C. Common claim form errors

## III. FILING CLAIMS

A. Electronic filing

1. Electronic data interchange (EDI)
2. CMS standards for EDI

B. Filing paper claims

1. Limited situations when paper claims may be used
2. Situations detailed in Administrative Simplification Compliance Act (ASCA)

C. Clearinghouses

1. Serve as middleman between providers and payers
2. Ensure that claims are complete and in correct format for payers

### IV. CLAIMS TRACKING

A. Method of monitoring outstanding claims

B. Electronic claims tracking

1. Available with most practice management software
2. Many advantages of electronic claims tracking

C. Manual claims tracking less common today

D. Delinquent claims

1. Follow up if claim has not been paid in an appropriate time period
2. Electronically submitted claims: follow up after three weeks
3. Paper claims: follow up after six weeks

### V. INSURANCE PAYMENTS

A. Explanation of benefits (EOB) and remittance advice (RA)

1. Sent by insurance companies to patients
2. Details how much was paid on a claim

B. Apply insurance payments and adjustments (Procedure 17–2)

### VI. BILLING SECONDARY INSURANCE

A. More common today with dual income earners in households

B. Once payment is received from primary insurance, new bill is created for secondary insurance

C. Attach copy of EOB to claim

D. Secondary insurance often pays remainder of claim

## CHAPTER ACTIVITIES

1. Supply students with a folder of chart notes for several different patients. The students should locate the diagnosis and complete CMS-1500 forms for each patient.
2. Have the students identify common errors in insurance claim submissions.
3. Provide for student review improperly completed CMS1500 forms and have them identify the errors.

## ANSWERS TO CHECK YOUR KNOWLEDGE QUESTIONS

1. What is the term that describes payment by someone other than the patient for services rendered?

   a. Remittance advice

   b. EOB

   c. Claims tracking

   **d. Third-party reimbursement**

2. The most common claim form used in the medical office is the:
   a. CMS-1450.
   **b. CMS-1500.**
   c. UB-04.
   d. CPT-1450.
3. Which of these claims would be considered delinquent?
   a. Electronically submitted claim after two weeks
   **b. Electronically submitted claim after three weeks**
   c. Paper claim after four weeks
   d. Paper claim after five weeks
4. What does the acronym NPI stand for?
   a. National provider identification
   **b. National provider identifier**
   c. National physician identifier
   d. National physician information
5. A company that often serves as the middleman between providers and billing groups, payers, and other health care partners for the transmission and translation of electronic claims information into the specific format required by payers is known as:
   **a. a clearinghouse.**
   b. electronic claims tracking.
   c. electronic data interchange.
   d. a remittance advice.

## PROCEDURE SCENARIOS

The following scenarios are provided for use with the Competency Checklists. They are optional; instructors may modify the scenarios or make up their own. Forms referenced can be downloaded from the students' Premium Website.

### Procedure 17–1

Students can download the following forms from the Premium Website to complete this activity and use as work product for this procedure:

- Procedure Form 17–1: CMS-1500 form

Provide the following information to the students for their completion of the CMS-1500 form for scoring of the Competency Checklist:

- Use yourself as the patient and your provider's name as the doctor. Use today's date.
- Your spouse is the insured policy holder.
- Signature on file.
- Diabetes mellitus, congestive heart failure, arthritis (hip)
- Seen in office on 05/03/XX for the following:

- Office visit, intermediate 65.00
- Blood drawing 30.00
- Urinalysis 25.00

**Procedure 17–2**

Students can download the following forms from the Premium Website to complete this activity and use as work product for this procedure:

- Procedure Form 17–2: Patient Ledger Card (*Note*: Some entries are already completed. Students must add entries and perform calculations.)

Use the following information to complete the insurance payment processing and insurance adjustment for scoring of the Competency Checklist:

- Use yourself as the patient and your provider as the doctor. Use today's date as date of payment.
- Insurance company is XYZ Insurance Company.
- The insurance payment check is for $75.00 (check number 1234).
- The insurance adjustment check is for $5 (check number 1235) for a procedure.

Procedure 17–2 Answer Key

# PATIENT LEDGER

**Date:**

**MR#:** **Address** **Provider:**

**Name:** **City/State/Zip:** **Date of Birth:** **Sex:**

## Charges

| *Date of Service:* | *Procedure:* | *Description:* | *Diagnosis Codes* | *Amount* |
|---|---|---|---|---|
| 2/1/20XX | 70373 | X-Ray | 052.9 354.0 503 847.2 | $75.00 |
| 2/1/20XX | 29130 | App. of Finger Splint | 052.9 354.0 503 847.2 | $30.00 |
| 2/1/20XX | 99204 | Office Visit New | 052.9 354.0 503 847.2 | $75.00 |
| 3/1/20XX | J1820 | Inj, Insulin, Up to 100 Units | 052.9 354.0 503 847.2 | $20.00 |
| | | | **Total:** | **$200.00** |

## Insurance Payments

| *Date of Payment:* | *Payment Code:* | *Line Description:* | *Transaction Description:* | *Amount* |
|---|---|---|---|---|
| 2/1/20XX | XP | XYZ Insurance Payment | XYZ | ($40.00) |
| 2/1/20XX | XP | XYZ Insurance Payment | XYZ | ($20.00) |
| **X/X/20XX** | | **XYZ Insurance Payment** | **XYZ Check #1234** | **($75.00)** |
| | | | **Total:** | **($135.00)** |

## Insurance Adjustments/Other Credits & Adjustments

| *Date of Payment:* | *Payment Code:* | *Line Description:* | *Transaction Description:* | *Amount* |
|---|---|---|---|---|
| 5/1/20XX | MED ADJ | Medicare Writeoff | Adjustment | ($10.00) |
| 5/1/20XX | MED ADJ | Medicare Writeoff | Adjustment | ($10.00) |
| **X/X/20XX** | **Procedure ADJ** | **XYZ Insurance** | **Adjustment Check #1235** | **($5.00)** |
| | | | **Total:** | **($25.00)** |

## Patient Payments

| *Date of Payment:* | *Payment Code:* | *Payment Description:* | *Transaction Description:* | *Amount* |
|---|---|---|---|---|
| 2/1/20XX | COCHECK | Copay Check Payment | | ($20.00) |
| 3/1/20XX | CCARDCOP | Credit Card Copay | | ($20.00) |
| | | | **Total:** | **($40.00)** |
| | | | **Total Payments** | **($200.00)** |
| | | | **Amount Due:** | **$ 0** |

# CHAPTER 18 Patient Billing, Posting Patient Payments, and Collecting Fees

## ABHES Curriculum

| | |
|---|---|
| MA.A.1.7.b | Identify and properly use office machines, computerized systems, and medical software such as: (2) Apply computer application skills using a variety of electronic programs, including both practice management software and EMR software |
| MA.A.1.8.i | Perform billing and collection procedures |
| MA.A.1.8.n | Process credit balances |
| MA.A.1.8.o | Process refunds |
| MA.A.1.8.p | Post nonsufficient funds (NSF) |
| MA.A.1.8.q | Post collection agency payments |

## CAAHEP Core Curriculum

| | |
|---|---|
| VI.C.9 | Explain both billing and payment options |
| VI.C.11 | Discuss procedures for collecting outstanding accounts |
| VI.C.12 | Describe the impact of both the Fair Debt Collection Act and the federal Truth in Lending Act of 1968 as they apply to collections |
| VI.C.13 | Discuss types of adjustments that can be made to a patient's account |
| VI.P.2 | Perform accounts receivable procedures, including: (c) perform collection procedures; (e) process a credit balance; (f) process refunds; (g) post nonsufficient fund [NSF] checks; (h) post collection agency payments |

# LESSON OUTLINE

## I. PATIENT BILLING

A. Patient account statements

B. Billing may be outsourced

## II. METHODS OF BILLING

A. Monthly billing

B. Cycle billing

C. Computerized billing

D. Practice management software (PMS) systems

1. Might integrate with an electronic medical record (EMR) system
2. Ability to post procedures and payments to patient ledger (account history)
3. Ability to generate encounter forms and electronic claims
4. Ability to generate various reports
    a. Daily journal
    b. Year to date
    c. Aging account reports

## III. PATIENT PAYMENTS

A. At time of service (ATOS): best time for collection
B. Precautions for accepting checks (see Chapter 19 for more information)
C. Posting payments to patient accounts
D. Procedure for handling nonsufficient fund checks (Procedure 18–1)
E. Procedure for handling collection agency payments (Procedure 18–1)

## IV. CREDIT BALANCES AND REFUNDS (PROCEDURE 18–2)

## V. COLLECTING FEES

A. Aging accounts
B. Accounts are current within 30 days
C. Each practice has guidelines for when account considered delinquent

## VI. COLLECTION LAWS

A. Truth in Lending Act
B. Fair Debt Collection Practice Act
C. Statute of limitations laws

## VII. STRATEGIES FOR COLLECTION

A. Making collection call
B. Setting up payment schedules
C. Collection letters
D. Collection agencies

## VIII. SPECIAL COLLECTION CIRCUMSTANCES

A. Skip patients
B. Bankruptcy
C. Estate claims
D. Exceptions to usual billing procedures

# CHAPTER ACTIVITIES

1. Role play how the students should appropriately encourage patients to pay on their accounts.
2. Assign an Internet activity for the students to research the Fair Debt Collection Act and prepare a report on acceptable practices.

# ANSWERS TO CHECK YOUR KNOWLEDGE QUESTIONS

1. In this billing system, accounts are divided into groups to correspond to the number of times you will be billing.
   a. Computerized billing
   b. Monthly billing
   **c. Cycle billing**
   d. Electronic billing
2. What is PMS?
   a. Practice monitoring software
   **b. Practice management software**
   c. Payment management software
   d. Payment management system
3. All the following bits of information are required to post a payment to a patient account, except:
   a. date of payment.
   **b. time of payment.**
   c. payment amount.
   d. form of payment.
4. When is the best opportunity for collecting patient fees?
   **a. When the patient is in the office**
   b. Over the phone
   c. When the patient declares bankruptcy
   d. With a collection agency
5. A patient's account history is also referred to as a:
   a. monthly summary.
   b. fee statement.
   c. patient journal.
   **d. patient ledger.**
6. Of the following terms, which word should be avoided when composing a collection letter?
   a. Missed
   **b. Neglected**
   c. Overlooked
   d. Forgotten

# PROCEDURE SCENARIOS

The following scenario is provided for use with the Competency Checklists. It is optional; instructors may modify the scenario or make up their own. Forms referenced can be downloaded from the students' Premium Website.

## Procedure 18–1

Students can download the following forms from the Premium Website to complete this activity and use as work product for this procedure:

- Procedure Form 18–1 (Patient Ledger)

Your office recently placed several accounts with an outside collection agency the practice uses for collection efforts when the practice has been unsuccessful in collecting the debt from the patient. One of the accounts was turned over to the agency because the patient had a habit of presenting checks that bounced due to lack of funds in the account to cover the amount the checks were issued for. Today, you received another NSF check written for payment on this patient's account. You also received the first collection agency payment on this same account.

- Use yourself as the patient and your provider's name as the doctor.
- Use today's date.
- The NSF check amount is for the $20 co-pay check payment accepted on 2/1/20XX as listed on the patient ledger.
- Collection agency payment is for $15.

Procedure 18–1 Answer Key

# PATIENT LEDGER

**Date:**

| **MR#:** | **Address:** | **Provider:** | |
|---|---|---|---|
| **Name:** | **City/State/Zip:** | **Date of Birth:** | **Sex:** |

## Charges

| ***Date of Service:*** | ***Procedure:*** | ***Description:*** | ***Diagnosis Codes*** | ***Amount*** |
|---|---|---|---|---|
| 2/1/20XX | 70373 | X-Ray | 052.9 354.0 503 847.2 | $75.00 |
| 2/1/20XX | 29130 | App. of Finger Splint | 052.9 354.0 503 847.2 | $30.00 |
| 2/1/20XX | 99204 | Office Visit New | 052.9 354.0 503 847.2 | $75.00 |
| 3/1/20XX | J1820 | Inj, Insulin, Up to 100 Units | 052.9 354.0 503 847.2 | $20.00 |
| **Today's date** | | **NSF from 2/1/20XX** | **Copay check** | **$20.00** |
| | | | **Total:** | **$220.00** |

## Insurance Payments

| ***Date of Payment:*** | ***Payment Code:*** | ***Line Description:*** | ***Transaction Description:*** | ***Amount*** |
|---|---|---|---|---|
| 2/1/20XX | XP | XYZ Insurance Payment | XYZ | ($40.00) |
| 2/1/20XX | XP | XYZ Insurance Payment | XYZ | ($20.00) |
| | | | **Total:** | **($60.00)** |

## Insurance Adjustments/Other Credits & Adjustments

| ***Date of Payment:*** | ***Payment Code:*** | ***Line Description:*** | ***Transaction Description:*** | ***Amount*** |
|---|---|---|---|---|
| /1/20XX | MED ADJ | Medicare Writeoff | Adjustment | ($10.00) |
| /1/20XX | MED ADJ | Medicare Writeoff | Adjustment | ($10.00) |
| **Today's date** | | **Collection Agency Payment** | **Adjustment** | **($15.00)** |
| | | | **Total:** | **($35.00)** |

## Patient Payments

| ***Date of Payment:*** | ***Payment Code:*** | ***Payment Description:*** | ***Transaction Description:*** | ***Amount*** |
|---|---|---|---|---|
| /1/20XX | COCHECK | Copay Check Payment | | ($20.00) |
| /1/20XX | CCARDCOP | Credit Card Copay | | ($20.00) |
| | | | **Total:** | **($40.00)** |
| | | | **Total Payments** | **$135.00)** |
| | | | **Amount Due:** | **($85.00)** |

## Procedure 18–2

Students can download the following forms from the Premium Website to complete this activity and use as work product for this procedure:

- Procedure Form 18–2a (Patient Ledger)
- Procedure Form 18–2b (Blank Check)
- Use yourself as the patient and your provider's name as the doctor.
- Use today's date.
- The co-payment was discovered by the medical assistant to be $10 rather than the accepted check for $20. The overpayment amount is for $10 from the $20 co-pay check payment accepted on 2/1/20XX as listed on the patient ledger.

1490 BAL. BRO'T FOR'D

*Today's date* 20__

TO *Student name*

DEPOSITS

FOR *Overpayment refund*

| | | |
|---|---|---|
| TOTAL | 10 | 00 |
| THIS CHECK | | |
| BALANCE | | |

1490

*Today's date* 20 *XX* 25-64/440

PAY TO THE ORDER OF *Student name* $ *10.00*

*Ten dollars and 00/100* DOLLARS

THE NEVER FAIL BANK
ANYWHERE, U.S.A 00000 7-88-25

FOR *Overpayment refund* *Doctor's signature*

|:00006 7894|: 12345678;' 01490 ;0000039158;

Procedure 18–2 Answer Keys

# PATIENT LEDGER

**Date:**

**MR#:** **Address:** **Provider:**

**Name:** **City/State/Zip:** **Date of Birth:** **Sex:**

## Charges

| *Date of Service:* | *Procedure:* | *Description:* | *Diagnosis Codes* | *Amount* |
|---|---|---|---|---|
| 2/1/20XX | 70373 | X-Ray | 052.9 354.0 503 847.2 | $75.00 |
| 2/1/20XX | 29130 | App. of Finger Splint | 052.9 354.0 503 847.2 | $30.00 |
| 2/1/20XX | 99204 | Office Visit New | 052.9 354.0 503 847.2 | $75.00 |
| 3/1/20XX | J1820 | Inj, Insulin, Up to 100 Units | 052.9 354.0 503 847.2 | $20.00 |
| | | | **Total:** | **$200.00** |

## Insurance Payments

| *Date of Payment:* | *Payment Code:* | *Line Description:* | *Transaction Description:* | *Amount* |
|---|---|---|---|---|
| 2/1/20XX | XP | XYZ Insurance Payment | XYZ | ($40.00) |
| 2/1/20XX | XP | XYZ Insurance Payment | XYZ | ($20.00) |
| | | | **Total:** | **($60.00)** |

## Insurance Adjustments/Other Credits & Adjustments

| *Date of Payment:* | *Payment Code:* | *Line Description:* | *Transaction Description:* | *Amount* |
|---|---|---|---|---|
| 5/1/20XX | MED ADJ | Medicare Writeoff | Adjustment | ($10.00) |
| 5/1/20XX | MED ADJ | Medicare Writeoff | Adjustment | ($10.00) |
| **Today's date** | **Cred ADJ** | **Overpayment from 2/1/20XX** | **Refund Adjustment** | **($10.00)** |
| | | | **Total:** | **($30.00)** |

## Patient Payments

| *Date of Payment:* | *Payment Code:* | *Payment Description:* | *Transaction Description:* | *Amount* |
|---|---|---|---|---|
| 2/1/20XX | COCHECK | Copay Check Payment | | ($20.00) |
| 3/1/20XX | CCARDCOP | Credit Card Copay | | ($20.00) |
| | | | **Total:** | **($40.00)** |
| | | | **Total Payments** | **($130.00)** |
| | | | **Amount Due:** | **$70.00** |

# UNIT 9 BANKING AND ACCOUNTING PROCEDURES
# CHAPTER 19 Banking Procedures

## ABHES Curriculum

| | |
|---|---|
| MA.A.1.8.g | Prepare and reconcile a bank statement and deposit record |
| MA.A.1.8.j | Perform accounts payable procedures (write a check) |

## CAAHEP Core Curriculum

| | |
|---|---|
| VI.C.3 | Describe banking procedures |
| VI.C.4 | Discuss precautions for accepting checks |
| VI.C.5 | Compare types of endorsements |
| VI.P.1 | Prepare a bank deposit |

## LESSON OUTLINE

### I. BANKING

A. Online banking
B. Mobile banking
C. Automated teller machines (ATMs)
D. Telephone banking
E. Mail banking
F. Types of bank accounts
   1. Checking
   2. Savings
   3. Overdraft checking
   4. Special checking
G. Checking and savings are most common

### II. CURRENCY

A. Paper bills and coins
B. Care must be taken to secure currency in the office

### III. CHECKS

A. Types of checks
   1. Cashier's check
   2. Certified check
   3. Electronic check
   4. Limited check
   5. Money order
   6. Postdated check
   7. Stale check
   8. Traveler's check
   9. Voucher check

B. Check components
   1. Date
   2. Words of negotiability
   3. Payee
   4. Numeric amount
   5. Written amount
   6. Drawee financial institution
   7. Signature
C. Other features of a check
   1. Name and address of maker
   2. Chronologic check number
   3. Check routing symbol or ABA number
   4. MICR numbers
   5. One rough or perforated edge
D. Check endorsement
   1. Signature on the back of the check
   2. Blank endorsement
      a. Signature only
      b. Should not be used until check is about to be cashed
   3. Restrictive endorsement
      a. Used to endorse checks when they are received
      b. "Pay to the Order of"
E. Accepting checks from patients
   1. Do not accept third-party checks
   2. Do not accept overpayment
   3. Do not accept a check marked "paid in full"
   4. Do not accept a postal money order with more than one endorsement
F. Common check writing errors
   1. Written and numeric amounts do not match
   2. Wrong date
   3. Unsigned check
   4. Signature does not match
   5. Alterations or modifications
G. Preparing checks (Procedure 19–1)
   1. Five essential factors
      a. Date
      b. Payee
      c. Numeric amount
      d. Written amount
      e. Payer signature
   2. Completing the check register

## IV. BANK DEPOSITS

A. Sort and total currency

B. Sort and enter checks

C. Prepare the deposit slip (Procedure 19–2)

D. Other types of deposits

   1. Direct deposit

   3. Wire transfers

   4. Deposits by mail

E. Stop payment on checks

## V. BANK STATEMENTS

A. Summary of financial transactions

B. Mailed or emailed to account holder each month

C. Reconciling bank statements (Procedure 19–3)

# CHAPTER ACTIVITIES

1. Have students make up flash cards for each of the following from this chapter:
   - Types of bank accounts
   - Types of checks
   - The seven features of checks
2. Have students research three local banks and determine the charges for the following services: certified checks, cashier's checks, traveler's checks, stop payment, insufficient funds, overdraft protection, money orders.
3. Have students research a local bank and gather information about the types of checking accounts it offers. The student should choose one account and explain all the features it offers.

# ANSWERS TO CHECK YOUR KNOWLEDGE QUESTIONS

1. A ____________ increases the balance of an account, whereas a _________________ decreases the balance.

   **a. deposit, withdrawal**

   b. withdrawal, deposit

   c. transaction, withdrawal

   d. deposit, transaction

2. The person to whom the check is written is the:

   a. payer.

   **b. payee.**

   c. maker.

   d. third party.

3. Which person signs the front side of the check?

   **a. Payer**

   b. Payee

   c. Receiver

   d. Endorser

4. All the following are essential factors that must be included when writing a check, except:
   a. payee.
   b. numeric amount.
   c. written amount.
   **d. endorsement.**
   e. date.
5. To make sure the office and the bank agree on the amount in the account, a(n) _______________ is performed.
   a. audit
   **b. reconciliation**
   c. trial balance
   d. accounts receivable

## PROCEDURE SCENARIOS

The following scenarios are provided for use with the competency checklists. They are optional; instructors may modify the scenarios or make up their own. The following forms can be downloaded from the student's Premium Website.

### Procedure 19–1

Write checks to the following suppliers of goods and services provided to the medical office, using the checks provided in Procedure Form 19–1. Use the current date and sign the checks with the provider's name provided, with your name below the line. Complete the stub end, subtracting each subsequent check with the initial total starting balance being $10,000. (Extra check are provided in case you make an error.)

| | |
|---|---|
| Clinical Laboratory Services | $987.45 |
| Brown Office Equipment | $535.90 |
| Spencer Building Maintenance | $1,248.75 |

Students can download the following forms from the Premium Website to complete this activity and use as work product for this procedure:

- Procedure Form 19–1: Blank checks and check stubs

## Answer Key for Procedure Form 19–1

**Check 1491 — Stub**

| 1491 | BAL. BRO'T FOR'D | 10000 | 00 |
|---|---|---|---|
| Current date 20 | | | |
| TO Clinical Laboratory Services | DEPOSITS | | |
| FOR | | | |
| | TOTAL | 10000 | 00 |
| | THIS CHECK | 987 | 45 |
| | BALANCE | 9012 | 55 |

**Check 1491**

ELIZABETH R. EVANS, M.D.
SUITE 205 100 E. MAIN ST.
YOURTOWN, US 98765-4321

1491
Current date 20 25-64/440

PAY TO THE ORDER OF Clinical Laboratory Services $ 987.45
nine hundred eighty seven and 45/100 DOLLARS

THE NEVER FAIL BANK
ANYWHERE, U.S.A 00000
7-88-25

FOR Elizabeth R. Evans M.D.

|:00006 7894|: 12345678;' 01491 ;0000039158;

**Check 1492 — Stub**

| 1492 | BAL. BRO'T FOR'D | 9012 | 55 |
|---|---|---|---|
| Current date 20 | | | |
| TO Brown Office Equipment | DEPOSITS | | |
| FOR | | | |
| | TOTAL | 9012 | 55 |
| | THIS CHECK | 585 | 90 |
| | BALANCE | 8426 | 65 |

**Check 1492**

ELIZABETH R. EVANS, M.D.
SUITE 205 100 E. MAIN ST.
YOURTOWN, US 98765-4321

1492
Current date 20 25-64/440

PAY TO THE ORDER OF Brown Office Equipment $ 585.90
five hundred eighty five and 90/100 DOLLARS

THE NEVER FAIL BANK
ANYWHERE, U.S.A 00000
7-88-25

FOR Elizabeth R. Evans M.D.

|:00006 7894|: 12345678;' 01492 ;0000039158;

**Check 1493 — Stub**

| 1493 | BAL. BRO'T FOR'D | 8426 | 65 |
|---|---|---|---|
| Current date 20 | | | |
| TO Spencer Building Maintenance | DEPOSITS | | |
| FOR | | | |
| | TOTAL | 8426 | 65 |
| | THIS CHECK | 1248 | 75 |
| | BALANCE | 8277 | 90 |

**Check 1493**

ELIZABETH R. EVANS, M.D.
SUITE 205 100 E. MAIN ST.
YOURTOWN, US 98765-4321

1493
Current date 20 25-64/440

PAY TO THE ORDER OF Spencer Building Maintenance $ 1248.75
one thousand two hundred forty eight and 75/100 DOLLARS

THE NEVER FAIL BANK
ANYWHERE, U.S.A 00000
7-88-25

FOR Elizabeth R. Evans M.D.

|:00006 7894|: 12345678;' 01493 ;0000039158;

**Check 1494 — Stub**

| 1494 | BAL. BRO'T FOR'D | | |
|---|---|---|---|
| 20 | | | |
| TO | DEPOSITS | | |
| FOR | | | |
| | TOTAL | | |
| | THIS CHECK | | |
| | BALANCE | | |

**Check 1494**

ELIZABETH R. EVANS, M.D.
SUITE 205 100 E. MAIN ST.
YOURTOWN, US 98765-4321

1494
20 25-64/440

PAY TO THE ORDER OF $
DOLLARS

THE NEVER FAIL BANK
ANYWHERE, U.S.A 00000
7-88-25

FOR

|:00006 7894|: 12345678;' 01494 ;0000039158;

**Check 1495 — Stub**

| 1495 | BAL. BRO'T FOR'D | | |
|---|---|---|---|
| 20 | | | |
| TO | DEPOSITS | | |
| FOR | | | |
| | TOTAL | | |
| | THIS CHECK | | |
| | BALANCE | | |

**Check 1495**

ELIZABETH R. EVANS, M.D.
SUITE 205 100 E. MAIN ST.
YOURTOWN, US 98765-4321

1495
20 25-64/440

PAY TO THE ORDER OF $
DOLLARS

THE NEVER FAIL BANK
ANYWHERE, U.S.A 00000
7-88-25

FOR

|:00006 7894|: 12345678;' 01495 ;0000039158;

## Procedure 19–2

You are responsible for depositing money in the bank and must complete a deposit slip for the coin, currency, and checks. Use the following list of cash and check payments to prepare a bank deposit slip.

Currency/coin: $35.50, $40.00, $50.75, $25.00, $15.75

| Checks | Holley | Check #134 | $40.00 |
|---|---|---|---|
| | Segal | Check #285 | $25.00 |
| | Gomez | Check #596 | $55.00 |
| | Schmidt | Check #436 | $38.00 |
| | Moriarty | Check #1073 | $47.00 |
| | Kostrevski | Check #735 | $150.00 |
| | Kendrix | Check #489 | $145.00 |

Money orders Li, $45.00; Jackson, $55.00

Students can download the following forms from the Premium Website to complete this activity and use as work product for this procedure:

- Procedure Form 19–2: Blank deposit slip

## Answer Key for Procedure Form 19–2

I.M. Healthy, M.D.
101 Fitness Lane
Anywhere, U.S.A. 00000

DATE *Today's date* 20____

The Never Fail Bank
Anywhere, U.S.A.

| | | |
|---|---|---|
| CASH CURRENCY | 165 | 00 |
| CASH COIN | 2 | 00 |
| LIST CHECKS SINGLY | | |
| | | |
| | | |
| TOTAL FROM OTHER SIDE | 600 | 00 |
| TOTAL | 667 | 00 |
| LESS CASH RECEIVED | | |
| NET DEPOSIT | 667 | 00 |

USE OTHER SIDE FOR ADDITIONAL LISTING

BE SURE EACH ITEM IS PROPERLY ENDORSED

⑆044000024⑆ 0289411086⑈

CHECKS AND OTHER ITEMS ARE RECEIVED FOR DEPOSIT SUBJECT TO THE PROVISIONS OF THE UNIFORM COMMERCIAL CODE OR ANY APPLICABLE COLLECTION AGREEMENT

| CHECKS LIST SINGLY | DOLLARS | CENTS |
|---|---|---|
| 1 *Kostrevsky#735* | 150 | 00 |
| 2 *Kendrix#489* | 145 | 00 |
| 3 *Gomez# 596* | 55 | 00 |
| 4 *Monarty#1073* | 47 | 00 |
| 5 *Holley#134* | 40 | 00 |
| 6 *Schmidt#436* | 38 | 00 |
| 7 *Segal#285* | 25 | 00 |
| 8 *Jackson* | 55 | 00 |
| 9 *Li* | 45 | 00 |
| 10 | | |
| 11 | | |
| 12 | | |
| 13 | | |
| 14 | | |
| 15 | | |
| 16 | | |
| 17 | | |
| 18 | | |
| 19 | | |
| TOTAL | 860 | 00 |

ENTER TOTAL ON THE FRONT OF THIS TICKET

## Procedure 19–3 Scenario

You are responsible for reconciling the monthly bank statement with the office checkbook. Use the following information to reconcile the bank account on Procedure Form 19–3.

## CCOUNT STATEMENT

***THE NEVER FAIL BANK***
ANYWHERE BRANCH
0000 THIS STREET
ANYTOWN, STATE 00000-0000
CUSTOMER SERVICE 24 HOURS A DAY, 800-000-0000

| | ACCOUNT |
|---|---|
| ANE D. CUSTOMER | 12345-678910 |
| 234 HOME STREET | STATEMENT PERIOD |
| NYTOWN, STATE 00000-0000 | 1-1-20XX TO 2-1-20XX |

**CCOUNTS SUMMARY**

| CHECKING | | SAVINGS |
|---|---|---|
| EGINNING BALANCE | 2,999.55 | |
| EPOSITS | 6,466.00 | |
| HECKS PAID | 7,929.24 | |
| TM & DEBIT CARD WITHDRAWALS | 400.00 | |
| ERVICE CHARGES/FEES | 6.00 | |
| NDING BALANCE | 1,130.31 | |

**HECKING ACTIVITY**

| EPOSITS POSTED | AMOUNT | DESCRIPTION |
|---|---|---|
| -05 | 1,500.00 | ATM DEPOSIT |
| -15 | 765.50 | ATM DEPOSIT |
| -18 | 600.00 | DIR DEPOSIT |
| -20 | 2,200.00 | DEPOSIT |
| -22 | 1,400.00 | DEPOSIT |

| HECKS PAID CHECK # | PAID | AMOUNT |
|---|---|---|
| 01 | 1-2 | 632.75 |
| 02 | 1-4 | 35.98 |
| 04 | 1-6 | 72.43 |
| 05 | 1-8 | 2,000.00 |
| 06 | 1-10 | 500.00 |
| 09 | 1-15 | 3,000.00 |
| 1 | 1-16 | 210.00 |
| 2 | 1-17 | 1,100.00 |
| 3 | 1-20 | 200.43 |
| 5 | 1-22 | 63.70 |
| 6 | 1-28 | 98.40 |
| 7 | 1-29 | 15.55 |

| ITHDRAWALS POSTED | AMOUNT | DESCRIPTION |
|---|---|---|
| 01 | 80.00 | ATM WITHDRAWAL |
| 14 | 20.00 | ATM WITHDRAWAL |
| 16 | 100.00 | ATM WITHDRAWAL |
| 30 | 200.00 | ATM WITHDRAWAL |

**HECKING SERVICES CHARGE AND FEE SUMMARY**

| MOUNT | DESCRIPTION |
|---|---|
| 00 | MONTHLY SERVICE CHARGE |

## CHECKBOOK (REGISTER)

Ending balance: $2,066.18

Checks written during the month:

| Check # | Amount | √ | Check # | Amount | √ |
|---|---|---|---|---|---|
| 101 | 632.75 | | 110 | 58.50 | |
| 102 | 35.98 | | 111 | 210.00 | |
| 103 | 102.75 | | 112 | 1,100.00 | |
| 104 | 72.43 | | 113 | 200.43 | |
| 105 | 2,000.00 | | 114 | 300.15 | |
| 106 | 500.00 | | 115 | 63.70 | |
| 107 | 400.00 | | 116 | 98.40 | |
| 108 | 207.56 | | 117 | 15.55 | |
| 109 | 3,000.00 | | 118 | 101.17 | |

Deposits made during the month:

| Deposit Date | Amount | √ |
|---|---|---|
| 1-05 | 1,500.00 | |
| 1-15 | 765.50 | |
| 1-18 | 600.00 | |
| 1-21 | 2,200.00 | |
| 1-22 | 1,400.00 | |
| 1-29 | 1,000.00 | |
| 1-30 | 1,200.00 | |

Withdrawals made during the month:

| Withdrawal Date | Amount | √ |
|---|---|---|
| 1-01 | 80.00 | |
| 1-14 | 20.00 | |
| 1-16 | 100.00 | |
| 1-30 | 200.00 | |
| 1-31 | 100.00 | |
| | | |
| | | |

## nswer Key for Procedure Form 19–3

ECONCILING THE BANK STATEMENT

ank Statement Balance $**1,130.31**

+) Plus Deposits not shown

**$1,000**

**$1,200**

otal **$2,200** $ **3,330.31**

-) Less Outstanding Checks

\# **103 $102.75**

\# **107 $400.00**

\# **108 $207.56**

\# **110 $58.50**

\# **114 $300.15**

\# **118 $101.17**

\# **ATM 1/31 $100.00**

otal **$1270.13** $ **2,060.18**

| ORRECTED BANK STATEMENT BALANCE | $ **2,060.18** |
|---|---|

heckbook Balance $ **2,066.18**

-) Less Bank Charges $ **6.00**

| ORRECTED CHECKBOOK BALANCE | $ **2,060.18** |
|---|---|

# CHAPTER 20 Accounts Payable and Accounting Procedures

## ABHES Curriculum

| | |
|---|---|
| MA.A.1.8.j | Perform accounts payable procedures |
| MA.A.1.8.l. | Establish and maintain a petty cash fund |

## CAAHEP Core Curriculum

| | |
|---|---|
| VI.C.1 | Explain basic bookkeeping computations |
| VI.C.2 | Differentiate between bookkeeping and accounting |
| VI.C.6 | Differentiate between accounts payable and accounts receivable |
| VI.C.8 | Describe common periodic financial reports |
| VI.C.13 | Discuss types of adjustments that can be made to a patient's account |

## LESSON OUTLINE

### I. ACCOUNTS PAYABLE

A. Amounts owed by the practice to suppliers and other service providers

B. Abbreviated A/P

C. Qualities of A/P personnel

1. Highly organized
2. Attentive to details
3. Good communication skills

### II. PURCHASING SUPPLIES AND EQUIPMENT

A. Expenditure: acquired material, property, and labor in exchange for money

B. Elements of an invoice

1. Company details
2. Invoice number
3. Dates
4. Client dates
5. Fees
6. Payment terms

### III. PETTY CASH (PROCEDURE 20–1)

### IV. ACCOUNTING

A. Difference between bookkeeping and accounting

B. Operational information

C. Managerial accounting information

D. Basic accounting formula (assets – liabilities = net worth)

E. Accounts receivable ratio (current A/R balance ÷ average months gross production)

F. Collections ratios

1. Gross collection ratio (total payments ÷ total charges)
2. Net collection ratio (total payments ÷ total charges, minus write-offs)
3. Types of write-offs
   a. Anything deemed uncollectable
   b. Bad debt
   c. Professional courtesy discount
   d. Contractual discounts

G. Cost ratio (total expenses ÷ number of procedures)

H. Cost–benefit analysis

1. Identify costs
2. Identify benefits
3. Compare costs against methods

### V. FINANCIAL RECORDS

A. Income statements

1. Demonstrates profit and expenses for a given month
2. Most commonly generated year-end report

B. Balance sheets

1. Statement of financial position
2. Displays assets as well as liabilities and owner's equity
3. Different ways to format and display a balance sheet

## CHAPTER ACTIVITIES

1. Have students make flash cards of the types of ratios and their specific formulae. On one side, write the word components and, on the other side, record the meanings of each.
2. Have students search the Internet to find a WEBSITE that automatically calculates their net worth. Forms are also available to complete this process manually, and students may alternatively download one of these forms to complete this activity.

## ANSWERS TO CHECK YOUR KNOWLEDGE QUESTIONS

1. The R in A/R stands for __________ and the P in A/P stands for __________.
   a. receipts, purchases
   b. receipts, payable
   **c. receivable, payable**
   d. receivable, purchases
2. This type of accounting is the study and analysis of financial data as it applies to operational issues within a company.
   **a. Managerial accounting**
   b. Operational accounting

c. Cost ratio accounting
d. Expenditure accounting

3. All the following is information contained on an invoice, except:
   a. company details.
   b. invoice details.
   **c. packing slip.**
   d. fees.
4. Another term for net worth is:
   **a. owner's equity.**
   b. assets.
   c. financial position.
   d. gross collections.
5. This ratio is calculated by dividing the total payments for a specific period of time by the total charges, *with* the write-offs deducted from the total charges.
   a. Cost ratio
   b. Accounts receivable ratio
   c. Gross collection ratio
   **d. Net collection ratio**
6. This demonstrates the profit and expenses for a given month and includes year-to-date information for a given year.
   a. Balance sheet
   **b. Income statement**
   c. Cost–benefit analysis
   d. Net worth
7. These are debts or accounts payable (A/P) owed by the business.
   a. Assets
   **b. Liabilities**
   c. Owner's equity
   d. Cost ratio

## ROCEDURE SCENARIOS

ne following scenarios are provided for use with the competency checklists. They are optional; instructors may modify the enarios or make up their own. The following forms can be downloaded from the students' Premium Website.

### rocedure 20–1

se Procedure Form 20–1 and the following amounts to establish and maintain a petty cash fund. The petty cash fund was ened on 2/15 (current year) with an opening balance of $25.00. When the petty cash fund decreases below $5.00, a new check ould be written to bring the fund back up to the $25.00 level.

a. #1 voucher: $5.00 donation, 2/20
b. #2 voucher: $3.75 parking, 2/21
c. Bill: $3.80 package shipping, 2/25
d. #3 voucher: $9.00 Girl Scout cookies, 2/27

e. Bill: $1.39 mailing envelope, 3/1

f. #4 voucher: $10 gift card, 3/1

Students can download the following forms from the Premium Website to complete this activity and use as work product for this procedure:

- Procedure Form 20–1: Petty Cash form

Answer Key for Procedure Form 20-1

| PETTY CASH FORM | | | |
|---|---|---|---|
| **Date** | **Bill/Voucher Description** | **Amount** | **Balance** |
| **2/15** | **Fund established** | **$25.00** | **$25.00** |
| **2/20** | **Voucher #1: Donation** | **$5.00** | **$20.00** |
| **2/21** | **Voucher #2: Parking** | **$3.75** | **$16.25** |
| **2/25** | **Bill: Package shipping** | **$3.80** | **$12.45** |
| **2/27** | **Voucher #3: Girl Scout cookies** | **$9.00** | **$3.45** |
| **2/27** | **New check: replenish petty cash to $25** | **$21.55** | **$25.00** |
| **3/1** | **Bill: Mailing envelope** | **$1.39** | **$23.61** |
| **3/1** | **Voucher #4: Gift card** | **$10.00** | **$13.61** |
| | | | |

# UNIT 10 MANAGING THE MEDICAL OFFICE ENVIRONMENT
# CHAPTER 21 Facilities Management and Emergency Preparedness

## ABHES Curriculum

| | |
|---|---|
| MA.A.1.5.a | Define and understand abnormal behavior patterns |
| MA.A.1.8.x | Maintain medical facility |
| MA.A.1.8.z | Maintain inventory equipment and supplies |
| MA.A.1.9.i | Use standard precautions |
| MA.A.1.10.c | Disposal of biohazardous materials |
| MA.A.1.11b(2) | Demonstrate professionalism by: Exhibiting a positive attitude and a sense of responsibility |
| MA.A.1.11b(6) | Demonstrate professionalism by: Adapting to change |

## CAAHEP Core Curriculum

| | |
|---|---|
| III.P.2 | Practice Standard Precautions |
| III.P.3 | Select appropriate barrier/personal protective equipment (PPE) for potentially infectious situations |
| V.P.10 | Perform an office inventory |
| XI.C.2 | Identify safety techniques that can be used to prevent accidents and maintain a safe work environment |
| XI.C.3 | Describe the importance of Materials Safety Data Sheets (MSDS) in a healthcare setting |
| XI.C.4 | Identify safety signs, symbols and labels |
| XI.C.7 | Describe fundamental principles for evacuation of a healthcare setting |
| XI.C.8 | Discuss fire safety issues in a healthcare environment |
| XI.C.9 | Discuss requirements for responding to hazardous material disposal |
| XI.C.11 | Discuss critical elements of an emergency plan for response to a natural disaster or other emergency |
| XI.C.12 | Identify emergency preparedness plans in your community |
| XI.C.13 | Discuss potential role(s) of the medical assistant in emergency |
| XI.P.1 | Comply with safety signs, symbols and labels |
| XI.P.2 | Evaluate the work environment to identify safe v. unsafe working conditions |
| XI.P.3 | Develop a personal (patient and employee) safety plan |
| XI.P.4 | Develop an environmental safety plan |
| XI.P.5.b | Demonstrate proper use of the following equipment: fire extinguishers |
| XI.P.6 | Participate in a mock environmental exposure event with documentation of steps taken |
| XI.P.7 | Explain an evacuation plan for a physician's office |
| XI.P.8 | Demonstrate methods of fire prevention in the healthcare setting |
| XI.A.1. | Recognize the effects of stress on all persons involved in emergency situations |
| XI.A.2 | Demonstrate self awareness in responding to emergency situations |

## LESSON OUTLINE

### OPENING THE OFFICE (PROCEDURE 21-1)

A. The surroundings set the tone for the office and the first impression and level of professionalism anticipated.

B. A checklist, specific to your office, should be created and followed to ensure you cover all daily functions of opening, operating, and closing the office.

C. Security in the medical office

D. Evaluating the reception area

1. Condition of the furniture
2. Lamps and electrical cords
3. Floors for carpet wrinkles or tears, or anything lying on the floor

E. Preparing the front desk

1. Turn on computers, scanners, printers (and other electronic equipment).
2. Retrieve telephone messages.
3. Retrieve and sort faxes.
4. Retrieve and sort printed lab and hospital reports.
5. Place charts for check in.
6. Prepare sign-in sheets, cash balance forms, etc.

F. Inspecting examination rooms and lab areas

1. Replace examining paper and be certain waste receptacles are emptied.
2. Observe room temperature and plug in any disconnected electrical equipment.
3. Be certain everything is in working condition.
4. Restock supplies so that needed materials are available.
   a. Maintain an inventory control sheet (check list)

G. Check common work areas.

1. Check the water level in the autoclave and turn it on.
2. Be sure hazardous waste disposal containers are available for use in all areas where needed.

H. Supply Inventory (Procedure 21-2)

1. Maintain an inventory of clinical and administrative supplies.
2. Duties may include inventory and ordering of office (clerical) supplies, clinic supplies (exam room orders), and medication orders.
3. Do not want to run out of needed supplies, yet also do not over-order items, especially since many may have an expiration date and are often quite costly.

## II. CLOSING THE OFFICE (PROCEDURE 21-3)

A. Exam rooms should be restocked and cleaned, and discarded material should be placed for pick-up.

B. Charts must be collected, checked for completeness, and filed in a locked cabinet.

1. If there is not time to file, place charts in a separate folder of "charts to be filed" and place in the cabinet to be filed the next day.
2. Some doctors may dictate their notes, which must first be typed onto the chart before it can be filed.

C. All electrical appliances and the autoclave must be turned off, including computers.

D. Receipts collected during the day can be taken to the bank for deposit or locked in the office safe.

E. Tidy the reception area and sanitize (if you have a cleaning service, be sure to inspect for proper cleaning of entire office suite and report any deficiencies).

F. Pull and prepare charts for the next day.

G. Place lab, consultations, and hospital reports with the chart and then place at the front desk (reception area) for check in.

H. Walk through the office to complete your checklist of things to do.

## III. SAFETY IN THE MEDICAL OFFICE

A. Federal and state regulations
   1. OSHA
   2. CDC
   3. ADA
   4. CLIA
   5. Fire regulations

B. Safety signs, symbols, and labels

C. MSDS

D. Cleaning Spills and Dropped Objects (Procedure 21–4)
   1. Follow proper procedure and clean up immediately.
   2. Use universal precautions.

E. Personal Safety
   1. Developing personal safety plans.
   2. Infection control and personal safety.

## IV. FIRE PREVENTION

A. Fire triangle: heat, fuel, and oxygen.

B. Fire causes and how they can be prevented

C. Using a fire extinguisher (Procedure 21–5)
   1. PASS acronym

## V. EMERGENCY PREPAREDNESS AND EVACUATION

A. Routine fire and weather drills.

B. Those who are prepared have a greater chance of surviving a crisis than those who do not know what to do or how to act.

C. Keep calm and confident in times of emergency to reduce panic and irrational behavior.

D. Each member of the office team should be assigned specific duties and know how to carry out duties safely and efficiently.

E. Post emergency phone numbers by all phones.

# CHAPTER ACTIVITITES

1. Invite a Practice Manager to class to explain safety, policies, and procedures.
2. Have students research OSHA and CLIA Websites to determine regulations that apply to the health care office.
3. Log in to United States Department of Homeland Security Website (www.ready.gov) and have class create emergency preparedness plans (see downloads).
   a. www.ready.gov/business/_downloads/computerinventory.pdf
   b. www.ready.gov/business/_downloads/sampleplan.pdf
   c. www.ready.gov/business/_downloads/emergency_supplies.pdf
   d. www.ready.gov/business/_downloads/insuranceform.pdf
   e. www.ready.gov/business/_downloads/readybusiness-brochure.pdf

# ANSWERS TO CHECK YOUR KNOWLEDGE QUESTIONS

1. Preparing to open the office involves creating a checklist and performing which of the following functions?
   a. Check the waiting room temperature.
   b. Perform a visual check of electrical devices, furniture, floors, and lighting.
   c. Lock the outside access doors.
   d. All of the above
   **e. a and b only**
2. To prepare the front desk for opening the office, which of the following is NOT a function?
   a. Retrieve faxes
   b. Retrieve messages
   **c. Retrieve superbills**
   d. Turn on computers and office equipment.
3. Inspection of the examination rooms entails which of the following responsibilities?
   a. Replace examining paper
   b. Plug in electrical equipment
   c. Restock supplies
   **d. All of the above**
   e. a and b only
4. Which of the following is NOT part of the inventory supply duties?
   **a. Printed schedule of patient appointments**
   b. Medication
   c. Office (clerical) supplies
   d. Laboratory
   e. Checklist of exam room supplies
5. Safety in the medical office is regulated and promoted by which of the following agencies?
   a. Occupational Health and Safety Administration (OSHA)
   b. Drug Enforcement Agency (DEA)
   c. American with Disabilities Act (ADA)
   d. Center for Medicare and Medicaid Services (CMS)
   e. All of the above
   **f. a, b, and c**
6. Which agency created the guidelines called universal precautions?
   **a. Centers for Disease Control and Prevention (CDC)**
   b. Occupational Health and Safety Administration (OSHA)
   c. Drug Enforcement Agency (DEA)
   d. Center for Medicare and Medicaid Services (CMS)
7. The objective of the Clinical Laboratory Improvement Amendments (CLIA) is?
   a. To receive Medicare payments
   **b. To ensure quality laboratory testing**
   c. To promote Universal Precautions
   d. To comply with OSHA regulations

8. Proper use of Safety Signs, Symbols, and Labels would be used in which of the following?
   a. A refrigerator used to store reagents, test kits, or biological specimens are labeled with a biohazard symbol and bear the legend "Not for storage of food or medications."
   b. Biohazard waste receptacles bear the biohazard symbol and are lined with red plastic bags. Biohazard waste is not disposed of in inappropriate receptacles.
   c. Chemicals and reagents are evaluated for hazard category classification and labeled with the National Fire Association's color and number coding.
   d. Signs are clearly posted in appropriate places for where smoking is allowed, and where to eat or drink.
   e. All of the above
   **f. a, b, and c**
9. In response to a fire, your responsibility is to?
   a. Wedge open doors
   b. Warn others in a frantic tones
   c. Evacuate patients and staff using the closest elevator.
   **d. Sound the alarm**
   e. All of the above
10. When closing the office, it is your responsibility to?
   a. Cancel appointments
   b. Turn off fax machine
   **c. Deposit receipts (cash) to bank or in safe**
   d. Collect charts for review the following day
   e. All of the above

# CHAPTER 22 Managing the Office

## ABHES Curriculum

| | |
|---|---|
| MA.A.1.1.b | Compare and contrast the allied health professions and understand their relation to medical assisting |
| MA.A.1.8.e | Locate resources and information for patients and employers |
| MA.A.1.8.dd | Serve as a liaison between provider and others |

## CAAHEP Core Curriculum

| | |
|---|---|
| IV.P.2 | Report relevant information to others succinctly and accurately |

## LESSON OUTLINE

### I. RESPONSIBILITIES TO EMPLOYEES

A. The manager in large practices often has the following responsibilities related to the support staff employees:
   1. Interview, hire, discipline, and terminate employees in coordination with providers.
   2. Supervise or personally train employees. This applies to new personnel as well as to updating current staff.
   3. Conduct staff meetings to inform, discuss, and exchange information.
   4. Create, implement, and enforce work schedules.
   5. Arrange vacation schedules and coverage.
   6. Conduct performance evaluations, establishing probationary periods as deemed necessary.
   7. Consult providers concerning performance evaluations, salary increases, and benefits. (In a larger group practice or association with health care facility, the HR department might set the policy for salary increase, probationary periods, and benefits.)

B. HIPAA and office policy
   1. The manager has the responsibility to ensure compliance in all HIPAA-related areas.
   2. One method is to conduct audits and present an analysis of PHI security.
   3. The manager must review policy and procedure, update if necessary, and develop training materials and implement training and education for employees as needed.
   4. HIPAA discussions should be included at every staff meeting to heighten awareness.
   5. Enforcement of policies, including disciplinary action for HIPAA violations, is another responsibility of the practice manager.
   6. An office manual can include policies on such topics as:
      a. Absenteeism
      b. Paid time off (PTO)
      c. Harassment
      d. Confidentiality
      e. Continuing education
      f. Chain of command
      g. Expected performance
      h. Employment evaluation
      i. Information technology

C. Office procedure manual—An office procedure manual will identify the common procedures performed in the office. The manual may include such procedures as:
    1. Opening and closing the office
    2. Laboratory tests
    3. Documentation requirements
    4. OSHA and CLIA requirements
    5. Basic clinical procedures
    6. Basic administrative procedures
    7. Emergency procedures

D. Employee records
    1. All employees in a medical office must have a Social Security number, the nine-digit number obtained from the Social Security Administration.
    2. Each employee must also complete an Employee's Withholding Allowance Certificate (W-4 form) indicating the number of exemptions claimed (refer to Figure 22–3).
    3. Federal legislation requires employees to complete an Employment Eligibility Verification, Form I-9 (refer to Figure 22–4).
        a. The form is issued by the Department of Justice, Immigration and Naturalization Service.
        b. Its purpose is to ensure that all employed persons are United States citizens, lawfully admitted aliens, or aliens authorized to work in the United States.
        c. By law, this form must be completed before an individual can be officially hired.
        d. Payroll will not be issued to individuals who do not have an I-9 form on file.

E. Employee payroll (see Procedure 22–1)
    1. The medical office must have a federal tax reporting number (called the Employer Identification Number [EIN]), which is obtained from the Internal Revenue Service.
    2. In states that require employer reports, a state employer number must also be obtained.
    3. When payroll checks are prepared, a record must be kept showing Social Security, federal taxes, any state and city taxes, and insurance amounts deducted from earnings.
    4. Employees may be paid an hourly wage or a salary (a fixed amount paid on a regular basis for a prescribed period of time).
    5. The Federal Fair Labor Standards Act regulates the minimum wage and requires overtime to be paid to hourly wage earners at a minimum rate of one and one-half times the regular rate for hours above 40 hours per week.
    6. It is necessary to keep records of hours worked, total pay, and all deductions withheld for all employees.
    7. All employees are expected to work the assigned number of hours per day, week, and month.
    8. Any time off must be reconciled on the payroll records and the wages adjusted according to office policy.

F. Benefits
    1. Full-time medical office employees can expect benefits in addition to their wages.
    2. Benefits vary according to the size of the practice.
    3. The following are examples of benefits that might be offered.
        a. Paid time off (PTO
        b. Vacation
        c. Holidays
        d. Sick time (if not included as part of your PTO or vacation)

e. Personal time

f. Bereavement time

g. Jury duty

h. Health insurance

i. Disability insurance

j. Life insurance

k. Profit sharing (retirement)

G. Office liability insurance

1. Risk management is a fundamental component of the medical practice.
2. The individual provider or the providers within a group practice will purchase insurance to protect their personal and professional assets in case they are found liable for some action or lack of action (commonly referred to as malpractice insurance).
3. Cost of such coverage varies greatly in relation to the type of practice.
4. Other types of insurance need to be in place, including, general liability coverage, workers' compensation insurance, and structure coverage (from loss due to theft, fire, or other damage).
5. If, as manager, you must acquire necessary insurance coverage, it is imperative to find a reputable insurance broker, experienced in medical practices.
6. If your practice is part of a medical group, the risk management and quality assurance departments will most likely handle all insurance and claims on behalf of the practice.

H. Staff meetings

1. The office manager is responsible for setting staff meeting schedule and agenda and conducting the meetings but will often delegate and rotate this responsibility with office staff, which promotes shared responsibility and teamwork.
2. Staff meetings should last from 30 minutes to one hour and be held at least once a month.
3. Meetings are often held during lunch time or before patient hours to use time more effectively.
4. Employees should receive pay for staff meeting time.
5. To have a successful meeting, create the agenda to organize the topics to be covered and distribute to staff in advance.
6. If decisions are made that will affect office operation, be sure a written record in the form of minutes is kept so there is a reference for any necessary changes in the policy and procedure manual.
7. The meetings should be informative and beneficial and should concern the operation of the office.
8. The meeting should never be allowed to turn into a gripe session.
9. Discussing personal issues associated with individual employees should be avoided when the total staff is present.

I. Employee evaluation and review

1. Most employers require employees to have regular, routine, or periodic reviews or evaluations regarding their work performance.
2. The time schedule can vary from place to place, but usually there is a probationary review at 90 days and then annual reviews thereafter.
3. A review may be scheduled more often if there is a problem. (Often, a performance improvement plan is developed and implemented with a specific time frame for progress to be attained.)

4. Evaluations should be regarded as an opportunity to share views on performance and expectations.
5. Some employers might ask each employee to submit a self-evaluation and peer evaluations.

J. Terminating employment

1. There are many reasons an employee might leave his or her job: relocation, advancement to a more responsible position, a higher-paying job, illness, educational pursuits, pregnancy, or a change in lifestyle.
2. There is, however, a major responsibility by the employee to give as much advance notice as possible but no less than two weeks.

## II. RESPONSIBILITIES TO PROVIDERS

A. Providers need to be kept informed and aware of conditions affecting the practice, including finances, staffing, legal issues, budgets, security, and technology support.

B. The manager has a great deal of obligation to the providers and must at all times listen to their concerns.

C. Provider's professional meetings (see Procedure 22–2)

1. The provider might ask the manager for assistance with all office scheduling, including travel arrangements to attend or make presentations at professional meetings.
2. The schedule can be marked (blocked) so that no patients are booked if it is known far enough in advance.
3. If patients have already been scheduled, they will have to be contacted and offered alternative times.
4. Providers can also want another provider contacted to cover during their absence.
5. When providers practice within a group, it is usually possible to schedule patients with another group member.
6. If arranging travel, ask the provider for personal preferences.

## III. RESPONSIBILITIES FOR THE FACILITY

A. The physical structure of the office must be observed and maintained. The manager assumes responsibility for:

1. Maintenance of office services such as cleaning and laundry.
2. Subscriptions to magazines and health-related literature.
3. Monitoring and paying utilities.
4. Suggesting improvements: repairs, decorating, and organization of rooms.
5. Security (locks, alarm, and so on), privacy, and HIPAA-compliant staff and vendors.
6. Information technology support: hardware and software (security and operability).
7. Grounds and parking maintenance (unless included in building lease; if so, responsibility can include lease negotiations for the facility).
8. OSHA and other regulatory compliance of the facility.
9. Proper licensing and insurance of the facility.
10. Handling renewals of business and professional insurance policies (given to a manager who has served successfully in the position).

B. Practice information brochure

1. The office manager might be asked to compose an information brochure (also known as a patient information booklet).
2. The brochure can be created using work processing, graphic design, or publishing software. It should be printed on good-quality paper and, if the practice has a logo, it could be placed on the cover of the brochure.

3. The brochure must be updated as providers or services are added or deleted from the practice.
4. The brochure may also contain some of the following information:
   a. Brief overview of the practice (name, address, phone and fax numbers, email address, and Website)
   b. Brief description of provider's education and practice interests
   c. Hospital affiliation
   d. Practice information and policies
   e. Office hours
   f. After-hours policy (nonemergency care)
   g. Appointment policy (missed and cancellation)
   h. Financial and payment policies
   i. Referrals

C. Daily and monthly account records
   1. Medical offices use a variety of bookkeeping and accounting systems to maintain a sense for fiscal status.
   2. Identify expenditures and income totals to ensure that the practice is earning sufficient income to meet office expenses, employee salaries, taxes, insurance premiums, benefits payments, and an income for the provider.
   3. In addition, it is necessary to build assets for equipment purchases, investments, and perhaps the hiring of additional employees when needed.

D. Fee schedules
   1. The office manager may be asked to research fee schedules for patient care.
   2. You must have a continuing awareness of the costs involved for the provider to perform certain diagnostic studies, and the costs associated with products and supplies. The CMS Website will provide updated information regarding approved procedures and reimbursement rates for your reference and guidance.

E. Patient accounts
   1. Many medical offices have outside billing services to handle patient accounts.
   2. It is the responsibility of the provider and office staff to ensure accurate ICD and CPT coding.
   3. The office (provider, manager, or staff) will be responsible for recoding rejected claims.
   4. The practice is required to collect current insurance and demographic information from patients and update on a regular basis.
   5. If your office bills directly, then as manager, you must follow billing guidelines.

F. Patient refunds
   1. Managers usually assume the responsibility of verifying overpayment to a patient's account before approving reimbursement.
   2. This situation occurs when both the patient and the insurance company pay the provider or an error in the amount due is made and a refund is due the patient.

G. Missed or late cancelled appointments
   1. A missed-appointment policy should be distributed in new-patient packets either prior to or during the first office visit.
   2. If a patient does not show or cancels late, the provider or practice receives no payment for that scheduled time of the day.
   3. Another patient who needed to see the provider was either scheduled at another time or referred out if necessary.

H. Preparing for site reviews
   1. It is the responsibility of the manager to prepare the office for site visits, which might need to be delegated to the office staff.
   2. Many insurance companies announce their visits in advance.
   3. Inspections for compliance with regulations (such as CLIA, OSHA, and boards of health) do not always give advance notification. It is imperative for the office manager to be familiar with the latest guidelines and regulations.
   4. Keep current handbooks, licenses, policies, and procedure manuals up to date and readily accessible.
   5. Good teamwork is essential when preparing for site visits.

I. Moving the office
   1. Medical offices change locations for many reasons.
      a. Some offices outgrow their space.
      b. Others find a facility that is more economical or in a better and more convenient location.
   2. The office manager is usually the one who coordinates the move.
   3. Prior to the change, communication with the practice owner is essential.
   4. Goals must be clearly defined.
   5. When the date of the move is known, patient schedules should be adjusted to allow for any last-minute changes.
   6. It is also recommended to reduce schedules to 50 percent for the first day at the new office because, often, there are technical issues with equipment, computers, EHR programs, software, hardware, and so on (refer to Table 22–2).

J. Preparing the new facility
   1. Many things must be coordinated to prepare the new facility.
   2. There will be construction contractors, IT consults, wiring, and regulatory compliance concerns.
   3. All necessary building permits must be obtained and signed off as being code compliant before the practice moves.
   4. New equipment, furniture, window coverings, and so on must be ordered and installed.
   5. Coordination of the provider schedule and patient notification are required for a smooth and seamless transition.

K. The day of the move
   1. You might want to divide the staff (between the old and new offices), assigning responsibilities for the move.
   2. Arrange (in advance) professional movers (HIPAA-compliant) to move the bulk of the office.
   3. Have utility companies on standby and have the IT department on site to address any functionality issues with electronic equipment.

# CHAPTER ACTIVITIES

1. Research the Internal Revenue Service Website and locate the forms referred to in this chapter (W-2, W-9, I-9, 941, and 940) and determine the maximum number of deductions a single person, a married person, a married person without children, and married with children can claim. Also determine the dollar amount allowed for each deduction. Determine the appropriate amount of taxes withheld from employee payroll and complete forms 941 and 940.
2. Search the Internet and determine what the current minimum wage is for your state as well as the requirements for paying overtime.
3. Ask a certified public accountant (CPA) to visit the class for a presentation on payroll and bookkeeping methods, including accounts payable (AP), accounts receivable (AR), and general ledger (GL).
4. Contact a local health care provider and ask the practice manager or HR department representative to visit the class and explain management duties (responsibilities to employees, providers, and facility).
5. Have students prepare an office brochure, using templates available from Microsoft, HP, or Apple.

# ANSWERS TO CHECK YOUR KNOWLEDGE QUESTIONS

1. The manager has the following responsibilities?
   a. Conduct staff meetings to inform, discuss, and exchange information
   b. Create, implement, and enforce work schedules
   c. Arrange vacation schedules and coverage
   d. Conduct performance evaluations, establishing probationary periods as deemed necessary
   e. a, b, and d
   **f. All of the above**
2. Ensuring compliance with HIPAA regulations is the manager's responsibility by:
   a. Discussing HIPAA at providers' meetings.
   b. Discussing HIPAA at staff meetings.
   c. Conducting an audit of PHI.
   d. Updating computer passwords.
   e. b, c, and d.
   **f. b and c.**
3. The office policy manual does NOT include:
   a. Paid time off (PTO).
   b. Harassment.
   c. Information technology.
   **d. Opening and closing the office.**
4. The office procedure manual includes procedures regarding:
   a. confidentiality.
   b. continuing education.
   c. employment evaluation.
   **d. emergency procedures.**
5. All employees should have the following documents or information available when filling out initial payroll forms.
   a. Driver's license or other state picture identification
   b. Major credit card
   c. Social Security card and a copy of Social Security numbers of all dependents
   d. All the above
   **e. a and c**
6. Documentation needed for personnel files include:
   a. immunization record.
   b. copies of any professional license, registration, degree, diplomas, or certification.
   c. verification of Occupational Safety and Health Administration and Clinical Laboratory Improvement Amendments (OSHA and CLIA) training.
   **d. all of the above.**
7. When preparing a payroll check, which of the following should NOT be included?
   a. Date of check
   **b. Employee telephone number**
   c. Gross salary

   d. Individual deductions: federal income tax, Social Security tax, state tax, local tax, insurance, and other deductions
   e. Net pay (the actual amount of the paycheck after deductions)

8. In addition to wages, employees can often expect to receive which of the following benefits?
   a. Paid time off (PTO)
   b. Health insurance
   c. Auto insurance
   d. All of the above
   **e. a and b**
9. Staff meetings are a method to accomplish what?
   a. Personality conflict resolution
   b. Employee evaluations
   **c. Policy implementation**
   e. Employee salaries
10. Employee evaluations achieve which of the following?
    a. Two-week termination notice
    b. Performance goals
    c. Achievement recognition
    d. Necessary improvements
    e. All of the above
    **f. b, c, and d**
11. Responsibilities to the providers do NOT include:
    **a. Grounds maintenance.**
    b. Financial and budgeting issues.
    c. Staffing.
    d. Security.
    e. Technology support.
12. Responsibilities to the facility include which of the following?
    a. Monitoring and paying (approving) bills
    b. Staff meetings
    c. OSHA and other regulatory compliance
    **d. a and c**

# SECTION 3 STRUCTURE AND FUNCTION OF THE BODY

# UNIT 11 ANATOMY AND PHYSIOLOGY OF THE HUMAN BODY

# CHAPTER 23 Anatomical Descriptors and Fundamental Body Structure

*Note:* This unit contains 13 chapters discussing the structure and function of the body's 10 systems. The ABHES Curriculum components and CAAHEP Core Curriculum plan pertaining to Anatomy and Physiology applies to all 13 chapters. Therefore, they will be identified only once here, before we begin Chapter 23.

## ABHES Curriculum

| | |
|---|---|
| MA.A.1.2.b | Identify and apply the knowledge of all body systems; their structure and functions; and their common diseases, symptoms, and etiologies |
| MA.A.1.2.c | Assist the physician with the regimen of diagnostic and treatment modalities as they relate to each body system |
| MA.A.1.3.c | Understand the various medical terminology for each specialty |

## CAAHEP Core Curriculum

| | |
|---|---|
| I.C.1. | Describe structural organization of the human body |
| I.C.2. | Identify body systems |
| I.C.3. | Describe body planes, directional terms, quadrants, and cavities |
| I.C.4. | List major organs in each body system |
| I.C.5. | Describe the normal function of each body system |
| I.C.6. | Identify common pathology related to each body system |
| I.C.7. | Analyze pathology as it relates to the interaction of body systems |
| I.C.8. | Discuss implications for disease and disability when homeostasis is not maintained |
| I.C.9. | Describe implications for treatment related to pathology |
| I.C.10. | Compare body structure and function of the human body across the life span |
| I.C.11. | Identify the classifications of medications, including desired effects, side effects and adverse reactions |
| I.C.12. | Describe the relationship between anatomy and physiology of all body systems and medications used for treatment in each |

## LESSON OUTLINE

### I. ANATOMY AND PHYSIOLOGY DEFINED

A. Anatomy is the study of the physical structure of the body and its organs

B. Physiology is the science of the functions of cells, tissues, and organs

C. Anatomy fields of study

1. Gross anatomy
2. Microscopic anatomy
    a. Cytology
    b. Histology

## II. ANATOMICAL DIRECTIONAL TERMS

A. Median or sagittal plane
   1. An imaginary line dividing the body vertically down the front
   2. Divides the body into right and left halves
      a. Medial refers to anything located toward the midline
      b. Lateral refers to anything away from the midline

B. Proximal and distal
   1. Terms used to describe the relationship of the extremities (arms or legs) to the trunk of the body
      a. Proximal indicates nearness to the point of attachment
      b. Distal indicates distance away from the point of attachment

C. Frontal or coronal plane
   1. An imaginary line that divides the body into front and back sections
   2. Anterior or ventral refers to anything located in the front section
   3. Posterior or dorsal refers to anything located in the back section

D. Transverse plane
   1. An imaginary horizontal line that divides the body into top and bottom halves
   2. Superior refers to anything located above the line
   3. Inferior refers to anything located below the line
   4. Use of terms depends on where the "line" is drawn, e.g., the chest is superior to the abdomen, but inferior to the head

## III. BODY CAVITIES

A. Two main cavities

B. Dorsal or posterior cavity is divided into two sections
   1. Cranial cavity contains the brain
   2. Spinal cavity contains the spinal cord

C. Ventral or anterior cavity is divided by the diaphragm
   1. Thoracic cavity
      a. The chest
      b. Contains heart, lungs, and great blood vessels
      c. Protected by the ribs
   2. Abdominopelvic cavity has three parts
      a. Upper abdominal portion contains the stomach, small intestine, large intestine, liver, spleen, pancreas, and gallbladder
      b. Lower pelvic portion contains the bladder, part of the large intestine, and the internal reproductive organs
      c. Retroperitoneal cavity contains the kidneys

D. Cranial cavity provides protection for the brain

E. Spinal cavity contains the spinal cord

F. Orbital cavity contains the eyes

G. Nasal cavity contains the structures of the nose

H. Buccal cavity contains the mouth

## IV. ABDOMINAL REGIONS

A. Abdomen is divided into regions for purposes of identification or reference

B. Quadrant method of division

1. Right upper quadrant (RUQ)
2. Left upper quadrant (LUQ)
3. Right lower quadrant (RLQ)
4. Left lower quadrant (LLQ)

C. Nine-region method more exacting division

1. Epigastric region is in upper center region above the stomach
2. Umbilical region is in middle center region by umbilicus
3. Hypogastric or pubic region is in lower center region
4. Hypochondriac regions (right and left) are on either side below the ribs
5. Lumbar regions (right and left) are on either side by large bones of spinal cord
6. Iliac or inguinal regions (right and left) are on either side by the groin

## V. THE CELL

A. The basic building block of life

B. Microscopic image of the body

1. Takes in food and oxygen
2. Produces heat and energy
3. Gives off waste products
4. Reproduces itself
5. Performs specific duties

C. Body contains 75 trillion cells

D. Cells vary in shape, size, and activities

E. Cell parts

1. Cytoplasm
   a. Sticky semifluid
   b. Contains water, protein, lipids, carbohydrates, minerals, and salts
2. Cell membrane
   a. Outer protective covering of cell
   b. Controls what enters and leaves the cell
3. Organelles
   a. Nucleus
      i. Dense mass within the cytoplasm
      ii. Controls center of the cell
         (a). Regulates chemical reactions
         (b). Regulates mitosis

b. Chromosomes
  i. Located within the nucleus
  ii. Human beings have 23 pairs
    (a). 22 pairs are autosomes
    (b). One pair are sex chromosomes—either both X, female; or X and Y, male
  iii. Contain deoxyribonucleic acid (DNA), which contains genes
    (a) Carries genetic coding
    (b). Structure determine heredity factors
    (c). Segments of DNA molecules on chromosomes
    (d). Act in pairs
    (e). 35,000–45,000 genes

c. Nucleolus
  i. Located inside the nucleus
  ii. Where ribonucleic acid (RNA) is assembled with proteins to make subunits of ribosomes

d. Centrioles
  i. Two cylinder-shaped organelles
  ii. Active during mitosis

e. Endoplasmic reticulum
  i. Serves as a passageway for the transportation of materials in and out of the nucleus
  ii. Grouped together can store large amounts of protein
  iii. Ribosomes attached to membrane give it rough appearance, called rough endoplasmic reticulum

f. Mitochondria
  i. Round or rod-shaped organelles
  ii. Supply cell's energy

g. Golgi apparatus
  i. Stack of membrane layers
  ii. Synthesizes carbohydrates and combines them with proteins

h. Lysosomes
  i. Round or oval structures
  ii. Serve as centers of cellular digestion

i. Pinocytic vesicles
  i. Pocket-like formations
  ii. Used in transport of large particles into a cell
  iii. Endocytosis (phagocytes)
  iv. Exocytosis

## VI. PASSING MOLECULES THROUGH CELL MEMBRANES

A. Diffusion is the process whereby gas, liquid, or solid molecules distribute themselves evenly through a medium
  1. In alveolus
  2. Internal respiration

B. Osmosis
   1. A process of diffusion of water or a solvent through a selected permeable membrane (Figure 23-9)
   2. Osmotic characteristics of solutions are classified by their effect on red blood cells (Figures 23-10 and 23-11)
      a. Isotonic is having the same concentration of salt as found in blood cell
      b. Hypotonic is having a lower concentration of salt than found in a red blood cell
      c. Hypertonic is having a higher concentration of salt than found in a red blood cell

C. Filtration is the movement of solutes and water across a semipermeable membrane as a result of a force (Figure 23-12)

D. Active transport is movement across a membrane from an area of low concentration to an area of higher concentration due to presence of adenosine triphosphate (ATP), a carrier molecule

E. Phagocytosis is known as "cell eating"; WBC become phagocytes (Figure 23-13)

## II. SHOW MEDIA LINK: "ANATOMY OF A TYPICAL CELL"

## III. BIOCHEMISTRY

A. Elements
   1. Substances in their simplest form
   2. 92 natural elements
   3. 13 manmade elements
   4. 20 elements are needed to sustain life
      a. Carbon, oxygen, hydrogen, and nitrogen are most common; 97% of living matter
      b. Four are called trace elements

B. Compounds
   1. Two or more elements combined
   2. Classification
      a. Acid
         i. Positively charged ions of hydrogen
         ii. Negatively charged ions of another element
         iii. Sour taste
      b. Base or alkali
         i. Negatively charged ions of hydroxide
         ii. Positively charged ions of a metal
      c. Salt and water
         i. Results from combination of acid and base
         ii. When water evaporates, salt remains
      c. pH determines acidity or alkalinity of a solution
         i. pH value of 7.0 is neutral
         ii. pH value < 7.0 is acid
         iii. pH value > 7.0 is base

## X. CELLULAR DIVISION

A. Mitosis occurs when a cell reproduces by dividing into two identical cells (Figure 23-15)

B. Meiosis is the process by which the ovum and spermatozoon reduce their respective 46 chromosomes to 23

## X. HOMEOSTASIS IS A STABLE CONDITION OF AN INTERNAL ENVIRONMENT

A. Intracellular

B. Extracellular

C. Dysfunction causes illness, death

## XI. MUTATIONS AND TRAITS

A. DNA is code

B. Mutation from copy error

C. Internal/external factors

D. Traits

1. Dominant gene
2. Recessive
   a. Carriers
3. X-linked
4. Multifactoral, genes, and environment
   a. Combined influences of factors above a threshold
5. Chromosomal abnormalities

## XII. GENETIC CELLULAR CHANGE

A. Improper sex division at time of fertilization

B. Altered gene or genes from inheritance

## XIII. GENETIC AND CONGENITAL DISORDERS

1. Cleft lip
2. Cleft palate
3. Color vision deficiency
4. Cystic fibrosis
5. Down syndrome
6. Dwarfism
7. Galactosemia
8. Hemochromatosis
9. Hemophilia
10. Klinefelter's syndrome
11. Phenylketonuria (PKU)
12. Spina bifida
13. Talipes
14. Turner's syndrome

## XIV. SYSTEM INTERACTION

A. Cystic fibrosis–endocrine, digestive, and respiratory

B. Hemochromatosis–circulatory, musculoskeletal, integumentary, and reproductive

## XV. AGE-RELATED BODY CHARACTERISTICS

## XVI. DISCOVERIES IN HUMAN GENETICS

A. Human Genome Project
  1. Sequencing of DNA
  2. Location of genes
  3. Genetic map
  4. First drafts published in 2001
  5. About 26,000–40,000 genes
  6. 3 billion code of DNA
  7. Providing information, cancer therapy

B. Disease identification and treatment

C. Employment and insurance considerations
  1. Discrimination
  2. Pre-existing classifications

D. Predicting disease

E. BRAC analysis

F. Psychological effects

G. Ethical, legal, social questions

## XVII. GENETIC TECHNIQUES

A. Polymerase chain reaction

B. DNA fingerprinting

C. Genetic counseling

D. Gene therapy

E. Genetic engineering
  1. Oncogenes

F. Manipulating cellular structure controversy

## XVIII. STEM CELL RESEARCH

A. Scientists believe tissue could be regenerated

B. Stem cells can be embryonic or adult
  1. Embryonic
    a. Obtained from inner cell mass of embryo
    b. Potential to develop into all or nearly all tissues of the body
  2. Adult
    a. Unspecialized
    b. Can renew themselves
    c. Can become specialized to yield cells from original tissue
    d. Induced pluripotent stem cells are adult cells which have the potential to develop into all or nearly all of the tissues of the body

## XIX. TISSUES

A. Cells of the same type joined together for a common purpose

B. Made up of 60–99% water, with various substances dissolved in it

1. Dehydration is an insufficient amount of tissue fluid
2. Edema is an excess amount of tissue fluid, causing puffiness

C. Four main types

1. Epithelial tissue
    a. Covers surface of the body
    b. Forms body glands
        i. Endocrine
        ii. Exocrine
    c. Forms lining of body cavities
2. Connective tissue
    a. Supporting structure of the body
    b. Soft tissue
        i. Fat or adipose tissue
            (a) Stores fat as reserve of food
            (b) Fills in between tissue fibers
            (c) Insulates the body
            (d) Acts as padding
            (e) Subcutaneous skin layer
        ii. Dense connective tissue
            (a) Tendons, ligaments, and organ capsules
            (b) Soft and dense
            (c) Supports and protects organs
            (d) Lends elasticity to arterial walls
        iii. Blood and lymphatic vessels, lymph, blood, and blood cells
            (a) Role in repairing body tissue
            (b) Scar tissue development
            (c) Keloid tissue
    c. Hard tissue
        i. Cartilage
            (a) Tough, elastic material found between bones of spine and at end of long bones
            (b) Acts as a shock absorber
            (c) Found also in ear, nose, and voice box, providing shape
        ii. Bone (osseous tissue)
            (a) Living material
            (b) Easily repairs itself when damaged
3. Nerve tissue
    a. Made up of neurons

b. Types

i. Sensory neuron picks up and sends stimulus toward spinal cord and brain

ii. Interneuron carries impulse from one neuron to another

iii. Motor neuron receives an impulse and sends a message, which causes a reaction

c. Makes up nerves, brain, and spinal cord

d. Clusters form nerve tissue

i. Spinal cord

ii. Peripheral nerves

(a) Myelin sheath

(b) Neurilemma

iii. Surgical repair if sheathed

iv. Brain, spinal cord, eye, and ear are not sheathed or repairable by surgery

4. Muscular tissue

a. Contracts on stimulation

b. Types

i. Voluntary is skeletal

ii. Involuntary is cardiac and visceral (smooth)

## XX. ORGANS

A. Two or more tissues working together to perform a specific function

## XXI. SYSTEMS

A. Organs of the body that join together for a particular function

B. Types

1. Digestive
2. Integumentary
3. Skeletal
4. Muscular
5. Respiratory
6. Circulatory
7. Urinary
8. Nervous
9. Endocrine
10. Reproductive
11. Immune

# CHAPTER ACTIVITIES

1. Demonstrate the different planes by cutting a piece of fruit into appropriate sections.
2. Demonstrate diffusion by placing a cube of sugar in a cup of coffee. *Note:* Cup should be made from clear glass.
3. Have students practice identifying organs and describing their locations using illustrations or an anatomical model.
4. Ask students to work in pairs to identify directional terms on each other.

5. Draw two outlines of a body torso on a sheet of paper, duplicate copies, and have students illustrate and label the four and nine anatomical divisions of the abdomen.
6. Assign oral reports on individual genetic defects. When the students present their findings, everyone has an opportunity to hear and learn.

## ANSWERS TO CHECK YOUR KNOWLEDGE QUESTIONS

1. The science of the function of cells, tissues, and organs of the body is called:
   a. anatomy.
   **b. physiology.**
   c. pathophysiology.
   d. homeostasis.
2. An individual is standing erect, with arms down to the sides and the palms of the hands facing forward. What is this position?
   a. Midsagittal
   b. Frontal
   **c. Anatomic**
   d. Anterior
3. What are the names of the two main cavities of the body?
   a. Abdominal and pelvic
   b. Abdominal and ventral
   c. Anterior and ventral
   **d. Anterior and posterior**
4. RUQ, RLQ, LUQ, and LLQ refer to what?
   **a. The abdominal quadrants**
   b. The regions of the abdomen
   c. The thoracic cavity
   d. The abdomenopelvic cavity
5. Diffusion is:
   a. the movement of water or a solvent through a selected permeable membrane.
   **b. the movement of solutes and liquid molecules evenly within a medium.**
   c. the engulfing of bacteria or damaged cells.
   d. the movement of water across a membrane as a result of gravity or pressure.
6. When the internal environment is functioning properly and all the organs and tissues of the body are performing their appropriate tasks, this is known as:
   a. mutation.
   b. osmosis.
   **c. hemostasis.**
   d. equilibrium.

7. What are the four main types of tissues?

    **a. Epithelial, connective, nerve, and muscular**

    b. Endocrine, exocrine, muscular, and nerve

    c. Muscular, bone, nerve, skin

    d. Connective, osseous, nerve, muscular

# CHAPTER 24 The Nervous System

## LESSON OUTLINE

### I. THE NERVOUS SYSTEM

A. Organizes and coordinates all the body's functions

B. Two main divisions

1. The central nervous system (CNS) consists of the brain and the spinal cord
2. The peripheral nervous system includes all nerves that connect the CNS to every organ and body area

### II. THE NERVE CELL OR NEURON

A. The basic functioning unit of the nervous system

B. Sensory neurons receive stimuli

C. Connecting neurons, also called associative or internuncial neurons, transmit impulses

D. Motor neurons deliver response actions to muscles and glands

E. Parts of the neuron

1. Cell body
2. Nucleus
3. Nerve fibers
    a. Dendrites carry impulses toward the cell body
    b. An axon is a single nerve fiber that carries impulses away from the cell body
    c. Schwann cells around axons of peripheral nerves form the myelin sheath
    d. Nerve from sense organs to brain is a sensory or afferent nerve
    e. Nerve from brain or spinal cord to muscle or organ is a motor or efferent nerve
    f. Nerve with both fibers is a mixed nerve

### III. MEMBRANE EXCITABILITY

A. Process in which electrical charges create impulses in nerves

1. A chemical process produced by the exchange of potassium and sodium ions across the neuron membrane (sodium-potassium pump)
2. A stimulus increases the permeability of the neuron to positive sodium ions, leaving a slight excess of negative ions outside the membrane, producing the beginning of the nerve impulse

B. Synaptic cleft is the minute space between axon terminal and dendrite

C. Neurotransmitters

1. Chemical compounds released from an axon that stimulate the dendrite (Figure 24-1)
2. Mental disorders; Prozac action, SSRIs, SSNRIs
3. Tetanus is a disease condition produced by *Clostridium tetani*
    a. Neurotoxin release by the bacteria is toxic to motor neurons
    b. Produces excessive contraction of muscles
4. Show Media Link, "Firing of a Neuron"

## IV. PERIPHERAL NERVOUS SYSTEM

A. 12 pairs of cranial nerves
   1. Connect brain directly to the sense organs
   2. Can have both sensory and motor nerves
B. 31 pairs of spinal nerves
   1. Mixed nerves
   2. Enter and leave the spinal column
   3. Function is to conduct impulses necessary for sensations and voluntary movements
C. Simple reflex action involves impulses going to spinal cord and back
D. Complex reflex action relays impulse to spinal cord, brain, and then back down spinal cord and out to appropriate nerves

## V. AUTONOMIC NERVOUS SYSTEM

A. Regulates the body's automatic or involuntary functions
B. Prepares the body in "flight-fright" mechanism
C. Has two divisions working together to maintain homeostasis in the body
   1. Sympathetic nervous system
      a. Accelerates the activity in the smooth, involuntary muscles
      b. Increases heart rate and respirations
      c. Raises blood pressure
      d. Slows activity in the digestive tract
   2. Parasympathetic nervous system
      a. Counters the actions of the sympathetic system
      b. Has two important nerves
         i. Vagus, which extends from the brain to the neck, chest, and upper abdominal organs
         ii. Pelvic nerve, which exits the spinal cord around hip area and branches into lower abdominal and pelvic organs

## VI. CENTRAL NERVOUS SYSTEM

A. The brain
   1. Mass of over 100 billion nerve cells
   2. Weighs about 3 pounds
   3. Groups of specialized cells produce memory, language, emotion, perception
   4. Discoveries
B. The structure and function of the brain
   1. Protected by meninges and cranium
   2. Two hemispheres
   3. Five brain divisions
      a. Cerebrum
         i. Largest part
         ii. Frontal lobe

(a) Responsible for emotions, personality, and intellectual functions

(b) Controls speech

iii. Occipital lobe

(a) Responsible for vision by transmitting the nerve impulses via the optic nerve to the occipital lobe from the eye

iv. Parietal lobe

(a) Between frontal and occipital lobes

(b) Responsible for many sensory and motor actions

v. Temporal lobe

(a) auditory nerve; sense of hearing

(b) olfactory area; sense of smell

b. Cerebellum

i. Located below the back of the cerebrum

ii. Controls smooth muscle movements to maintain balance, posture, and muscle tone

C. Brain stem

1. Medulla oblongata

a. Adjoins the spinal cord

b. Influences the heart, lungs, and blood pressure

2. Pons

a. Located above medulla

b. Conducts reflex actions with chewing, tasting, and secreting saliva; helps regulate breathing

3. Midbrain

a. Superior to pons

b. Controls eye movements

4. Thalamus relays impulses to and from brain

5. Hypothalamus

a. Located below the thalamus

b. Connected to the pituitary gland, midbrain, and thalamus

c. Major center for controlling the autonomic nervous system

i. Controls most of the functioning of internal organs

ii. Controls appetite, body temperature, wakefulness, and certain emotions

6. Other structures

a. Meninges is made up of three layers

i. Pia mater

(a) Innermost layer

(b) Nourishes nerve tissue

ii. Arachnoid

(a) Middle layer

(b) Delicate, lacelike membrane

iii. Dura mater

(a) Outer layer

(b) Protects the CNS

iv. Subdural and subarachnoid spaces

b. Cavities of the brain and spinal cord

i. Four ventricles are interconnected

ii. Filled with cerebrospinal fluid

(a) Acts as a shock absorber

(b) Transports nutrients to the brain and spinal cord

## VII. DIAGNOSTIC TESTS

A. Arteriogaphy

B. Coma scale

C. Computerized axial tomography

D. Electroencephalography

E. Electromyography and nerve conduction studies

F. Lumbar puncture

G. Magnetic resonance imaging, MRI

H. Myelography

I. Positron emission tomography

J. Skull X-ray

## VIII. DISEASES AND DISORDERS (CONSULT TEXT)

A. Alzheimer's disease

1. Progressive, degenerative disease affecting the brain
2. Gradual memory loss, personality change
3. Cause unknown
4. No known cure
5. Eight steps to reduce risk
6. Alzheimer's Association 10 warning signs
7. Genetic possibilities

B. Amyotrophic lateral sclerosis

1. Lou Gehrig's disease
2. Causes degeneration of the upper motor nerves in the medulla oblongata and the lower nerves of the spinal cord
3. Weakness, speech problems
4. No effective treatment

C. Bell's palsy

1. Disease of the seventh cranial nerve
2. Causes weakness or paralysis of one side of face, drool, cannot close eye
3. Steroids are used in treatment

D. Cerebral palsy

1. Common crippler of children
2. No cure, only supportive treatment

E. Encephalitis
   1. Severe brain inflammation
   2. Many different disease vectors
F. Epilepsy
   1. Abnormal electrical impulses from the neurons of the brain
   2. Characterized by either petit or grand mal seizures
   3. Treatment is drug therapy to control seizures
G. Essential tremor
   1. Involuntary shaking
   2. Differentiate from Parkinson's
   3. Unknown etiology
   4. Treat with Inderal or Mysoline
H. Headaches
   1. Most common are vascular, muscle contraction (tension), or traction-inflammatory
   2. Migraine is severe throbbing vascular headache caused by initial constricting then dilation of blood vessels
   3. Medications are preventive, abortive, and rescue
I. Herpes zoster (shingles)
   1. Acute inflammation of the dorsal root ganglion
   2. Herpes virus also causes chickenpox
J. Hydrocephalus
   1. Excessive accumulation of cerebro-spinal fluid (CSF) within the ventricles of the brain
   2. Surgery is only treatment
K. Meningitis
   1. Bacterial-induced inflammation of the meninges
   2. Bacterial meningitis mortality is 70–100% if untreated
   3. Treatment consists of antibiotics, medication to reduce cerebral edema, pain relievers, and an anticonvulsant
   4. Age-related body characteristics related to bacterial meningitis
L. Multiple sclerosis
   1. The demyelination of the white matter of the brain and spinal cord
   2. Cause unknown
   3. Treatments relieve symptoms and may hasten remission
M. Neuralgia
   1. Cutting pain along course of nerve
   2. Term used to describe general nerve pain
N. Paralysis
   1. Temporary or permanent loss of function
   2. Two divisions
      a. Spastic—upper motor neurons
      b. Flaccid—lower motor neurons
   3. Important to prevent damage to brain and spinal cord
   4. Reduce probability of stroke
   5. Prevent injuries

O. Hemiplegia is paralysis on one side of the body due to damage on the opposite side of the brain

P. Paraplegia is motor or sensory loss in the lower extremities due to spinal cord injury

Q. Quadriplegia is paralysis of the arms, legs, and body below an injury to the cervical spinal cord

R. Parkinson's disease

1. Condition characterized by severe muscle rigidity
2. No cure

S. Reye's syndrome

1. Childhood disease causing fatty infiltration of the liver and increased intracranial pressure (ICP)
2. Prognosis depends on degree of CNS depression from ICP

T. Sciatica

1. Inflammation of the sciatic nerve
2. Treatment is or cold applications, heat, and use of traction

U. Spinal cord defects

1. Result from failure of tissues to properly close during first three months of development
2. Folic acid deficiency
3. Types are spina bifida, meningocele, and myelomeningocele

V. Subarachnoid hemorrhage is a collection of blood in the subarachnoid space

W. Subdural hematoma is a collection of blood in the subdural space

X. Tourette syndrome

1. Neurological disorder characterized by "tics"
2. Usually facial tic first; often voice, limbs
3. Indefinite cause
4. Psychotherapy and medication

Y. Transient ischemic attack (TIA)

1. Warning sign of impending thrombotic cerebrovascular accident (CVA)
2. Aspirin is used to reduce blood clot formation

Z. Trigeminal neuralgia

1. Disorder of the 5th cranial nerve
2. Episodes of excruciating facial pain
3. Treatment may be medication to deaden the nerve or surgical procedure to sever the nerve

AA. Tumor

1. Malignant brain tumors especially difficult to treat
2. Common cause of death from cancer in children
3. Cause changes in the CNS
4. Unknown cause
5. Treated with resection if possible

## IX. SYSTEM INTERACTION

A. Cerebral palsy

B. Spina bifida

## CHAPTER ACTIVITIES

1. Demonstrate simple reflex behaviors: patellar tendon reflex, Achilles tendon reflex, plantar reflex (firm stroking of lateral surface of dorsum of foot), Babinski reflex (pathological after age 1), and ciliospinal reflex (touch back of neck with ice and observe pupils).
2. Demonstrate the knee jerk test using a percussion hammer. Have students divide into pairs and, under supervision, administer the test to each other.
3. When discussing the autonomic nervous system, suddenly startle a student without warning. Immediately ask the student to describe his or her awareness of heart and lung activity. Hopefully, the heartbeat will be rapid and bounding and the respiration rate increased.
4. Assign additional oral reports on any of the diagnostic tests, diseases, or disorders.
5. Visit a radiology department to view X-ray equipment, scanning devices, and a CAT scanner. Ask the X-ray technician to show examples of different radiological study films.

## ANSWERS TO CHECK YOUR KNOWLEDGE QUESTIONS

Select the most appropriate answers to the following multiple choice questions:

1. The space between a neuron dendrite and the next neuron axon is called:
   a. membrane potential.
   **b. synapse.**
   c. axon terminal.
   d. neurotransmitter.
2. A ganglion is:
   a. a collection of nerve endings.
   b. a type of nerve cell.
   c. part of the gray matter of the spine.
   **d. a group of sensory nerve cell bodies.**
3. The autonomic nervous system (ANS) includes all but:
   a. the sympathetic division.
   b. the parasympathetic division.
   c. nerves, ganglia, and plexuses.
   **d. motor and sensory nerves.**
4. The largest part of the brain is:
   a. the cerebellum.
   **b. the cerebrum.**
   c. the frontal lobe.
   d. the parietal lobe.
5. The outermost meninges is:
   a. the arachnoid.
   b. the pia mater.
   c. the duramoid.
   **d. the dura mater.**

6. The cavities and hollow spaces within the brain are called the:

   **a. ventricles.**

   b. subarachnoid space.

   c. subdural space.

   d. hypothalamus.

7. Electroencephalography:

   a. measures peripheral muscle activity.

   b. shows irregularities of the spinal cord.

   c. measures the level of spinal fluid.

   **d. measures the brain's electrical signals.**

8. Alzheimer's disease is characterized by:

   **a. gradual memory loss, personality change, inability to care for self.**

   b. wasting away of the muscles.

   c. a sudden onset with weakness or paralysis.

   d. involuntary shaking of the hands and head.

9. Multiple sclerosis is the result of:

   a. abnormal brain chemistry, premature birth or brain injury.

   b. acute inflammation of the dorsal root ganglion.

   **c. destruction of the myelin sheath of the nerves.**

   d. excessive accumulation of cerebral spinal fluid.

10. Parkinson's disease causes:

    a. severe headache, sensitivity to light, and nausea.

    b. permanent muscle contracture and underdevelopment.

    **c. muscle rigidity, drooling, and hand tremors.**

    d. weakness and paralysis on one side of the face.

# CHAPTER 25 The Senses

## LESSON OUTLINE

### I. SENSES

A. Allow human beings to interact with and react to the environment through the ability to see, hear, taste, smell, and touch

B. Requires brain, cranial nerves, and sense organs

C. Receptors

1. Composed of nerve endings

2. Respond to stimuli

    a. Environmental chemical energy by chemoreceptors with sense of taste and smell

    b. Mechanical energy by mechanoreceptors with sense of hearing and touch

    c. Photoreceptors in eyes with sense of sight

    d. Thermoreceptors of skin and connective tissue

3. Stimuli produce action potential in nerve

### II. THE EYE AND THE SENSE OF SIGHT

A. Works like a camera

B. Protected by a bony socket in the skull

C. Sclera

1. Tough outermost layer

2. The "white" of the eye

3. Maintains the shape of the eyeball

D. Extraocular or intrinsic muscles

1. Contract and relax to move eye

2. Permits large field of vision

E. Choroid covering is a collection of blood vessels that form the blood supply to the retina.

F. Focusing the image

1. The retina is the innermost layer of the eye that acts like the surface of film in a camera

2. The crystalline lens of the eye focuses light rays onto the retina

3. Ciliary body muscles change shape of lens for accommodation

G. Controlling light

1. The iris acts like the aperture in a camera

2. The iris is the colored portion of the eye

3. The pupil is the hole in the center of the iris

4. Melanin determines color

5. Controls light with muscle fibers

H. Cornea

1. Transparent extension of sclera in front of pupil

2. Has pain and touch receptors

3. Curvature corrects portion of vision
4. Abnormal shape causes astigmatism

I. Surface membranes

1. Conjuctiva
    a. Mucous membrane that lines the inner surface of the eyelids and causes sclera
    b. Protects the eye
2. Lacrimal glands secrete tears to moisten and clean the eye

J. Cavities and humors

1. Two main areas
    a. Anterior chamber, between iris and cornea
    b. Posterior chamber, between iris and lens
2. Aqueous humor
    a. A salty, clear fluid
    b. Circulates between chambers.
    c. Maintains curvature of cornea
    d. Assists in the refraction process
3. Vitreous humor
    a. Fills cavity behind the lens
    b. Jellylike substance
    c. Aids in the refraction process
    d. Maintains shape of eyeball
    e. Loss of humor may result in enucleation, the removal of eye

K. Retina

1. The inside layer of multilayered nervous tissue
2. Cones
    a. Sensitive to colors
    b. Function best in well-lighted areas
    c. Located mostly in the fovea centralis
3. Rods
    a Very sensitive to light
    b Used for dark or dim light vision
4. Optic disc (blind spot) is where the optic nerve exits the retina

L. The path of light

1. Light passes through the parts of the eye that refract the light rays (cornea, aqueous humor, pupil, lens, vitreous humor, and retina)
2. Light is focused on the retina
3. Transformed into nerve impulses and sent to brain to interpret the signals

M. Refraction error occurs if the rays are not refracted properly; vision is distorted (Figure 25–3)

1. Myopia is nearsightedness
2. Hyperopia is farsightedness
3. Refractive errors can be corrected by glasses

## III. DISEASES AND DISORDERS OF THE EYE

A. Age-related macular degeneration (AMD) is a disease affecting retina and alters the visual field
    1. Leading cause of blindness in United States.
    2. Dry type
    3. Wet type
    4. Possible help from artificial retina
B. Amblyopia occurs when one eye does not develop properly, causing blurring of vision
C. Arcus senilis is a condition accompanying normal aging
D. Blepharitis is the inflammation from excess secretion by the sebaceous glands
E. Cataracts occur from the gradual development of opacity (cloudiness) of the lens
F. Conjunctivitis (pinkeye) is an inflammation of the conjunctiva by bacteria or a virus
G. Corneal abrasion is a scratch or trauma to the cornea
H. Corneal ulcers develop from an infection infiltration of the cornea
I. Diabetic retinopathy is a vascular retinopathy from juvenile or adult-onset diabetes
J. Glaucoma
    1. Excessive intraocular pressure resulting in atrophy of the optic nerve
    2. Result of too much aqueous humor or blocked drainage
    3. Chronic open-angle from blockage of aqueous flow
        a. Insidious symptoms of painless, loss of peripheral vision, seeing halos, and difficulty seeing at night
        b. Increased IOP destroys nerve fibers causing "cupping."
        c. Treat with eye drops or laser. Trabeculectomy if treatments insufficient.
    4. Acute close-angle from anatomical obstruction
        a. Rapid onset where pain, emergency
        b. Treated with aggressive drugs and peripheral iridotomy.
        c. Bilateral treatment to prevent attack in other eye.
        d. Blindness if not treated within a few days
K. Hordeolum (stye) is a localized infection of a gland of the eyelid
L. Iritis is an inflammation of the iris from illness or trauma
M. Myopia, also called nearsightedness, due to large eye, longer
    1. Radial keratotomy procedure, rare
    2. Eximer
    3. Lens extraction
    4. With IOL installed
N. Presbyopia
    1. Loss of elasticity causing the lens not to focus properly
    2. Part of normal aging
    3. Correct with eyeglasses or contact lenses
O. Ptosis is drooping of the upper eyelid
P. Retinal detachment is the separation of the retina from the choroid layer
    1. Three main types
    2. Treated with laser

3. Cold and gas treatment
4. Scleral buckle
5. Virectomy

Q. Strabismus occurs when one eye deviates from normal gaze

## IV. EYE PROTECTION

A. Goggles and safety glasses of impact-resistant glass

B. First aid with injury

C. Prompt medical attention

## V. SHOW MEDIA LINK: "VISION"

## VI. THE EAR AND THE SENSE OF HEARING

A. The ear controls the functions of hearing and balance

B. Three main sections

1. Outer ear
    a. Pinna or auricle
        i. Visible part of the ear
        ii. Picks up vibration
    b. External auditory canal
        i. Tube or canal from outer ear to tympanic membrane
        ii. Sound waves travel through the canal
    c. Tympanic membrane
        i. Separates outer ear from middle ear
        ii. Vibrates when sound hits it
2. Middle ear
    a. Malleus bone vibrates from tympanic membrane
    b. Incus is in turn vibrated by malleus
    c. Stapes
        i. Is moved by incus
        ii. Pushes against fluid in vestibule of inner ear
    d. Eustachian tube
        i. Connects middle ear to the throat
        ii. Equalizes air pressure in middle ear
        iii. Pathway for ear infections
3. Inner ear
    a. Vibrations continue to the cochlea
        i. Shaped like a snail's shell
        ii. Contains the organ of Corti
            (a) Receptor for sound waves
            (b) Transmits the impulses to auditory nerve that goes to the brain

b. Three semicircular canals are responsible for maintaining equilibrium
c. Carries out functions of hearing and balance

## VII. DIAGNOSTIC TESTS (REFER TO CHAPTER 40)

A. Audiometry, Weber, and Rinne
B. Ventronystagmograph (VNG), measures eye movement to evaluate balance
C. MRI

## VIII. DISEASES AND DISORDERS OF THE EAR

A. Auditory canal obstruction occurs when a foreign object or cerumen (ear wax) blocks the canal
B. Hearing loss is due to lack of sound conduction or nerve loss, or both
   1. Sensorineural
   2. Conductive
   3. Presbycusis
C. Ménière's disease is the degeneration of the hair cells in the inner ear
   1. Vertigo
   2. Tinnitus
D. Motion sickness results from excessive stimulation of the inner ear receptors or confusion between the visual stimulus and movement perception
E. Otitis externa is a bacterial infection of the external auditory canal
F. Otitis media is an infection of the inner ear due to respiratory infection or obstruction of the eustachian tube
G. Otosclerosis
   1. Most common cause of conductive deafness
   2. Results from formation of spongy bone that immobilizes the stapes
H. Presbycusis is hearing loss due to the effect of aging

## X. THE NOSE AND THE SENSE OF SMELL

A. Smell is due to the olfactory receptors in the upper part of the nasal cavity
   1. Chemoreceptors are stimulated by molecules that are dissolved by the mucous secretions
   2. Carried to the brain by the olfactory nerve

## X. DISEASES AND DISORDERS OF THE NOSE

A. Epistaxis is a nosebleed
B. Nasal polyps are benign growths that may obstruct the airways
C. Rhinitis (allergic) is a reaction to airborne allergens

## XI. THE TONGUE AND THE SENSE OF TASTE

A. Taste is dependent on receptors on the tongue
B. All substances must be moistened to be tasted

## XII. DISEASES AND DISORDERS OF THE MOUTH AND TONGUE

A. Candidiasis, also called thrush, is a fungal infection of the mucus membranes

B. Glossitis is an inflammation of the tongue

C. Oral cancer can be due to chewing tobacco or snuff

## XIII. THE SKIN AND THE SENSE OF TOUCH

A. Contact receptor on the body

1. Pain
2. Touch
3. Heat
4. Pressure
5. Traction
6. Cold
7. Tickle

B. Protects by allowing the body to react to its environment

# CHAPTER ACTIVITIES

1. Have students dry their tongues thoroughly, then sprinkle a few grains of salt or sugar on their tongues. Have them describe the taste of these materials without saliva.
2. Provide each student with a flashlight and dim the room lights. Instruct the students to concentrate on the reaction of the pupil to light.
3. Have students observe the inability to see colors well in dim light.
4. Have students move the eyes in inner, outer, upward, and downward positions and observe the feeling of tension in the muscles of the eye.
5. Demonstrate sensory perceptions to blindfolded student volunteer(s). Present different familiar objects to be tested by the senses:

SMELL: Wave each of the following under the nose: garlic bud, vanilla, chocolate, perfume, soap, alcohol.

TASTE: Drop each of the following on the tongue: lemon juice, salty water, almond extract, sugar water.

Try an experiment: Grasp and hold the tongue with a gauze pad. Thoroughly dry it with another gauze pad, then place a drop of lemon juice on the sweet area of the tongue, to test the student's ability to perceive. Try sweet on sweet, sweet on the sour area, etc. Be sure the student does not know what you are using.

TOUCH: Place familiar objects into a paper sack and allow a student to put a hand into the sack and determine, by feel, what the objects are. (Be sure to keep the objects out of sight.) Use a coin, paper clip, safety pin, button, grape, rubber band, and other familiar objects.

HEARING: Place objects producing sound near the ear to be identified, such as the ticking of a watch, the stapling of paper, crumpling of paper, snapping of fingers, and striking of a match (usually results in the student moving away and pulling off the blindfold).

# ANSWERS TO CHECK YOUR KNOWLEDGE QUESTIONS

1. The outside of the eye is covered with a tough membrane called the:
   a. retina.
   b. sclera.
   **c. choroid.**
   d. cornea.
2. When the ciliary body focuses the lens for near or far vision, it is known as:
   a. refraction.
   b. astigmatism.
   c. ciliary contraction.
   **d. accommodation.**
3. The amount of light entering the eye is controlled by the muscles of the:
   **a. iris.**
   b. cornea.
   c. lens.
   d. pupil.
4. The area of the retina where vision is sharpest is called the:
   a. optic disc.
   **b. fovea centralis.**
   c. vision receptor.
   d. myopia.
5. When a cataract develops,
   a. a grayish-white circle appears around the cornea.
   **b. the lens becomes cloudy.**
   c. the macula has thinned.
   d. the pupil dilates.
6. Glaucoma is the result of:
   a. improper drainage of the vitreous humor.
   b. increased pressure against the sclera.
   **c. increased interocular pressure.**
   d. excessive of blood supply to the eye.
7. The middle ear contains the:
   a. tympanic membrane, malleus, and stapes.
   b. cochlea, malleus, and incur.
   c. malleus, stapes, and semicircular canals.
   **d. malleus, incus, and stapes.**
8. Meniere's disease is characterized by:
   **a. ringing in the ears and vertigo.**
   b. pain and redness of the tympanic membrane.
   c. loss of hearing.
   d. motion sickness.

9. The most common cause of conductive deafness is:
   a. presbycusis.
   b. otitis media.
   c. tinnitus.
   **d. otosclerosis.**
10. Nasal polyps are:
    a. developed from infected hair follicles.
    **b. benign growths in the nose.**
    c. malignant growths in the nose.
    d. the main cause of nosebleeds.
11. Candidiasis:
    a. can lead to oral cancer.
    b. causes a red, swollen, and painful tongue.
    c. interferes with the sense of taste.
    **d. causes cream-colored patches of exudate on the tongue.**
12. Oral cancer may be caused by:
    a. use of alcohol and cigarettes.
    **b. use of chewing tobacco, snuff, and alcohol.**
    c. eating spicy foods.
    d. the lack of vitamins C and E.
13. A trabeculoplasty:
    a. instills a tiny tube through the tympanic membrane.
    b. reshapes the trabecula of the eye.
    c. removes the lens of the eye.
    **d. makes an opening to drain aqueous tumor.**
14. The videonystagmograph diagnostic test:
    **a. evaluates balance.**
    b. determines the need for a hearing aid.
    c. measures the intraocular pressure.
    d. determines the strength of the impulse in the auditory nerve.
15. Diabetic retinopathy involves the:
    a. sense of vision and muscular system.
    b. sense of vision and urinary system.
    **c. sense of vision and endocrine system.**
    d. sense of vision and respiratory.

# CHAPTER 26 The Integumentary System

## LESSON OUTLINE

### I. SKIN

A. Both a body system and an organ

B. 3,000 square inches

C. 15% of body weight

D. Essential to life

E. Continuous external and internal covering

### II. FUNCTIONS

A. Protection when intact

1. A barrier against bacteria
2. Protects from the sun
3. Protects from loss of fluids

B. Perception occurs when receptors register pain, heat, cold, and pressure

C. Temperature control

1. Works with the blood vessels to dilate or constrict
2. Sweat glands produce sweat that cools the skin surface

D. Absorption

1. Through hair follicles and glands
2. Useful to treat certain conditions with medications
   a. Time release of drug
   b. No digestive side effects

E. Excretion occurs when waste products, salt, and excess water are eliminated

### III. STRUCTURE OF THE SKIN

A. Epidermis

1. Top layer
2. Ridges that fit over papillae of dermis form whorls that make fingerprints
3. Cells constantly flake off and are replaced every 30–45 days

B. Dermis

1. Contains blood vessels, nerves, hair follicles, and sweat and oil glands
2. "True skin"
3. Papillae create uneven surface

C. Subcutaneous

1. Innermost layer of skin
2. Filled with fat globules, blood vessels, and nerves

D. Characteristics
   1. Keratin, collagen, and fat in young skin
   2. Loss of fat and elastic fibers cause wrinkles
E. Sweat glands are tiny coiled tubes in the dermis leading to the surface
F. Sebaceous glands (oil)
   1. Located in or near hair follicles
   2. Produce oil to prevent hair or skin from being dry and brittle
   3. Plugged oil glands produce a blackhead or pimple, resulting in acne
G. Hair
   1. Each has a root, a follicle, and a hair shaft
   2. Attached to each follicle is an involuntary muscle that reacts to emotion or coldness, called goose flesh
   3. Pigment
      a. Gives hair its color
      b. White hair is caused by air in cells rather that pigment
H. Hair and nails are composed of hard keratin
   1. Does not slough
   2. Requires cutting

## IV. SKIN COLOR

A. Determined by pigments in epidermis
   1. Melanin is produced by melanocytes
      a. Brownish-black pigment
      b. Protect against ultraviolet light
   2. Erythema (sunburn), reddened skin color due to dilation of superficial blood vessels
   3. Freckles are melanin pigment
   4. Birthmarks
   5. Moles
   6. Albino
      a. Little or no pigment in the skin
      b. Eyes very sensitive to light due to lack of pigment

## V. THE SKIN AS A DIAGNOSTIC TESTING SITE

A. Usually for testing of allergies
B. Helps in identifying causative substances and treating allergic disorders

## VI. SKIN LESIONS

A. Refer to Table 26–1

## VII. SHOW MEDIA LINK: "THE SKIN"

## VIII. DISEASES AND DISORDERS OF THE SKIN

A. Acne vulgaris is the inflammation of the follicles of sebaceous glands
B. Alopecia is the loss of hair
   1. Scarring
   2. Non-scarring
   3. Physiologic
   4. Areata (idiopathic)
   5. Trichotillomania
   6. Chemotherapy related
C. Cancer
   1. Basal cell carcinoma
      a. Nodulo-ulcerative lesions appear yellow to white and waxy
      b. Superficial
      c. Sclerosing
   2. Squamous cell carcinoma is predisposed by sunlight, premalignant lesions, X-ray therapy, and environmental carcinogens
   3. Malignant melanoma
      a. Develops from pigment-producing melanocytes
      b. Four types
         i. Superficial spreading
         ii. Nodular
         iii. Lentigo maligna
         iv. Acral lentiginous
      c. Major cause is exposure to the sun
      d. Surgery and/or chemotherapy and radiation
D. Cellulitis
   1. Diffuse inflammation of the skin
   2. Caused by streptococcus or staphylococcus
E. Dermatitis is an inflammation of the skin
F. Eczema is noncontagious, dry, red, itchy, and scaly skin in acute and chronic types
G. Folliculitis results from staphylococcal infection of the hair follicle
H. Furuncles (boils)
I. Carbuncule
J. Herpes simplex (cold sores)
K. Herpes zoster
   1. Acute infectious process
   2. Called shingles
L. Hirsutism is excessive body hair growth in women and children

M. Impetigo
   1. Caused by either streptococcal or staphylococcal infection
   2. Contagious, superficial skin infection in young children

N. Keloid is a scar with excessive dense tissue

O. Lyme disease is caused by a spirochete-infested deer tick
   1. Careful removal
   2. Testing
   3. Bull's eye rash

P. Pediculosis is from parasitic lice
   1. Capitis, head lice, are found primarily among children
   2. Corporis, body lice, live in clothing seams and feed on the host
   3. Pubis, commonly called crabs, in pubic area

Q. Poison ivy is a dermatitis caused by contact with the plant
   1. Itching and burning
   2. Blisters that break and lose serum

R. Psoriasis
   1. Chronic disease
   2. Itching and red papules covered with silvery scales
   3. Cannot be cured

S. Ringworm
   1. Caused by a fungus
   2. Three types
      a. Tinea capitis (scalp)
      b. Tinea corporis (body)
      c. Tinea pedia (athlete's foot)

T. Rosacea
   1. Chronic skin eruption
   2. Dilation of small blood vessels
   3. Exact cause unknown

U. Scabies is a skin infection caused by the itch mite

V. Urticaria
   1. Hives
   2. Self-limiting reaction to allergens

W. Verrucae are warts, a benign viral infection
   1. Genital warts require prompt treatment

X. Wrinkles are due to environmental exposure and decrease in collagen
   1. Dermabrasion is a controlled scraping of the skin
      a. Microdermabrasion
   2. Chemical peel is chemosurgery with acid to remove skin
      a. Light, medium, and deep
   3. Laser resurfacing uses a controlled laser beam to vaporize skin surface

Y. Plastic surgery used to reshape the facial features
   1. Quadrilateral blepharoplasty to eyes
   2. Face lift to raise sagging features

## IX. AGE-RELATED BODY CHARACTERISTICS

A. Infants and small children
B. Teenagers
C. Aging adults
D. Aged

## X. SYSTEM INTERACTION

A. Lyme disease
B. Hirsutism

# CHAPTER ACTIVITIES

1. Have each student examine his or her own hair and nails and identify their parts.
2. Have students paint an area of iodine on the inner aspect of the arm and a small region on the palm of the hand, avoiding the creases. Let the areas dry. Place a square of bond paper over each iodine-painted area. Secure the paper with tape and leave for one hour. Remove the paper. The blue-black dots represent active sweat glands. Ask the students why one area has more than the other.
3. Have students observe their skin using a magnifying glass. See if they can determine the few surfaces where there are no hair follicles (palms, soles, and distal phalanx of fingers).
4. Instruct students to apply a hot, wet cloth to the inner surface of a partner's arm for two minutes and then remove it. Have them record their observations as to the skin color and note when the skin returns to normal. Have them describe what happened and explain why. Next, conduct the same experiment with ice wrapped in a wet cloth. *Note:* If skin color is dark, results may be difficult to observe.
5. If you have access to a microscope, have students obtain samples of skin flakes and hair to observe under the lens.
6. Using fingerpaint, have each student put the right thumbprint on the same piece of paper and observe the differences in patterns.
7. Demonstrate the skin's ability to perceive by blindfolding a student volunteer and touching the forearm with something hot, cold, and sharp, pinching the surface, pinching and retracting the skin, and tickling it.
8. Demonstrate the skin's ability to absorb by instructing the students to apply a specified amount of cream to a partner's forearm.

# ANSWERS TO CHECK YOUR KNOWLEDGE QUESTIONS

1. Giving medication by applying it to the skin is called:
   a. intramuscular.
   b. subcutaneous.
   c. intradermal.
   **d. transdermal.**

2. Which of the following cannot pass through the skin?
   a. Oxygen
   **b. Carbon monoxide**
   c. Vitamins
   d. Sex hormones
3. Which layer of skin contains blood vessels, nerves, hair follicles, sweat, and oil glands?
   a. Subcutaneous
   b. Epidermis
   c. Hypodermia
   **d. Dermis**
4. Patchy hair loss due to the pulling out of hair from a compulsive behavior is:
   a. alopecia.
   b. areata.
   c. physiologic loss.
   **d. trichotillomania.**
5. Which description does not reflect melanoma?
   a. Asymmetry
   **b. Defined border**
   c. Irregular pigmentation
   d. A diameter larger than 6 mm
6. Herpes simplex refers to lesions that:
   a. spread around one side of the body.
   b. are located in the genital area.
   c. are located on mucous membranes.
   **d. are located around the nose and mouth.**
7. A disease caused by a tick is:
   a. pediculosis.
   b. scabies.
   **c. Lyme disease.**
   d. ringworm.
8. Verrucae is the medical term for:
   a. ringworm.
   b. hives.
   c. shingles.
   **d. warts.**
9. Skin wrinkles are not the result of which of the following?
   a. Loss of collagen
   b. Increased size of elastic fibers
   c. Environmental exposure
   **d. Excessive rubbing of the skin**

10. A temporary red, itchy spot caused by an allergic reaction or an insect bite is called a:
    **a. wheal.**
    b. whorl.
    c. bulla.
    d. vesicle.
11. Elderly persons have skin that is:
    a. full of collagen.
    b. supple.
    c. excessively oily.
    **d. easily damaged.**
12. Hirsutism involves the:
    a. urinary, muscular, and reproductive systems.
    **b. integumentary, muscular, and reproductive systems.**
    c. muscular, nervous, and integumentary systems.
    d. skeletal, reproductive, and integumentary.

# HAPTER 27 The Skeletal System

## ESSON OUTLINE

### THE SKELETAL SYSTEM

A. Consists of organs called bones

B. Made up of two sections

1. Axial skeleton
    a. Spinal column
    b. Skull
    c. Rib cage
2. Appendicular skeleton
    a. Arms
    b. Hands
    c. Legs
    d. Feet
    e. Shoulders
    f. Pelvis

C. Primary purpose is to support the body

### . BONE STRUCTURE

A. Over 20% water

B. Main minerals

1 Calcium

3. Phosphorus

4. Magnesium

C. Organic matter

1. Primarily collagen
2. Forms matrix

### I. LONG BONES

A. Articulating surfaces at joints

B. Cancellous bone

C. Red marrow

D. Yellow marrow

E. Periosteum membrane

### '. NUMBER OF BONES

A. 270 at birth

B. 206 at adulthood

C. Difference between number at birth and adulthood due to fusion of bones

D. Smallest bones are malleus, incus, and stapes of middle ear

## V. FUNCTIONS OF THE SKELETON

A. Provides the framework to support the body's fat, muscles, and skin

B. Protects the body's vital organs

C. Serve as points of attachment for skeletal muscles

D. Gives shape to the body

E. Forms red and white blood cells and platelets

F. Stores most of the body's calcium supply

## VI. SPINAL COLUMN

A. Vertebrae
   1. Support head
   2. Keep the trunk erect
   3. Protect the spinal column

B. Sections
   1. Cervical has seven neck vertebrae
   2. Thoracic has 12 chest vertebrae
   3. Lumbar has five back vertebrae
   4. Sacral has one large vertebrae fused from five original bones
   5. Coccyx is four fused bones

C. Intervertebral cartilage disks
   1. Separate vertebrae
   2. Absorb shock
   3. Allow vertebrae to bend or twist

## VII. SKULL

A. Consists of a cranial and facial portion

B. Cranium
   1. Protects the brain from injury
   2. Composed of the fusion of eight cranial bones; main bones are:
      a. Frontal
      b. Two parietal bones
      c. Two temporal
      d. Occipital
   3. Facial bones
      a. Mandible
      b. Maxillae
      c. Zygomatic
      d. Other small bones
   4. Fontanels

a. Unossified space or "soft spot" located between the cranial bones

b. Allow for molding of skull during birth and for enlargement of skull as growth occurs

i. Found in newborn and infancy

ii. Close by second year

## III. SHOW MEDIA LINK: "HEAD INJURIES"

## X. RIB CAGE

A. 12 pairs of long slender bones attached to thoracic vertebrae and sternum (breast bone)

B. Top 10 pairs also attached to sternum by cartilage for flexibility to breathe

C. Two pairs floating

D. True ribs

1. First seven pairs of ribs

2. Attached directly to sternum and posterior to spine

E. False ribs

1. Last five pairs of ribs

2. Attached anteriorly to cartilage of rib above or have no anterior attachment

F. Xiphoid is attached to inferior edge of sternum

G. Other bones of rib cage

1. Clavicle (collar bone)

2. Scapula (shoulder blade)

3. Xiphoid process of sternum

## . LONG BONES

A. Bones of the extremities

B. Parts

1. Diaphysis is the main shaft

2. Epiphyses are the two ends

3. Metaphysis

C. Bones of the arm

1. Humerus is found in the upper arm

2. Radius

a. Found in lower arm

b. On thumb side

3. Ulna

a. Found in lower arm

b. On little finger side

D. Bones of the leg

1. Femur

a. Longest bone in body

b. Thigh bone

2. Tibia

a. Shin bone
b. Supporting bone of lower leg

3. Fibula is the smaller bone of lower leg
4. Patella is the kneecap

## XI. BONES OF THE HANDS

A. Carpals are the eight bones of the wrist
B. Metacarpals are the five bones forming each palm
C. Phalanges are the 14 bones of the fingers of each hand
   1. Form fingers and thumb
   2. Phalanx
      a Two sections on thumb
         i. Distal
         ii. Proximal
      b. Three sections on fingers
         i. Distal
         ii. Medial
         iii. Proximal

## XII. BONES OF THE FEET

A. Tarsals are the seven bones of the ankle
B. Metatarsals are the five bones forming the instep
C. Phalanges are the 14 bones of the toes of each foot
   1. Form the toes and big toe
   2. Phalanx
      a. Two sections on big toe
         i. Distal
         ii. Proximal
      b. Three sections on toes
         i. Distal
         ii. Medial
         iii. Proximal

## XIII. PELVIC GIRDLE

A. Provides structure of hip area
B. Os coxae are two large bones that are joined posteriorly at the sacrum
   1. Ilium is the top blade-staped portion
   2. Pubis is the anterior lower portion
      a. Attachment called symphysis pubis
   3. Ischium is the posterior lower portion
C. Acetabulum is the socket where the head of the femur fits

## XIV. JOINTS

A. Place where two or more bony parts join together

B. Ligaments are bands of connective tissue that hold long bones together at joints

C. Joint classification

1. Diarthrosis/synovial
    a. Movable
    b. Knee or elbow, which has action like that of hinge
    c. Shoulder or hip, which has action like that of ball and socket
2. Amphiarthrosis/cartilaginous
    a. Partially movable
    b. Vertebrae
3. Synarthrosis/fibrous
    a. Immovable
    b. Cranial suture
4. Diarthrotic joints
    a. Articular cartilage provides slippery surface
    b. Bursa, a saclike capsule
    c. Synovial cavity that secretes synovial fluid to lubricate joint
    c. Synovial membranes around and between tendons to lubricate and reduce friction
5. Synovial joints copied in devices
    a. Desk pen
    b. Hinges

## XV. FRACTURES

A. Types

1. Greenstick is a bone that cracks but doesn't break
2. Simple or closed
    a. Complete break
    b. No skin involvement
3. Compound or open
    a. Complete bone break
    b. Bone protrudes through skin
4. Impacted occurs when the broken ends are jammed into each other
5. Comminuted
    a. More than one fracture
    b. Bone fragments
6. Depressed occurs when a broken piece of skull is driven inward
7. Spiral occurs when the break winds around the bone
8. Colles fracture
    a. fracture of distal end of radius and/or ulna

B. Treatment

1. Immobilization of the affected part
2. Prevention of shock
3. Elevate
4. Coldpack or ice
5. Reducing the fracture
    a. Setting the bone after alignment
    b. Splint or cast keeps bone immobilized
6. Open reduction is a surgical procedure to achieve alignment of the bone and repair tissues and skin

C. Healing process
1. Callus
    a. Fibrous bridge around a fracture
    b. Accumulates calcium
    c. Becomes catilage
    d. Later becomes true bone
2. Embolus complication
    a. Mass of foreign material in blood vessels
        i. Fat droplets released from marrow
        ii. Catecholamines activate fatty acids
        iii. Fatty acids develop into embolus
    b. Can cause an infarction
        i. Blocked blood vessel
        ii. Can cause death
    c. Complication of healing process

## XVI. AMPUTATION

A. Loss of an extremity due to injury or disease
B. Phantom limb is the sensation that missing limb is present
C. Prosthesis is an artificial limb

## XVII. DIAGNOSTIC EXAMINATIONS

A. Arthroscopy permits visual inspection of a joint
B. Bones scan uses radioactive material and a scintillation camera
C. Computerized tomography (CT scan) allows three-dimensional views
D. Magnetic resonance imaging (MRI)
E. X-ray

## XVIII. DISEASES AND DISORDERS (SEE TEXT)

A. Arthritis
1. Osteoarthritis is the progressive deterioration of joint cartilage
2. Rheumatoid arthritis is chronic inflammatory disease attacking joints and surrounding tissue
3. Juvenile rheumatoid arthritis

B. Bursitis
   1. Inflammation of the bursa, a sac located around a joint containing lubricating fluids
   2. Occurs most often at the hip, shoulder, or knee
C. Carpal tunnel syndrome is the compression of the median nerve at the wrist
D. Congenital hip dysplasia
   1. Abnormality of the hip joint
   2. Present at birth
E. Dislocation is the displacement of bones at joint
F. Epicondylitis
   1. Tennis elbow
   2. Inflammation of the forearm extensor tendon at its attachment to the humerus
G. Gout is a metabolic disease resulting in severe joint pain
   1. Caused by urate deposits
   2. Drug induced
H. Hallux valgus
   1. Lateral deviation of the great toe with enlargement of the first metatarsal head
   2. Bunion formation, which is a bursa with a callus formation
I. Herniated disk is a soft gel-like material within an intervertebral disk that has been forced through its outer surface
   1. Spinal fusion
J. Kyphosis
   1. Roundback, humpback
   2. Bowing of the back at the thoracic level
   3. Adolescent and adult
K. Lordosis
   1. Swayback
   2. Abnormal anterior convex curvature of the lumbar spine
L. Lumbar myositis is an inflammation of the lumbar region muscles
M. Osteoporosis
   1. Metabolic bone disorder
   2. Loss of bone mass
   3. Porous, brittle, prone to fracture
   4. DEXA
   5. NTX
   6. National Osteoporosis Foundation risk analysis
N. Scoliosis
   1. Lateral curvature of the spine
   2. "S" curve appearance
   3. Infant, juvenile, and adolescent
O. Sprain
   1. Complete or incomplete tear of the ligaments of a joint
   2. R.I.C.E. treatment
      a. Rest

b. Ice
c. Compression
d. Elevation

P. Subluxation is the partial or incomplete dislocation of the articulating surfaces of joint bones

Q. Temporomandibular disorder (TMD) feels as though jaw is unhinged

### XIX. REPLACING BONE AND JOINTS

A. Injury

B. Cancer

C. Disease process

D. Borrow bone from own body, cadavers, or ocean coral

### XX. SYSTEM INTERACTION

A. Rheumatoid arthritis

B. Osteoporosis

## CHAPTER ACTIVITIES

1. Using a skeleton model, have students identify the bones of the body. This can be a game when students call out the bone and are given points for correct identification.
2. Using an anatomical chart, have students identify bones of the body.
3. Contact an orthopedic physician, nurse, or medical assistant who works in orthopedic practice, to discuss the common diseases and disorders of the skeletal system usually encountered in the office.
4. Contact an orthopedic physician or radiologist to obtain X-rays of fractures.
5. Visit a supplier of artificial limbs to observe the different types available and learn about the process of fitting a prosthesis.

## ANSWERS TO CHECK YOUR KNOWLEDGE QUESTIONS

1. An adult has how many bones?
   a. 207
   b. 270
   **c. 206**
   d. 260
2. The bone covering is called:
   a. marrow.
   b. cancellous.
   c. cortical.
   **d. periosteum.**
3. Sacral vertebrae are located in the:
   a. neck.
   b. chest.
   c. back.

**d. posterior pelvic girdle.**

4. The place where two or more bony parts join together is called a(n):

   a. diarthrosis.

   b. bursa.

   c. amphiarthrosis.

   **d. articulation.**

5. Arthroscopy is:

   **a. a surgical procedure to view inside a joint.**

   b. the injection of radioactive substance into a vein.

   c. a special X-ray of a joint.

   d. an imaging test using radio waves.

6. Rheumatoid arthritis is caused by:

   **a. a fault in the immune system.**

   b. a virus.

   c. an injury to the joint.

   d. wear and tear on the joint.

7. Carpal tunnel syndrome:

   a. develops after acute bursitis.

   **b. causes symptoms in the thumb and first two fingers.**

   c. causes deformities of the joint.

   d. is an inflammation of the forearm extensor tendon.

8. Lordosis refers to:

   a. the bowing of the back at the thoracic level.

   b. a lateral curvature of the spine.

   c. a backward curvature of the cervical area.

   **d. the abnormal anterior convex curvature of the lumbar spine.**

9. Subluxation is:

   a. a feeling the jaw is unhinged.

   **b. the incomplete dislocation of a joint.**

   c. the incomplete tear in the supporting ligaments of a joint.

   d. the deposit of urates at a joint.

10. Bones of the spinal column are separated by:

    a. marrow.

    b. ligaments.

    c. synovial fluid.

    **d. cartilage disks.**

11. Osteoporosis involves:

    a. skeletal, circulatory, and immune systems.

    **b. skeletal, digestive, and reproductive.**

    c. Immune, digestive, and skeletal.

    d. digestive, circulatory, and skeletal.

# CHAPTER 28 The Muscular System

## LESSON OUTLINE

### I. APPROXIMATELY 600 MUSCLES IN THE BODY

A. Muscles are composed of bundles of muscle fibers

B. After stimulation by the nerves, muscles contract

1. Motor unit
2. Twitch
3. Contraction causes movement
4. Repeated stimulation causes muscle cramps and spasms
5. Muscle recruitment

C. Glycogen changes to glucose to provide fuel for muscles and produce heat

### II. FUNCTIONS OF MUSCLES

A. Attach to bones to provide movement

B. Provide heat and energy

C. Keep body upright

D. Protect some internal organs, blood vessels, nerves

E. Provide protective padding

F. Add shape to the body

G. Aid in the return flow of blood

### III. MUSCLES GROW IN RELATION TO THE STRUCTURES TO WHICH THEY ARE ATTACHED

### IV. MUSCLE TYPES

A. Skeletal

1. Attached to bones
2. Permit movement
3. Also called voluntary muscle
4. Bundles and sheaths

B. Smooth

1. Found in internal organs except for the heart
2. Also called involuntary muscle

C. Cardiac

1. Found in heart
2. Involuntary control
3. Structure does not permit independent cell contraction
4. Produces heartbeat

### V. SKELETAL MUSCLE ACTION

A. Flexor

1. Bends a joint
2. Example is the biceps

B. Extensor
   1. Straightens a joint
   2. Example is the triceps
C. Muscle team
   1. Different muscles work together to produce movement
   2. Adduction is moving a body part toward midline
   3. Abduction is moving a body part away from midline

## VI. MUSCLE TONE

A. Muscles are partially contracted at all times even though they may not be in use
B. Loss of muscle tone
   1. Atrophy
      a. Muscles are not used for a long period
      b. Muscle becomes useless
   2. Contracture
      a. Flexor muscle becomes shorter
      b. Results in a permanently bent joint

## VII. MUSCLE ATTACHMENT

A. Tendon
   1. Strong fibrous structure attaches muscle to bone
   2. Do not stretch
   3. Achilles tendon is thickest and strongest tendon in body; attaches gastrocnemius to heel
B. Ligaments
   1. Connect bone to bone at joints
   2. Stretch
C. Fascia
   1. Sheetlike tough membrane
   2. Covers and protects the muscle tissue
   3. Aponeurosis
D. Origin or insertion
   1. Origin
      a. End that does not move
      b. Bone is the anchor
      c. Proximal
   2. Insertion
      a. End that moves bone when muscle contracts
      b. Distal

## II. SHEATHS

A. Protect muscles and tendons from friction

B. Bursa is a sac-shaped sheath

   1. Filled with fluid

   2. Acts as a cushion

      a. Elbow

      b. Knee

      c. Shoulder

## . MAJOR SKELETAL MUSCLES

A. Diaphragm

B. Obicularis oculi and orbicularis oris

C. Sternocleidomastoid

D. Trapezius

E. Pectoralis major

F. Intercostal

G. Abdominal muscles

   1. External oblique

   2. Internal oblique

   3. Transversus abdominus

   4. Rectus abdominus

H. Latissimus dorsi

I. Deltoid

J. Gluteus maximus

K. Sartorius

L. Quadriceps femoris

M. Tibialis anterior

N. Hamstring group

   1. Biceps femoris

   2. Semitendinosus

   3. Semimembranosus

   4. Portion of adductor magnus

O. Gastrocnemius

P. Achilles tendon

## MUSCLE STRAIN AND CRAMPS

A. Strain

   1. Results from overstretching or injury

   2. Recovers after a period of rest

B. Muscle cramp

   1. Caused by a muscle that has contracted and cannot relax

   2. Treated by stretching the muscle or causing it to bear weight

C. Muscle fatigue
    1. Caused by lack of sufficient oxygen to muscle and accumulated lactic acid
    2. Results in being unable to react to stimulus
    3. Deep breathing will relieve the oxygen debt

## XI. SMOOTH MUSCLE ACTION

A. Controlled by autonomic nervous system
B. Found in internal organs and structures
    1. One muscle contracts and narrows opening
    2. Another layer contracts and shortens the length
    3. Producing a wave motion, called peristalsis, that moves food through digestive tract
C. Lower esophagus and stomach action

## XII. SPHINCTERS

A. Doughnut-shaped muscles that can pinch shut
B. Found in digestive system and blood vessels

## XIII. DISORDERS AND DISEASES

A. Bursitis is an inflammation of the bursa
B. Tendonitis is an inflammation of a tendon
C. Epicondylitis
    1. Tennis elbow
    2. Inflammation of a forearm tendon
D. Fibromyalgia is a chronic musculoskeletal condition
E. Muscular dystrophy is a group of congenital disorders resulting in progressive wasting away of skeletal muscles
    1. Duchennes
    2. Erb's
F. Torticollis is a neck deformity caused by shortening or spasm of the sterno-cleidomastoid neck muscle
G. System interaction
    1. Fibromyalgia

# CHAPTER ACTIVITIES

1. Have the class divide into pairs and identify muscles on an anatomical model or chart.
2. Assign students to work in pairs to follow the directions on a lab exercise sheet, with one student reading and the other performing the activity. Prepare a list of activities such as:
   Adduct fingers
   Flex right forearm
   Adduct arm
   Flex leg
   Flex thigh
   Adduct leg
   Flex fingers

Extend leg

Flex toes

Extend arm

Contract diaphragm

Contract orbicularis oris

Contract orbicularis oculi

Flex foot

Extend foot

Contract pectoralis major

Contract gastrocnemius

Contract tibialis anterior

Contract quadriceps

Contract biceps

Contract abdominal muscles

Contract sartorius

Contract gluteus maximus

Contract trapezius

Contract deltoid

3. Use a tape measure to determine the size of relaxed biceps and a contracted biceps.
4. Dissect a turkey leg to show muscle groups, membranes, sheaths, ligaments, and tendons.
5. Using an oral thermometer, take a student's temperature at rest. Have the student exercise for 15 minutes. Take the temperature again. Why is there a difference?

## NSWERS TO CHECK YOUR KNOWLEDGE QUESTIONS

1. Tendonitis is:
   a. an inflammation of the coverings of the muscles and tendons at a joint.
   b. a tear in the tendon atachment.
   c. a chronic condition of the joint structures.
   **d. an inflammation of the tendon–muscle attachment.**
2. Bursitis is:
   a. an inflammation of the tendon–muscle attachment.
   **b. an inflammation of the coverings of the muscles and tendons at a joint.**
   c. an inflammation of the smooth muscle.
   d. the result of misaligned posture.
3. Epicondylitis is:
   a. inflammation of the condyles at the knee.
   b. widespread pain in muscles.
   **c. inflammation of the forearm tendon at the elbow.**
   d. a congenital muscle disease.

4. Muscular dystrophy is:
   a. a temporary muscle disorder.
   b. a group of muscles that are inflamed.
   **c. a muscle-wasting disorder.**
   d. characterized by trigger points.
5. The Achilles tendon:
   a. attaches the quadriceps femoris to the knee.
   b. permits a person to sit cross-legged.
   c. permits flexion of the biceps.
   **d. attaches the gastrocnemius to the heel.**
6. A sphincter is:
   a. the permanent flexor muscle shortening.
   b. a painful muscle contracture.
   c. a smooth muscle found in the opening of the heart.
   **d. a circular-shaped muscle.**
7. Food is moved throughout the body by:
   a. contracture.
   **b. peristalsis.**
   c. the conversion of glycogen to ATP.
   d. intercostal muscle contractions.
8. The term *flexor* refers to:
   a. straightening a joint.
   b. bringing the legs together.
   c. raising the arm at the side of the body.
   **d. bending the joint.**
9. Abduction means to:
   **a. move an extremity away from the body's center.**
   b. move an extremity toward the body's center.
   c. flex the muscle to bend a joint.
   d. flex muscles to straighten a joint.
10. Hiccoughs are caused by:
   a. a lack of oxygen.
   b. the contraction of the intercostal muscles.
   **c. spasmotic contractions of the diaphragm and vocal cord space.**
   d. the rhythmic contraction of the muscles of the throat.
11. Fibromyalgia syndrome involves:
   a. nervous, respiratory, and urinary systems.
   b. reproductive, nervous, and muscular systems.
   c. digestive, circulatory, and muscular systems.
   **d. muscular, urinary, and digestive systems.**

# CHAPTER 29 The Respiratory System

## LESSON OUTLINE

### I. $O_2$/$CO_2$ CYCLE

A. Plants use sun, water, and carbon dioxide and release oxygen

B. Humans and animals breathe oxygen and release water and carbon dioxide

### II. RESPIRATORY SYSTEM

A. Responsible for taking in oxygen

B. Responsible for removing carbon dioxide from blood

C. Adult human carries 2 quarts of oxygen; adequate for 4 minutes

### III. PATHWAY OF OXYGEN

A. Nose

1. Air flows into nose, which is divided by cartilage called the nasal septum
2. Nasal cavities
   a. Abundant blood supply, warming the air
   b. Lined with mucus-producing epithelium
      i. Add moisture in the air
      ii. Traps pathogens and dirt
3. Cilia
   a. Tiny hairlike structures in nostrils
   b. Trap dirt and other particles as they enter nose
4. Mucus
   a. Dilutes irritant
   b. Sneezing, runny nose
   c. Mucus streaming

B. Pharynx serves as a passageway for air and food

C. Epiglottis is a cartilage "lid" that prevents food from going into larynx

D. Larynx

1. Voice box
2. Lies between pharynx and trachea
3. Framework
   a. Nine cartilages
   b. Thyroid cartilage is largest and forms the Adam's apple
4. Lined with mucous membrane, forming the vocal cords
   a. Air from the lungs causes cords to vibrate to produce sound
   b. Degree of tension and length of cords determine pitch of voice
   c. Air pressure determines volume

5. Intubation
   a. Indicated when mucous membranes become swollen and prevent respiration
   b. Passing of a tube through the mouth into larynx
6. Tracheotomy
   a. Making an external opening into the trachea
   b. Inserting tube in opening permits air to enter

E. Trachea
1. The windpipe
2. Carries air into the bronchi
3. Held open by a series of C-shaped cartilage rings

F. Bronchi
1. Two sections, the right and left bronchi
2. Bronchi continue to divide into smaller bronchi
3. Smallest bronchi are called bronchioles

G. Alveoli
1. Air sacs located at the end of bronchioles
2. Resemble a bunch of grapes
3. Contain a rich network of blood capillaries

## IV. RESPIRATION PROCESS

A. Inspiration
1. Air enters body
2. Diaphragm and the muscles of the rib contract
   a. Produces a vacuum
   b. Air is sent to the alveoli, where oxygen is released into capillaries

B. Expiration
1. Air leaves lungs
2. Diaphragm relaxes, air is forced out of body
3. Carbon dioxide leaves the capillary and enters alveoli to exit body

C. External respiration is the process by which oxygen goes to the alveolus and into the capillary, and carbon dioxide is picked up and exhaled from the body

D. Internal respiration
1. Process of gas exchange in the circulatory system
2. At the cell level

## V. LUNGS AND THE PLEURA

A. Contain the bronchi and alveoli

B. Surfactant
1. Fatty molecule that maintains inflation of the lungs at birth
2. Lack of sufficient amounts causes respiratory distress syndrome (RDS)

C. Right lung has three sections (lobes)
   1. Upper
   2. Middle
   3. Lower
D. Left lung has two sections (lobes)
   1. Upper
   2. Lower
   3. Cardiac notch is where the heart lies
E. Pleura
   1. Visceral pleura is the membrane that encloses the lungs
   2. Parietal pleura
      a. Lines the thoracic cavity
      b. Space is called pleural cavity
      c. Contains lubricating fluid

## VI. THE MUSCLES OF BREATHING

A. Controlled by the respiratory center in the brain
B. Lungs alone are not capable of breathing action
   1. Contraction of the diaphragm produces a vacuum that draws air in
   2. Relaxation of the diaphragm forces the air out of the lungs
C. Altered breathing patterns
   1. Coughing
   2. Hiccoughs
   3. Sneezing
   4. Yawning
   5. Crying or laughing
D. Show Media Link: "Respiration"

## VII. DIAGNOSTIC EXAMINATIONS

A. Arterial blood gases
   1. Blood taken from artery
   2. Evaluates the exchange of oxygen and carbon dioxide
B. Bronchoscopy is when an instrument is used to view the bronchial tree
C. Chest CT scan
D. Chest X-ray is a radiological examination of the lungs
E. CT scan of pulmonary arteries
F. CT-guided needle biopsy
G. Lung perfusion scan is an examination of the lung with a radioactive contrast medium
H. Lung ventilation scan is a test to indicate areas of lung that are ventilated during respiration
I. PET scan
J. Pulmonary angiography/arteriography
   1. A radiological examination of the pulmonary circulation system

2. Requires injection of radiopaque iodine

K. Pulmonary function tests measure normal lung volume and capacity

L. Pulse oximeter

1. Measures amount of oxygen in the blood

2. Small electronic device that fits over finger

M. Sputum analysis is the laboratory examination of material coughed up from lungs

N. Thoracentesis

1. Withdrawal of fluid from pleural space

2. Analysis to determine various disorders

## VIII. DISEASES AND DISORDERS

A. Allergic rhinitis is a reaction to airborne allergens

B. Asthma is a chronic allergic disorder from sensitivity to allergens

C. Atelectasis is the lack of air in the lungs due to the collapse of the microscopic structures of the lung

D. Bronchitis is an acute or chronic inflammation of bronchial walls

E. Chronic obstructive pulmonary disease

1. Characterized by chronic obstruction of the airways resulting from various disorders

F. Emphysema

1. Irreversible enlargement of the air spaces due to destruction of the alveoli wall

2. Inability to exchange oxygen and carbon dioxide

G. Epistaxis is a nosebleed

H. Histoplasmosis is a fungal infection occurring in three forms

I. Influenza

1. Flu: Types A, B, and C

2. Highly contagious upper respiratory infection

3. Avian flu (bird flu)

4. 2009 H1N1 virus vaccine recommendation

J. Laryngectomy is the surgical removal of the larynx

K. Laryngitis is an inflammation of the vocal cords

L. Legionnaires' disease

1. Acute bronchopneumonia

2. Transmitted through water

M. Lung cancer

1. Leading cause of cancer deaths

2. Preventable

3. Attributed to inhalation of carcinogens in tobacco and the environment

4. Four types

N. Pleurisy is an inflammation of the pleura or parietal pleura

O. Paroxysmal nocturnal dyspnea

1. Symptom of heart disease or chronic lung disease

2. Individuals awaken with a feeling of suffocation

P. Pleural effusion is the presence of excess fluid in the pleural space

1. Causes hypoxia
2. From empyema

Q. Pneumoconiosis is a group of lung diseases developed after years of contact with causative agents
1. Silicosis occurs from exposure to silica sand dust
2. Asbestosis occurs from exposure to asbestos fibers
3. Black lung disease occurs from exposure to coal dust

R. Pneumonia
1. Acute infection of the lung
2. Classifications
a. Microbiological origin
b. Location
i. Bronchus
ii. Lobar
iii. Lobular
c. Type
i. Primary is caused by inhaled pathogen
ii. Secondary is caused by inhaled chemicals or infection spread from another area

S. Pneumothorax is the collapse of lung tissue due to air or gas between the parietal and visceral pleura
1. Spontaneous
2. Traumatic
3. Tension

T. Pulmonary edema is the accumulation of fluid within the tissues of the lungs

U. Pulmonary embolism is the obstruction of a pulmonary artery or arteriole by a blood clot or another substance

V. Respiratory distress syndrome
1. Immature alveolar and bronchiolar development
2. Occurs in premature infants
3. Characteristic grunting

W. Snoring
1. Obstructive air flow
2. Sleep apnea
3. Causative factors

X. Sinusitis is the inflammation of the paranasal sinus cavities

Y. Sudden infant death syndrome
1. Cause unknown
2. Suspected to be caused by prolonged periods of apnea
3. Back to Sleep program

Z. Tuberculosis
1. Acute or chronic infection causing nodular lesions and patchy infiltrations of the lung tissue
2. Bacteria induced

AA. Upper respiratory infection
1. Caused by a virus
2. Common cold

3. Allergy

## IX. AGE-RELATED CHARACTERISTICS OCCURRING WITH ASTHMA

## X. SYSTEM INTERACTION

A. Interaction of respiratory, circulatory, digestive and muscular systems with COPD

# CHAPTER ACTIVITIES

1. Invite a guest speaker from the American Lung Association to discuss the work of the organization.
2. Ask the local telephone company to discuss the artificial larynx and the TDD service (telecommunication devices for the deaf that are also used by speech-impaired persons).
3. Invite a person who has had a laryngectomy to speak to the class. (Contact a local support group or a thoracic surgeon for a referral.)
4. Assign students to prepare individual oral reports on the more common respiratory diseases. Sharing their findings in class will acquaint all students with the disease.
5. Measure everyone's vital capacity. Compare the smokers to the nonsmokers and people who exercise regularly to those who do not.
6. Use two panes of glass to explain the physiology of the thoracic cavity. Wet one pane, then lay the other on top. The cohesiveness demonstrates how the lungs adhere to the chest cavity.

# ANSWERS TO CHECK YOUR KNOWLEDGE QUESTIONS

1. Mucus streaming is:
   a. what makes your nose run.
   b. the cause of post-nasal drip.
   c. watery discharge after breathing in an allergen.
   **d. propelling particles upward past the epiglottis.**
2. The epiglottis:
   a. vibrates to make speech.
   b. is attached to the upper pharynx.
   **c. covers the opening to the larynx when swallowing.**
   d. is above the tongue.
3. The bronchoscope can be used for all the following except:
   a. removing a foreign body.
   **b. delivering oxygen into the lungs.**
   c. obtaining a sample tissue of secretion.
   d. viewing the airways.
4. The pulse oximeter:
   **a. measures the amount of oxygen in the blood.**
   b. measures pulse.
   c. determines the rhythm of the pulse.
   d. can detect pulse irregularities.

5. Emphysema causes:

   **a. enlarged alveolar spaces in the lungs.**

   b. large amounts of mucus.

   c. slower respirations due to enlarged alveoli.

   d. more efficient exchanges of oxygen and carbon dioxide.

6. Which of the following is not a symptom of influenza?

   **a. Vomiting and diarrhea**

   b. Chills and fever

   c. Coughing

   d. Fever

7. A pneumothorax is:

   a. the collection of air in the lungs.

   b. air in the thorax.

   **c. air in the pleural space.**

   d. air between the lung and the diaphragm.

8. Pulmonary edema occurs when:

   **a. fluid accumulates within the tissues of the lung.**

   b. the pulmonary artery becomes enlarged.

   c. blood pressure decreases within the blood vessels.

   d. tissue fluids leak out of the alveoli.

9. A pulmonary embolus is:

   a. a mysterious condition that kills healthy infants.

   **b. a blood clot obstructing an arteriole in the lungs.**

   c. the result of years of smoking.

   d. something that can occur after an extended period of running.

10. The incidence of tuberculosis is increasing because of all of the following except:

    a. its relationship with AIDS.

    b. an influx of immigrants.

    **c. the organism mutating to a stronger strain.**

    d. the use of drugs.

11. Asthma:

    a. primarily affects adults.

    **b. can progress to a condition similar to COPD.**

    c. is not affected by environmental conditions.

    d. is not associated with the incidence of bronchitis and pneumonia.

12. COPD involves:

    a. respiratory, skeletal, and immune systems.

    b. muscular, circulatory, and urinary systems.

    **c. respiratory, digestive, and circulatory systems.**

    d. circulatory, muscular, and endocrine systems.

# CHAPTER 30 The Circulatory System

## LESSON OUTLINE

### I. THE CIRCULATORY SYSTEM IS A TRANSPORTATION SYSTEM

A. Transports oxygen and nutrients to the body's cells

B. Transports carbon dioxide and waste materials away from body cells

C. Blood is the transportation vehicle

### II. COMPOSED OF FOUR MAIN PARTS

A. Heart

B. Blood vessels

C. Blood

D. Lymphatic system

### III. HEART

A. The pump of the body

  1. Muscles contract and blood is squeezed out, which is called the systole phase

    a. Produces the beat heard in the stethoscope and felt as a pulse

    b. Top number of the blood pressure reading, greatest pressure on the blood

  2. Muscles relax and blood flows into heart, which is called the diastole phase

    a. Cannot be felt as a pulse

    b. Bottom number of the blood pressure reading, period of least pressure on blood

B. Muscular, hollow organ, the size of a clenched fist, behind sternum

C. External heart structures

  1. Pericardium

    a. Double-layered sac

    b. Parietal layer lines the sac and visceral layer, which covers the heart

    c. Blood supply to heart structure provided by small blood vessels called coronary arteries and veins

  2. Myocardium

    a. Muscular middle layer of the heart

    b. Thickest layer

D. Internal heart structures

  1. Endocardium

    a. Lines the interior surface of the heart

    b. Allows for the smooth flow of blood

  2. Septum

    a. Muscular wall

      i. Separates the heart into left and right parts

      ii. Prevents the blood on the right side from mixing with the left

    b. Right and left upper chambers are called atria

    c. Right and left lower chambers are called ventricles

3. One-way valves in chambers keep the blood flowing in the right direction
    a. Tricuspid valve
        i. Found between the right atrium and ventricle
        ii. Closes when the right ventricle contracts and pushes blood to lungs through semilunar valve of pulmonary artery
        iii. Prevents blood from reentering the atrium
    b. Mitral valve
        i. Located between the left atrium and ventricle
        ii. Closes when the left ventricle contracts and pushes blood through semilunar valve of aorta
        iii. Prevents blood from flowing back into left atrium
    c. Semilunar valves
        i. Located between the ventricles and aorta and pulmonary arteries
        ii. Closes after the ventricles contract, preventing blood from flowing back into the ventricles

E. Pulmonary circulation
    1. Blood from body enters the right atrium
    2. The right atrium contracts and pushes blood through tricuspid valve into the right ventricle; valve closes
    3. Right ventricle contracts, sending blood out through the semilunar valve into the pulmonary artery; valve closes
    4. Pulmonary artery carries blood into the lungs to be oxygenated
        a. Arteries carry blood from heart
        b. Deoxygenated blood gives up carbon dioxide and picks up oxygen in alveoli of lungs
    5. Pulmonary veins carry oxygenated blood back into the heart
        a. Veins carry blood to heart
        b. Oxygenated blood empties into left atrium
    6. Left atrium contracts, forcing blood through mitral valve into the left ventricle; valve closes
    7. Left ventricle contracts, sending blood out through semilunar valve into the aorta; valve closes
    8. Right and left sides of the heart work together to function properly

F. Heart sounds
    1. With stethoscope, two distinct sounds are heard, called the lubb dupp sounds
        a. Lubb sound (or $S_1$), produced by the valves slamming shut between the atria and ventricles
        b. Dupp sound (or $S_2$), produced by the semilunar valves closing in the aorta and pulmonary arteries
        c. $S_3$: ventricular gallop
        d. $S_4$: atrial gallop

G. Pacemaker
    1. Sinoatrial (SA) node produces the electrical impulse to start the contraction of the heart
    2. Atrioventricular (AV) node produces the contraction of the ventricles
    3. Bundle of His in septum
    4. Purkinje fibers in muscle

H. Rhythm disorders
    1. Heart will continue to beat as long as it is supplied with the necessary nutrients
    2. Abnormal rhythm patterns can be viewed on electrocardiograph (ECG)
    3. Heart block
        a. The impulse from the SA node is not transmitted properly to the AV node

b. First-degree block is characterized by a momentary delay at AV node

c. Second-degree block can be of two forms

d. Third-degree block

i. Complete heart block

ii. Ventricles contract at about half the atrial rate

4. Arrhythmias

a. Deviation from normal rhythm

b. Three types

i. Atrial

(a) Premature atrial contractions

(b) Usually no clinical significance

ii. AV junctional

(a) Premature junctional contractions

(b) Usually no clinical significance

iii. Ventricular

(a) Premature ventricular contractions

(i) Bigeminal

(ii) Trigeminal

(b) Can be deadly

c. Artificial pacemaker is a battery-powered pulse generator

d. Fibrillation

i. Rhythm breaks down and muscle fibers of ventricles contract at random without coordination

ii. Can be life threatening

iii. Defibrillator

iv. Implantable cardioverter defibrillator

v. Automatically shocks heart at adequate amount

5. Controlling the rate

a. Vagus nerve slows down the heart rate

b. Accelerator nerve increases the heart rate

c. Tachycardia

d. Bradycardia

## V. SHOW MEDIA LINK: "THE HEART"

## . BLOOD VESSELS

A. Three main types

1. Arteries

a. Carry oxygenated blood away from the heart with the exception of the pulmonary artery

b. Have elastic fibers in their walls, which expand and recoil to make the pulse

c. Major arteries
   i. Aorta largest artery in the body
   ii. Arteries branch into smaller arteries
   iii. Arterioles
      (a) Smallest branches of arteries
      (b) Join with capillaries

2. Capillaries
   a. Have thin walls that contain only one layer of cells
   b. Oxygen and nutrients pass through to the cells
   c. Carbon dioxide and waste products from the cells enter the capillaries
   d. Connect arterioles with venules, the smallest branches of the veins

3. Veins
   a. Have thinner walls than arteries
   b. Do not have an elastic layer
   c. Have valves to assist in the return flow of blood
   d. Action of leg muscles "pumps" blood
   e. Major veins
   f. Carry deoxygenated blood back to the heart
   g. Venules
      i. Smallest branches of veins
      ii. Connect with the capillaries
      iii. Join together to form veins
   h. Superior and inferior vena cava
      i. Largest veins
      ii. Superior vena cava brings the blood from the upper part of the body to right atrium
      iii. Inferior vena cava brings the blood from the lower part of the body to right atrium

## VI. SYSTEMIC CIRCULATION

A. The process of carrying blood through the circulatory system
   1. Exits heart at the left ventricle to aorta
   2. Exits aorta to arteries
   3. Arteries branch to all systemic arteries
   4. Systemic arteries subdivide until they become arterioles
   5. Arterioles
      a. Join the capillaries
      b. Deliver oxygen, water, and nutrients
   6. Capillaries
      a. Join the venules
      b. Pick up carbon dioxide and wastes
   7. Venules become veins

8. Veins enter into inferior vena cava or superior vena cava
9. Inferior vena cava and superior vena cava empty into the right atrium of the heart

## VII. PORTAL CIRCULATION

A. The passage of blood through the organs of the body
B. Each organ receives substances on which it reacts
C. Leave organs to portal vein
D. Flows through liver for treatment
E. Goes to inferior vena cava

## VIII. LYMPHATIC SYSTEM

A. Lymph
  1. Thin watery fluid
  2. Composed of blood plasma, lymphocytes, hormones, and other substances
  3. Fills the spaces between the cells
  4. Called interstitial fluid
B. Lymph vessels
  1. Similar to veins
  2. Located throughout the body
  3. Have valves to prevent backflow
  4. Absorb fluid and other substances and return them to the circulatory system via a one-way system
  5. Lymph capillaries become small lymph vessels
  6. Lymph vessels become lymphatics
  7. Lymphatics form two main ducts
    a. Right lymphatic duct
    b. Thoracic duct
C. Lymph nodes
  1. Small round or oval structures located along lymph vessels
  2. Lymph vessels bring lymph to the nodes
  3. Filter lymph to remove bacteria or malignant cells
  4. Contain lymphocytes, a type of white blood cell
  5. Contain phagocytes, another type of white blood cell
  6. Become swollen and tender during infection because of the increase in cells and filtered substances
  7. Are indicators of cancer prognosis
D. Spleen
  1. Organ composed of lymphatic tissue
  2. Located on the left side in back of the upper part of the stomach
  3. Functions
    a. Produces lymphocytes
    b. Stores red blood cells

c. Keeps the appropriate balance between cells and plasma in the blood

d. Removes and destroys old, worn-out blood cells

## IX. BLOOD

A. Life-giving fluid of the body

B. About 8–10 pints in the average adult

C. Circulates throughout the body continually

D. Transports

1. Oxygen from lungs to body cells
2. Carbon dioxide from body cells to the lungs
3. Nutrients from the digestive system to the cells
4. Cellular wastes from the cells to organs of excretion
5. Hormones excreted from endocrine glands to the body's organs
6. Minerals necessary for homeostasis of the body

E. Blood composed of two main parts

1. Plasma

a. Straw-colored liquid

b. Makes up one-half of the volume of blood

c. 90% water

d. Other substances

i. Electrolytes

(a) Minerals

(b) Play major role in maintaining acid-base balance

ii. Vitamins

iii. Hormones

iv. Enzymes

v. Nutrients from the digestive system

(a) Glucose

(b) Fatty acids

(c) Amino acids

vi. Gases

(a) Oxygen

(b) Carbon dioxide

vii. Metabolic and waste products

viii. Fibrinogen and prothrombin, which are needed to form clots

ix. Serum albumin, which aids in maintaining blood pressure

x. Serum globulin, which is needed for the formation of antibodies

2. Cells

a. Cellular portion of the blood

b. Three main types

i. Erythrocytes or red blood cells; 5M per cm of blood

(a) Produced in the bone marrow

(b) Contain hemoglobin

(i) Carries oxygen and carbon dioxide

(ii) Gives cells their red color

(iii) If blood contains a lot of oxygen, it is bright red

(iv) If there is less oxygen, the color changes to a dark reddish blue

ii. Leukocytes or white blood cells; 5,000–9,000 per cm of blood

(a) Twice the size of erythrocytes

(b) Not as numerous as erythrocytes

(c) Main function is to fight infection

(d) Granulocytes are produced in red bone marrow

(i) Neutrophils phagocytize bacteria

(ii) Eosinophils consume toxic substances in tissue

(iii) Basophils phagocytize bacteria

(e) Agranulocytes

(i) Lymphocytes are produced in bone marrow and lymphoid tissues, and develop antibodies

(ii) Monocytes are formed in bone marrow and assist with phagocytosis

(iii) Exudate

iii. Platelets; 200,000–400,000 per cm of blood

(a) Smallest of blood cells

(b) Contain thromoboplastin

(i) Triggers the clotting process

(ii) Bleeding time is the length of time required for blood to clot from induced puncture wound

F. Blood types

1. Four main types

a. Type A

i. Can receive A or O

ii. Can donate to A or AB

b. Type B

i. Can receive B or O

ii. Can donate to B or AB

c. Type AB

i. Universal recipient

ii. Can donate to AB

d. Type O

i. Can receive O

ii. Universal donor

e. Blood typed and cross-matched

2. Rh factor

a. Antigen in blood (Rh+)

b. Antigen absent (Rh–)
c. Causes an antibody response
d. Can cause serious problems with pregnancy

## X. SHOW MEDIA LINK: "THE BLOOD"

## XI. CARDIOVASCULAR TESTS

A. Arteriograph is a radiological examination of an artery with a contrast medium
B. Cardiac catheterization is when a catheter is used to permit visualization of the heart's circulation
C. Doppler ultrasonography is when sound waves are used to determine various disorders
D. Echocardiograph uses ultra-high frequency sound waves to detect valve irregularities and defects of the heart
E. Electrocardiograph (ECG)
   1. Commonly called EKG
   2. Graphic recording of the electrical activity of the heart
   3. Holter monitor—ambulatory ECG
F. Heart scan is a high-speed CT scan using an electron beam tomography scanner. It can detect calcified plaque in the coronary arteries
G. MUGA scan is a test to evaluate the condition of the myocardium of the heart using isotopes
H. Myocardial perfusion imaging measures the passage of blood through the coronary arteries. The test uses medication to stress the heart by dilating the arteries. Radioactive material is injected to identify the blood flow
I. Persantine thallium—stress test without exercise
J. Stress thallium ECG is a test to evaluate myocardial blood flow and the condition of the cells
K. Transesophageal echocardiography involves placing a transducer in the esophagus behind the heart to get clearer pictures
L. Ultrasound (see echocardiograph)
M. Venogram is a radiographic examination to determine the condition of the deep veins of the legs

## XI. DISEASES AND DISORDERS

A. Anemia occurs when the red blood cell count is low due to
   1. Iron deficiency
   2. Aplastic
   3. Acute blood loss
B. Aneurysm is a weak section in the walls of the artery that has ballooned out
   1. Cerebral
   2. Aortic
   3. Abdominal
C. Angina is severe chest pain that radiates down the inner surface of the left arm
   1. Nitroglycerin tablets and patch
   2. Enhanced external counterpulsation
D. Arrest is a complete, sudden cessation of heart action
E. Arrhythmia is any abnormal change in the heart rhythm
F. Arteriosclerosis is known as "hardening" of the arteries
G. Atherosclerosis is a condition characterized by the deposit of fatty material along the linings of the artery

H. Athletic heart syndrome is an enlargement of the heart due to strenuous exercise

I. Carditis—Inflammation of the heart
   1. Pericarditis is the inflammation of the pericardium
   2. Myocarditis is the inflammation of the myocardium
   3. Endocarditis is the inflammation of the endocardial lining

J. Cerebrovascular accident (CVA)
   1. Commonly known as a stroke
   2. A sudden impairment of the flow of blood to the brain
   3. Transient ischemic attacks (TIA)
   4. Called "a brain attack"
   5. Warning strokes
   6. Differentiate between ischemic and hemorrhagic stroke
   7. Treat ischemic within three hours
   8. Hemorrhagic treatment
   9. Use of enzyme-blocking drugs
   10. Prevention is best

K. Congestive heart failure (CHF) includes a group of dysfunctions, resulting in poor performance of the heart
   1. Left-sided heart failure
   2. Right-sided heart failure
   3. Treat with ACE inhibitors
   4. Use diuretics

L. Coronary artery disease
   1. Disease of the arteries that surround the heart
   2. Volume of blood flow is reduced
   3. Arteriograph
   4. Angioplasty
      a. Balloon
      b. Atherectomy
      c. Stent
         i. Brachytherapy
         ii. Coated stents

M. Embolism is foreign matter that enters and circulates in the bloodstream
   1. Blood
   2. Exudate
   3. Fat
   4. Air

N. Heart failure
   1. Dilated cardiomyopathy
   2. Leaking valves

3. Treat with heart strengthers and diuretics
4. Replacement valves

O. Heart replacement
1. When transplant not possible
2. Physical and mental considerations
3. Artificial hearts

P. Hypertension is high blood pressure
1. Essential
2. Secondary
3. Benign
4. Malignant

Q. Hypertrophic cardiomyopathy
1. Thickened ventricles
2. Affects athletes
3. Unknown cause or gene defect

R. Hypotension is low blood pressure

S. Leukemia is a malignant disease of the bone marrow or lymphatic tissue
1. Acute
2. Chronic

T. Murmur is an abnormal sound of blood flowing through a heart valve

U. Myocardial infarction (MI) is commonly known as a heart attack

V. Phlebitis is a localized inflammation of a vein

W. Sickle cell anemia is a congenital anemia occurring primarily among African Americans

X. Stasis ulcer is a secondary condition resulting from chronic venous insufficiency

Y. Thrombophlebitis
1. An acute condition in which the lining of the vein wall becomes inflamed
2. Thrombus blood clot forms

Z. Varicosities are veins that become dilated, twisted, and inefficient

## CHAPTER ACTIVTIES

1. Give students a sample of unknown blood to determine its type.
2. Have students identify the structures of the heart on an anatomical model.
3. Have students trace the flow of blood on an anatomical chart, naming all the structures through which it passes.
4. Assign students to work in pairs. Instruct one to place pressure on the proximal ends of the visible blood vessels on the back of the partner's hand or on the inner surface of the wrist. With the fingers of the other hand, press and slid the finger distal to the point where the blood flow is shut off. Have them observe and explain what happens and wh Then tell them to put pressure at the distal end and slide the fingers toward the body. Again, tell them to explain wh they saw and why it happened. They should be able to detect branching veins, which are filled from other veins, ev though return blood is shut off. Try to get the students to realize the veins are returning blood and that is why they stay empty when held in the second position. If the vessels were arteries, the opposite action would be observed.

5. Contact a surgeon who implants pacemakers to arrange to obtain one that has been removed or one that is nonfunctional to show to your students.
6. Using a blood sample in a test tube, allow the cells to settle to illustrate the plasma-to-cell proportion.
7. The muscle action of the veins to move blood uphill can be demonstrated by holding a piece of flexible rubber tubing vertically over a pan of water in which the end of the tube is immersed. With both hands, alternately squeeze and release the tubing, moderately fast. The water will soon squirt out the top of the tubing each time you squeeze. (Practice before you show your class. If tubing is too long, it may not work.)
8. Obtain 5-quart or 5-liter containers. Fill each of them with red-colored water to illustrate five liters of blood.

## NSWERS TO CHECK YOUR KNOWLEDGE QUESTIONS

1. Cholesterol is:

   **a. a by-product of fat metabolism in the blood.**

   b. caused by being overweight.

   c. developed from a lack of exercise.

   d. due to decreased blood flow in the arteries.

2. Triglycerides:

   a. are common with diabetes.

   **b. are believed to contribute to the thickening of arterial walls.**

   c. are beneficial in high levels.

   d. are a combination of three fats high levels.

3. A heart catheterization can:

   **a. permit visualization of the coronary arteries.**

   b. measure the amount of oxygen in the heart.

   c. remove blood for analysis.

   d. accurately measure electrical activity of the heart.

4. The Dobutamine stress test:

   a. is done on a treadmill.

   **b. uses a drug to stress the heart.**

   c. allows visualization of the coronary arteries.

   d. requires instillation of a radioactive material and a special camera.

5. The Doppler ultrasound:

   a. can diagnose coronary artery disease.

   b. determines leaking heart valves.

   c. measures cardiac output.

   **d. evaluates disease in major blood vessels.**

6. Arrhythmia is a term that can mean any of the following except:

   **a. absence of heartbeat.**

   b. a rhythm with extra beats.

   c. a rhythm with missed beats.

   d. the presence of delayed beats

7. Atherosclerosis is the:
   a. replacement of muscular artery tissue by fibrous tissue and calcification.
   **b. presence of fatty deposits on the artery lining.**
   c. scarring of the arterial lining.
   d. thickening of the lining of the arterial wall.
8. A cerebrovascular accident is not caused by:
   a. high blood pressure rupturing and artery.
   b. athersclerosis occluding an artery.
   c. a thrombus that clogs an artery.
   **d. an accidental injury to the cerebral artery.**
9. A heart murmur is:
   a. an additional flutter of the heart valves.
   b. a soft, barely audible extra heartbeat.
   c. a sound caused by inadequate blood flow.
   **d. an abnormal sound of blood flowing through a closed valve.**
10. What will most likely contribute to death when an MI occurs?
   a. Taking an aspirin tablet
   **b. Waiting to see if the symptoms improve**
   c. Taking a dose of nitroglycerin
   d. Taking a strong pain medication
11. Collateral circulation:
   a. is absent at birth.
   b. increases more rapidly in the aged.
   c. is between arteries and veins.
   **d. is best in young and middle aged.**
12. Leukemia affects:
   **a. circulatory, integumentary, and immune systems.**
   b. circulatory, digestive, and respiratory systems.
   c. digestive, respiratory, and urinary systems.
   d. respiratory, urinary, and circulatory systems.

# CHAPTER 31 The Immune System

## LESSON PLANS

### I. THE IMMUNE SYSTEM

A. Group of special cells and organs essential to the health and well-being of the body

B. Environment of antigens, nonself things

C. Three lines of defense

1. Anatomic barriers
    a. Skin and mucous membrane
    b. Biochemical barriers
    c. Sebaceous glands
    d. Tears, perspiration, and saliva
    e. Glandular secretions
    f. Mechanical barriers
        i. Sloughing skin
        ii. Vomiting
        iii. Urinating
2. Inflammatory process after barrier penetrated
    a. Begins within seconds of injury
    b. Results in symptoms of infection
3. Antibody defense
    a. Involves specific cells
    b. Immunity, last line of defense

### II. FUNCTION OF IMMUNE SYSTEM

A. To create effective immune response and continually defend the body

1. Identify self and destroy nonself
2. Maintain homeostasis
3. Conduct continual surveillance

### III. ORIGIN OF CELLS

A. Blood cells originate in the bone marrow and develop from stem cells

B. Types of cells

1. Erythrocytes
    a. Develop from erythroid stem cells
    b. Mature in bone marrow
2. Granulated white blood cells
    a. Develop from myeloid stem cells
    b. Mature into
        i. Eosinophils

ii. Neutrophils

iii. Basophils

c. Functions

i. Neutrophils carry granules with potent chemicals to destroy microorganisms

ii. Eosinophils and basophils release chemicals to affect cells or microbes

3. Granulated lymphocytes

a. Develop from a lymphocyte stem cell

b. Two major classes

i. B cells mature in the bone marrow

ii. T cells mature in the thymus

4. Monocytes

a. Develop from mononuclear phagocyte stem cells

b. Enlarge into macrophage

i. Effectively fight infection

ii. Act as phagocytes engulfing and destroying antigens

iii. Can phagocytize large organisms and some parasites

5. Neutrophils

a. Phagocytes with potent granules to destroy small antigens

b. Are 40–60% of all white blood cells

c. Also called segmentals or polymorphonuclear neutrophils

d. Attack and destroy bacteria, viruses, and other antigens

6. Eosinophils

a. Are about 2–3% of total white blood cells

b. Weak phagocytes during common infections but are produced in large amounts to fight parasites

c. Are present with inflammation

7. Basophils release heparin and histamine for inflammation process

## IV. ORGANS OF THE IMMUNE SYSTEM

A. Lymphoid organs promote growth development and activity of lymphocytes

1. Bone marrow
2. Thymus
3. Lymph nodes
4. Spleen
5. Tonsils
6. Adenoids
7. Appendix
8. Peyer's patches

## V. CELLULAR ACTIVITY

A. B cells and T cells exit capillaries and enter extracellular fluid to patrol

B. Lymph carries lymphocytes, macrophages, and antigens into lymph capillaries and vessels

C. Clusters of lymph nodes along lymphatic vessels
   1. Store B and T cells in compartments
   2. Incoming antigens trapped and destroyed
   3. B and T cells return to lymph nodes and blood
   4. Nodes swell and become tender
   5. Nodes lose cells, which metastasize new sites
      a. Extent of cancer determined by number of involved nodes, size of tumor, and metastatic progress; assessment is called staging

## I. CELL MARKERS

A. Major histocompatibility complex (MHC)
   1. Group of genes in a specific chromosome
   2. Allows immune cells to recognize and communicate with each other
   3. Attacks any cell that is not marked as "self"
   4. Maintains steady state called homeostasis
   5. Performs surveillance
   6. Removes abnormal cells

## II. LYMPHOCYTES

A. Small white blood cells with immune functions
B. 80% of lymphocytes are T lymphocytes
   1. Act directly through cell-mediated immunity
   2. Are helper, suppresser, memory, and killer Ts
C. 20% of lymphocytes are B lymphocytes
   1. Act by producing antibodies
   2. About 100,000 antibodies

## III. ANTIBODIES

A. Produce five classes of immunoglobulins (Table 31–1)
B. Measured by serum protein electropheresis test

## . COMPLEMENT SYSTEM

A. Antibody-mediated response or humoral immunity
   1. Group of about 25 inactive enzyme proteins
   2. Are activated when in contact with antibody-antigen complex
      a. Produces lethal chemicals to attract phagocytes
      b. Coats the target cell
      c. Destroys the antigen by puncturing its membrane
      d. Antibody and complement system response is humoral immunity
   3. Develops an inflammatory response
      a. Basophils and mast cells release histamine. Dilation of blood vessels occurs, making them more permeable

i. Slows down blood flow and allows fluid to seep into surrounding tissues
ii. Results in warmth, redness, and swelling
iii. Complement proteins leave blood vessels and attract phagocytes

## X. CYTOKINES ARE NON-ANTIBODY PROTEINS THAT REGULATE THE IMMUNE RESPONSE

A. Lymphokines
  1. Produced by T cells
B. Monokines
  1. Produced by monocytes and macrophages
C. Lymphotoxin
  1. Produced by lymphocytes
  2. Kills tumor cells
D. Tumor necrosis factor
  1. From macrophages
  2. Inhibits viruses
  3. Measures effectiveness of chemotherapy

  See text, pp. 619–622, for a summary of the 14 groups of cytokines included in the components of the immune system color-treated section

## XI. NATURAL KILLER (NK) CELLS

A. Non-T and non-B lymphocytes
B. Kill cancer cells and virus-infected cells
  1. Don't need antibodies or prior exposure
C. Contain potent chemical granules
D. Function can be enhanced with alpha interferon

## XII. IMMUNE RESPONSES

A. Primary antibody-mediated response
  1. Meets with B cell, processed
  2. Helper T combines, interleukins released
  3. Other cells being engulfed and displayed
  4. Interleukins cause rapid growth of B cells and produce clones
  5. Antibodies release to combine with antigens to be destroyed
  6. Some B cells become memory cells and go to lymphoidal tissue
  7. Immunoglobulins activate other cells and substances
  8. Response requires five to six days
  9. Acts against bacteria and extracellular viruses, fungi, and parasites *outside* cell's cytoplasm
B. Secondary response
  1. Requires only two to three days
  2. Clonal lymphocytes with memory attack antigen
  3. Immediate antibodies are produced

C. Primary cell-mediated response
   1. T cells quick and direct
   2. Help B cells make antibodies
   3. Identify antigens trapped by macrophages
   4. Process antigens
   5. Helper Ts secrete interleukin to activate killer Ts
   6. B cells carry out humoral immunity
   7. Macrophages are recruited and cause inflammation
   8. NK cells directly destroy cancer and virus-infected cells
   9. Some T cells also develop memory and stay in reserve
   10. Intracellular response attacks viruses, fungi, protozoa, cancer cells, and transplant tissue
   11. Destroys any cell with MHC marker and an antigen

D. Responses stopped by suppressor T cells

## XIII. SHOW MEDIA LINK: "THE IMMUNE SYSTEM"

## X. IMMUNIZATION

A. Vaccine causes the production of antigen-antibody complex followed by memory cells

B. Active immunity develops when recipients make their own immunity

C. Passive immunity
   1. Antibodies developed in another individual's immune system are injected into nonimmune individual
   2. Immunity is short-lived

## X. DISEASES AND DISORDERS

A. Acquired immunodeficiency syndrome (AIDS)
   1. Caused by human immunodeficiency virus (HIV)
      a. Is a retrovirus, with RNA genetic material, not DNA
   2. Found in many body fluids, mainly in blood, semen, and vaginal secretions
   3. Invades T helper cells and macrophages rendering both T and B immune response ineffective
      a. Hides for months or years, average about 10 years
      b. Depletes T helper cells
      c. Vulnerable to opportunistic diseases
   4. Conditions for acquiring HIV
   5. Transmission misconceptions
   6. Signs and symptoms
      a. None at first
      b. Flulike
      c. Highly contagious
   7. Later signs and symptoms
      a. May be 10 years later
      b. Declining CD+4 counts and other symptoms.
   8. Late signs and symptoms

   a. Affects of infections and cancer identify AIDS

9. Diagnosis of HIV
   a. Blood or saliva test for antigens or antibodies
   b. Elisa and Western Blot tests
   c. Coulter HIV-p24
   d. Home testing kits
   e. Measure risk of progression to AIDS

10. Diagnosis of AIDS
    a. Confirmed HIV test and at least one of the three conditions.

11. AIDS prevention
    a. Practice personal measures
    b. Sexual abstinence or monogamous relationship
    c. Avoid high-risk sexual activities
    d. Use latex condom properly

12. Treatment of AIDS
    a. Medications
    b. Numerous side effects

13. Treatment of opportunistic infections and cancer
    a. At least 22 approved drugs
    b. HIV vaccines
    c. Search Internet for latest information

B. Allergies

1. Hypersensitivity to harmless environmental antigens
   a. Immediate response involves humoral immunity
   b. Delayed allergic responses involve cell-mediated immunity and may cause exaggerated reactions
   c. Caused by substances, emotions, air pressure, and infections
   d. Diagnosed with blood counts, chest X-ray, pulmonary function tests, and skin tests
   e. Treated by eliminating cause, desensitizing shots, antihistamines, bronchial dilators, and corticosteroids

C. Cancer

1. Large group of diseases characterized by uncontrolled growth and spread of abnormal cells, the result of the mutation of cells
2. Second-leading cause of death among adults and children ages 1 to 14
   a. Best treated by specialists
3. Characteristics of cancer cells
   a. Neoplasm means new growth
      i. Benign are slow growing, non-spreading
      ii. Malignant differ
4. Classifications
   a. Carcinomas from epithelial tissue
   b. Sarcomas from connective tissue
   c. Leukemia from blood-forming organs
   d. Lymphomas from lymph tissues

5. Differentiation
   a. Well-differentiated is very abnormal
   b. Poorly differentiated
   c. Graded I to IV by degrees of differentiation
6. Staging
   a. Identifies extent of disease process
   b. Provides description for treatment and clinical trials
   c. Called TNM system and combines with tumor size, node involvement, and metastasis; combines with staging classification letters c, p, r, and a
7. Signs and symptoms
   a. Differ according to type (Table 31–8 and Table 31–9)
8. Cause
   a. Cellular mutation
   b. Abnormal activation of genes controlling growth and division
      i. Oncogene in "on" position
      ii. Tumor suppressor in "off" position
      iii. Only small fraction of mutated survive
      iv. (a) Probability of mutation increases due to carcinogens
9. Reasons for failure of immune system
   a. Decrease in antibodies and lymphocytes
   b. Stress
   c. Severe systemic infection
   d. Cancer effects
   e. Increased infection due to radiation, drugs, marrow suppression
   f. Cellular marker confusion
10. Diagnostic tests
    a. Indicated with positive screening or symptoms
    b. Goals to obtain diagnosis
       i. Primary site
       ii. Identify tissue type
       iii. Grade
       iv. Stage
    c. Types of tests
       i. Biopsy: needle, excisional, aspiration, sentinel node, and stereotatic breast
       ii. Laboratory tests: markers, genetic testing (BRAC1, 2)
       iii. Tumor imaging: X-ray, CT scan, MRI
       iv. Endoscopic: bronchoscopy, sigmoidoscopy, colonoscopy
       v. Ultrasound
       vi. Nuclear medicine imaging: PET scan, radiolabeled monoclonal antibodies (Posta-scint), radiolabeled peptides

11. Treatment based on type, grade, stage, and probability of recurrence
    a. Goals of therapy: cure, control, or palliation
    b. Local surgery or systemic chemotherapy and radiation
        i. Surgery in about 60% to diagnose, treat, or palliate symptoms
    c. Radiation by X-ray or gamma rays to damage cancer cells
        i. External beam through skin
        ii. Brachytherapy using radioactive isotopes on or near tumor
        iii. Interstitially by implanting "seeds"
    d. Chemotherapy affects both normal and cancer cells
        i. Oral
        ii. Intravenous
        iii. Subcutaneous
        iv. Intramuscular
        v. Intraarterial
        vi. Topical
        vii. Intraperitoneal
        viii. Intrathecal
    e. Biologic response modifiers (BRM)
        i. Alter immune system
        ii. Direct antitumor activity
        iii. Other biological effects
    f. Colony-stimulating factor (CSF)
        i. Cytokines; granulocyte colony, erythropoietin, interferon
        ii. Interleukins; interleukin-2
    g. Monoclonal antibodies directed at specific antigens
    h. Alternative therapies such as laetril, shark cartilage, megadoses of vitamins, immunoaugmentation therapy, and herbal supplements
    i. Complementary therapies such as massage, relaxation, biofeedback, etc.
12. Cancer vaccine
    a. Leukopheresis
    b. Additional treatment option
    c. HPV vaccine
13. Clinical research trials
    a. Testing of a treatment regime after laboratory and animal studies
    b. Specific patients receive new therapy

D. Chronic fatigue syndrome is a debilitating disorder, perhaps genetically related
1. Signs and symptoms
    a. Affects twice as many women as men
    b. Etiology appears genetic
    c. Also theories suggesting viral, bacterial, allergen, or environmental
2. Treatment primarily symptomatic and avoiding stress

E. Lupus erythematosus
   1. Chronic disease of unknown cause
   2. Causes inflammation of various parts of the body
   3. Can be life-threatening
   4. Antibodies react against the person's own tissue
   5. Types
      a. Discoid or cutaneous is confined to the skin
      b. Systemic lupus erythematosus
         i. Inflames the organs of the body
         ii. Has periods of remission
      c. Drug-induced lupus
         i. Caused by certain medications
         ii. Symptoms fade when drugs are stopped
         iii. General and suggestive symptoms
         iv. Diagnosed from symptoms and blood tests
            (a) Antibody test (ANA) is diagnostic
         v. Etiology unknown
         vi. Treated with rest, exercise as able, anti-inflammatories and analgesics
         vii. New treatments of self-antigens, immunoreplacements, and plasmaphoresis

F. Lymphedema
   1. Accumulation of lymphatic fluid
   2. Often follows removal of nodes and radiation
   3. Treat with massage, exercise, and compression bandages or clothing
   4. Precautions reduce risk

G. Rheumatoid arthritis
   1. Chronic systemic inflammatory autoimmune disease
   2. Affects joints and surrounding muscles, tendons, ligaments, and blood vessels
   3. Connection to immune system
   4. Suggestive link to genetic defect
   5. Autoantibody rheumatoid factor affects synovial membranes causing inflammation
      a. Inflammatory response dilate blood vessels, fluids accumulates, causing joint membranes to thicken; eventual joint destruction
   6. Treat with salicylates to reduce inflammation, corticosteroids, and other anti-inflammatories

## HAPTER ACTIVTIES

1. Have students research and report on past epidemics and on the AIDS epidemic. Discuss how these events are similar and how they are different.
2. Have a presentation of standard precautions.
3. Obtain literature on AIDS from a local health department or contact the Centers for Disease Control and Prevention in Atlanta. There is much available to educators.
4. Ask the individual responsible for infection control in your local or state health department to speak to your class.

5. Invite an HIV-positive person to talk with your class. (Contact a local support group.)
6. Obtain literature from the American Cancer Society to use as resource materials or arrange to have a speaker talk with your class.
7. Invite a medical oncologist, hematologist, or surgeon to share case studies with your students.
8. Obtain literature from the Lupus Foundation to supplement your information, or invite an individual with lupus to talk about the disease.
9. Obtain literature from the Arthritis Foundation.

## ANSWERS TO CHECK YOUR KNOWLEDGE QUESTIONS

1. Persons diagnosed with cancer are best treated by a(n):
   a. personal family practice physician.
   b. internist.
   c. cytologist.
   **d. oncologist.**
2. A clinical trial is:
   a. a test performed in a physician's office.
   b. the discussion of a treatment by a group of attorneys.
   c. the testing of a new product to be used in a clinic.
   **d. a research study to determine the effectiveness and safety of a treatment.**
3. Tumor markers can:
   a. help locate sentinel lymph node.
   **b. help diagnose a tumor and its response to treatment.**
   c. mark the best location for focusing radiation.
   d. assist the surgeon to locate the tumor for removal during surgery.
4. A biopsy can be any of the following except:
   a. withdrawing a tissue sample through a needle.
   b. excising the whole tumor.
   c. removing a piece of the tumor by incision.
   **d. focusing a laser beam on the tumor to destroy a small part at a time.**
5. Genetic testing is appropriate when:
   **a. a person is at high risk for developing inherited cancers.**
   b. a patient wants to see if he has cancer.
   c. you want to determine if all the cancer has been removed.
   d. you need to see if a treatment has been effective.
6. Brachytherapy refers to:
   **a. treatment that places radioactive material at the tumor.**
   b. a treatment used only with patients who have the BRCA genes.
   c. an intravenous therapy given through the brachial artery.
   d. the administration of the drug Brachysone DX.

7. Which of the following statements does not refer to lupus?
   **a. It cannot be detected by a blood test.**
   b. It causes changes in the immune system.
   c. It is an autoimmune disease.
   d. It affects women more than men.
8. Lymphedema:
   a. results from the weakening of the immune system.
   **b. is swelling of the tissues by accumulated lymph fluid.**
   c. can be confirmed by a blood test.
   d. requires the removal of lymph nodes to stop the symptoms.
9. Rheumatoid arthritis:
   a. occurs primarily after age 65.
   b. is the wearing of cartilage at the joints.
   c. is treated with braces and splints to prevent joint movement.
   **d. is an insidious chronic autoimmune disease.**
10. Cancer vaccine:
    **a. can make cells visible to the immune system.**
    b. will eliminate all cancer cells in the body.
    c. can be developed quickly.
    d. is primarily directed toward people with BRCA1 gene mutation.
11. Immunity is strongest:
    a. in the aged.
    b. after recovering from the illness.
    **c. during infancy.**
    d. at 18 months of age.
12. Lupus:
    a. is a contagious disease.
    b. is limited to females only.
    c. occurs primarily after age 50.
    **d. is an autoimmune disease.**

# CHAPTER 32 The Digestive System

## LESSON OUTLINE

### I. GASTROINTESTINAL (GI) TRACT

A. Responsible for the physical and chemical breakdown of food so that it can be used by the body's cells

B. Alimentary canal is the connecting chain of organs

### II. DIGESTIVE PROCESS

A. Ingestion

B. Digestion

C. Absorption

D. Elimination

### III. MAIN ORGANS OF SYSTEM

A. Mouth

B. Pharynx

C. Esophagus

D. Stomach

E. Small intestine

F. Large intestine

### IV. ACCESSORY ORGANS

A. Teeth

B. Tongue

C. Salivary glands

D. Liver

E. Gallbladder

F. Pancreas

### V. DIGESTIVE PROCESS REQUIRES COOPERATION

A. Nervous system

B. Muscular system

C. Circulatory system

D. Endocrine system

### VI. BODY NUTRITIONAL NEEDS

A. Carbohydrates supply two-thirds of the needed energy calories per day

B. Fats

1. Stored if not used

2. Excellent source of energy

C. Proteins

1. Obtained from plant and animal sources

2. Not stored by the body
3. Used to build and repair cells and tissue

D. Vitamins are regulating chemicals

E. Minerals

## VII. MOUTH RECEIVES THE FOOD INTO THE SYSTEM

A. Teeth
1. Break down the food physically
2. Types
    a. Deciduous teeth
        i. Baby teeth
        ii. 6 months to 6 years
    b. Permanent teeth
3. Different teeth have specific duties
    a. Incisors bite
    b. Canines or cuspids puncture and tear
    c. Premolars or bicuspids, and molars, grind and crush

B. Tongue
1. A muscle
2. Moves the food around
3. Contains the taste buds

C. Salivary glands
1. Three pairs
    a. Parotid
    b. Sublingual
    c. Submandibular
2. Saliva
    a. Produced by the glands
    b. Provides moisture for taste buds
    c. Contains ptyalin, an enzyme that begins the breakdown of food
    d. Aids in cleansing the teeth
    e. Keeps surfaces moist and flexible
    f. Aids with speech
    e. When combined with food, it forms a bolus

## VIII. PHARYNX OR THROAT

A. Carries food to the esophagus

B. Carries air to the trachea

## IX. ESOPHAGUS

A. Has two layers of involuntary muscles

B. Peristalsis occurs when the circular and longitudinal muscles alternately contract and relax to move the bolus in one direction toward the stomach

## X. STOMACH

A. Cardiac sphincter
   1. Circular muscle at the upper opening of stomach
   2. Closes after food enters, preventing it from going back into esophagus
B. J-shaped organ that is 10 inches long
   1. Rugae
      a. Mucous membrane folds
      b. Straightens out as stomach fills
   2. Three layers of muscle aid in digestion, providing a churning action that further breaks down food
C. Gastric glands aid a chemical process to break down food
   1. Secrete hydrochloric acid
      a. Excess acid may cause a gastric/peptic ulcer
      b. Ammonia is secreted to counteract the acid
   2. Secrete enzymes
      a. Rennin curdles milk
      b. Lipase splits certain fats
      c. Pepsin digests the milk curds
D. Chyme is the semiliquid state of digested food
E. Pyloric sphincter
   1. Located between the stomach and small intestine
   2. Allows the chyme to leave the stomach
F. Emesis or vomiting occurs when pressure and reverse peristalsis push the stomach contents out through the mouth

## XI. SMALL INTESTINE

A. Coiled section
B. 20 feet in length and 1 inch in diameter
C. Completes digestion by secreting intestinal juices and receiving secretions from the accessory organs
   1. Liver
   2. Gallbladder
   3. Pancreas
D. Absorbs nutrients from the chyme
E. Three sections
   1. Duodenum
      a. 9 inches long
      b. Has highest concentration of acid
      c. Connecting link between the stomach and the remainder of the system
   2. Jejunum
      a. 8 feet in length
      b. Most nutrients are absorbed here

3. Ileum
    a. Last segment
    b. 12 feet in length

F. Mesentery
    1. Fan-shaped fold of tissue
    2. Supports the jejunum and ileum

G. Ileocecal valve
    1. Circular muscle separates the ileum and cecum
    2. Allows chyme to enter the cecum
    3. Prevents food from returning to ileum

## XII. LIVER

A. Largest gland in the body

B. Accessory organ for the digestive tract

C. Located under the diaphragm mostly in the upper-right quadrant of the abdomen

D. Function
    1. Secretes bile and breaks down fats
    2. Stores sugar in the form of glycogen, which can be converted to glucose as needed
    3. Processes proteins
    4. Burns or stores fats
    5. Produces blood proteins used in blood-clotting process
        a. Fibrinogen
        b. Prothrombin
    6. Produces antibodies
    7. Neutralizes poisons
    8. Stores large quantities of blood and body fluids

## XIII. GALLBLADDER

A. Small muscular sac

B. Receives bile from liver
    1. Stores and concentrates bile
    2. Releases concentrated bile through the cystic duct, into the common bile duct, where it is released into the duodenum
    3. Cholelithiasis can obstruct
    4. Jaundice
    5. Laparoscopic cholecystectomy and ERCP

## XIV. PANCREAS

A. Located behind the stomach

B. Functions as an exocrine gland by secreting pancreatic digestive juices

  1. Enters duodenum through pancreatic duct
  2. Contain three powerful enzymes to digest food

C. Functions as an endocrine gland by secreting insulin directly into the bloodstream

## XV. ABSORPTION FUNCTION

A. Villi

  1. Fingerlike projections lining wall of small intestine
  2. Keep chyme moving and mixed
  3. Contain blood capillaries that absorb nutrients and carry them to liver
  4. Lacteals
     a. Intestinal lymphatic capillary
     b. Pick up most digested fats, processing and returning them to the circulatory system

## XVI. LARGE INTESTINE

A. Also called the colon

B. Final section

C. About 5 feet long and approximately 2 inches in diameter

D. Functions

  1. Absorption of excess liquid
  2. Forms any indigestible materials into feces
  3. Eliminates the leftover waste products

E. Sections

  1. Cecum
     a. First section
     b. Connects with ileum
     c. Veriform appendix extends
        i. Worm-shaped structure
        ii. Appendicitis
           (a) Inflammation of the appendix
           (b) Appendectomy is the surgical procedure to remove the appendix
  2. Ascending colon to hepatic flexure
  3. Transverse colon to splenic flexure
  4. Descending colon
  5. Sigmoid is S-shaped
  6. Rectum
     a. 6–8 inches long
     b. Collecting area for the remains of digestion
     c. Eliminates its contents when an appropriate amount has been accumulated

7. Anal canal is the narrow passageway extending from the rectum to the anus
    a. About 1 inch long
    b. Controlled by sphincter muscles at each end
        i. Internal anal sphincter is an involuntary muscle
        ii. External anal sphincter is a voluntary muscle
8. Anus is the opening from the body at the end of digestive tract
    a. Incontinence
    b. Fecal impaction
9. Show Media Link: "Digestion"

## XVII. DIAGNOSTIC EXAMINATIONS

A. Colonoscopy is an examination to view the entire large intestine using a flexible fiberoptic scope

B. Gastrointestinal series includes radiological studies of the GI tract
    1. Upper GI series
    2. Lower GI series

C. Gastroscopy
    1. Viewing the esophagus, stomach, and upper duodenum
    2. Use of a flexible scope, which is lighted by fiberoptics

D. Nuclear medicine study
    1. Scanning of structures such as the liver or spleen
    2. Use of radioactive materials

E. Occult blood test is the analysis of the feces for blood

F. Proctoscopy
    1. Examination of the lower rectum and anal canal
    2. Use of proctoscope

G. Sigmoidoscopy
    1. Examination of the sigmoid
    2. Use of sigmoidoscope

H. Ultrasound uses high-frequency sound waves to study the liver, gallbladder, or pancreas

## XVIII. DISORDERS AND DISEASES

A. Anorectal abscess is a localized infection due to a collection of exudate in the soft tissue adjacent to the anus or rectum

B. Appendicitis is the acute inflammation of the appendix

C. Cirrhosis is a chronic disease of the liver that destroys liver cells

D. Colitis is an inflammatory disease of the colon

E. Colorectal cancer is a malignancy of the colon or rectum

F. Colostomy is an artificial opening of the colon, allowing fecal material to be excreted from the body

G. Constipation is the inability to expel fecal material, note constipation in infants

H. Crohn's disease is inflammation of the GI tract

I. Diarrhea is characterized by frequent liquid stools

J. Diverticulosis is the presence of bulging pouches in the wall of the GI tract

K. Esophageal varices are dilated, tortuous veins in the lower section of the esophagus
L. Fissure of the anus is a crack or tear in the lining of the anus
M. Gastroenteritis is an inflammation of the stomach and intestines
N. Gastroesophageal reflux (GERD) is a backflow of stomach contents into the esophagus
O. Hemorrhoids are enlarged veins in the anal canal
P. Hepatitis
    1. Type A is called infectious hepatitis
    2. Type B is called serum hepatitis
    3. Type C is the silent form
    4. Identified types D, E, and G
    5. Transmission varies with type
        a. Practice standard precautions
        b. Virus very contagious
    6. Results in liver destruction and death
    7. Symptoms vary with type and include fatigue, malaise, headache, loss of appetite, light sensitivity, sore throat, cough, nausea, vomiting, fever, and jaundice
    8. Disease progresses through stages
    9. Diagnosed with history and blood test for antigens
    10. HCV spread through contact with blood, shared needles, other sexual activity
    11. Vaccine available for types A and B
    12. Treatment varies with type from bed rest, to diet, to antiviral drugs.
Q. Hernia
    1. The protrusion of an internal organ through a natural opening in the body wall
    2. Hiatus
        a. A defect in the diaphragm
            i. Sliding
            ii. Rolling or paraesophageal
            iii. Mixed
    3. Inguinal
    4. Femoral
    5. Umbilical
    6. Incisional
R. Ileostomy is a surgical opening of the ileum, allowing the chyme of the small intestine to empty through the abdominal wall
S. Irritable bowel syndrome is alternating diarrhea and constipation
T. Oral cancer
U. Pancreatitis is the inflammation of the pancreas
V. Paralytic ileus is a physiological intestinal obstruction
W. Peptic ulcer is an encircled lesion caused by contact with gastric juices
X. Polyp is a mass of tissue in the GI tract
Y. Pruritus ani is itching of the area surrounding the anus
Z. Pyloric stenosis

1. Narrowing of the pyloric sphincter
2. Interferes with the emptying of the stomach

AA. Spastic colon is a condition characterized by alternating periods of constipation and diarrhea

BB. Ulcerative colitis is an inflammatory disease of the colon

### XIX. AGE-RELATED BODY CHARACTERISTICS

A. GERD in infants

B. GERD in adults

### XX. SYSTEM INTERACTION

A. GERD–Digestive, respiratory

B. Hepatitis–Digestive, circulatory, integumentary, senses

## CHAPTER ACTIVTIES

1. With a lab partner, listen with a stethoscope as a gulp of water is swallowed. Place the stethoscope below the xiphoid process. There should be two sounds, one when the water reaches the cardiac sphincter and one when the peristaltic waves begin and the sphincter opens.
2. Obtain gallstones from a local hospital or surgeon to show to the students.
3. Give student volunteers different sour or bitter foods to demonstrate the action of the salivary glands. Foods such as lemons, limes, sour candies, and almond extract will work.
4. Identify the organs of digestion on an anatomical model or chart.
5. Ask adult students to voluntarily take a healthy dose of Pepto-Bismol and report to the class any changes they see in their stool. (Stool should be very dark or black.)
6. Have students work in pairs using stethoscopes to listen to the bowel sounds.
7. Request X-rays from an upper and lower GI series and gallbladder studies to show to students.
8. Obtain brochures, pamphlets, and patient information sheets about the digestive system from hospitals and physicians' offices.

## ANSWERS TO CHECK YOUR KNOWLEDGE QUESTIONS

1. Cholecystography can detect:
   a. a properly functioning gallbladder.
   b. a non-functioning gallbladder.
   c. cholelithiasis.
   d. bile duct operation.
   **e. all of the above.**
2. Barium swallow can detect all of the following except:
   a. condition and function of esophagus.
   b. esophageal varices.
   c. hiatal hernia.
   d. esophegeal stricture.
   **e. cholelithiasis.**

3. Upper GI series can detect a:
   a. gastric ulcer.
   b. tumor of the stomach.
   c. polyp of the colon.
   **d. both a and b.**
   e. both b and c.
4. Lower GI series can detect all of the following except:
   **a. a duodenal ulcer.**
   b. tumors of the colon.
   c. polyps.
   d. ulcerative areas.
   e. diverticula.
5. Gastroscopy makes it possible to:
   a. view growth for biopsy.
   b. remove foreign objects.
   c. obtain cells for study.
   d. both a and c.
   **e. all of the above.**
6. Nuclear and ultrasonography studies can:
   **a. screen for disease processes.**
   b. obtain cells for study.
   c. locate cysts and tumors.
   d. both a and b.
   e. both a and c.
7. Occult blood test will:
   a. detect mucus in feces.
   **b. detect blood in feces.**
   c. determine location of bleeding.
   d. determine enzymes in stool.
   e. all of the above.
8. Proctoscopy will permit viewing of:
   **a. hemorrhoids.**
   b. colitis.
   c. polyps of the sigmoid.
   d. gastric ulcers.
   e. diverticula.
9. Sigmoidoscopy will permit viewing of:
   a. duodenal ulcers.
   b. condition of ileocecal valve.
   **c. tumor of the lower colon.**
   d. gastric ulcers.
   e. both a and b.

10. Cirrhosis is a disease of the:
    a. stomach.
    b. pancreas.
    **c. liver.**
    d. gallbladder.
11. Colitis disease effects primarily the:
    a. appendix.
    b. stomach.
    c. liver.
    **d. ileum.**
12. The prime symptom of ulcer colitis is:
    a. jaundice.
    **b. bloody diarrhea.**
    c. constipation.
    d. hunger.

# CHAPTER 33 The Urinary System

## LESSON OUTLINE

### . FUNCTIONS OF THE URINARY SYSTEM

A. Excretion is the removal of waste products and other elements from the blood

B. Secretion is the production of urine

C. Elimination is the emptying of urine from the bladder

D. Interaction of circulatory, digestive, muscular, nervous, endocrine, and respiratory systems

### I. ORGANS OF THE URINARY SYSTEM

A. Kidneys

1. Two bean-shaped organs
2. Located on either side of the vertebral column, behind the upper part of the abdominal cavity, and separated from the cavity by parietal peritoneum
3. A heavy cushion of fat protects and keeps the kidneys in their proper position
4. Covered with capsule
5. Hilum
    a. Renal artery
    b. Renal vein
    c. Ureter
6. Internal structure
    a. Cortex is the outer layer
    b. Medulla
        i. Inner layer
        ii. Pyramids
            (a) Triangular divisions of medulla
            (b) Renal papillae
            (c) Empty into the calyces
    c. Calyces are the cavities of the renal pelvis
7. Nephron units
    a. Microscopic filtering units
    b. Over 1 million in each kidney
    c. Renal corpuscle
        i. Bowman's capsule
            (a) Cup-shaped top of the nephron
            (b) Surrounds the glomerulus
        ii. Glomerulus
            (a) Network of about 50 blood capillaries
            (b) Filters fluid and other useful substances out of the blood into Bowman's capsule
                (i) Afferent arteriole
                (ii) Efferent arteriole

d. Renal tubule

i. Proximal convoluted tubule is the first twisted section of renal tubule

ii. Loop of Henle descends into medulla with descending and ascending limbs

iii. Distal convoluted tubule

(a) Twisted section of renal tubule returning into cortex

(b) Empties into a collecting tubule, which empties into the calyx

8. Formation of urine

a. Filtration

i. Blood enters the capsule by way of the afferent arteriole

ii. Glomerular blood pressure causes fluid to filter out and enter the Bowman's capsule

b. Reabsorption

i. Return of about 99% of filtered substances from renal tubules into blood via peritubular capillaries

ii. About 80% of water, as well as other nutrients and ions, is reabsorbed in the proximal tubule

iii. Depending on the body's need, the remaining 10–15% of water may be reabsorbed in distal tubule

c. Secretion

i. Movement of substances from blood directly into urine

ii. Elements are selectively secreted to maintain the body's acid–base balance

d. Urinary output

i. Increase in blood volume in the capillaries increases the urine output

ii. Decrease in blood volume in the capillaries decreases urine output

iii. Amount of solutes affects output

e. Show: Media Link: "Urine Formation"

B. Ureters

1. Two muscular tubes approximately 10–12 inches long

2. Function is to drain urine from calyces through renal pelvis to urinary bladder

3. Peristaltic waves move urine through ureters

4. Renal calculi from solutes

C. Urinary bladder

1. Collapsible, muscular sac, with folds in lining

2. Located behind the symphysis pubis

3. Function

a. Serves as reservoir for urine

b. Urge to void is felt when bladder contains 250 ml of urine, although it can hold in excess of 1,000 ml of fluid

c. Catheterization to remove urine

D. Urethra

1. Narrow tube leading from bladder to exterior

2. External opening is called the urinary meatus

3. Function

a. Carries urine to outside

b. In males, also carries semen

4. External urethral sphincter permits voluntary control of bladder

## III. TERMS

A. Anuria is the absence of urine

B. Dysuria is painful urination

C. Hematuria is blood in urine

D. Nocturia is having to urinate at night

E. Oliguria is scanty urinary output

F. Polyuria is excessive urination

G. Incontinence is involuntary urination

H. Dribbling is the involuntary loss of drops of urine

I. Frequency is the necessity to void often

J. Hesitancy is difficulty in initiating

K. Urgency is a sudden need to void

## IV. DIALYSIS

A. Mechanical process of removing waste products from the blood

B. Hemodialysis

1. Purifying blood by allowing waste products to diffuse into dialysate solutions
2. Dialyzer is "artificial kidney"
3. Patient connected to machine by needles and tubing
4. Fistulas and grafts for sites
5. Avoid B/P measurement in arm with dialysis access
6. Permacath with double lumen; surgically inserted into jugular or subclavian vein

C. Continuous ambulatory peritoneal dialysis

1. Dialysate is introduced into the peritoneal cavity
2. Four to six hours later the dialysate and waste products are drained into a bag
3. Continuous cycler-assisted peritoneal dialysis
   a. Performed at night
   b. Well-suited for children
4. Nocturnal intermittent peritoneal dialysis
5. Peritonitis complication

## V. KIDNEY TRANSPLANT

A. Usually the donor is a family member

B. Body may reject organ

## VI. DIAGNOSTIC EXAMINATIONS

A. Analysis of blood determines levels of uric acid and urea nitrogen present

B. Urinalysis determines presence of blood cells, bacteria, acidity level, specific gravity, and physical characteristics, such as color, clarity, and odor

C. Noninvasive procedures are used to evaluate urinary output
    1. Intake/output
    2. Routine urine specimen
    3. Clean catch specimen
    4. 24-hour specimen
    5. X-ray and fluoroscopy
    6. KUB series
    7. Ultrasound

D. Invasive procedures involve entering the body to perform the test
    1. Intravenous pyelography
    2. Cystourethroscopy
        a. Kidney catheterization
        b. Tumor biopsy
        c. Calculi removal
        d. Sterile specimen studies
    3. Catheterization
    4. Retrograde ureteropyelography
    5. Fluoroscopy

## VII. DISEASES AND DISORDERS

A. Cystitis is an inflammation of the bladder

B. Glomerulonephritis is the inflammation of the glomerulus of the nephron
    1. Acute is caused by delayed immune response to a strep infection
    2. Chronic is slow and progressive

C. Incontinence
    1. Stress
    2. Overflow
    3. Urge
    4. Kegel exercises
    5. Incontinence pads, garments
    6. Medications
    7. Collagen injections
    8. Surgery and artificial sphincter, sling

D. Nephrotic syndrome (nephrosis)
    1. Noninflammatory disease of the glomerular membrane
    2. Results in large amount of water being retained

E. Polycystic kidney disease
    1. Inherited disease
    2. Bilateral, grapelike clusters of fluid-filled cysts around the kidney

F. Pyelonephritis
   1. Common kidney disease
   2. Caused by bacteria normally found in the intestines
G. Renal calculi are kidney stones
   1. Lithotripsy (ESWL), water tank, special table
H. Renal failure
   1. Acute results in the sudden cessation of kidney function
   2. Chronic occurs as an end result of the progressive loss of kidney function
I. Stricture is a narrowing of a passage that interferes with the movement of substances through its interior
   1. Treatment with
   2. Laser treatment
   3. Excision treatment
J. Uremia is the presence in the blood of products normally found in urine

### VIII. AGE-RELATED CHARACTERISTICS ASSOCIATED WITH INCONTINENCE

### IX. SYSTEM INTERACTION

A. Chronic glomerular nephritis
B. Renal failure

## CHAPTER ACTIVITIES

1. Obtain kidney stones from a local hospital or urologist and discuss their formation and removal. Or, ask a urologist to speak about kidney diseases and bring some calculi that have been removed from patients. (They can be very interestingly shaped and colored.)
2. Have each student keep a record of the amount of fluid taken in and the amount excreted for one day. Compare the intake to the output.
3. Have a guest speaker discuss dialysis. If possible, visit a dialysis center.
4. Obtain X-ray films from a KUB, IVP, and retrograde studies.
5. Obtain brochures and pamphlets from the Kidney Foundation.
6. Get sample patient information sheets on diagnostic tests from hospitals and physicians' offices.
7. Assign reports on the more common renal diseases and conditions.
8. Have students provide a service for faculty in your building. Place numbered specimen cups in the teachers' rest rooms. Instruct teachers to collect a specimen and place it in a designated area within the bathroom. Remind them to make a note of their numbers. At a specified time collect and analyze the samples. Post the results by number in the faculty rest rooms. If a significant finding occurs, leave a note requesting that #— see the instructor.

## ANSWERS TO CHECK YOUR KNOWLEDGE QUESTIONS

1. Which of the following diagnostic procedures is not noninvasive?
   **a. Catheterization**
   b. Ultrasound
   c. KUB series
   d. Fluoroscopy

2. A clean catch specimen is not
   **a. a sterile specimen.**
   b. caught in midstream.
   c. collected by the patient.
   d. obtained after careful cleaning.
3. An intravenous pyelography
   a. requires catheterization.
   **b. is an X-ray study with contrast media.**
   c. is a noninvasive procedure.
   d. allows visualization of the bladder interior.
4. Which of the following terms does not refer to a type of incontinence?
   a. Stress
   b. Overflow
   c. Urge
   **d. Pressure**
5. Polycystic kidney disease is characterized by
   a. a large number of protein molecules in the urine.
   **b. fluid-filled structures within the kidney tissue.**
   c. a history of a systemic infection.
   d. rapidly developing symptoms.
6. Which of the following is the basic cause of renal calculi?
   a. Drinking hard water
   b. A habit of delaying passing urine
   c. Getting too much calcium in the diet
   **d. Crystals formed from chemicals in the urine**
7. Acute renal failure may result in all the following except:
   a. uremia.
   b. death.
   c. sudden kidney failure.
   **d. progressive loss of kidney function.**
8. A long-term treatment for uremia is
   **a. a kidney transplant.**
   b. antibiotics.
   c. radiation.
   d. blood transfusions.
9. Which of the following is not a type of incontinence?
   **a. Retention**
   b. Stress
   c. Overflow
   d. Urge

10. Hemodialysis can be achieved through all the following except

    a. arteriovenous fistula.

    **b. indwelling urinary catheter.**

    c. synthetic graft.

    d. Permacath.

# CHAPTER 34 The Endocrine System

## LESSON OUTLINE

### I. ENDOCRINE SYSTEM

A. Group of ductless glands

B. Secretes hormones directly into the blood capillaries

1. Chemical messengers that produce changes on various organs
2. Perform various functions
   a. Regulate growth and development
   b. Regulate metabolism
   c. Stimulate other endocrine glands
   d. Control sexual processes

### I. EXOCRINE GLANDS SECRETE INTO DUCTS

### II. TYPES OF GLANDS

A. Pituitary

B. Thyroid

C. Parathyroid

D. Pancreas

E. Adrenals

F. Ovaries

G. Testes

H. Thymus

I. Pineal body

### V. PITUITARY GLAND

A. Master gland of the body

B. Sits under the brain in a small bony depression called the sella turcica

C. Secretes nine known hormones

D. Divided into two lobes that produce specific hormones

1. Anterior lobe
   a. Growth hormone (GH) is essential for normal growth of body's tissues
      i. Gigantism occurs from overproduction in childhood
      ii. Dwarfism occurs from underproduction in childhood
      iii. Acromegaly occurs from overproduction in adulthood
   b. Thyrotropin (TSH) increases the production of thyroid hormone
   c. Adrenocorticotropic hormone (ACTH) stimulates the cortex of the adrenal gland
   d. Melanocyte-stimulating hormone (MSH) increases skin pigmentation
   e. Prolactin (PR)
      i. Breast development
      ii. Production of milk

f. Gonadotropic hormones control the development of reproductive system

i. Follicle-stimulating hormone (FSH)

(a) Stimulation produces estrogen in females

(b) Stimulation produces sperm in males

ii. Luteinizing hormone (LH)

(a) Produces progesterone in females

(b) Produces testosterone in males

2. Posterior lobe

a. Oxytocin stimulates the contractions of the uterus and flow of milk from breast

b. Vasopressin or anti-diuretic hormone (ADH), concentrates urine to conserve water and constricts blood vessels

## V. THYROID GLAND

A. Located in front of the upper part of the trachea

B. Has two lobes

1. One on each side of the larynx
2. Connected by isthmus

C. Produces three hormones

1. Thyroxin ($T_4$)
2. Triiodothyronine ($T_3$)
3. Calcitonin

D. Thyroid activity

1. Hypothyroidism occurs when underproduction causes decreased metabolic rate
2. Hyperthyroidism occurs when overproduction causes increased metabolic rate

a. Exophthalmia

b. Thyrotoxic crisis

E. Requires iodine to produce hormones, results in goiter, the enlargement of the gland due to feedback mechanism

1. Lack of iodine
2. Thyroidectomy

## VI. PARATHYROID GLANDS

A. Two pairs of glands

B. Located on posterior surface of the thyroid gland

C. Regulates the amount of calcium in the blood

D. Secretes parathormone

E. Disorders

1. Hyperparathyroidism

a. Increased level of calcium in the blood

b. Results in kidney stones and a decalcification of bones

2. Hypoparathyroidism
    a. Results in a low level of calcium in the blood
    b. Causes a series of muscle twitchings called tetany

## VII. ADRENAL GLANDS

A. Called suprarenal glands
B. Located above each kidney
C. Two parts
    1. Medulla (inner tissue)
        a. Principal hormones
            i. Adrenaline (epinephrine)
            ii. Norepinephrine
        b. "Fight-or-flight" hormone
    2. Cortex (outer tissue)
        a. Principal hormones
            i. Mineral corticoids (aldosterone)
            ii. Glucocorticoids
            iii. Sex steroids (androgens)
            iv. Excess may cause external genitalia abnormalities
        b. Essential to life

## VIII. PANCREAS

A. Both an exocrine and endocrine gland
B. Located behind the stomach
C. Four types of cells
    1. The B cells of Islands of Langerhans secrete insulin
        a. Hyperglycemia is an elevated blood sugar level
            i. Glycosuria
            ii. Diabetes mellitus
        b. Hypoglycemia is an abnormally low level of blood sugar
    2. The A cells secrete glucagon
    3. C cells
    4. D cells

## IX. THYMUS

A. Two-lobed structure under sternum
B. Primarily composed of lymphoid tissue
C. Atrophies during puberty
D. Produces thymosin, which affects immunity

## X. PINEAL BODY

A. Small mass of tissue in brain

B. Believed to produce melatonin, which combines with a hypothalmic substance to regulate puberty

## XI. GONADS (TESTES AND OVARIES)

A. Ovaries

1. Sex glands of female
2. Located in pelvic cavity
3. One on each side of the uterus
4. Hormones
    a. Estrogen
    b. Progesterone
    c. Regulate sexual characteristics of the female

B. Testes

1. Sex glands of the male
2. Located in the scrotum
3. Produce testosterone
    a. Regulates sexual characteristics of the male
    b. Stimulates maturation of sperm cells

## XII. INTERRELATIONSHIP OF THE GLANDS

A. Regulated by a feedback mechanism

B. Production of some hormones affect the secretion of hormones from other glands

C. As hormone levels rise, the production of the stimulating hormone stops

1. Gland secretion is slowed down
2. As levels drop, the stimulating hormone again is produced

## XIII. DIAGNOSTIC EXAMINATIONS

A. Blood sugar is used to assess the function of the pancreas

B. $T_3$, TSH, and $T_4$ measure thyroid hormone levels

C. Urine human chorionic gonadotropin (HCG) is a pregnancy test

D. Glucose tolerance test is the measure of the body's ability to process a large dose of glucose

E. Glucohemoglobin or hemoglobin A1C (Hgb A1c) measures control of glucose level over four to six weeks

F. Scanning tests

1. Radioactive iodine uptake test
2. Thyroid scan
3. Ultrasound

## IV. DISEASES AND DISORDERS

A. Acromegaly
   1. Uncommon hormonal disorder
   2. Occurs when the pituitary gland produces excess growth hormone during adulthood
   3. Results in overgrowth of connective tissue
B. Addison's disease
   1. Results from a deficiency of adrenal hormones from the cortex of the adrenal gland
   2. Causes metabolic changes
C. Cretinism results from the lack of thyroxine in the early stages of life, which leads to retarded mental and physical development
D. Cushing's syndrome
   1. Excess in adrenal cortex hormones
   2. Results in hypertension, obesity, and moon-faced appearance
E. Diabetes mellitus
   1. Chronic disease of insulin deficiency or resistance
   2. Interferes with metabolism of carbohydrates, proteins, and fats
   3. Insulin assists sugar to enter cells
   4. Body's program stores energy
   5. Types of diabetes
      a. Type 1 or insulin-dependent considered to be genetic or autoimmune disorder
      b. Type 2 adult-onset form
   6. Symptoms are fatigue, polyuria and dehydration of cells, and thirst
   7. Treat with diet, exercise, drugs, and insulin injections
      a. Use of multi-drug approach
      b. Anticipate information from genome project will help
   8. Diabetic coma and insulin shock
F. Graves' disease
   1. Overproduction of the thyroid gland
   2. Exophthalmus
G. Myxedema
   1. Caused by hyposecretion of the thyroid gland in adulthood
   2. Alters metabolism and vital functions

## V. AGE-RELATED BODY CHARACTERISTICS

A. Change in lens, retinopathy
B. Neuropathy
C. End-stage kidney disease
D. Infection, amputation

## VI. SYSTEM INTERACTION

A. Diabetes–Endocrine, urinary, circulatory, senses, integumentary, nervous
B. Grave's disease–Endocrine, circulatory, muscular, nervous, senses

## CHAPTER ACTIVITIES

1. Invite an endocrinologist to discuss patients with endocrine disorders.
2. Assign students reports on endocrine disorders.
3. Obtain brochures and pamphlets from the American Diabetes Association.
4. Invite a person with diabetes mellitus to talk about the changes the disease has made in his or her lifestyle. Have the person demonstrate self-injection of insulin if the time can be arranged.
5. Ask a nurse clinician who specializes in diabetes mellitus to talk about the importance of diet, drug and insulin therapy, and the testing for glycosuria or blood sugar.

## ANSWERS TO CHECK YOUR KNOWLEDGE QUESTIONS

1. An endocrine gland:
   **a. secretes substances into the bloodstream.**
   b. secretes substances into a duct.
   c. secretes substances into the lymph vessels.
   d. secretes substances into the stomach.
2. All of these statements are true except:
   a. insulin is secreted by the islets of Langerhans.
   **b. hyperglycemia refers to too much insulin.**
   c. insulin is an endocrine secretion from the pancreas.
   d. insulin is necessary to metabolize carbohydrates.
3. Which of the following statements is not true?
   a. Type I diabetes is called juvenile diabetes
   b. Type 2 diabetes develops from insulin resistance
   c. Type 1 diabetes is an autoimmune disease
   **d. Hypoglycemia is the main symptom of diabetes**
4. The following statements about the thymus gland are true except:
   a. it gets smaller as we age.
   b. it causes certain T cells to mature.
   **c. it is located in the brain.**
   d. it produces peptides.
5. Progesterone is a hormone secreted by the:
   **a. ovaries.**
   b. testes.
   c. pituitary gland.
   d. pineal gland.
6. A test that measures glucose levels of four to six weeks is:
   a. glucose tolerance.
   b. human chorionic gonadotropin.
   c. fasting blood sugar.
   **d. hemoglobin A1c.**

7. A moon face and a buffalo hump are symptoms of:
   a. Addison's disease.
   c. Myxedema.
   b. Graves' disease.
   **d. Cushing's syndrome.**
8. Enlarged thyroid, nervousness, and weight loss are symptoms of:
   a. Addison's disease.
   **b. Graves' disease.**
   c. Myxedema.
   d. Cushing's disease.
9. The following are symptoms of hypoglycemia except:
   a. nervousness.
   b. paleness.
   c. full bounding pulse.
   **d. dry skin.**
10. Escalated hyperthyroidism may develop into:
    a. cardiomegaly.
    b. generalized paralysis.
    c. exophthalmus.
    **d. a thyroid storm.**
11. Diabetes causes:
    a. obesity.
    **b. hyperglycemia.**
    c. hypoglycemia.
    d. urinary retention.

# CHAPTER 35 The Reproductive System

## LESSON OUTLINE

### I. REPRODUCTIVE SYSTEM FUNCTION IS THE CREATION OF NEW LIFE

A. Two types of reproduction
  1. Asexual occurs when an organism reproduces by dividing into two cells
  2. Sexual requires a male and female cell to unite into one single cell
    a. Each sex has special sex glands or gonads that produce sex cells called gametes
      i. Spermatozoan in males
      ii. Ovum in females
    b. Union of gametes produces zygote, which undergoes mitosis repeatedly to form a new individual

### II. DIFFERENTIATION OF REPRODUCTIVE ORGANS

A. Organs develop from the same embryonic tissue
B. Presence of androgens and müllerian inhibitor produces sex differentiation
C. Medulla of the gonad develops into testes
D. Cortex of the gonad develops into ovaries
E. The tubercle becomes the glan penis in males and the clitoris in females
F. The folds become the penile shaft in males and the labia minora in females
G. The swelling develops into the scrotum in males and the labia majora in females
H. Wolffian ducts become the epididymis, vas deferens, and ejaculatory duct in males and the embryonic müllerian ducts degenerate
I. The müllerian ducts become the fallopian tubes, uterus, and part of the vagina in females and the wolffian ducts degenerate

### III. MALE REPRODUCTIVE ORGANS

A. Development
  1. Develop in fetal abdomen
  2. Descend through inguinal canal during eighth and ninth month
  3. Inguina hernia from relaxed structure
  4. Undescended testicle is cryptorchidism
B. Testes
  1. Suspended in the scrotum
  2. Two male gonads
  3. Produce sperm and testosterone, causing primary and secondary male characteristics
    a. Longer, heavier bones
    b. Larger muscles
    c. Deep voice
    d. Growth of body hair
    e. Development of external genitalia

f. Increased metabolism

g. Sexual desire

C. Epididymis

1. Coiled tube about 20 feet long
2. Receives, stores, and matures the sperm from the testes
3. Produces a fluid secreted during ejaculation

D. Vas deferens

1. Passageway for sperm and fluid from the epididymis
2. Joins each epididymis
   a. Extends up into the abdominal cavity
   b. Curves to base of the urinary bladder
   c. Joins with seminal vesicle and forms the ejaculatory duct

E. Seminal vesicles

1. Pair of small tubes behind bladder
2. Secrete fluid
   a. Provides nutrition for the sperm
   b. Fluid makes up a large part of the semen

F. Prostate gland

1. Doughnut-shaped gland with urethra passing through center
2. Located below the urinary bladder
3. Secretes prostatic alkaline liquid
   a. Stimulates sperm motility
   b. Neutralizes the acidity in the vagina
4. Muscular tissue contracts during ejaculation to empty semen into the urethra

G. Bulbourethral glands

1. Also called Cowper's glands
2. Produce a fluid
   a. Serve as a lubricant for intercourse
   b. Are alkaline and aids in movement of sperm

H. Urethra

1. Carries urine from the urinary bladder
2. Carries semen from the reproductive tubes

I. Semen is combined secretion of all glands and ducts of the male reproductive system

1. 5% fluids from the testes and epididymis
2. 30% fluid from the seminal vesicles
3. 60% fluid from the prostate gland
4. 5% fluid from the bulbourethral glands

J. Penis

1. Glans
   a. Enlarged structure at distal end

b. Foreskin or prepuce

i. Circular fold of skin that covers glans

ii. Circumcision is the surgical removal of the foreskin

iii. Phimosis of foreskin

2. Constructed of three columns of spongy erectile tissue

a. During sexual arousal, the spaces in the tissue become filled with blood

b. Squeezed veins prohibit venous return

c. Orgasm is the forceful release of semen and fluids

d. Engorgement subsides after orgasm

K. Vasectomy

L. Show Media Link: "Male Reproductive System"

## V. DIAGNOSTIC EXAMS AND TESTS OF THE MALE REPRODUCTIVE SYSTEM

A. Chromosomal analysis

B. Digital rectal examination

C. Hormonal studies

D. Prostatic specific antigen (PSA)

E. Semen analysis

F. Testicular biopsy

G. Testicular self-examination

## V. DISEASES AND DISORDERS OF THE MALE REPRODUCTIVE SYSTEM

A. Epididymitis is an infection of the epididymis

B. Erectile dysfunction is the inability to have or sustain an erection

1. Primary

2. Secondary

C. Hydrocele is the presence of an excessive amount of normal fluid within the scrotum

D. Prostatic hypertrophy is an enlargement of the prostate gland

1. Prostatectomy, robotic

2. Transurethral

3. PSA blood test

4. PCPT

5. Cryosurgery

6. Radioactive seeds

## I. FEMALE REPRODUCTIVE SYSTEM

A. Ovaries

1. Female gonads

2. Small, almond-shaped glands

3. Located in pelvic cavity and attached to the uterus

4. Two main roles
    a. Produce ovum, the sex cell
    b. Secrete the hormones estrogen and progesterone
        i. Estrogen produces the secondary sex characteristics
            (a) Broadening of pelvis
            (b) Epiphysis becomes bone and growth ceases
            (c) Soft, smooth skin
            (d) Pubic hair
            (e) Breasts develop
            (f) Deposits of fat in buttocks and thighs
            (g) Sexual desire
            (h) Ovulation
            (i) Menstruation, menarche
        ii. Progesterone develops mammary glands and aids in maintaining pregnancy

B. Primary follicles
1. Contain immature ova
2. Thousands are in the ovaries
3. Mature under influence of FSH and LH, then release ovum
4. Graafian follicle
5. Corpus luteum

C. Fallopian tubes
1. Attached at superior lateral surface of uterus
2. Serve as a passageway for ovum to reach the uterus
3. Conception takes place in outer third of tube
4. Ectopic pregnancy

D. Uterus
1. Thick-walled, hollow, muscular organ
2. Located behind urinary bladder but in front of rectum
3. Divided into three parts
    a. Fundus
        i. Top section
        ii. Where fallopian tubes attach
    b. Body or middle portion
    c. Cervix
        i. Narrow bottom section that opens into the vagina
        ii. Has internal and external opening
4. Has three layers
    a. Endometrium
    b. Myometrium has three muscle layers
    c. Serous membrane
5. Capable of great expansion to allow for the development and growth of fetus
    a. Contracts to aid in expulsion of fetus during birth

6. Uterine positions
   a. Anteflexed
   b. Anteverted
   c. Mid-position
   d. Retroverted
   e. Retroflexed

E. Vagina
1. Collapsible muscular tube connecting cervix with the outside
2. Functions
   a. Passageway for the menstrual flow
   b. Birth canal
   c. Organ of sexual intercourse
3. Lined with mucous membrane
4. Cul-de-sac
5. Muscular sphincter
6. Opens at perineum
7. External opening called hymen

F. Vulva comprises the structures that form the external female genital area
1. Mons pubis
   a. Lies over the pubic area
   b. Covered with large pad of fat
2. Labia majora
   a. Pair of rounded folds of skin on each side of vulva
   b. Covered with hair on outer surface
3. Labia minora
   a. Two smaller folds of tissue
   b. Located within the labia majora
4. Bartholin's glands secrete a fluid lubricant during intercourse
5. Vestibule

G. Clitoris is made up of two small columns of erectile tissue
1. Produces sexual arousal when stimulated
2. Is involved in the orgasmic response

H. Perineum
1. Area between the vagina and anus in the female
2. Childbirth may cause tear or a need to perform episiotomy
3. Can be used to describe the entire pelvic floor in both the male and female

I. Mammary glands
1. Secondary sexual structures that develop and function only in females
2. Provide milk for infant

## VII. MENSTRUAL CYCLE

A. When ova is not fertilized, the uterine lining deteriorates and is discharged from body

B. Process begins with menarche and ends with menopause

C. Lunar month schedule

D. Caused by hormones

E. Four phases

1. Follicular phase
    a. Pituitary secretes high levels of FSH to stimulate the follicles
    b. One follicle matures, bringing about ovulation and secreting estrogen
    c. LH begins affecting the follicle and the endometrium thickens (proliferation)
2. Ovulation
    a. Matured ovum released
    b. Estrogen level is high
    c. FSH is reduced
    d. Release of LH causes rupture of follicle
    e. Endometrium continues to thicken
3. Luteal
    a. Follicle changes into a corpus luteum under the influence of LH, producing progesterone as well as estrogen
    b. Endometrium secretes nourishment for the egg
    c. Progesterone levels rise and LH is inhibited and levels drop
        i. Corpus luteum disintegrates
        ii. Progesterone and estrogen levels drop
4. Menstruation
    a. In the absence of hormones
        i. Endometrium deteriorates
        ii. Is expelled with a small amount of blood as the menstrual flow
    b. Estrogen and progesterone levels low
    c. FSH begins to rise to start the next cycle
5. Show Media Link: "Female Reproductive System"

## VIII. FERTILIZATION

A. Millions of sperm are deposited in female vagina

B. Travel to outer third of fallopian tube

C. Meet ovum and penetrate the corona radiata

1. Zygote is formed and genetic determination is complete
2. Zygote starts to travel to uterus and implants in uterus
3. Hormones support zygote
4. HCG is detectable

## X. PREGNANCY

A. Length of pregnancy or gestation period for humans is about 39 weeks

B. Embryonic state extends from fertilization to the end of week 8

C. Fetal state extends from week 8 to 39

D. Growth processes

1. Cell differentiation
2. Cell multiplication
3. Growth
4. Rearrangement

E. Signs of pregnancy

F. Naegele's rule

G. Incidence of Down syndrome

H. Edema and weight gain

G. IOM recommendations

## . BIRTH PROCESS

A. Called parturition

B. Fetus takes head-down position against the cervix

C. Irregular contractions begin

D. Amniotic sac ruptures

E. Labor begins

F. Stages of labor

1. Stage one
    a. Regular uterine contractions
    b. Cervical dilation and effacement
2. Stage two
    a. Complete dilation
    b. Head or other part enters vagina
    c. Crowning
    d. Delivery
        i. APGAR scoring system
            (a) One minute
            (b) Five minutes
3. Stage three
    a. Placenta detaches
    b. Afterbirth expelled
4. Cesarean section
    a. Inadequate outlet
    b. Breech
    c. Large baby
    d. Ineffective labor

e. Complications
f. Vaginal birth after cesarean (VBAC)

## XI. INFERTILITY

A. Causes are numerous
B. Solutions
    1. Artificial insemination
    2. In vitro fertilization
    3. Gamete intrafallopian transfer
    4. Intracytoplasmic sperm injection (ICSI)
    5. Zygote intrafallopian transfer (ZIFT)

## XII. CONTRACEPTION

A. Birth control practiced for many reasons
    1. Avoiding health risk to the woman
    2. Avoiding babies with birth defects
    3. Limiting family size
    4. Permitting woman to develop career
    5. Spacing pregnancies
    6. Delaying pregnancy early in marriage
    7. Avoiding pregnancy among unmarried couples
    8. Curbing population growth
B. Forms of contraception (Table 35–3)
    1. Abstinence
    2. Sterilization
    3. DPMA
    4. Birth control pills
    5. Contraception patch
    6. Contraception ring
    7. IUD
    8. Diaphragm
    9. Condom
    10. Cervical cap
    11. Female condom
    12. Spermicides
    13. Douching
    14. Withdrawal
    15. Rhythm

## III. PREGNANCY TERMINATION

A. Abortion

1. Spontaneous
2. elective
3. Therapeutic

## IV. DIAGNOSTIC AND SCREENING TESTS IN PREGNANCY

A. Alpha-fetoprotein screening blood test to detect multiple births, birth defects, etc.
B. Amniocentesis
C. Chorionic villi sampling
D. Gestational diabetes screening
E. Group B streptococcus (GBS)
F. Routine pregnancy screening tests

## V. DIAGNOSTIC TESTS OF THE FEMALE REPRODUCTIVE SYSTEM

A. Colposcopy is the examination of the cervix using a colposcope to rule out cancer
B. Hysteroscopy is used to look at the endometrium
C. Mammogram is an X-ray of the breast
D. Maturation index is a means of determining hormonal level
E. Papanicolaou smear (Pap smear)
F. Pregnancy test determines presence of human chorionic gonadotropin
G. Ultrasonography is a test for malignancy

## VI. DISEASES AND DISORDERS OF THE FEMALE REPRODUCTIVE SYSTEM

A. Cervical erosion is the ulceration of the cervix
B. Cervicitis is an inflammation of the cervix
C. Cystic breast disease is the presence of lumps within breast tissue
D. Cystocele is the bulging of the anterior vaginal wall and bladder into the vagina; use of pessary
E. Dysmenorrhea is lower abdominal and pelvic pain associated with menstruation
F. Endometriosis is the presence of endometrial tissue outside the uterus
G. Fibroids are benign, smooth tumors formed of muscle cells (leiomyomas)
H. Embolization procedure to treat leiomyomas
I. Hysterectomy is the surgical removal of uterus

1. Abdominal
2. Vaginal
3. Endometrial ablation

J. Ovarian cyst is a sac of fluid on an ovary
K. Premenstrual syndrome (PMS) is a combination of characteristics preceding menstruation
L. Polyp is a growth attached by a slender stem to the membrane
M. Rectocele is the bulging of the posterior vaginal wall and rectum into the vagina; use of pessary
N. Vaginitis is inflammation of vaginal mucosa

## XVII. MALIGNANCY OF THE FEMALE REPRODUCTIVE ORGANS

A. Breast
   1. Number two cause of death in females
   2. Warning signs
      a. A lump or mass in breast tissue
      b. Change in breast size or shape
      c. Change in appearance of the skin
      d. Change in skin temperature
      e. Drainage or discharge from a non-nursing woman
      f. Change in the nipple
         i. Itching
         ii. Burning
         iii. Erosion
         iv. Retraction
   3. Inflammatory breast cancer
B. Cervical
   1. Most common form
   2. Can be detected by a Pap smear
   3. Pap smear recommendations
C. Ovarian
   1. Common cause of death from cancer
   2. Early diagnosis difficult
D. Uterus
   1. Uterine enlargement
   2. Unusual bleeding
E. Vaginal
   1. Discharge
   2. Bleeding
   3. Ulcerated, firm lesion
F. Vulva
   1. Pruritus
   2. Bleeding
   3. Small surface ulcer

## XVIII. SEXUALLY TRANSMITTED DISEASES

A. Acquired immunodeficiency syndrome (AIDS) is a viral disease that suppresses the body's immune system (Unit 9)
B. Chlamydia is caused by a specialized bacterium
C. Gonorrhea is caused by the gonococcus bacterium
D. Herpes is a chronic viral infection
E. Human papillomavirus (HPV) infection is a group of related viruses and one of the most common sexually transmitted diseases

F. Nongonococcal urethritis (NGU) (NSU) is a bacterial infection

G. Pelvic inflammatory disease (PID)

1. Acute or chronic infection of the reproductive tract
2. Caused by an aerobic or anerobic organisms

H. Pediculosis pubis (pubic lice) are little, yellowish-gray insects that attach themselves to pubic hair roots

I. Syphilis is caused by a spirochete bacterium; VDRL and RPR test

1. Disease has four stages

J. Trichomoniasis is an inflammation caused by the single-celled parasitic organism called *Trichomonas vaginalis*

## XIX. AGE-RELATED BODY CHARACTERISTICS

A. Ovarian hormone effects

B. Menarche

C. Pregnancy

D. Menopause

## XX. SYSTEM INTERACTION

A. Pregnancy

B. Premenstrual syndrome

# CHAPTER ACTIVITIES

1. Depending on local policies, contact Planned Parenthood to discuss and show methods of contraception.
2. Ask a person who instructs Lamaze classes to share with the class the purpose and use of this technique.
3. Invite a speaker to discuss sexually transmitted diseases.
4. Obtain a film showing the birth of a baby. (In secondary settings, be certain to check with school administration and policy regarding such material.)
5. Invite a pregnant woman to talk to the class about her body changes and concerns with approaching delivery. If possible, and if she is willing, allow students to listen to the fetal heartbeat. (Appropriateness depends on makeup of class and is probably good only with students who have not experienced pregnancy.)
6. Invite a gynecological physician, nurse, or medical assistant to discuss the importance of the prenatal period.

# ANSWERS TO CHECK YOUR KNOWLEDGE QUESTIONS

1. Sperm are produced in the:

   a. epididymis.

   **b. seminiferous tubules.**

   c. vas deferens.

   d. seminal vesicles.

2. The prostate gland is located:

   a. in the testes.

   b. just above the bladder.

   c. in the penis.

   **d. just below the bladder.**

3. Which of the following is not a treatment for prostate cancer?
   a. Cryosurgery
   b. Radioactive seeds
   c. Female hormones
   **d. Prosthesis implant**
4. The corpus luteum is a(n):
   a. mature ova.
   b. immature graafian follicle.
   c. primary follicle.
   **d. follicle after ovulation occurs.**
5. The fallopian tubes are all the following except:
   a. a passageway for sperm.
   b. a passageway for ova.
   c. attached to the uterus.
   **d. attached to the ovaries.**
6. Which of the following terms does not refer to a uterine position?
   a. Anteflexed
   b. Retroflexed
   c. Retroverted
   **d. Antelapsed**
7. The perineum refers to the area:
   a. around the urinary meatus.
   b. within the labia minora.
   c. adjacent to the clitoris.
   **d. between the vagina and anus.**
8. Menarche means the:
   **a. beginning of menses.**
   b. end of menses.
   c. highest point in the menstrual cycle.
   d. period of ovulation.
9. Amniocentesis is done to:
   a. determine the sex of the baby.
   b. rule out multiple births.
   c. check for gestational diabetes.
   **d. check for chromosomal abnormalities.**
10. A colposcope is an instrument used to:
    **a. view the cervix.**
    b. view the uterus.
    c. evaluate fallopian tubes.
    d. observe the fetus in utero.

# SECTION 4 THE BACK OFFICE

# UNIT 12 PREPARING FOR CLINICAL PROCEDURES

# CHAPTER 36 Infection Control and Medical Asepsis

## ABHES Curriculum

| | |
|---|---|
| M.A.A.1.2.b | Identify and apply the knowledge of all body systems; their structure and functions; and their common diseases, symptoms, and etiologies |
| M.A.A.1.4.f | Comply with federal, state, and local health laws and regulations |
| M.A.A1.9.b | Apply principles of aseptic techniques and infection control |
| M.A.A.1.9.h | Wrap items for autoclaving |
| M.A.A.1.9.i | Use Standard Precautions |
| M.A.A.1.9.r | Teach patients methods of health promotion and disease prevention |
| M.A.A.1.10.c | Dispose of biohazardous materials |

## CAAHEP Core Curriculum

| | |
|---|---|
| I.C.6 | Identify common pathology related to each body system |
| III.C.1 | Describe the infection cycle, including the infectious agent, reservoir, susceptible host, means of transmission, portals of entry, and portals of exit |
| III.C.2 | Define asepsis |
| III.C.3 | Discuss infection control procedures |
| III.C.4 | Identify personal safety precautions as established by the Occupational Safety and Health Administration (OSHA) |
| III.C.5 | List major types of infectious agents |
| III.C.6 | Compare different methods of controlling the growth of microorganisms |
| III.C.7 | Match types and uses of personal protective equipment (PPE) |
| III.C.8 | Differentiate between medical and surgical asepsis used in ambulatory care settings, identifying when each is appropriate |
| III.C.11 | Describe Standard Precautions, including: (a) Transmission based precautions, (b) Purpose, (c) Activities regulated |
| III.C.12 | Discuss the application of Standard Precautions with regard to: (a) All body fluids, secretions and excretions, (b) Blood, (c) Non intact skin, (d) Mucous membranes |
| III.C.13 | Identify the role of the Center for Disease Control (CDC) regulations in healthcare settings. |
| III.P.1 | Participate in training on Standard Precautions |
| III.P.2 | Practice Standard Precautions |
| III.P.3 | Select appropriate barrier/personal protective equipment (PPE) for potentially infectious situations |
| III.P.4 | Perform hand washing |
| III.P.5 | Prepare items for autoclaving |
| III.P.6 | Perform sterilization procedures |
| IX.P.6 | Complete an incident report |
| XI.C.1 | Describe personal protective equipment |
| XI.C.2 | Identify safety techniques that can be used to prevent accidents and maintain a safe work environment |
| XI.C.9 | Discuss requirements for responding to hazardous material disposal |

# LESSON OUTLINE

## I. THE INFECTION CYCLE AND DISEASE TRANSMISSION

A. Common communicable diseases: their means of transmission, incubation times, symptoms, and treatments (Table 36–1)

B. Microorganisms

1. Disease-producing microorganisms (pathogens)
2. Normal flora providing balance and destroying pathogens
3. Growth requirements of microorganisms
   a. Aerobes need oxygen
   b. Anaerobes grow without oxygen
   c. Average body temperature (37ºC or 98.6ºF)
   d. Moisture inside the body
   e. Neutral pH, the normal body pH
   f. Nutrients—body's membranes
   g. Darkness inside the body

C. Stages of infection cycle (chain of infection, Figure 36–1)

1. Infectious agents
   a. Bacteria
      i. Unicellular microorganisms that vary in morphology
      ii. Many pathogenic to humans and animals
      iii. Examples: *Escherichia coli* causes UTIs and other illnesses, *Bordetella pertussis* causes the droplet infection called whooping cough (airborne particles are breathed in by organism), and *Vibrio cholerae* causes cholera in humans who ingest contaminated food and water.
   b. Viruses
      i. Smallest living microorganisms and can be viewed only with electron microscope
      ii. Classified by the type of DNA or RNA or by the clinical properties
      iii. Reproduce only within a host
      iv. Examples: HIV/AIDS, herpes, chickenpox, hepatitis, the common cold, and influenza
   c. Fungi
      i. Depend on other life forms for a nutritional source
      ii. Molds: multicelled fungi and reproduce by spore formation
      iii. Yeasts: single-celled fungi and reproduce by budding
      iv. Examples of pathogenic fungal conditions are *Histoplasmosis* (a lung infection passed on by droppings of certain birds or bats), *Candida albicans* (yeast infection), and *Tinea pedis* (athlete's foot)
   d. Parasites
      i. Organisms that depend on another living organism for nourishment
      ii. Classified as protozoa, metazoa, and ectoparasites
      iii. Characteristics of protozoa (single-celled) such as hair-like projections (flagella) and tails determine the classification
      iv. Common diseases caused by protozoa include malaria, toxoplasmosis, and *trichomonas vaginalis*
      v. Metazoa (multicelled) causes pinworms, hookworms, and tapeworms
      vi. Ectoparasites (multicelled) cause scabies and lice

- e. Rickettsiae
  - i. Known as obligate parasites and depend completely on their host for survival
  - ii. Larger than viruses and can be seen by conventional microscopes when stained
  - iii. Generally caused by fleas, ticks, and mice
  - iv. Common diseases include Lyme disease, Rocky Mountain spotted fever, and typhus

2. Reservoir or source
   - a. Person or object that becomes infected
   - b. Where the pathogen can survive, grow, and multiply
   - c. People, equipment, food, water, and insects are all examples
3. Portal of exit from reservoir or source—Following invasion of the host, transmission of the pathogen occurs through secretions, excretions, and body fluids from body openings to another person, either by direct or indirect contact
4. Means of transmission
   - a. How microorganism travels from reservoir and portal of exit to a susceptible individual
   - b. Direct contact: eating, drinking, kissing, touching, sexual intimacy
   - c. Indirect contact: inhaling contaminated air from a cough or sneeze, handling a fomite, ingestion, airborne, and vector
5. Portals of entry—Enters new host through body cavities: mouth, nose, throat, eyes, ears, intestinal, urinary and respiratory tracts, and breaks in skin.
6. Susceptible host
   - a. One capable of being infected by the pathogen
   - b. Ability to fight off disease is low
   - c. poor health, nutritional habits, or hygiene
   - d. elderly, frail, immunosuppressed, or those with chronic diseases

## I. INFECTIOUS DISEASE PROCESS

A. Incubation

B. Prodromal

C. Acute

D. Declining

E. Convalescent

## II. DEFENSE MECHANISMS

A. Immunity best when body is in state of good physical, emotional, and mental condition

B. Stress patient education: promote circulation, reduce stress, and maintain the immune system

C. Practice good health habits of proper rest, diet, exercise, nutrition, and hygiene

D. Respiratory tract

1. Hair-like cilia filter out invading pathogens
2. Coughing and sneezing rid body of invaders
   - a. Tears, sweat, urine, and mucus wash out pathogens from body
   - b. Low pH discourages bacterial growth
   - c. Hydrochloric acid in stomach has low pH and discourages growth of pathogens

## IV. INFECTION CONTROL AND DISEASE PREVENTION

A. Provide a safe and comfortable environment for patients and staff

B. Provide patient education

C. Ensure proper cleaning

D. General guidelines for safety and prevention—Discuss and demonstrate as necessary the 12 guidelines presented in the text

E. Practice and apply prevention techniques

F. Universal precautions

G. Standard precautions

H. OSHA guidelines

1. Written statement in each POL signifying compliance with OSHA regulations
2. The blood-borne pathogen standard
    a. Exposure control plan—Completing an Exposure Report (Procedure 36–1)
    b. Reporting exposure incidents
    c. Needlesticks and other sharps
    d. Blood spill cleanup and disposal of hazardous waste materials
    e. Regulated waste
    f. Incineration

## V. MEDICAL ASEPSIS

A. Hand Washing (Procedure 36–2)

1. Most effective way to eliminate many diseases
2. Hand washing/gloving throughout day—i.e., breaks, lunch, using rest room, before and after wearing gloves
    a. Discuss appropriate times to perform hand washing
    b. Effect of jewelry
    c. Differentiate between routine hand washing and surgical scrub
    d. Protecting the skin
    e. Alcohol-based rub

B. Gloving (Procedure 36–3)

1. Necessary when cleaning up blood or bodily fluid
2. Provide protection as a barrier and prevent contamination
    a. Reduce the possibility of transfer of pathogens from you to another
    b. Diminish the chance of pathogens transmitted to you from another
3. Not a substitute for hand washing
    a. Glove imperfections (i.e., holes, tears, and so on)
    b. Ill-fitting gloves
4. Latex allergies

C. Applying Other PPE (Procedure 36–4)

D. Sanitization (Procedure 36–5)

1. Washing and scrubbing to remove materials, such as blood, body tissue, or other contaminants
2. Must glove when sanitizing items to prevent skin damage

3. Rinse in cool water
4. Soak in detergent solution for about 20 minutes
5. Wash with brush
6. Rinse thoroughly and dry

E. Disinfection

1. Process by which disease-producing microorganisms are killed by placing items in solutions such as zephirin chloride or chlorophenyl
2. Used on objects only

F. Sterilization

1. Necessary to kill spores (capsules formed by bacteria that grow and multiply when conditions are favorable; not killed by antiseptics or disinfectants)
   a. Sterile means free from all living microorganisms
   b. Autoclaving
   c. Shelf life
   d. Rotating stock
2. Wrapping Items for Autoclaving (Procedure 36–6)
   a. Items must be wrapped in double thickness of a special autoclave paper or cloth (after being properly sanitized) or in envelopes with identification of contents, date, and your initials
   b. Must use indicator tape or device to ensure proper temperature for sterilization, indicating the color change on the tape that shows sterilization has been achieved
   c. View the Media Link on the Premium WEBSITE, "Wrapping Items for Autoclaving"
3. Using the Autoclave (Procedure 36–7)
   a. Steam under pressure
   b. Only method that kills spores (15 lbs. of steam under pressure per square inch at a temperature between 250°F/121°C and 270°F/132°C, with the steam flowing through the items to destroy all microorganisms and spores)
   c. Follow autoclave manufacturer's instructions for operation and care
   d. Proper temperature and amount of time must be observed for sterilization to take place
4. Chemical Sterilization (Procedure 36–8)
   a. For sharp items and instruments that would dull with sterilization or rubber or vinyl items that cannot withstand heat of sterilization
   b. Items must be completely covered
   c. Minimum of 10 hours or manufacturer's recommendation
   d. Follow manufacturer's guidelines for strengths and disposal
5. Dry Heat Sterilization
   a. Useful to sterilize sharp instruments
   b. Time-consuming process, taking one to two hours at a temperature of 350°F/176.6°C

## CHAPTER ACTIVITIES

1. Have students bring in newspaper and magazine articles about communicable diseases and report to the class.
2. To make students aware of how disease can be transmitted from one person to another, have the students role-play a though one student has a communicable disease. Using a hand-glo product, have the students with the mock disease apply the hand-glo and thoroughly rub into hands, then have that person shake hands with another student, who in turn shakes hands with another, and so on, until the whole class is "infected." The class can see how the transmissio occurs by using a black light. Discuss the infection cycle and how to break the cycle, starting with proper, frequent hand washing. Then have students wash their hands, using medical asepsis technique, and reuse the black light to se whether they are using good washing technique.
3. Direct class discussion in the importance of personal hygiene and cleanliness.
4. Have students wash, dry, and wrap (for autoclaving) specified instruments and label the packages properly.
5. Have students make 5" x 7" cards with the names of diseases, the symptoms, treatment, means of transmission, and incubation periods. Have them submit the cards to you for checking. Allow them to use the cards to quiz each other.
6. Invite a speaker from the health department to talk to the class about community health issues and concerns.
7. Practice applying and removing a variety of PPE (gloves, gowns, masks, and eyewear). Discuss various procedures and what PPE would be appropriate.
8. As a class, assign individual sections for each student or group of students to obtain and compile an exposure contro manual.
9. Have students write their own blood-borne pathogen or other OPIM exposure scenario and fill out the OSHA incident report Form 301 completely and accurately.
10. Assign students a communicable disease from Table 36–1 and have them prepare a 5–10 minute presentation, educating the class about the disease, means of transmission, incubation, symptoms, and treatment.

## ANSWERS TO CHECK YOUR KNOWLEDGE QUESTIONS

1. An example of a disease that must be reported to the National Notifiable Diseases Surveillance System of the CDC is:
   a. *herpes simplex* virus.
   b. impetigo.
   c. pediculosis.
   **d. meningitis.**
2. When the infection cycle is broken:
   a. an individual becomes susceptible.
   **b. the spread of disease is prevented.**
   c. an individual becomes infected.
   d. disease can be transferred from one person to another.
3. An infectious agent that can be viewed only with an electron microscope and can reproduce itself only within a hos is known as:
   a. bacteria.
   **b. a virus.**
   c. fungi.
   d. a parasite.

4. The stage of infection when the first onset of signs and symptoms of infection occur is the:
   a. incubation stage.
   **b. prodromal stage.**
   c. acute stage.
   d. convalescent stage.
5. Which of the following organizations established the bloodborne pathogen standard?
   **a. OSHA**
   b. CDC
   c. CLIA
   d. EPA
6. Contaminated surfaces must be cleaned with a ___________ bleach solution.
   a. 1:100
   b. 100:1
   **c. 1:10**
   d. 10:1
7. Standard precautions should be used:
   a. only if the infectious status of the patient is unknown.
   b. only if the patient is known to have HIV.
   **c. with all patients at all times.**
   d. for self-protection rather than for the protection of the patient.
8. An exposure control plan should include:
   a. engineering controls.
   b. work practice controls.
   c. PPE.
   **d. all of the above.**
9. Sharps containers should be:
   a. odor-proof.
   **b. puncture proof.**
   c. white in color.
   d. red in color.
10. According to CDC standards, vigorous hand washing should be done for at least __________ before and after seeing each patient.
    a. 15 minutes
    b. 30 seconds
    **c. 15 seconds**
    d. 60 seconds
11. Gloves are worn to:
    **a. prevent contamination of the hands when touching blood or body fluids.**
    b. increase the possibility of transferring pathogens on your hands to another.
    c. protect hands by reducing the amount of hand washing needed.
    d. all of the above.

12. The process that destroys all forms of microorganisms is known as:
    a. Disinfection
    **b. Sterilization**
    c. Sanitization
    d. Both a and b are correct
13. Autoclaved items have a shelf life of ___________ days if items are kept dried and intact.
    a. 10
    b. 20
    **c. 30**
    d. 45

## PROCEDURE SCENARIOS

The following scenario is provided for use with Procedure 36–1 Competency Checklist. It is optional; instructors may modify th scenario or make up their own. Forms that follow can be downloaded from the student's Premium Website.

### Procedure 36–1

Students can download the following forms from the Premium Website to complete this activity and use as work product for thi procedure:

- Procedure Form 36–1: OSHA Form 301

### Scenario

Today's Date: Monday, June 5, 20XX

Roberta Gonzalez is a medical assistant working for Dr. Tammy Smith in a busy family practice clinic. Dr. Smith has complete an office visit that included removing skin tags from a patient's neck. Roberta is in charge of cleaning up the instruments an supplies used for the procedure. Roberta sorts the instruments, rinses them, and places the contaminated forceps and scissors in the sanitization container to be scrubbed. While scrubbing the scissors, she accidentally pokes her hand, which punctures her gloved hand. She immediately removes her gloves and washes the area with soap and water and reports the incident to th nursing supervisor, Jim Clark. Together, they fill out the incident report form. Roberta is counseled by Dr. Smith. They obta consent from the patient and both Roberta and the patient proceed to the clinic's laboratory where they will leave a blood sample for further testing.

| **Employee Information:** | | **Employer Information:** | |
|---|---|---|---|
| Name: | Roberta Gonzalez | Name: | Wichita Family Practice |
| Address: | 231 Birch St | Address: | 100 Libby Avenue |
| | Wichita KS, 55119 | | Wichita KS, 55119 |
| DOB: | 05/25/1991 | Phone: | (563)555-1234 |
| Hire date: | 09/15/2010 | | |

**Case number from the log:** 2

# HAPTER 37 The Medical History and Patient Screening

## BHES Curriculum

MA.A.1.4.a Document accurately

MA.A.1.8.aa Are attentive, listen, and learn

MA.A1.8.bb Are impartial and show empathy when dealing with patients

MA.A.1.8.cc Communicate on the recipient's level of comprehension

MA.A.1.8.dd Serve as liaison between physician and others

MA.A.1.8.ff Interview effectively

MA.A.1.8.gg Use pertinent medical terminology

MA.A.1.8.hh. Receive, organize, prioritize, and transmit information expediently

MA.A.1.8.ii Recognize and respond to verbal and nonverbal communication

MA.A.1.8.jj Perform fundamental writing skills including correct grammar, spelling, and formatting techniques when writing prescriptions, documenting medical records, etc.

MA.A.1.8.kk Adapt to individual needs

MA.A.1.9.a Obtain chief complaint, recording patient history

MA.A.1.9.g Maintain medication and immunization records

MA.A.1.11.b(3) Demonstrate professionalism by: Maintaining confidentiality at all times

MA.A.1.11.b(8) Demonstrate professionalism by: Being courteous and diplomatic

## AAHEP Core Curriculum

I.P.6 Perform patient screening using established protocols

I.A.1 Apply critical thinking skills in performing patient assessment and care

I.A.2 Use language/verbal skills that enable patients' understanding

I.A.3 Demonstrate respect for diversity in approaching patients and families

IV.C.4 Identify techniques for overcoming communication barriers

IV.C.6 Differentiate between subjective and objective information

IV.C.7 Identify resources and adaptations that are required based on individual needs, i.e., culture and environment, developmental life stage, language, and physical threats to communication

IV.P.1 Use reflection, restatement, and clarification techniques to obtain a history

IV.P.2 Report relevant information to others succinctly and accurately

IV.P.3 Use medical terminology, pronouncing medical terms correctly, to communicate information, patient history, data, and observations

IV.A.1 Demonstrate empathy in communication with patients, family, and staff

IV.A.2 Apply active listening skills

IV.A.3 Use appropriate body language and other nonverbal skills in communicating with patients, family and staff

IV.A.4 Demonstrate awareness of the territorial boundaries of the person with whom communicating

IV.A.7 Demonstrate recognition of the patient's level of understanding in communications

IV.A.8 Analyze communications in providing appropriate responses/feedback

IV.A.9 Recognize and protect personal boundaries in communicating with others

IV.A.10 Demonstrate respect for individual diversity, incorporating awareness of one's own biases in areas including gender, race, religion, age, and economic status

IX.P.7 Document accurately in the patient record

IX.A.1 Demonstrate sensitivity to patient rights

# LESSON OUTLINE

## I. PATIENT SCREENING

A. Screening is the process of obtaining information from patients to determine who will be the most beneficial to handle their needs.

1. Types
    a. Phone screening (see Chapter 9 for an in-depth discussion of phone screening)
    b. In-person screening
2. Triage
    a. Concept developed by the military
    b. Particularly applicable to trauma and disaster situations
    c. Term used in prioritizing the conditions of the injured following a disaster
    d. Rules dictating that those who have emergent conditions should be given first priority, conditions that are not life-threatening can wait a short time.
    e. The word *screening* has replaced the term *triage* because it is more appropriate for the process used in the medical office

B. In-person screening

1. In-person screening is the first step taken between the patient and you to make his or her experience at the office beneficial.
2. Requires professional communication skills and the assurance of privacy
3. Performed in a private area or examination room
4. All the data obtained is subject to legal and ethical considerations and must remain confidential. Patients are entitled to certain rights that must be enforced. (Refer to Unit 3 for a comprehensive understanding of the Patient Bill of Rights.)
    a. Patients have certain rights that they are entitled to, and these rights must be enforced
5. Goals of in-person screening
    a. Determine why the patient is seeking health care
    b. Determine what the patient sees as his or her main problem
    c. Note any other concerns he or she may have
    d. Find out what, if anything, he or she has done about it
6. Purpose of screening
    a. Help patients focus on their main concern, called the chief complaint (CC), and its related symptoms
    b. Obtain and record other health concerns
    c. Establish an accurate database
7. HIPAA considerations
    a. Following the privacy standards, be sure to get the patient's approval to involve another person in the discussion of their private health information
    b. Document the permission; without documentation, it is considered "not permitted"

C. Factors influencing screening
 1. Ensure privacy
 2. Be aware of your biases
 3. Establish a nonthreatening, relaxed atmosphere
 4. Be aware of your own nonverbal messages
 5. Be sure the patient understands
 6. Allow the patient to do most of the talking.
 7. Listen attentively to what the patient says
 8. Pay attention to the patient's nonverbal communication
 9. Use open-ended questions
 10. Focus on the interview
 11. Conclude the screening portion of the interview with a summary

D. Conducting the in-person screening (Procedure 37–1)
 1. Unique to each medical office
 2. Patients complete preliminary health history form
 3. Introduce yourself to the new patient and request the patient's assistance with the interview
 4. Be open when approaching patients; there is no room in the medical office for prejudice
 5. Treat all patients with respect, regardless of their financial status, race, religion, age, or station in life

E. Developing the chief complaint
 1. Ask what brought the patient to the office today
 2. Record CC in the patient's own words, on the chart or enter in the EHR
 3. Add descriptive information
  a. When the problem started
  b. What the patient has done for the condition
  c. Whether any over-the-counter (OTC) medications or home remedies were tried
  d. What they were and whether they were effective
  e. Ask patient to describe characteristics regarding symptoms
 4. Summarize results of your screening
 5. Ask patient whether there is anything else to add
 6. View the Media Link , "Developing the Chief Complaint," on the Premium Website.

## . THE HEALTH HISTORY

A. The purpose of the medical history
 1. A comprehensive medical history that includes information about the patient and the patient's family
 2. Information incorporated in the history includes previous illnesses, medications, allergies, and surgical history
 3. Basis for understanding present health status
 4. Basis for all treatment provided by the health care provider—helpful when patients are seen by a provider who is not their primary provider or when referred to a specialist
 5. Helps guide treatment for the patient
 6. Can provide statistical data to research companies, the health department, and insurance data
 7. The health history is acquired when the patient is new to the facility

8. All patients are asked to complete a health history form at their initial visit to a physician's office
   a. Some are mailed prior to the appointment; others are completed in the office prior to the provider's examination
   b. Standard paper and electronic versions
      i. Paper version can be as short as one page or many pages long; depends on provider's preference
      ii. Electronic version can be completed in the comfort of the patient's home, if he or she has access to a computer, or by a kiosk inside of the facility prior to the appointment
      iii. Most of the electronic versions of the health history forms have drop-down lists within the system, making it quicker and easier for the patient to fill in the information
      iv. These systems are also easier to update if changes need to be made rather than having the patient fill out an annual paper form
   c. You may need to assist in the completion of the history
      i. There are unfamiliar medical terms and some confusing questions with which the patient may need help
      ii. There may be language, literacy, cultural, and other barriers that prevent completion

B. Reviewing the patient's health history—prepare for the patient. (Refer to Procedure 37–2, "Obtain and Record a Patient Health History"; View Media Link, "Reviewing a Patient's Health History," on the Premium Website.)
   1. Prepare the exam room, ensuring that all supplies are available
   2. Review the patient chart
   3. Review the history to be certain that the data collected is complete
   4. Introduce yourself and use clear communication skills
      a. Determine whether any assistance is needed for the patient
      b. Provide any necessary assistance
         i. Accompany the patient from the reception area to the area in which the interview will take place (generally the exam room)
         ii. Seat the patient comfortably and sit face to face to begin interview
         iii. Build rapport with the patient
         iv. Use the patient's name often
   5. Reviewing the information
      a. Review provided information with patient for clarity and completeness
      b. Patient's health history may identify areas where educational materials may be helpful
      c. Be prepared to answer any questions from the patient

C. Sections of the form
   1. Chief complaint (CC)
      a. The reason that the patient is being seen currently in the office
      b. Should be short and written with precision and conciseness
      c. Should contain the subjective and objective data that the patient discusses
         i. Subjective symptoms or sensations are those that only the patient can perceive, such as pain, dizziness, itching, or numbness
         ii. Objective findings are information or symptoms that can be observed, such as swelling, bruising, vital signs and physical examination findings
   2. Present illness (PI) and history of present illness (HPI)—detailed information about the chief complaint

3. Medical history and past medical history (PMH)
    a. Used to identify all surgeries and health problems, illnesses, or disorders ever diagnosed.
    b. Includes present and past *diseases* and *disorders*
    c. Usual childhood diseases (UCHD) are also included
    d. Some questions are gender specific
    e. Includes serious illnesses and hospitalizations
    f. Current medications, including prescription, OTC, and herbal supplements
    g. Any known allergies, including medications, food, and environmental factors
4. Family health history
    a. Health status of the immediate family members—forewarn and possibly prevent future conditions that tend to develop within families
    b. Ages and status of health or age and cause of death for immediate family members
    c. Family members should include siblings, parents, grandparents (maternal and paternal), aunts, uncles, and children
    d. Providers who treat familial disorders and diseases may also use another type of history form called a genogram.
        i. Most genograms include at least three generations
        ii. Provides visual information helpful in determining chances of developing a disease that has genetic tendencies
5. Social and occupational history
    a. Patient's personal or lifestyle habits—may be sensitive in nature
    b. Includes drug usage, both prescribed and illegal
    c. Work history
    d. Additional questioning on the patient's living environment, firearm practices, hobbies, sexual practices, diet, and exercise
6. Review of Systems
    a. After the history is completed
        i. Patient is weighed and measured and the vital signs obtained and recorded
        ii. Prepare patient accordingly
        iii. Patient is ready for the physician's examination
    b. The Review of Systems (ROS) is performed by the provider during the physical examination.
        i. An orderly and systematic check of each of the body systems is recorded.
        ii. Essential in the current diagnostic state of the patient as well as information used as a baseline for subsequent visits
        iii. Provider documents all findings during the ROS, whether positive or negative on the health history form
        iv. If the patient responds positively to an area, the provider will then ask the patient to elaborate.

## HAPTER ACTIVITIES

1. Have students look up medical history form terms in reference books and write the definitions and other information in a notebook.

2. Make flash cards with medical history form terms and definitions and have students quiz each other in pairs or small groups.

3. Make copies of several types of medical history forms. (Obtain them from local medical offices or clinics or download them from online.) Have students role-play as medical assistant and patient in completing the forms, using good communication and active listening skills, and then reverse roles. Give students a stopwatch or other timepiece to record how long it actually takes to obtain the requested information accurately and legibly.

4. Have students complete a medical history form on a variety of students such as students from your school's English as a second language program, someone for whom English is not the primary language, students who are hearing impaired, or students with cultural or ethnic differences. Have students focus on any communication issues that might occur and role-play on how to overcome any major obstacles they may encounter.

5. Have students practice appropriate communication skills with a child, facing them at eye level, using simple terms. Ask the child to explain in his or her own words what you have said, either via role-play or with an actual child.

6. In pairs, have students role-play, demonstrating the ability to communicate with a teenager, a geriatric patient, and a patient with limited mental capacity.

7. Using local biases, have students role-play a scenario in which these biases interfere with patient care. Have students describe why it is important to the staff and patient for these to be addressed prior to providing care to ensure quality care.

8. Have students pair up with a classmate to practice recording a history. The one who is the patient can identify a disease and pretend to have the symptoms. (Refer to Unit 11 for ideas.) The medical assistant can conduct the interview and obtain the chief complaint and secondary concerns. Ask him or her to anticipate and write down what type of examination and testing the physician may need to do.

9. Have students prepare a 3" × 5" card with all their personal health information. Have them keep this card in their purse or folded in their wallet. It will be very useful to have the information handy if they have to visit a new physician or the emergency department or are admitted to a hospital. The card should include:

   - Family physician's name, address, and phone
   - Family members' ages or age at death, health state, or cause of death
   - Student's past serious illnesses, diagnoses, and dates
   - Past surgical procedures and dates
   - Dates of hospitalizations
   - Current list of prescription and OTC drugs and dosage
   - If female, age at first and last menstrual period
   - If female, dates of all births

## ANSWERS TO CHECK YOUR KNOWLEDGE QUESTIONS

1. The purpose of screening in today's medical office is to:
   a. prioritize the condition of the injured following a disaster.
   b. tag the victims requiring immediate attention.
   c. sorting and assess soldiers' injury.
   **d. determine who will be the most beneficial to handle the patient needs.**

2. An example of an open-ended question would be:
   a. "How long have you had the pain?"
   b. "Does strenuous activity increase your symptoms?"
   c. "How would you describe your pain?"
   **d. "Do you have pain now?"**
3. Information collected in the health history includes:
   a. medications.
   b. allergies.
   c. previous illness.
   **d. all of the above.**
4. When a medical office has the patient fill out the health history form, areas that are incomplete may indicate the following:
   a. laziness.
   b. language problem.
   c. reading problem.
   **d. both b and c.**
5. A genogram is used to determine genetic tendencies and covers how many generations?
   **a. Three**
   b. Four
   c. Two
   d. Five
6. Questions regarding alcohol and tobacco use would be found under the following section of the health history form:
   a. family health history.
   b. review of systems.
   **c. social and occupational.**
   d. medical history.
7. Where on the health history form is a systematic check of all the body systems recorded?
   a. Medical history
   **b. ROS**
   c. EHR
   d. Present illness
8. Having the patient elaborate on his or her present illness by asking him or her, "What makes the symptoms better?" would cover the following aspect while screening the chief complaint:
   a. aggravating factors.
   **b. alleviating factors.**
   c. associated symptoms.
   d. severity.

# HAPTER 38 Vital Signs and Measurements

## BHES Curriculum

| | |
|---|---|
| MA.A.1.4.a | Document accurately |
| MA.A.1.8.cc | Communicate on the recipient's level of comprehension |
| MA.A.1.8.jj | Perform fundamental writing skills including correct grammar, spelling, and formatting techniques when writing prescriptions, documenting medical records, etc |
| MA.A.1.9.c | Take vital signs |

## AAHEP Core Curriculum

| | |
|---|---|
| I.C.4 | List major organs in each body system |
| I.C.8 | Discuss implications for disease and disability when homeostasis is not maintained |
| I.P.1 | Obtain vital signs |
| I.A.1 | Apply critical thinking skills in performing patient assessment and care |
| I.A.2 | Use language/verbal skills that enable patients' understanding |
| IX.P.7 | Document accurately in the patient record |

# ESSON OUTLINE

## BODY MEASUREMENTS

A. Referred to as mensuration, meaning the process of measuring
   1. Height and weight—For adults, abnormal changes could indicate the presence of a disease or disorder
   2. In infants, length of extremities and the circumference of head, chest, or abdomen; in infants and children to ensure there is proper growth and development
   3. Become the baseline for all measurements that follow
   4. Measurements can also provide information regarding treatment
   5. Measurements are obtained at the beginning of the patient's visit
   6. The measurement performed and frequency will largely be determined by the patient's condition

B. Height and weight measurements—Measurements are important to patients for many reasons
   1. The young adult may be very interested in his or her height, especially to those who wish to play certain sports
   2. Elderly are concerned about the loss of height
   3. Athletes may have to gain or lose a certain amount of weight to meet regulations or goals
   4. People of all ages are struggling to lose excess pounds
   5. Some fight eating disorders and struggle to gain a pound or two

C. Height—To measure an adult patient's height, you will need a height apparatus
   1. Most of the balance beam scales have one attached to them
   2. Stand-alone devices that can be mounted to a wall
   3. Be familiar with how to read the height scales
      a. Height bar is calibrated in inches
      b. By quarter-inch markings
   4. Height should be measured to the nearest quarter of an inch

5. Can be recorded in total inches or converted to feet and inches
6. Obtained by dividing the inches by the number 12

D. Weight—Obtaining the patient's weight using a balance beam scale
1. Manipulate the two weights until the pointer rests in the middle
2. Must be sure the scale is calibrated
    a. Performed by setting both of the weights at zero
    b. Make sure the pointer floats in the middle
    c. Screw at the end that needs to be adjusted to get the scale to balance
3. The bottom large weight is calibrated in 50-pound increments—Place the large weight into the groove you estimate closest to the weight of the patient
4. Move the smaller weight until you have added enough weight to balance the beam
5. Estimate too high or low, readjust the weights
6. When the beam balances, add two measurements and record the patient's weight

E. Measuring and weighing the patient
1. Instruct him or her to remove shoes
2. Remove items from pockets
3. Measure height and weight (Procedure 38–1)

F. Body mass index
1. Numerical correlation between patient's height and weight
2. Calculated by the medical assistant
3. Documented in the patient's record along with the height and weight
4. Number of ways to determine the patient's BMI

## II. VITAL SIGNS

A. Vital signs identify measurement of body functions essential to life
1. Four vital indicators are temperature, pulse, respiration, and blood pressure
    a. Commonly referred to as TPR and B/P
        i. Indicate the body's ability to control heat
        ii. Rate, volume, and rhythm of the heart
        iii. Rate and quality of breathing
        iv. Force of the heart and condition of the blood vessels
    b. Give provider an assessment of the status of the brain, the autonomic nervous system, the heart, and the lungs
    c. The correct measurement of vital signs is extremely important
        i. Proper technique and attention to details are essential
        ii. Findings should be recorded immediately following measurement to avoid a memory error
        iii. Repeat the procedure if you think you have made a mistake in measuring or recording
        iv. Never estimate the measurement

B. Temperature
1. Indicates the amount of heat produced by the activity of changing food into energy
2. The body loses heat through perspiration, breathing, and the elimination of body wastes
3. The balance between heat production and heat loss determines the body's temperature

4. Conditions affecting body heat
    a. Metabolic rate
    b. Time of day
    c. Amount of activity
        i. Body temperature usually lower in the morning
        ii. Afternoon and evening, body temperature rises
    d. Not all people have the same normal oral temperature (refer to Table 38–1)
        i. A person with a temperature above normal is said to be febrile or to have a temperature elevation
        ii. A person with a temperature that is normal or subnormal is said to be afebrile

C. Controlling body temperature
1. The temperature-regulating center in the body is located in the hypothalamus of the brain
2. The action of the hypothalamus can be compared with a thermostat
3. The brain, autonomic nervous system, blood vessels, and skin cooperate to regulate temperature
    a. Achieved through a feedback mechanism from temperature receptors
    b. One section of hypothalamus has many heat-sensitive neurons
        i. Increase their output of impulses when temperature rises
        ii. Decrease their output when it drops
    c. During an infectious process, microorganisms cause pyrogens to be secreted
        i. Raise the set point of the hypothalamic thermostat
        ii. Pyrogens are toxins from bacteria or a by-product of degenerating tissues
        iii. Set point is higher than normal, the body's heat production and conservation processes are activated
        iv. Surface blood vessels constrict, person feels cold even though the temperature is above normal
        v. No sweat is secreted
        vi. Increased white blood cell activity produces heat
        vii. Chills and shivering begin; until the temperature reaches higher set point, hypothalamus continues to operate until infectious process is reversed
        viii. Hypothalamic thermostat is reset to a lower or normal value; body's temperature reduction results in profuse sweating and hot, red skin
        ix. Temperature will begin to fall
    d. Refer to Table 38–2

D. Thermometer types and designs
1. Body temperature measured by means of a thermometer
2. Thermometers are of the following main types
    a. Disposable, in form of plastic strips
    b. Battery-operated electronic
    c. Self-contained digital
    d. Tympanic infrared
    e. Temporal artery
3. Large variety of thermometers; advantages and disadvantages (refer to Table 38–3)

E. Measuring oral temperatures
1. Measuring body temperature by mouth (refer to Procedure 38–2)

2. Contraindications to oral temperature measurement
   a. Infants and young children
   b. Patients with respiratory complications that result in mouth breathing or use of supplemental oxygen
   c. Confused, disoriented, or emotionally unstable patients
   d. Patients with oral injuries or dental problems such as diseased gums or abscesses
   e. Patients with recent oral surgery
   f. Patients with facial paralysis
   g. Patients with nasal obstruction, sinus congestion, or colds

F. Measuring rectal temperatures
   1. Rectal temperature is a very accurate measurement
   2. Rectal measurement appropriate with babies and young children who have not yet learned how to keep oral thermometer in place
   3. The provider usually has policy and recommendations for rectal temperatures
   4. When recording a rectal measurement, place letter *R* in parentheses following reading
   5. Normal rectal temperature is 37.5°C or 99.6°F, one full degree above normal oral temperature
   6. Refer to Procedure 38–3 for detailed steps on measuring with a rectal temperature

G. Measuring axillary temperatures
   1. Least accurate method
   2. Axillary measurement appropriate when oral and rectal temperatures are undesirable or contraindicated
   3. Normal axillary temperature is36.4°C or 97.6°F, one full degree *below* normal oral temperature
   4. When recording the axillary temperature, place letters *Ax* in parentheses following reading
   5. Refer to Procedure 38–4 for obtaining an axillary temperature

H. Measuring tympanic (aural) temperatures
   1. Tympanic membrane thermometers are easy, safe, and fast to use.
   2. Refer to Procedure 38–5 for obtaining a temperature using a tympanic thermometer

I. Measuring temporal artery temperatures
   1. TA measurement provides results more closely related to true internal body temperature measured in major artery than any other method
   2. Normal TA measurement is equivalent to a rectal temperature; therefore, approximately one degree higher than oral measurement
   3. When recording on the chart, put (TA) after the temperature to indicate the method used
   4. Measuring temperature by using a TAT has several advantages:
      a. Appropriate for all ages, infants through elderly
      b. Convenient, easily accessible, and fast
      c. Comfortable and safe for the patient
      d. Proven highly accurate
      e. No danger from contact with mucous membranes
      f. Reading not affected by oral factors such as hot and cold fluids, mouth breathing, oral surgery, or injury
      g. Can be sanitized between patients like a stethoscope, with an antiseptic wipe; or clinical models have covers, caps, and sheaths if desired
   5. Refer to Procedure 38–6 to obtain a temporal artery temperature

J. Temperature conversions

1. Temperature can be converted from one scale to another by mathematical calculation
2. Refer to Table 38–4

K. Pulse

1. Each time heart beats, blood is forced into aorta, temporarily expanding its walls and initiating wavelike effect
2. Wave continues through all body's arteries, causing alternating expansion and recoil of arterial walls
3. Palpated (felt) in the arteries close to body surface and lie over bone or firm structures
4. Artery is pressed against the underlying structure to feel rhythmic pulsation, known as pulse
5. Pulse sites; pulse can be felt in several locations on the body
   a. Radial pulse is located on the thumb side of the inner surface of the wrist, lying over the radius bone—Site used most frequently when measuring pulse rate
   b. Brachial artery pulse location is on the inner medial surface of the elbow, at the antecubital space (crease of elbow)—Site is used to palpate and auscultate (listen to) blood pressure
   c. Carotid pulse can be felt in the carotid artery of the neck when pressure is applied to the area at either side of the trachea—Palpated during the cardiopulmonary resuscitation (CPR) life-saving maneuver
   d. Femoral pulse, located midway in the groin where the artery begins its descent down the femur—Palpated to evaluate circulation in the lower extremities
   e. Dorsalis pedis, on the instep of the foot—Palpated to evaluate circulation in the lower extremities
   f. Popliteal, at the back of the knee—Palpated to evaluate circulation in the lower extremities
   g. Pulse sites of the upper and lower extremities and the neck (refer to Figure 38–19)
6. Pulse rate
   a. The average adult pulse range is 60 to 100 beats per minute
   b. The pulse rate is recorded as beats per minute preceded by a capital *P* (i.e., P. 72)
   c. The rate of the pulse is influenced by several factors
      i. Exercise or activity
      ii. Age
      iii. Gender of the patient
      iv. Size
      v. Physical condition of the body
7. Pulse characteristics
   a. Two other characteristics must be observed and recorded
      i. The force or strength of the pulse is referred to as its volume; normal, full or bounding, weak, and thready
      ii. The quality of rhythm of the pulse refers to its regularity or the equal spacing of the beats
   b. Arrhythmia refers to a pulse that lacks a regular rhythm
   c. Intermittent and occasionally skip or insert beats—Caffeine or nicotine react on the heart to cause irregularity and increased rate
8. Measuring the radial pulse—Refer to Procedure 38–8 on how to obtain a radial pulse (with respirations)
9. Measuring the apical pulse
   a. When measuring heart rate by the radial pulse, is not appropriate
   b. Listen to heart at its apex with a stethoscope
   c. Accurate method of measuring pulse rate
   d. Both contraction phases are counted as only one beat

e. Whenever measured at a site other than the radial, location should be noted (e.g., P. 97 [Ap])

f. Apical pulse is counted for a full minute, so possible to record an uneven number

g. Locating the apex

i. The bottom or lower edge of the heart is apex

ii. Palpated at the left fifth intercostal space in line with the middle of the left clavicle

iii. Located by pressing the fingertips between the ribs and counting down five spaces on the left chest wall (Figure 38–21 A)

iv. Often, beat at apex can be felt with fingertips

v. Quicker method for estimating the location of the apex

vi. Place outstretched left hand on the chest wall with the tip of the middle finger in the suprasternal notch and the thumb at a 45-degree angle (Figure 38–21 B); end of thumb is approximately over apex

h. Obtaining an apical pulse (refer to Procedure 38-7)

10. Apical indications

a. Apical pulse measurement is indicated for infants and small children

b. Patients with heart conditions, especially if being medicated with cardiac drugs

c. Difficulty feeling a radial pulse and believe you may be missing beats

d. Excessively rapid or slow rate or a thready or irregular quality

L. Pulse oximetry—Device that can be used to obtain patient's pulse and arterial oxygen saturation in blood

1. Small handheld unit that has a clip attached to it that is usually applied to the patient's middle finger

2. Clip uses an infrared light to measure the pulse and oxygen levels

3. If pulse is outside of the normal range it should be taken manually for confirmation

M. Respiration

1. One respiration is the combination of total inspiration (breathing in) and total expiration (breathing out)

2. Other frequently used terms are *inhale* and *exhale*

3. Respirations are usually measured as one part of total vital signs assessment

4. Because patients can voluntarily control the depth, rate, and regularity of their breathing to some extent, it is important for them not to be aware the procedure is being done—Common practice to observe and measure respiration immediately after assessing the radial pulse while maintaining your fingers at the radial pulse site

5. Quality of respiration

a. Respirations should be quiet, effortless, and regularly spaced

b. Breathing should be through the nose with the mouth closed

c. Excessively fast and deep breathing, commonly associated with hysteria, called hyperventilation

d. Difficult or labored breathing called dyspnea—Frequently accompanied by discomfort and anxious expression caused by fear of being unable to breathe.

e. Presence of rales (noisy breathing) usually indicates constricted bronchial passageways or collection of fluid or exudate—Rales may be present with pneumonia, bronchitis, asthma, and other pulmonary diseases

f. Respirations should be observed for the depth of inhalation

i. Three words used to describe this quality: *normal*, *shallow*, or *deep*

ii. Depth of inhalation determined by watching rise and fall of chest

g. Rhythm of respirations must also be assessed—Quality can be described as regular or irregular

h. Absence of breathing known as apnea

i. Breathing pattern called Cheyne-Stokes occurs with acute brain, heart, or lung damage or disease and with intoxicants

ii. Characterized by slow, shallow breaths that increase in depth and frequency

iii. Followed by a few shallow breaths

iv. Followed by period of apnea for 10 to 20 seconds and often more (Figure 38–22)

iv. Breathing pattern frequently precedes death

6. Respiration rate

a. Normal respiration rate for adults 16 to 20 times per minute

b. Respiration rate in infants and children has greater range and fluctuates more during illness, exercise, and emotion than adult rates

c. In newborn, rate per minute can range from 30 to 60

d. In early childhood, from 20 to 40 and during late childhood from 16 to 26

e. Rate reaches adult normal range of 16 to 20 by age 16

f. Abnormally slow rate of respiration known as bradypnea

g. A faster than normal rate of respiration known as tachypnea

7. Counting respirations

a. Necessary to observe patient carefully while measuring respiration rate

i. If patient is lying on examination table, position patient's arm across upper abdominal area, placing your fingers over the radial pulse site; in this position, visualize and feel respiration

ii. With patient in sitting position, observe more carefully as you count respirations (Figure 38–23)

b. Refer to Procedure 38–8 on obtaining respirations

N. Blood pressure

1. Fluctuating pressure blood exerts against arterial walls as heart alternately contracts and relaxes

2. Measured in the brachial artery of the arm in the antecubital space

3. Maintaining blood pressure

a. Depends on two factors

i. Strong, effective heart

ii. Intact brain (and autonomic nervous system)

b. Both needed to maintain homeostasis

4. Blood pressure phases

a. Systole is the contraction phase, the period of greatest pressure

b. Diastole is the relaxation phase, the period of least pressure

5. Normal blood pressure

a. Measured with sphygmomanometer and stethoscope

b. Expressed as fraction with systolic pressure as numerator and diastolic pressure as denominator

c. Normal readings in adults

i. A systolic pressure 100–120 mm Hg

ii. A diastolic pressure between 60–80 mm Hg

d. Hypertension indicated by readings persistently above 140/90
   i. Caused by physical conditions
   ii. Stress
   iii. Obesity
   iv. Sedentary lifestyle
   v. Aging
e. Idiopathic (essential) hypertension is elevated blood pressure without apparent cause
f. Other types
   i. Primary
   ii. Secondary
   iii. Malignant
g. Hypotension indicated by blood pressure readings consistently below 90/60

6. Pulse pressure is the difference between the systolic and diastolic reading
7. Equipment factors
   a. Sphygmomanometers
      i. Must be in proper working order and calibrated
      ii. Aneroid dial
      iii. Electronic sphygmomanometer
   b. Cuffs
      i. Must be the correct size to obtain an accurate reading
      ii. If cuff too small, reading will be falsely high
      iii. If cuff too big, reading will be falsely low
      iv. Cuff should be approximately 20% wider than the arm
8. Measuring techniques (refer to Procedure 38–9, Measure Blood Pressure)
   a. Several factors affect accuracy
   b. Common error is to reinflate the cuff after partial deflation, causing false reading
   c. Auscultatory gap
      i. Silent interval between systolic and diastolic blood pressure
      ii. Source of serious under-measurement
9. Blood pressure in children
   a. Often omitted from physical examination because difficult to obtain
   b. Cuff size very important

## CHAPTER ACTIVITIES

1. Have students practice the height and weight of classmates. Record the measurements and practice converting height from inches into feet and inches and weight from pounds to kilograms; refer to Unit 17 for the pound-to-kilogram conversion.
2. With a partner, have students practice setting various weights and heights with the height bar on the balance beam scale and quizzing each other on the measurements.
3. Using proper technique, have students practice obtaining oral and axillary temperatures on each other with an electronic thermometer and document correctly on a mock patient chart or electronic medical record.

4. Using an electronic thermometer, have students explain to the instructor or demonstrate on a mannequin how to measure a rectal temperature by using proper technique and equipment. Be sure they choose the appropriate probe.
5. Using tympanic and temporal artery thermometers, have students practice obtaining temperatures on classmates and discuss issues that would cause inaccurate readings for each.
6. Have students practice pulse and respiration counts on classmates; when they feel they have the techniques down, have them use one student's arm and the instructor use the other and do comparisons.
7. Place students in groups of three, one being the patient. Practice locating the apex of the heart: Have one student check the apical pulse and the other the radial pulse on the patient, then rotate positions in the group.
8. Using a teaching stethoscope, have students practice blood pressures on classmates while the instructor listens; compare results.
9. Have students apply critical thinking skills in performing patient care by selecting the correct size blood pressure cuff for each patient and explaining why they would use that particular one.
10. Have students wrap their blood pressure cuff around a rolled-up towel and practice pumping it up and deflating. The cuff deflation needs to be at a rate of 2 to 4 mm Hg.
11. Have students examine the blood pressure equipment thoroughly. Point out the various sections, including the tubing connections, bulb valve directions, cuff construction, cuff measurement technique, and bladder section. Study the dial to become familiar with the calibrations.
12. Have students use the procedure checklists and, in pairs, practice performing procedures on each other.
13. Have students in pairs, one being the medical assistant the other the patient. Simulate obtaining all the patient's measurements and vital signs as if he or she were grooming a patient for an office visit.
14. Have students use a mock progress note, chart, or EHR software. Practice documenting all the measurements and vital signs they obtain on classmates.
15. Have students research a medical condition or disease of their choice that would require close monitoring of vital signs, measurements, or both and report to the class their findings. Have the class discuss each topic.

## ANSWERS TO CHECK YOUR KNOWLEDGE QUESTIONS

1. The process of measuring body measurements is referred to as:
   a. measuration.
   b. menstruation.
   **c. mensuration.**
   d. ministration.
2. Although the height bar is usually recorded in inches, you might need to convert into feet and inches by dividing the number of total inches by:
   a. 10.
   **b. 12.**
   c. 6.
   d. 5.
3. The four vital indicators that measure the body functions essential to life include:
   a. height, weight, temperature, and pulse.
   **b. temperature, pulse, respiration, and blood pressure.**
   c. temperature, pulse, respiration, and weight.
   d. height, weight, pulse, and blood pressure.

4. When measuring the oral temperature using an electronic thermometer, select the following probe:

   a. green.

   b. red.

   **c. blue.**

   d. black.

5. The radial pulse can be found:

   **a. on the thumb side of the inner surface of the wrist, lying over the radius bone.**

   b. on the pinkie side of the inner surface of the wrist, lying over the ulna bone.

   c. on the thumb side of the inner surface of the wrist, lying over the ulna bone.

   d. on the pinkie side of the inner surface of the wrist, lying over the radius bone.

6. Normal respiration rate in adults is:

   a. 16–26 times a minute.

   b. 20–40 times a minute.

   **c. 16–20 times a minute.**

   d. 30–80 times a minute.

7. The term *systole* refers to:

   a. noisy breathing.

   b. resting phase of the heart.

   **c. contraction phase of the heart.**

   d. absence of breathing.

8. This type of hypertension is caused by renal disease or another identifiable cause:

   a. primary.

   **b. secondary.**

   c. tertiary.

   d. malignant.

# CHAPTER 39 Preparing for Examinations

## ABHES Curriculum

| | |
|---|---|
| MA.A.1.9.b | Apply principles of aseptic techniques and infection control |
| MA.A.1.9.k | Prepare and maintain examination and treatment area |
| MA.A.1.9.l | Prepare patient for examinations and treatments |
| MA.A.1.9.m | Assist physician with routine and specialty examinations and treatments |

## CAAHEP Core Curriculum

| | |
|---|---|
| I.A.1 | Apply critical thinking skills in performing patient assessment and care |
| I.P.10 | Assist physician with patient care |
| III.C.3 | Discuss infection control procedures |

## LESSON OUTLINE

### I. PREPARING THE ROOM BEFORE THE EXAMINATION

A. Positioning the examination table appropriately

B. Preparing the room (Procedure 39–1)

1. Ensure that the room is clean and tidy
2. Temperature is comfortable
3. Clean surfaces with disinfectant
4. New paper on examination table
5. Check that supplies and equipment are present

### II. PREPARING AND ASSISTING THE PATIENT

A. Your role

1. Make patients feel as comfortable as possible
2. Medical assistant should remain in room when female patient is examined by male physician and vice versa

B. Patient instructions

1. Instruct patient to wear gown and apply drape
2. Allow patient time to empty his or her bladder and obtain a specimen if necessary
3. Provide footstool if exam table is too high
4. Never lift a patient who weighs more than you
5. Do not leave ill patients or small children alone on table before exam

C. Wheelchair transfers

1. Use proper technique for assisting patient from wheelchair to exam table (Procedures 39–2 and 39–3)
2. View Video Link on the StudyWARE CD for transferring a patient from an exam table to a wheelchair

### III. EXAMINATION POSITIONS

A. Anatomical or standing erect position

1. Arms at sides with the palms forward
2. Used for neurological examination, range of motion, and flexibility to instruct the patient about bending and walking

3. Well-patient examinations may begin this way, with patient sitting on the table with the legs over the side or at the end of the table

B. Horizontal recumbent or supine position (Procedure 39–4)
   1. Patient lies on the examination table on the back, with legs straight and arms at the sides of body
   2. For examination and treatment of the anterior surface of the body and for X-rays

C. Dorsal recumbent (Procedure 39–4)
   1. Indicates that the legs are flexed
   2. Allows for relaxation of abdominal muscles
   3. Position used for vaginal and rectal examinations

D. Prone position (Procedure 39–4)
   1. Patient lies on the stomach, face down
   2. Used in examination of the back or spine, with the gown open in back

E. Sims' position (Procedure 39–4)
   1. Patient lies on left side with the right knee drawn up to the waist level
   2. Used in examination and treatment of the rectal area and for enemas, rectal temperatures, and sigmoidoscopy

F. Knee-chest position (Procedure 39–4)
   1. Patient kneels with the body weight resting on the examination table on elbows and forearms
   2. Used for rectal and sigmoidoscopy examinations because the position straightens the S curve of the sigmoid colon and makes viewing easier with sigmoidoscope
   3. Because the position is difficult to maintain for a long period, be sure to assist the patient and help prevent a possible fall

G. Fowler's position (Procedure 39–4)
   1. Patient sits up
   2. Semi-Fowler's is at a 45° angle
   3. High Fowler's is at a 90° angle
   4. Used to help patients with dyspnea to breathe more easily
   5. Used for examinations of the trunk of the body, including the head, neck, and chest areas

H. Lithotomy position (Procedure 39–4)
   1. Patient lies on the back with the feet supported in stirrups and the knees bent
   2. Used for vaginal and rectal examinations and treatments
   3. Used for male genitalia examinations and for urinary catheterizations

I. Trendelenburg or shock position (Procedure 39–4)
   1. Patient lies on the back, with the feet elevated slightly
   2. Power table very helpful in tilting patient at an angle
   3. Used in critical care facilities and by EMS personnel
   4. Used as a simple test for incompetent valves in the legs of persons with varicose veins
      a. Placed in this position for a period of time
      b. Assisted to standing position
      c. Physician observes as veins fill from above or below

J. Jackknife or Kraske position
   1. Requires a power table or special manual table
   2. Patient's buttocks are elevated, with head lower than body

3. Used during sigmoidoscopy (covered in Chapter 40)
4. Used for examination and treatment of rectal and anal conditions

K. View the Media Link on the Premium Website for "Positioning the Patient"

## HAPTER ACTIVITIES

1. Simulate an exam room as if a patient had a complete physical performed by the provider; have students practice demonstrating the correct maintenance of exam room following the patient visit.
2. With a partner, have students practice instructing each other in the preparation for a physical exam and assemble equipment and supplies for assisting with a routine examination.
3. Using proper technique, have students practice positioning and draping each other into various examination positions. Have them refer to Chapter 56 for proper body mechanics.
4. Have students demonstrate the proper way to store and dispose of supplies and equipment according to standard precautions and OSHA guidelines.
5. Have students search the Web for various equipment and supplies and used for physical examinations. Have them compare costs for at least two supply companies.
6. Have students demonstrate on classmates the proper techniques for transferring a patient from a wheelchair to an exam table and vice versa.
7. Have students search the OSHA Website (www.osha.gov) and compile a list of safety requirements for products used to disinfect the examination room and equipment.
8. Have students apply critical thinking skills in performing patient care by selecting the correct position to assist the patient into according to what the provider is going to examine next.
9. If a power table is available, have students practice adjusting the table into the Trendelenburg, jackknife, and proctologic positions.
10. Have students use the procedure checklists and, in pairs, practice performing them on each other.

## NSWERS TO CHECK YOUR KNOWLEDGE QUESTIONS

1. The primary use of this position is for vaginal examinations of the female patient when a speculum is inserted, as when obtaining pap smears.
   a. Trendelenburg
   **b. Lithotomy**
   c. Fowler's
   d. Semi-Fowler's
2. These supplies are usually stored in the table drawers, while other supplies are kept in examination cabinet drawers or a supply cabinet.
   a. Tongue depressors
   b. Gauze squares
   **c. Gowns and drapes**
   d. Applicators
3. The lateral recumbent position is another term that may be used in describing the following position.
   **a. Sims'**
   b. Lithotomy

   c. Supine

   d. Prone

4. Which position would be used if a patient experiences or has symptoms of syncope?

   a. Prone

   **b. Trendelenburg**

   c. Sims'

   d. Anatomical

5. The horizontal recumbent or supine position is used for examination and treatment of the ____________ portion of the body, including the breasts and abdominal organs.

   a. Posterior

   b. Superior

   c. Inferior

   **d. Anterior**

6. Which position would be used for patients with respiratory or cardiovascular problems?

   **a. Fowler's**

   b. Prone

   c. Knee-chest

   d. Jackknife

# JNIT 13 ASSISTING WITH EXAMINATIONS
# 'HAPTER 40 The Physical Examination, Specialty Exams, and Procedures

## ABHES Curriculum

| | |
|---|---|
| MA.A.1.2.c | Assist the provider with the regimen of diagnostic and treatment modalities as they relate to each body system |
| MA.A.1.4.a | Document accurately |
| M.A.A.1.8.dd | Serve as a liaison between provider and others |
| MA.A.1.9.i | Use standard precautions |
| MA.A.1.9.k | Prepare and maintain examination and treatment area |
| MA.A.1.9.l | Prepare patient for examinations and treatments |
| MA.A.1.9.m | Assist provider with routine and specialty examinations and treatments |
| MA.A.1.9.o | Perform respiratory testing |
| MA.A.1.9.r | Teach patients methods of health promotion and disease prevention |

## 'AAHEP Core Curriculum

| | |
|---|---|
| I.P.4 | Perform pulmonary function testing |
| I.P.10 | Assist provider with patient care |
| I.A.1 | Apply critical thinking skills in performing patient assessment and care |
| III.P.2 | Practice standard precautions |
| III.P.4 | Perform hand washing |
| III.P.5 | Perform sterilization procedures |
| III.A.1 | Display sensitivity to patients' rights and feelings in collecting specimens |
| III.A.2 | Explain the rationale for performance of procedure to the patient |
| III.A.3 | Show awareness of patients' concerns regarding their perceptions of the procedure being performed |
| IV.P.5 | Instruct patients according to their needs to promote health maintenance and disease prevention |
| IV.P.6 | Prepare a patient for procedures, treatments, or both |
| IV.P.8 | Document patient care |

# LESSON OUTLINE

## . THE PHYSICAL EXAMINATION

A. The complete physical examination (Procedure 40–1)
   1. Purpose is to determine the general state of health and well-being of patient
   2. Covers all major organs and systems of the body
   3. Performed by the provider

B. The medical assistant's role
   1. Preparation of the room, exam equipment, and patient (Chapter 39)
   2. MA may scribe what the provider dictates during an examination
      a. Must have knowledge of medical terminology and anatomy and physiology
      b. Must have good spelling and writing skills

3. Some providers prefer to dictate into a recorder for transcription later or to enter findings directly into the patient's EMR.
4. CPEs do not follow an absolute pattern
5. MA should have a basic knowledge of all H and P procedures (Procedure 40–1)

C. Examination techniques
1. Inspection is evaluation by sight
2. Palpation is evaluation by touch
   a. Bimanual is using two hands
   b. Digital is using one finger
3. Percussion is producing sounds by tapping various body parts to determine size, density, and location of organs
   a. Refers to pitch, quality, duration, and resonance
   b. Immediate or direct percussion is done by striking a finger against the patient's body
   c. Mediate or indirect percussion is done by placing a finger on the patient's body and striking the finger with the finger of the other hand
4. Auscultation is evaluation by listening
   a. Indirect auscultation is listening to sounds made by the patient's body with a stethoscope
      i. Amplifies sounds from lungs, heart, and visceral organs
      ii. Sounds heard are bruits, murmurs, and rhythms
   b. Direct auscultation is done by placing the ear directly over the area
5. Mensuration is measurement
   a. Patient's chest and extremities are measured in centimeters and recorded
   b. Flexible tape measure is used
6. Manipulation is the passive movement of a joint to determine the range of extension and flexion

D. Physical examination format
1. General appearance—Inspection
2. Skin—Inspection, palpation
3. Neck—Inspection, palpation, auscultation, manipulation
4. HEENT
   a. Head, eye, ear, nose, throat
   b. Inspection/palpation
5. Chest—Inspection, palpation
6. Heart—Auscultation
7. Lungs—Auscultation, percussion
8. Breasts—Inspection, palpation
9. Abdomen—Auscultation, inspection, palpation, percussion
10. Back—Inspection, palpation, manipulation
11. Genitourinary and rectal (male and female)—Inspection, palpation
12. Extremities—Mensuration, manipulation
13. Muscle strength—Patient is asked to perform a set of movements that the provider counteracts with resistance
14. Reflexes—Percussion

15. Other evaluations
    a. Romberg balance test
    b. Coordination tests

F. Provider assessment and plan
1. Documentation of exam—In the POMR method, data is recorded in SOAP format
2. Provider makes decisions about the patient's condition, based on many sources
    a. Health history
    b. Examination findings
    c. Other procedures and laboratory tests
3. "Rule out" used to indicate there is not yet conclusive evidence to make a decision concerning a condition or in confirming a diagnosis
4. Provider makes a plan for management of the care of the patient
    a. Diet
    b. Exercise
    c. Physical therapy
    d. Medication
    e. Surgery
    f. Other
5. Check the patient chart for orders to perform any additional procedures or appointments with specialists

G. After the examination
1. Might need to perform or assist in additional screening tests
2. Help patient down from examination table
3. Assist patient in getting dressed if necessary
4. Answer questions about follow-up appointments or further studies
5. Let patient know how long to expect to wait for lab results

H. Patient follow-up (Table 40–1)

## I. EYE AND EAR EXAMINATIONS

A. Assist provider and patient with examinations
1. Hand instruments to provider in order of use
2. Clean and maintain instruments and supplies
3. Provide patient education and reassurance
4. Record procedure performed and results on patient's chart

B. Ear examinations
1. Equipment used
2. If ear is difficult to examine, the ear might require irrigation (lavage) (Procedure 40–2)—removes foreign objects (cerumen/wax in the ear)
3. Patient education related to the ear and hearing

C. Auditory acuity
1. Ear function can be impaired by disease or damage
2. Patients compensate for hearing loss by acquiring behaviors

3. Determine symptoms of hearing impairment and record behaviors on chart
4. Often, wax (cerumen) buildup is the cause of hearing loss
5. Specific complaints suggest auditory nerve damage—Need attention of provider

D. Hearing assessment

1. Audiometer
    a. Instrument used to measure one's hearing
    b. Determines hearing thresholds of pure tones of frequencies that are normally audible by an individual
        i. Threshold of hearing is the point at which a sound can barely be heard
        ii. Person with normal hearing should hear all frequencies up to 15 decibels, depending on surrounding noise levels
    c. Check performances and batteries periodically
    d. Keep operations manual on file for reference
    e. Attend in-service training to learn proper use of the equipment
    f. Instruct patients in use of controls
    g. File the printout of audiogram in chart and record observations of behavior, symptoms, and patient's complaints
2. Tympanometer
    a. Used to determine the ability of the middle ear to transmit sound waves
    b. Commonly performed on children to diagnose middle ear infections
    c. A probe is inserted into the ear canal
    d. Measures the air pressure of the ear canal in relation to the air pressure found in the middle ear
3. Tuning fork is two-pronged metal instrument that varies in size and tests hearing
    a. Rinne test
        i. Examiner strikes the fork against the palm and holds the shank (stem) against the patient's mastoid bone until the patient hears no more sound
        ii. Then prongs are placed near the opening of the ear and next to it
        iii. In normal hearing, sound is heard about twice as long by air conduction as by bone conduction
        iv. If hearing by bone conduction is greater, the result is recorded as a negative Rinne
    b. Weber Test
        i. The vibrating tuning fork is held against the vertex (crown) or against the skull or forehead in the midline
        ii. Sound is heard best by unaffected ear if deafness is due to disease of the auditory apparatus
        iii. Sound is heard best by the affected ear if deafness is due to obstruction of the air passages

E. Eye examinations

1. Provider will use an ophthalmoscope
2. Examine the internal structures of the eye
3. Visual examinations may be performed if a patient has an eye infection or injury or needs additional screening to check vision acuity or color vision

F. Eye irrigation (Procedure 40–3)

1. Soothes tissues
2. Relieves inflammation
3. Aids eye in draining

G. Visual acuity

1. Measuring should be done on first office visit

a. Perform in well-lighted room with no interruptions

b. Test patient with and without corrective lenses

c. Observe patient for visual disturbances and note on chart (Table 40–2)

2. Snellen chart for distance acuity (Procedure 40–4)

   a. Letter E chart for preschoolers and non-English speaking patients; kindergarten vision screening chart

   b. Written as a fraction, e.g., 20/100

3. Jaeger system for near-vision acuity (Procedure 40–5)

   a. Card held by patient 14"–16" from eyes, using a yardstick, meterstick, or tape measure to be sure distance is accurate

   b. Provides a series of text paragraphs in ascending sizes of type

      i. Type ranges from 0.37 mm to 2.5 mm

      ii. All paragraphs are different

      iii. Record the line number the patient can read easily

4. Electronic devices for screening both near and distance visual acuity available

5. Color vision acuity for determining accuracy of color perception

   a. Ishihara multicolored plates (Procedure 40–6)

   b. Arc numbers and letters (and curved lines and shapes for nonreaders) that are one color within another

   c. Patient may use a cotton applicator to trace the patterns of color

   d. Types of color blindness

      i. Daltonism

         (a) Person cannot tell difference between red and green

         (b) Hereditary disorder

      ii. Achromatic vision

         (a) Total color blindness

         (b) Rare condition

         (c) Person cannot recognize any color at all

      iii. Deuteranopia: when a person has trouble telling difference between greens, bluish reds, and neutral shades

      iv. Protanopia

         (a) Partial color blindness

         (b) Person has trouble with perception of reds and sometimes confuses yellows and greens

   e. Cause of color blindness is usually due to defective cones in the retina

   f. Patients with thyroid condition and Graves' disease should be screened routinely for color vision acuity

6. Contrast sensitivity screening

   a. Pelli–Robson chart

   b. Measures contrast sensitivity by determining faintest contrast an observer can see

   c. Aids in early detection of eye disease and treatment

7. Vector vision contrast sensitivity screening

   a. Especially useful for screening small children, international patients, people who cannot read

   b. Has a series of four groups of circles

   c. Instruct patient to look at first group and say which circles have lines in them

   d. Record the last correctly identified circle in each group

   e. Provider interprets screening results

## III. RESPIRATORY EXAMINATIONS

A. Provider will recheck the patient's breathing
   1. Determine whether there are any abnormalities that warrant any additional testing
   2. Many patients have risk factors or infections
   3. A variety of testing may be incorporated into the exam

B. Vital capacity tests
   1. Vital capacity is greatest volume of air that can be expelled during a complete, slow, unforced expiration following a maximum inspiration
   2. Should equal inspiratory capacity plus expiratory reserve
   3. Based on age, sex, and height of patient
   4. Indications for use
      a. To evaluate patients who are suspected of having pulmonary insufficiency
      b. To help determine the cause of dyspnea
   5. Spirometer (Procedure 40–7)
      a. Handheld version commonly used to test vital capacity
      b. Advise patients to eat lightly and not to smoke prior to test
      c. Demonstrate use of spirometer to patient and let patient practice
      d. Use disposable mouthpiece
      e. With actual test, encourage patient to expel all air out of lungs
         i. Be sure clip is on nose
         ii. Test and record three to five expirations
      f. Observe patient during and following procedure for dizziness
      g. Most spirometers have computerized printout of results to file in chart
      h. Results below 80% are abnormal

C. Peak flow testing (Procedure 40–8)
   1. Measures patient's ability to exhale
   2. A peak flow meter is a monitoring device that measures peak expiratory flow rate
   3. Peak flow testing may be used
      a. If a patient had an inconclusive or abnormal spirometry test
      b. To monitor the effectiveness of medications
      c. Determine whether another form of treatment should be tried
   4. Peak flow measurements can change over time
   5. Preferable to gauge asthma control by comparing daily peak flow readings with personal best reading
   6. Use peak flow meter for one or two weeks to arrive at personal best number
      a. Every effort must be made to maintain values within 80%
      b. Results between 50% and 70% indicate patient usually needs a quick-action inhaler
      c. Results below 50%: patient must seek emergency care

D. Pulse oximetry (Procedure 40–9)
   1. Noninvasive test that measures patient's pulse rate and oxygen saturation (SAT) in the blood
   2. To determine patient's oxygen status
   3. Many cardiopulmonary conditions could warrant provider seeking patient's oxygen saturation level

4. Small handheld devices that have a monitor and a sensor
5. Device measures amount of light absorbed by hemoglobin
6. Displayed as a percentage on the monitor
7. A normal pulse oximeter reading is 95% or higher

### V. PROCTOLOGICAL EXAMINATIONS

A. Proctoscope is an instrument used to examine the anus and interior of the rectum
B. Used when hemorrhoids, fissures, and ulcerations are suspected
C. See text for rectal setup and additional instruments used in rectal procedures
D. Patient preparation
   1. Advise patient to follow preparation prior to examination
   2. Enema is sometimes necessary for the successful completion of a sigmoidoscopy or other rectal examination; although not a common procedure in a medical office
E. Sigmoidoscopy
   1. Diagnostic examination of the interior of the sigmoid colon
   2. Useful in diagnosis of cancer of the colon, ulcerations, polyps, tumors, bleeding, and other lower intestinal disorders
   3. Metal and flexible scopes used
   4. Instruct and assist patient in positioning (Procedure 40–10)

## HAPTER ACTIVITIES

1. Ask students to write the method(s) of examination that are commonly used and state the reason for each.
2. Simulate an exam room as if a patient is having a complete physical performed by the provider; have students practice demonstrating assisting the patient and provider through the process.
3. Have students cut out pictures of instruments and items used in the physical examination and attach them to index cards. They can use these as flash cards to drill one another on spelling, usage, and care of the instruments and items.
4. Have students set up examination trays of instruments or other items for various types of examinations.
5. Place many instruments used in the physical examination into a large box. Have each student draw an instrument from the box without looking at it (so students cannot make a visual selection of a known instrument). Have each student identify the instrument, explain its use, and spell its name correctly. Use as an oral quiz or as a review for the entire class.
6. Ask a clinical supervisor or provider to speak to the class on the importance of efficient assisting, proper preparation of patients for examinations, the importance of being able to assess critically what to do next during the exam and related topics. This gives students firsthand information about their role in patient care.
7. Invite a speaker from the American Cancer Society to explain the importance of breast self-exams and testicular self-exams in detecting cancer.
8. Have students role play as medical assistant and patient. Medical assistants must explain diagnostic tests and procedures to the patient. This gives students valuable communications skill practice and helps them overcome shyness when talking about delicate matters.
9. Have students examine the eyes and ears of one another using the otoscope and ophthalmoscope.
10. Invite an ophthalmic assistant to speak to the class about procedures of the eye and an ENT specialist to speak about hearing and procedures of the ear.

11. Have students practice in pairs, performing audiometry and tympanometry screening on each other.
12. Have students practice using a tuning fork to check hearing acuity.
13. Have students simulate ear irrigations on a mannequin or ear simulator.
14. Have students determine distance, near, and color vision acuity with another student and record the results, including observations made.
15. Have students practice performing respiratory procedures on one another (spirometry, pulse oximetry, and peak flow measurement).
16. Have students role play teaching a patient how to perform peak flow measurement, including how to obtain his or her personal best.
17. Invite a respiratory therapist to class to discuss respiratory conditions and procedures.
18. Arrange to have a medical supply representative speak to the class about the latest equipment and supplies used in the diagnosis of colorectal disorders and diseases. The speaker might be able to show and explain to students the use operation, care, and cost of the items discussed in the presentation.

## ANSWERS TO CHECK YOUR KNOWLEDGE QUESTIONS

1. The following examination technique uses a means of producing sounds by tapping various parts of the body:
   a. inspection.
   b. palpation.
   **c. percussion.**
   d. manipulation.
2. Which examination technique must be used to detect sounds, including bruits, murmurs, rales, rhythms, and bowel sounds?
   **a. Auscultation**
   b. Inspection
   c. Mensuration
   d. Percussion
3. The Rinne and Weber tests are performed using the following piece of equipment:
   a. ophthalmoscope.
   b. otoscope.
   c. audiometer.
   **d. tuning fork.**
4. The breast examination is best done on the _______ days following the menstrual cycle of menstruating women.
   a. 21–28
   **b. 7–10**
   c. 5–10
   d. 7–14
5. At what age should men begin a routine testicular self-examination?
   a. 12
   **b. 15**
   c. 16
   d. 18

6. What is the name of the chart used most commonly for screening distance vision?

   a. Jaeger

   **b. Snellen**

   c. Ishihara

   d. Pelli–Robson

7. Which of the following devices are used to measure the capacity of the lungs?

   a. Spirometer

   b. Peak flow

   c. Tuning fork

   **d. Both a and b**

8. In the diagnosis of ulcerations, polyps, tumors, bleeding, cancer of the colon, and other lower intestinal disorders, the examination of the interior of the sigmoid colon can be done using a:

   a. proctoscope.

   b. rectal speculum.

   c. rectal snare.

   **d. sigmoidoscope.**

# HAPTER 41 OB/GYN Examinations

## BHES Curriculum

| | |
|---|---|
| MA.A.1.4.a | Document accurately |
| MA.A.1.8.dd | Serve as a liaison between provider and others |
| MA.A.1.9.i | Use standard precautions |
| MA.A.1.9.k | Prepare and maintain examination and treatment area |
| MA.A.1.9.l | Prepare patient for examinations and treatments |
| MA.A.1.9.m | Assist provider with routine and specialty examinations and treatments |
| MA.A.1.9.r | Teach patients methods of health promotion and disease prevention |

## AAHEP Core Curriculum

| | |
|---|---|
| I.P.10 | Assist provider with patient care |
| III.P.2 | Practice standard precautions |
| III.P.4 | Perform hand washing |
| III.A.2 | Explain the rationale for performance of procedure to the patient |
| III.A.3 | Show awareness of patients' concerns regarding their perceptions related to the procedure being performed |
| IV.P.5 | Instruct patients according to their needs to promote health maintenance and disease prevention |
| IV.P.6 | Prepare a patient for procedures, treatments, or both |
| IV.P.8 | Document patient care |

# ESSON OUTLINE

## OB/GYN EXAMINATIONS

A. Gynecological exam
   1. Gynecology practice addresses diseases and disorders of the female reproductive system
   2. Includes Pap smear
   3. Many women prefer to see a gynecologist for this type of examination

B. Pap Test
   1. Cytological screening is used to detect cancer of the cervix
      a. Developed by American provider George Papanicolaou in 1883
      b. Also used to screen for atypical cytology
      c. Routinely performed with CPE or by a gynecologist
      d. Females with a family history of cervical cancer should have it done more frequently
      e. Patient education (in text) is appropriate as patient is prepared for examination
   2. Patient preparation prior to office visit
      a. Do not use tampons, birth control foams, jellies, or other vaginal creams for 48 hours before the test
      b. Do not douche for 48 hours before the test
      c. Do not have sexual intercourse for 48 hours before the test
      d. Try to schedule the test at least five days after the menstrual period
      e. Avoid scheduling during period

3. Examination room preparation
    a. Exam table should have clean, protective covering
    b. Set out a gown and drape for patient
    c. Prepare the Mayo tray with instruments, supplies, and cover
    d. Attach requisition form label to ThinPrep collection bottle and place on Mayo stand
    e. Place exam lamp within reach at end of table
4. Patient preparation for examination
    a. Instruct patient to use the bathroom
    b. If specimen is to be obtained, provide instructions to patient
    c. Explain the procedure, making patient feel comfortable
    d. Instruct patient to undress and put on gown, assisting as needed
    e. Help patient onto exam table into sitting position
    f. Place a drape sheet on patient's lap
    g. Alert provider that the patient is ready to be seen
5. Assist with the examination
    a. Assist with breast examination if part of exam
    b. Provide patient education and instruction on BSE
    c. Position patient into lithotomy position during exam
    d. Assist provider as needed during pelvic examination and Pap test
6. After the examination
    a. Help patient off examination table
    b. Offer tissues to wipe off any excess lubricant and discard in appropriate waste container
    c. Ask patient to get dressed, assisting as needed
    d. Explain when to expect test results or report
    e. Assist in scheduling a follow-up appointment if necessary
    f. Clean exam room, restock supplies
    g. Place labeled specimen(s) and attached requisition form in appropriate area for pickup
7. Reporting Pap test results—most common is the Bethesda System

## II. OTHER GYNECOLOGICAL PROCEDURES

A. Done to make decisions regarding the condition of the uterus and cervix
    1. Uterine sounds are inserted into the uterus to explore the cavity and measure the depth
    2. Curettes are used to scrape the lining of the uterus for a specimen and to remove growths or remnants of an abortion
    3. Biopsy forceps permits taking a small piece of tissue for diagnostic examination

## III. OBSTETRIC PATIENTS

A. Obstetric patients
    1. Document information completely
    2. Stress compliance with checkups
    3. Provide patient education
    4. Answer any questions regarding pregnancy, labor, and delivery

5. Provider's visit to confirm pregnancy
   a. Prenatal health assessment and history
   b. Complete provider examination
   c. Laboratory tests
   d. Diagnostic tests as indicated

B. Estimating the date of delivery
1. Naegele's rule
   a. Formula for estimating date of delivery
   b. Take first day of last menstrual period, subtract three months, add seven days plus one year
2. Normal pregnancies are 37 to 41 weeks, so exact times are not possible
3. Infants born prior to 37 weeks are considered premature

C. The medical assistant's role
1. Encourage proper diet
2. Suggest attendance at prenatal and childbirth classes
3. Alert provider to any problems or concerns

D. Prenatal visits
1. Interview the patient to determine problems and record remarks and symptoms
2. Request first morning specimen or instruct patient to give a specimen
3. Measure and record the patient's weight and vital signs
4. Check the chart to be sure all lab reports from tests ordered since the last visit are provided
5. Check that any other studies or referral letters are included in the chart
6. Prepare patient for the provider's examination
   a. Have patient remove clothes and put on a gown
   b. Assist patient onto examination table into a sitting position
   c. Drape patient's legs
7. Notify provider that patient is ready for exam
8. Assist the patient into supine position for the provider's prenatal exam
9. Provide assistance to provider as appropriate
10. After exam is complete, assist patient to sitting position and instruct her to dress
11. Record appropriate information in patient's chart
12. Answer any questions
13. Assist patient to make a follow-up appointment
14. Clean exam room and restock supplies for next patient

## HAPTER ACTIVITIES

1. COMPETENCY PRACTICE: *Prepare the Patient for and Assist with a Gynecological Exam and Pap Test.* This Activity is printed in the Student Workbook for this chapter, in the Chapter Application section. In groups of four, role play preparing the patient and assisting the provider with a gynecological exam and Pap test. Assign each person in the group to one of the following roles: narrator, provider, MA, and patient. Using Procedure 41–1 and the group evaluation form (provided at the end of this Instructor's Manual chapter), evaluate the group's performance of the procedure (including completeness and preparedness) and communication skills (verbal and nonverbal). The final

calculated grade or evaluation will be determined by the students' self evaluations and your evaluation. *For a variation of this competency practice, try videotaping the groups and allowing them to watch and rate themselves.*

2. Arrange to take a tour of an OB/GYN clinic. Ask the tour guide whether it is possible to allow students to see the equipment and supplies used for gynecological examinations.
3. Divide into teams and set a time limit. Have the teams set up a Pap test and pelvic exam tray. At the end of the time limit, the instructor will check the setups and determine which team has the most correct one.
4. Have students demonstrate the correct maintenance of the examination room following each patient visit.
5. Have partners in pairs; prepare an exam room for an initial OB exam, a subsequent OB exam, and a gynecological exam with Pap test. One student should prepare the room, and the other should critique to see whether anything was left out; switch roles.
6. Place many instruments used in the gynecological examination into a large box. Have each person draw an instrument from the box without looking at it (so he or she cannot make a visual selection of a known instrument). Have each person identify the instrument, explain its use, and spell its name correctly. Use as an oral quiz or as a review for the entire class.
7. Have people role play acknowledging a patient's anxiety or embarrassment and respond appropriately when assistin with a gynecological exam and Pap smear.
8. Have people role play to provide patient education on the importance of health and wellness that is age appropriate for the patient. Provide brochure(s) to each other, pertaining to a particular condition and the importance of it in relation to that disease. (Use topic suggestions from the textbook.)
9. Invite a gynecologist or OB provider to speak to the class about procedures and conditions of the reproductive syste and prenatal issues.
10. Arrange to have a medical supply representative speak to the class about the latest equipment and supplies used in the diagnosis of reproductive disorders and diseases. The speaker may be able to show and explain to people the use operation, care, and cost of the items discussed in the presentation.

## ANSWERS TO CHECK YOUR KNOWLEDGE QUESTIONS

1. Over what age is it recommended that women start routine yearly mammograms?
   a. 21
   b. 30
   **c. 40**
   d. 50
2. All women should begin screening tests about three years after they begin having vaginal intercourse but no later than ______ years old.
   a. 16
   **b. 21**
   c. 18
   d. 40
3. The system most widely used to describe Pap test findings is the Bethesda System, which reports the test results using _______ general categories:
   **a. three**
   b. two

c. four

d. six

4. Which of the following gynecological instruments are inserted into the uterus to explore the cavity and measure the depth of the uterus?

a. Sims' uterine curette

b. Randall uterine curette

c. Toms-Gaylor uterine punch

**d. Sims' uterine sound**

5. During the 24th to 28th week of gestation, the following blood test is obtained from the mother:

a. Alpha-fetoprotein (AFP)

**b. Glucose tolerance test**

c. HIV

d. Hepatitis

6. Using Naegele's rule, the period of gestation (conception to birth) is determined by using the:

**a. first day of the last menstrual period (LMP), subtracting three months, and then adding seven days plus one year.**

b. last day of the last menstrual period (LMP), subtracting **three** months, and then adding **seven** days plus **one** year.

c. first day of the last menstrual period (LMP), subtracting **nine** months, and then adding **seven** days plus **one** year.

d. last day of the last menstrual period (LMP), subtracting **three** months, and then adding **seven** days plus **one** year.

## roup Project Evaluation Form

**Prepare the Patient for and Assist with a Gynecological Exam and Pap Test**

***Based on the performance, give feedback and rate the group according to the following scale:***

**1 = poor** **2 = fair** **3 = good** **4 = exceptional**

**rbal Communication** **1** **2** **3** **4**

- Communication was complete and concise with only necessary information given to the patient.
- The information given to the patient was clear (using good diction and enunciating each word distinctly). The message was audible. The MA did not use technical terms with patient.
- Patient was allowed time to process the message and verify its meaning.
- MA established rapport with the patient, acknowledging the patient by name.

**edback:**

__________________________________________

__________________________________________

__________________________________________

**nverbal Communication** **1** **2** **3** **4**

- MA smiled when greeting patient, used appropriate facial expression according to the situation, and maintained appropriate eye contact.

- Maintained a close but comfortable position facing the patient without standing over her; respected patient' personal space.
- Used appropriate gestures to enhance communication, used appropriate touch, and displayed empathy with the patient.
- Respected patient privacy by keeping patient covered during exam.

**Feedback:**

____________________________________________

____________________________________________

____________________________________________

**Performance** **1** **2** **3** **4**

- Group performed the procedure within 25 minutes.
- MA performed or role-played each step within Procedure 41–1. (Refer to competency assessment.)
- MA carried out each step correctly, including positioning the patient.
- Group members acted professionally.

**Feedback:**

____________________________________________

____________________________________________

____________________________________________

**Preparedness** **1** **2** **3** **4**

- Equipment and supplies were gathered prior to procedure.
- Group members seemed well-prepared.
- Procedure and scenario flowed naturally.
- Each member was aware of his or her role and responsibilities.

**Feedback:**

____________________________________________

____________________________________________

____________________________________________

**Final Score _______ / 16 pts**

# HAPTER 42 Pediatric Examinations

## BHES Curriculum

| | |
|---|---|
| MA.A.1.4.a | Document accurately |
| MA.A.1.4.f | Comply with federal, state, and local health laws and regulations |
| MA.A.1.5.b | Identify and respond appropriately when working with and caring for patients with special needs |
| MA.A.1.5.f | Identify and discuss developmental stages of life |
| MA.A.1.8.cc | Communicate on the recipient's level of comprehension |
| MA.A.1.8.dd | Serve as a liaison between provider and others |
| MA.A.1.9.g | Maintain medication and immunization records |
| MA.A.1.9.k | Prepare and maintain examination and treatment area |
| MA.A.1.9.l | Prepare patient for examinations and treatments |
| MA.A.1.9.m | Assist provider with routine and specialty examinations and treatments |
| MA.A.1.9.r | Teach patients methods of health promotion and disease prevention |

## AAHEP Core Curriculum

| | |
|---|---|
| I.P.10 | Assist provider with patient care |
| I.A.1 | Apply critical thinking skills in performing patient assessment and care |
| II.C.7 | Analyze charts, graphs, and tables in the interpretation of health care results |
| II.P.3 | Maintain growth charts |
| III.A.2 | Explain the rationale for performance of procedure to the patient |
| III.A.3 | Show awareness of patients' concerns regarding their perceptions of the procedure being performed |
| IV.P.5 | Instruct patients according to their needs to promote health maintenance and disease prevention |
| IV.P.6 | Prepare a patient for procedures, treatments, or both |
| IV.P.8 | Document patient care |
| IX.P.7 | Document accurately in the patient chart |

## ESSON OUTLINE

### PEDIATRICS

A. Pediatrics is a specialty medical practice dealing with children from birth through age 16–18 or high school graduation
B. Pediatric patients are examined more frequently than adults
C. Preventive care exam schedule
   1. American Academy of Pediatrics (AAP) "Recommendations for Preventive Pediatric Health Care" chart
   2. Medicaid's Early and Periodic Screening, Diagnosis, and Treatment (EPSDT) program

### PEDIATRIC GROWTH AND DEVELOPMENT

A. Must be monitored for growth and development
   1. Growth refers to changes in height and weight
   2. Development refers to the ability to control the body and use verbal and mental skills
B. Growth and Development Table 42–1

## III. PEDIATRIC MEASUREMENTS

A. Precise measurements are essential for monitoring growth and development

B. Measuring height or recumbent length

1. Measuring recumbent length of patient (Procedure 42–1)
2. Measuring height

C. Weighing the pediatric patient

1. Remove clothing and diaper
2. Calibrate scale
3. Various methods (Procedure 42–1)

D. Head circumference

1. Positioning
2. Method (Procedure 42–1)

E. Chest circumference—positioning (Procedure 42–1)

F. Growth charts and recording measurements

1. Graphs available from the National Center for Health Statistics (NCHS), a division of the Centers for Disease Control and Prevention (CDC), www.cdc.gov/growthcharts
2. Provider can compare measurements in relation to the percentiles of children the same age
3. Documenting (Procedure 42–2)
4. Failure to thrive (FTT)
   a. Poor physical and emotional environment
   b. Parent lack of knowledge
   c. Signs and symptoms

## IV. WELL- AND SICK-CHILD APPOINTMENTS

A. Pediatric practice will establish methods of handling well and sick patients

B. The pediatric office environment

1. Checking in and rooming the patient
2. Gain trust and cooperation
3. Maintaining the play area
4. Standard precautions
5. Handling illnesses

C. Medical assistant responsibilities

1. Assist in gathering data
2. Document information
3. Perform screening tests within your skill and ability level
4. Assist the patient
5. Assist the provider
6. Provide patient education
7. Liaison between parent and provider

D. Child neglect and abuse

1. Threats or acts that might cause physical or mental harm to a child must be reported
2. Law refers to suspicion of neglect of care as well as abuse

3. Symptoms of neglect and abuse (Table 42–2)

E. Establishing rapport

1. Establish cooperation
2. Treat pediatric patients as individuals and give them the same kindness and respect as any other patient

F. Exam preparation

1. Establish a good rapport
2. Discuss child's current health
3. Provide education

G. Assisting with the pediatric exam

1. Exam is similar to CPE for adults; provider examines from head to toe
2. Assist provider

### . IMMUNIZATIONS

A. Knowledgeable about vaccinations (Figure 42–13)

B. Patient and parent education

C. Vaccination information statements (VISs)

D. Immunization schedules from the CDC

1. 0–6 years
2. 7–13 years
3. Current year's schedule can be downloaded from CDC Website

E. More information on preparing injections in Chapter 53

### I. VISION SCREENING

A. Recommended by the American Academy of Pediatrics (Procedure 42–3)

B. Modified Snellen charts

1. Snellen big E chart requires child to identify which way the E is facing
2. Kindergarten version of chart uses shapes and symbols
3. Results are recorded on the last line correctly identified (same as adult Snellen chart)

### II. HEARING SCREENING

A. Observed by reaction to surrounding sounds

B. Pediatric specialist has instruments and skills to evaluate hearing

C. As child grows, an audiometer test can been given to screen hearing levels accurately

## HAPTER ACTIVITIES

1. Arrange for several people to bring in their infants and children of varying ages. Divide the class into teams and practice weighing and measuring the children and then compare the results. Have participants document their results in a mock patient chart or EMR and plot the information on a growth chart.
2. Practice testing for visual acuity on appropriately aged children from the previous exercise. Document the results.
3. Ask a clinical supervisor or provider to speak to the class on the importance of efficient assisting, proper preparation of patients for pediatric examinations, the importance of being able to assess critically what to do next during the exam and related topics. This gives the class members firsthand information about their role in patient care.

4. Invite a speaker from the Department of Health to explain the importance of infant and child immunizations and discuss the various types of immunizations, how to administer and document them, and precautions and reactions to watch for.
5. Have class members role play as medical assistant and patient. Medical assistants must explain diagnostic tests and procedures to the patient. This activity provides valuable communication skill practice and helps overcome shyness when talking about delicate matters.
6. Invite a pediatrician to class to discuss common pediatric conditions and procedures.

# ANSWERS TO CHECK YOUR KNOWLEDGE QUESTIONS

1. At which age will the infant begin the immunization schedule?
   a. 2 weeks
   **b. 2 months**
   c. 6 weeks
   d. 1 year
2. An infant or young child who is below the ___ percentile on standardized growth charts is said to be failing to thrive
   **a. third**
   b. fifth
   c. seventh
   d. tenth
3. Which of the following persons are obligated to report neglect or abuse to the proper authorities?
   a. Family members
   b. Healthcare workers
   c. Neighbors
   **d. All of the above**
4. Up until which age would you record the head circumference measurement?
   a. 12 months
   b. 24 months
   **c. 36 months**
   d. 48 months
5. Which measurement is taken and recorded in the patient's record but not on the growth chart?
   a. head circumference
   **b. chest circumference**
   c. height
   d. weight
6. The kindergarten version of the Snellen chart uses:
   **a. signs and symbols.**
   b. the capital letter *E*.
   c. letters.
   d. numbers.
7. When using the growth chart, each month is represented by a:
   a. dot.
   **b. square.**
   c. line.
   d. circle.

# NIT 14 LABORATORY PROCEDURES
# HAPTER 43 Blood Specimen Collection

## BHES Curriculum

MA.A.1.9.i Use Standard Precautions

MA.A.1.10.c Dispose of biohazardous materials

MA.A.1.10.d (1) Perform venipuncture

MA.A.1.10.d (2) Perform capillary puncture

## AAHEP Core Curriculum

I.P.2 Perform venipuncture

I.P.3 Perform capillary puncture

III.P.3 Select appropriate barrier and personal protective equipment (PPE) for potentially infectious situations

III.P.4 Perform hand washing

III.A.1 Use language and verbal skills that enable patients' understanding of the procedure being performed

III.A.2 Explain the rationale for performance of a procedure to a patient

III.A.3 Show awareness of patients' concerns regarding their perceptions of the procedure being performed

IX.A.1 Display sensitivity to patients' rights and feelings in collecting specimens

## ESSON OUTLINE

### SKIN PUNCTURE (PROCEDURE 43–1)

A. Also known as finger sticks

B. Capillary blood is obtained

1. Ideal for screening tests that require a small amount of blood
2. Just under the surface of the skin

C. Appropriate sites for capillary puncture

1. Ring finger
2. Great finger
3. Lateral sides of the heel on infants, also known as a heel stick
4. *Rarely* the earlobe

D. Make the skin punctures across the fingerprints, not parallel to them; making the puncture across the fingerprints makes blood collection easier

E. Sterile lancet is device used for finger sticks and heel sticks

1. Also considered a sharp
2. Comes in different sizes for different uses

### VENIPUNCTURE

A. Definition: Surgical puncture (incision) of a vein

B. Most common site for venipuncture is inner arm at bend of elbow (antecubital fossa)

## III. APPLYING THE TOURNIQUET

A. Must be placed on patient's arm about 3 inches above elbow or intended venipuncture site

B. Ask patient whether he or she has a preference for which to use

## IV. PERFORMING VENIPUNCTURE

A. Sterile needle and syringe method (Procedure 43–2)
   1. Used when very small veins are involved
   2. Size of syringe varies depending on how much blood specimen is required

B. Vacuum tube and sterile needle method (Procedure 43–3)
   1. Most popular method of collection
   2. Blood specimens enter directly into tubes

C. Butterfly needle method (Procedure 43–4) used when patient has small veins

## V. SPECIMEN COLLECTION

A. Test tubes are color coded for various hematology departments in the lab.

B. Red-stoppered tubes
   1. Range in size from 3 mL to 15 mL
   2. Use for whole blood collection and allowed to clot
   3. When clotted, blood is spun down and serum poured off

C. Red/black-stoppered tubes
   1. Efficient way to transfer serum from centrifuged tube because of SST
   2. SST separates red cells from serum

D. Lavender-stoppered tubes
   1. Contain EDTA
   2. Range in size from 5 mL to 10 mL
   3. Used in whole-blood collection

E. Gray-stoppered tubes
   1. Used in blood glucose tests
   2. Usually 5 mL
   3. Contains oxalate

F. Blue-stoppered tubes
   1. Must be completely full
   2. Usually 5 mL
   3. Used for testing prothrombin times

G. Green-stoppered tubes
   1. Usually 5 mL
   2. Contains heparin
   3. Used to determine several chemical constituents

## I. ORDER OF DRAW

A. Yellow

B. Red or red/black

C. Blue

D. Green

E. Lavender

F. Gray

## I. DOCUMENTATION FOR SPECIMEN COLLECTION AND SATELLITE LABORATORY PROCESSING

A. Date collected

B. Patient's full name, DOB, or records number

C. Date sent to lab

D. Test(s) requested

E. Date results received

F. Test results

G. Lab request form must be completed, sent with the specimens, and listed in the log book.

# HAPTER ACTIVITIES

1. Instruct students to develop sensitivity of touch in their fingertips by practicing palpation of veins in the antecubital are of several students, friends, and family members.
2. Have students draw a piece of paper out of a bucket that lists a common laboratory test in the POL. Student is then responsible for saying what the test is for and what color tube is needed for that test.
3. Have students practice venipuncture and capillary puncture methods on one another. Also have them practice spinning down the blood to draw off the serum and pouring into a transfer tube without causing hemolysis.
4. Conduct a field trip to a clinic laboratory and a satellite laboratory. After students go to both sites, have them compare and contrast the two.
5. Invite a laboratory technician to come into class and speak to students about his or her profession and how he or she interacts with medical assistants.

# NSWERS TO CHECK YOUR KNOWLEDGE QUESTIONS

1. Which are the most ideal areas for capillary puncture on the hand?

   **a. Ring finger and great finger**

   b. Great finger, ring finger, and thumb

   c. Pinky finger, thumb, and great finger

   d. Any of the five fingers

2. What should you do prior to applying a tourniquet to a patient's arm?

   a. Visually inspect one arm for the vein.

   b. Visually inspect both arms for the vein.

   c. Ask the patient which site is preferred or best site.

   **d. Both b and c**

3. To prepare the site for venipuncture, you should clean the site with alcohol and then do the following:
   a. fan the site to dry the alcohol.
   b. have patient blow on the site to dry.
   c. blow on the site to dry.
   **d. none of the above**
4. What is the first step for an MA to do if a patient faints when he or she is performing venipuncture?
   a. Remove the needle.
   **b. Remove the tourniquet.**
   c. Keep the needle and tourniquet on the arm and call for help.
   d. None of the above
5. Why must an MA check all blood collection supplies for expiration date?
   a. To remain in compliance with quality assurance
   b. To remain in compliance with quality control
   c. To remain in compliance to HIPAA
   **d. Both a and b**

# HAPTER 44 The Physician's Office Laboratory

## BHES Curriculum

MA.A.1.4.f Comply with federal, state, and local health laws and regulations

MA.A.1.8.y Perform routine maintenance of administrative and clinical equipment

## AAHEP Core Curriculum

III.C.III.4 Identify personal safety precautions as established by the Occupational Safety and Health Administration (OSHA)

III.C.III.7 Match types and uses of personal protective equipment (PPE)

V.P.V.9 Perform routine maintenance of office equipment with documentation

IX.C.IX.13 Discuss all levels of government legislation and regulation as they apply to medical assisting practice, including FDA and DEA regulations

X.C.XI.1 Describe personal protective equipment

X.C.XI.2 Identify safety techniques that can prevent accidents and maintain a safe work environment

## ESSON OUTLINE

### LABORATORY CLASSIFICATIONS AND REGULATIONS

A. POL falls under numerous regulatory bodies
   1. CLIA
   2. CMS
   3. OSHA
B. Categories of testing—complexity of lab tests performed determines the classification of POL
   1. Waived
      a. Certificate of waiver allows only those tests performed in a POL that are on list of waived tests
      b. Application obtained from CMS
      c. Lab tests on certificate of waiver list may be billed to Medicare and Medicaid for reimbursement
   2. Moderately complex
      a. Tests must be performed under more stringent regulations and a more expanded requirement of personnel
      b. Provider-performed microscopy procedures (PPMP) is a subcategory
   3. Highly complex
      a. Testing personnel must have specific and specialized training to perform these tests
      b. Testing would not typically be performed in a POL
      c. Usually found in hospital lab settings and reference labs
C. Quality assurance refers to evaluated services and the results compared to accepted standards
   1. Patient identification
   2. Patient preparation and specimen collection
   3. Specimen processing and transportation
   4. Instrumental and technical performance
   5. Safety
   6. In-service training and education of all health care personnel

D. Quality control
   1. A process of assessing testing procedures, reagents, and technique of individuals performing the test
   2. All labs required to follow QA programs
   3. Use of test kit control
      a. Value range of control
      b. Reagent strip test
E. POL guidelines for a well-managed and efficient POL
F. Safety in the POL with collecting and testing specimens
   1. Use of standard precautions essential
   2. Use of protective barriers especially in POL
      a. Properly sized gown, gloves
      b. Avoid touching items with contaminated gloves
   3. Maintain long hair up and away from face
   4. Jewelry items harbor organisms, can break and could cause injury
   5. Maintain personal immunizations
      a. Pneumonia and influenza optional
      b. HBV series necessary if in contact with patients
         i. Record maintained in personnel file
         ii. Waiver by employer possible if no patient contact, also kept in file
         iii. Can be declined, documented in file

## II. THE MICROSCOPE (PROCEDURE 44–1)

A. Used to examine and identify minute objects that cannot be seen with the naked eye
B. Fine and highly technical instrument that must be handled with great respect and care
   1. Carry microscope by grasping arm with one hand and placing other hand under base
   2. Have operations and care manual readily accessible for reference
C. Parts of microscope
   1. Arm supports eyepiece
   2. Eyepieces
   3. Binocular—meaning has two eyepieces
   4. Monocular—meaning has one eyepiece
   5. Eyepiece contains lens to magnify what is being examined
D. Body tube leads to revolving nosepiece, which has three or four small lenses called objectives
   1. Each has different magnifying power
   2. Low-power field (lpf) objective
      a. Has shortest lens and lowest power
      b. Objects 10 times larger
      c. Lens for scanning objects first
   3. High-power field (hpf) objective
      a. Magnifies objects 40 times
      b. Used for greater detail in viewing the specimen

4. Oil-immersion lens
    a. Has longest lens
    b. Magnifies objects 100 times
    c. With fine focus, objective will bring sharp definition to the object being viewed

E. Stage has two clips to hold the specimen to be viewed
    1. Substage under the stage is where condenser is located that directs light on specimen
    2. Shutter or diaphragm controls the amount of light desired
    3. Substage can be raised and lowered

F. Lens tissue paper should be kept near microscope
    1. Clean lenses after each use
    2. Eye secretions, makeup, oil, and dust can interfere with viewing through the lens and can be source of disease transmission

G. Eyeglasses not necessary to wear when using microscope; microscope can be focused to compensate for all visual defects except astigmatism

H. Requires much practice and patience to become proficient using a microscope

## CHAPTER ACTIVITIES

1. Have students obtain materials such as hair, saliva, and onion skin to view under the microscope, helping students gain proficiency in the use of the microscope.
2. Have students make safety posters from the guidelines for lab safety and present them to the class.
3. Invite a lab technician to speak to the class about the importance of safety in the lab, requirements of the profession, duties of a technician, and related topics.
4. Arrange a field trip to a local laboratory or the laboratory department of a local hospital. This helps students realize the importance of accuracy, proper labeling, and preparation of specimens.
5. Have students set up a mock clinic in the classroom and role-play how they will use their PPE for different exposure types.

## ANSWERS TO CHECK YOUR KNOWLEDGE QUESTIONS

1. The *waived* status is granted according to what?
    a. The tests cleared by the DFA
    b. That tests are manufactured for clinical use only
    **c. The difficulty in performing the diagnostic tests and whether they can be performed in a medical office following package insert directions**
    d. The amount of time it takes to perform the diagnostic tests
2. Which of the following properly describes inspections of laboratory facilities?
    a. May be made unannounced at any time
    b. A monetary fine per item may be assessed on the clinic if a violation is found.
    c. A monetary fine per employee is applied if a violation is found.
    **d. all of the above**

3. Why should the operation and care manual for the microscope be kept?

   a. It does not need to be kept.

   b. Only one needs to be kept because all microscopes are the same.

   c. It needs to be kept because it is a HIPAA standard.

   **d. It needs to be kept because all microscopes are slightly different.**

4. How many injections are involved with the hepatitis B vaccine?

   a. 2

   **b. 3**

   c. 4

   d. None of the above

5. High-power field, without oil submersion, magnifies objects by:

   **a. 40 times.**

   b. 50 times.

   c. 75 times.

   d. 20 times.

6. Low-power field magnifies objects by:

   a. 5 times.

   **b. 10 times.**

   c. 15 times.

   d. 20 times.

# CHAPTER 45 Diagnostic Testing

## ABHES Curriculum

MA.A.1.10.a Practice quality control

MA.A.1.10.b (2) Perform selected CLIA-waived tests that assist with diagnosis and treatment: hematology testing

MA.A.1.10.b (3) Perform selected CLIA-waived tests that assist with diagnosis and treatment: chemistry testing

MA.A.1.10.b (4) Perform selected CLIA-waived tests that assist with diagnosis and treatment: immunology testing

## CAAHEP Core Curriculum

I.C.9 Discuss quality control issues related to handling microbiological specimens

I.C.10. Identify disease processes that are indications for CLIA-waived tests

I.P.11. Perform quality control measures

I.P.12. Perform hematology testing

I.P.13. Perform chemistry testing

I.P.15. Perform immunology testing

I.P.16. Screen test results

I.A.2. Use language and verbal skills that enable patients' understanding

II.C.7. Analyze charts, graphs, and tables in the interpretation of health care results

II.P.2. Maintain laboratory test results by using flow sheets

II.A.2. Distinguish between normal and abnormal test results

III.A.1. Display sensitivity to patients' rights and feelings in collecting specimens

III.A.2. Explain the rationale for performance of a procedure to the patient

III.A.3. Show awareness of patients' concerns regarding their perceptions of the procedure being performed

## LESSON PLANNING

### I. QUALITY CONTROL AND QUALITY ASSURANCE

A. Quality assurance: evaluate services and the results compared to accepted standards
   1. Patient identification
   2. Patient preparation and specimen collection
   3. Specimen processing and transportation
   4. Instrumental and technical performance
   5. Safety
   6. In-service training and education of all health care personnel

B. Quality control: a process of assessing testing procedures, reagents, and technique of individuals performing the test

C. All labs required to follow QA programs

### II. HEMATOLOGY TESTING

A. Hemoglobin and hematocrit
   1. Screening tests that require a small amount of blood
   2. Most often capillary blood

3. Hemoglobin
    a. Normal range for males is 14–18 g/dL
    b. Normal range for females is 12–16 g/dL
4. Hematocrit
    a. Can use either capillary blood or venous blood
    b. Expressed as a percentage of total blood volume
    c. Normal range for males is 40–54%
    d. Normal range for females is 37–47%

B. Complete blood count
1. Common blood test ordered in health care provider's office
2. Automated instruments capable of measuring many values
    a. Total red blood cell count
    b. Total white blood cell count
    c. Total platelet count
    d. Hemoglobin
    e. Hematocrit
    f. Total granulocyte count
    g. Total lymphocyte and monocyte count
    h. Percentage of granulocytes
    i. Percentage of lymphocytes and monocytes
    j. Red blood cell indices

C. The WBC differential
1. Performed on 100 white blood cells
2. Numbers of neutrophils, eosinophils, basophils, monocytes, and lymphocytes counted
3. Physician reviews for abnormalities of the red blood cells
4. MAs do not perform these counts but should have idea of what report entails

D. Erythrocyte sedimentation rate (ESR)
1. Rate at which red blood cells settle in a calibrated tube within a given time
2. Gives provider an idea of how much inflammation is occurring in response to another disease condition
3. Common methods are Westergren and Wintrobe methods

## III. GLUCOSE TESTING

A. Glucose testing
1. Capillary blood samples usually used
2. Testing uses handheld meter with specially designed reagent strips to which blood is directly applied
3. Perform quality controls
    a. Perform controls at beginning of each day
    b. Log results prior to reporting any patient results

B. Glucose tolerance testing
1. Performed when a patient has consistently high fasting blood sugar
2. Test determines patient's ability to metabolize a glucose load within a prescribed amount of time

3. Patient education for GTT

C. Hemoglobin A1C

1. Also called glycohemoglobin
2. Modified form of hemoglobin elevated when blood glucose remains high
3. Provider commonly requests random blood sugar level with the hemoglobin A1C

D. Cholesterol testing—many CLIA-waived tests available for screening cholesterol in POL

## IV. IMMUNOLOGY

A. Immunology: study of the body's ability to prevent and fight off infection

B. Mononucleosis testing

1. Illness caused by Epstein-Barr virus
2. Extremely contagious

C. Allergy testing

1. Skin prick tests
   a. Desirable sites are arms and back depending on number of tests and patient's preference
   b. Patient comfort essential for compliance because patient must stay in same position for 20 minutes
   c. Small children should be restrained
   d. Tests should be numbered in pattern with washable ink
   e. Inform patient of temporary discomfort during test
   f. Instruct patient to tell of itching or swelling at injection site
   g. Instruct patient to avoid touching area
   h. Small drop of each extract can be applied to arm or back, in rows, with multiple applicator
   i. Skin wiped with alcohol prior to application
   j. Sterile needle or lancet used to tear skin surface to allow extract to enter the circulatory system
   k. Extracts at least 1 ½ to 2 inches apart to prevent solutions from running together
   l. Control used for comparison in interpreting results
   m. Reactions usually occur within first 20 minutes
   n. Severe reactions of swelling and itching, check with physician regarding the application of a cold pack or ice for temporary relief
   o. Physician may order return for recheck of reaction sites.
      i. In 24 hours for possible delayed reactions
      ii. Up to 48 hours from fungi and bacteria
2. Intradermal injections
   a. Also referred to as subcutaneous test
   b. Thought to be more accurate than scratch test
      i. Performed when scratch test is unclear or negative
      ii. Not advisable to perform this test on patients who have positive scratch tests
   c. Solutions about 100 times more dilute than those used for scratch tests because severe reaction can occur
   d. Tourniquet can be applied proximal to site when arm is used
   e. Epinephrine administered just above site if severe reaction occurs
   f. Sites spaced at intervals on forearm

g. Reaction time 15–30 minutes
h. Fine-gauge needle used (26G, ⅜–⅝ inches long); dosage 0.01–0.02 mL by sterile technique
i. Results read same as scratch tests
j. Serum or vaccine sometimes used in intradermal testing to help determine medication sensitivity and immunization needs

3. Skin patch tests
   a. To determine cause of contact dermatitis
   b. Patch of gauze square saturated with suspected substance placed on skin surface, usually arm, secured with nonallergenic tape
   c. Results read after 24 hours and then 48 hours
   d. Control placed near patch if substance not a known skin irritant
   e. Redness or swelling indicates reaction
4. Radioallergosorbent test (RAST)
5. Nasal smear
   a. Secretions examined to observe the eosinophil count
   b. Many present and clumped together indicate allergy

D. HIV testing
1. Screening tests are enzyme immunoassays
2. May have to draw blood for this screening

E. PKU testing
1. Screening test done with capillary blood from infant's heel
2. Required in all states and Canadian provinces
3. Drops of blood are soaked through outlined circles of treated paper, attached to health department's requisition
4. The form and PKU testing card mailed to state health department for processing

## V. TESTING OUTSIDE POL

A. Commonly ordered tests
B. Series of tests ordered are done as panels or profiles
C. MA's responsibilities
   a. Prepare specimens for sending
   b. Screen test results as they are returned to provider's office

## CHAPTER ACTIVITIES

1. Invite a lab technician to speak to the class about the importance of safety in the lab, requirements of the profession, duties of a technician, and related topics.
2. Give students 5" × 7" cards with orders for various blood tests. Have students describe what signs and symptoms a patient would have to warrant an order from the provider.
3. Have students do a presentation or group activity on the development of cells from stem cell to mature cells.
4. Ask a diagnostics company representative to speak to the class about the newest diagnostic products and procedures. If this is not a possibility, have students pick two diagnostic tests, do research on the products used to test, and present to their fellow classmates.

# ANSWERS TO CHECK YOUR KNOWLEDGE QUESTIONS

1. The medical assistant will be responsible for quality control and assurance. All the following are required components to be recorded in the log book *except*:
   a. patient's name.
   b. results of the test.
   **c. doctor's initials.**
   d. test performed.
2. Hemoglobin is an allosteric protein found in:
   a. monocytes.
   **b. erythrocytes.**
   c. lymphocytes.
   d. granulocytes.
3. Hemoglobin is responsible for transporting __________ to cells of the body.
   **a. oxygen**
   b. carbon dioxide
   c. iron
   d. vitamins and nutrients
4. Hematocrit is never expressed as a percentage.
   a. True
   **b. False**
5. If a patient has a rheumatoid arthritis, the provider will order which of the following tests to monitor inflammation?
   a. Hemoglobin
   b. CBC
   **c. ESR**
   d. Hemoglobin A1C
6. The forearm provides 14 prime sites for intradermal testing.
   **a. True**
   b. False
7. Which of the following are indicators of renal function?
   a. Triglycerides
   b. CK with PT
   c. Na with uric acid
   **d. BUN with creatinine**

# CHAPTER 46 Specimen Collection and Processing

## ABHES Curriculum

| | |
|---|---|
| MA.A.1.9.b | Apply principles of aseptic techniques and infection control |
| MA.A.1.9.f | Screen and follow up patient test results |
| MA.A.1.9.i | Use Standard Precautions |
| MA.A.1.9.k | Prepare and maintain examination and treatment area |
| MA.A.1.9.l | Prepare patient for examinations and treatments |
| MA.A.1.9.p | Advise patients of office policies and procedures |
| MA.A.1.10.a | Practice quality control |
| MA.A.1.10.b (1) | Perform selected CLIA-waived tests that assist with diagnosis and treatment: urinalysis |
| MA.A.1.10.b (5) | Perform selected CLIA-waived tests that assist with diagnosis and treatment: microbiology testing |
| MA.A.1.10.b (6) | Perform selected CLIA-waived tests that assist with diagnosis and treatment: kit testing |
| MA.A.1.10.b (6) (a) | Perform selected CLIA-waived tests that assist with diagnosis and treatment: pregnancy |
| MA.A.1.10.b (6) (b) | Perform selected CLIA-waived tests that assist with diagnosis and treatment: quick strep |
| MA.A.1.10.b(6)(c) | Perform selected CLIA-waived tests that assist with diagnosis and treatment: dip sticks |
| MA.A.1.10.d (3) | Collect, label, and process specimens: perform wound collection procedures |
| MA.A.1.10.d (4) | Collect, label, and process specimens: obtain throat specimens for microbiologic testing |
| MA.A.1.10.e | Instruct patients in the collection of a clean-catch midstream urine specimen |
| MA.A.1.10.f | Instruct patients in the collection of a fecal specimen |

## CAAHEP Core Curriculum

| | |
|---|---|
| I.C.5 | Describe the normal function of each body system |
| I.C.8 | Discuss implications for disease and disability when homeostasis is not maintained |
| I.C.9 | Describe implications for treatment related to pathology |
| I.P.11 | Perform quality control measures |
| I.P.12 | Perform hematology testing |
| I.P.13 | Perform chemistry testing |
| I.P.14 | Perform urinalysis |
| I.P.15 | Perform immunology testing |
| I.P.16 | Screen test results |
| I.A.2 | Use language and verbal skills that enable patients' understanding |
| II.A.2 | Distinguish between normal and abnormal test results |
| III.C.9 | Discuss quality control issues related to handling microbiological specimens |
| III.C.10 | Identify disease processes that are indications for CLIA-waived tests |
| III.P.2 | Practice Standard Precautions |
| III.P.3 | Select appropriate barrier and personal protective equipment (PPE) for potentially infectious situations |
| III.P.7 | Obtain specimens for microbiology testing |
| III.P.8 | Perform CLIA-waived microbiology testing |

| | |
|---|---|
| III.A.2 | Explain the rationale for performance of a procedure to the patient |
| III.A.3 | Show awareness of patients' concerns about the procedure being performed |

# LESSON OUTLINE

## I. URINE SPECIMENS

A. First morning specimen best for testing because it is most concentrated

B. Midstream clean-catch specimen (Procedure 46–1)

1. Partial voiding before specimen is collected
2. Midstream sample clears the urethra of contaminants that could adversely affect the results

C. 24-hour urine specimen

1. Provide patient with instructions for collection
2. Patient provided with a container in which to collect specimens over 24-hour period

D. Pediatric urine specimens

1. Special urine collection bags fit over the genital area
2. Infant's skin washed and dried thoroughly prior to affixing the bag

E. Urinary catheterization

1. Specialized type of urine collection
2. Reasons for catheterization
    a. Sterile specimen indicated for testing
    b. Patient unable to void
    c. Medication instilled in the bladder
3. Not performed routinely in most offices

F. Collection of specimens for substance abuse analysis and chain of custody

1. Detects presence of illegal drugs and chemical substances
2. Might prevent a person from obtaining or retaining a job
3. Chain-of-custody form informs patient of reason for test

G. Pregnancy testing (Procedure 46–2)

1. Measures amount of human chorionic gonadotropin in urine or blood
2. Home pregnancy tests and screening tests in POL are most commonly performed on urine specimens

H. Urinalysis

1. Physical
2. Chemical
3. Microscopic

I. Physical urinalysis

1. Color
2. Clarity
3. Volume
4. Odor
5. Specific gravity: Chemical reagent strips now include this parameter; offices no longer assessing specific gravity as a physical property but a chemical property

J. Chemical urinalysis (Procedure 46–3)
   1. Analyze specimens as soon as possible after collection
   2. If over an hour, allow specimen to return to room temperature
   3. Reagent strips provide qualitative and quantitative assessments
   4. Strips compared to known values on the bottle for reporting

K. Microscopic examination of urine
   1. Medical assistants may not read or interpret results of microscopic urine specimens
   2. Medical assistants may be asked to prepare the specimen for another to view slide and report results (Procedure 46–4)

L. Normal and abnormal values (Procedure 46–5)
   1. Protein (albumin)
   2. Ketone (acetone)
   3. Bilirubin
   4. Urobilinogen
   5. Hematuria
   6. Nitrite
   7. Leukocyte esterase
   8. Glucose
   9. Specific Gravity

## I. COLLECTING FECAL SPECIMENS

A. Fecal (stool) specimens
   1. Difficult for patients to collect properly
   2. Used to check for occult (hidden) blood, ova and parasites, bacterial and viral infections
   3. Patients instructed to obtain stool specimen at home and bring to lab for testing (Procedure 46–6)
   4. Patient education

B. Occult blood specimens (Procedure 46–7)
   1. Common screening tools for early detection of colon cancer
   2. Tests based on guaiac reagent

## II. COLLECTING SPUTUM SPECIMENS (PROCEDURE 46–8)

A. Sputum specimens indicated for diagnostic analysis when patient has unresolved cough with mucus production

B. Patient education for sputum collection

## V. COLLECTING BACTERIAL SPECIMENS

A. Bacterial specimen collection (Procedure 46–9)
   1. Bacteria, viruses, and fungi extracted from specimens for identification to provide appropriate medication to eliminate infection
   2. Culture commonly obtained from part of the body that appears to be infected

3. Culture sites
    a. Throat
    b. Mouth
    c. Ear
    d. Eye
    e. Nose
    f. Vagina
    g. Anus
    h. Infected wounds
4. Cultures collected in a culturette, a specialized container

B. Throat cultures (Procedure 46–10)
1. Obtained from patients complaining of sore throats, fever, swollen glands, and cough
2. Rapid Group A Strep kits provide results of swab in minutes (Procedure 46–11)
3. Patient education for obtaining a throat culture

C. Blood cultures
1. Blood drawn from patient directly into particular formulated broth in vacuum bottle
2. Culture and sensitivity testing

D. Culture media
1. Media, or agar a substance used to grow microorganisms for identification and sensitivity
2. Media comes in petri dishes, tubes, and broths
3. Primary media
4. Selective media
5. Inoculation of a plate not a common MA procedure

E. Gram staining and microbiological smears
1. Not usually performed by MAs
2. Important to understand reasons for testing and indications of various results

F. Morphologic shapes
1. Coccus
2. Bacillus
3. Spiral

## CHAPTER ACTIVITIES

1. Have students collect urine specimens from one another, perform a routine urinalysis, and record the results.
2. Have students look up the types of bacteria and draw, color, and label each one.
3. Have students take home a fecal occult testing kit and collect a three-day specimen. When completed, students can bring the kit back to the classroom and test the collected specimens.
4. Have students create pamphlets or brochures regarding the collection of:
    a. Fecal specimens
    b. Sputum specimens

    When completed, have students role-play with each other how they would present this to a patient.

# ANSWERS TO CHECK YOUR KNOWLEDGE QUESTIONS

1. Using the word *random* to describe a urine specimen means what?
   a. The provider has ordered a specimen that is collected in the morning.
   **b. They provider has ordered a specimen without specifying the time of collection.**
   c. The provider has ordered a specimen collected at bedtime.
   d. The provider has ordered a specimen to be collected at lunchtime.
2. There are special urine collection bags that fit over the genital area of an adult and are secured with adhesive.
   a. True
   **b. False**
3. All the following are portions of physical urinalysis testing *except:*
   a. color.
   b. clarity.
   **c. glucose.**
   d. specific gravity.
4. Which of the following components could be found in a patient's urine specimen when the patient has a urinary tract infection?
   a. Protein
   b. Nitrite
   c. Leukocytes
   **d. All of the above**
5. Which of the following is the normal value range for specific gravity?
   a. 1.015–1.025
   b. 1.005–1.020
   c. 1.010–1.025
   **d. 1.005–1.030**
6. Medical assistants are not allowed to read or interpret results of microscopic urine sediments according to OSHA.
   a. True
   **b. False**
7. Which color does the guaiac reagent turn when oxidized in the presence of blood?
   a. Purple
   b. Black
   **c. Blue**
   d. Yellow
8. Exudate is another word for:
   **a. drainage.**
   b. sputum.
   c. pus.
   d. blood.
9. When did Hans Christian Gram develop the staining technique?
   a. 1883
   **b. 1884**

   c. 1885

   d. 1886

10. Which disease does the bacterium *Bordetella pertussis* cause?

   a. Tuberculosis

   b. Anthrax

   c. Leprosy

   **d. Whooping cough**

# UNIT 15 CARDIOLOGY AND RADIOLOGY PROCEDURES
# CHAPTER 47 Cardiology Procedures

## ABHES Curriculum

| | |
|---|---|
| M.A.A.1.2.c | Assist the physician with the regimen of diagnostic and treatment modalities as they relate to each body system |
| M.A.A.1.4.a | Document accurately |
| M.A.A.1.9.f | Screen and follow up patient test results |
| M.A.A.1.9.l | Prepare patient for examinations and treatments |
| M.A.A.1.9.m | Assist provider with routine and specialty examinations and treatments |
| M.A.A.1.9.o (1) | Perform electrocardiograms |

## CAAHEP Core Curriculum

| | |
|---|---|
| I.C.8 | Discuss implications for disease and disability when homeostasis is not maintained |
| I.P.5 | Perform electrocardiography |
| I.P.10 | Assist provider with patient care |
| I.A.1 | Apply critical thinking skills in performing patient assessment and care |
| I.A.2 | Use language and verbal skills that enable patients' understanding |
| III.A.3 | Show awareness of patients' concerns about the procedure being performed |
| IV.P.6 | Prepare a patient for procedures or treatments |
| IV.P.8 | Document patient care |
| IX.P.7 | Document accurately in the patient record |

## LESSON OUTLINE

### I. ELECTROCARDIOGRAM (PROCEDURE 47–1)

A. Known also as an ECG or EKG
B. Recording of electrical impulses of the heart's activity (all muscle movement produces electrical impulses)
C. Path of electrical impulses
   1. Heart is four-chambered pump that produces minute electrical current by muscular contraction
   2. Electrical impulse originates in modified myocardial tissue of sinoatrial (SA) node
      a. Causes atria to contract
      b. Beginning of atrial depolarization of the first part of the cardiac cycle
      c. First impulse recorded is P wave
   3. Impulse continues through heart tissue to atrioventricular (AV) node, to bundle of His, to Purkinje fibers
      a. Causes ventricles to contract
      b. Produces the QRS complex of waves on the ECG paper
   4. T wave follows
      a. Represents the repolarization of the ventricles
      b. Recovery time before another contraction

D. Reasons for obtaining an ECG
   1. Detect heart damage and abnormalities
   2. Performed to determine a cardiac baseline

## II. ELECTROCARDIOGRAPH

A. Types
   1. Multichannel
   2. Computerized ECG machines
      a. Have simultaneous 12-lead interpretive analysis
      b. All 12 leads printed out onto one sheet of paper
   3. Single channel: mountings used for single-channel strip tracings for filing in patient's permanent record
B. Process
   1. Electrodes placed on the patient's extremities and chest to pick up electrical impulses
   2. Electrical impulses transmitted through patient cable wires attached to electrodes
   3. Current enters the ECG machine through wires, where the amplifier enlarges the impulses
   4. Galvanometer changes the impulse to mechanical motion
   5. Stylus imprints electrical activity on the tracing paper
C. Interpretation by provider
D. Electrocardiograph paper
E. Electrocardiograph leads
   1. The routine ECG consists of 12 leads
   2. Records the electrical activity of the heart from different angles
      a. First three leads
         i. Called standard or bipolar leads
         ii. Labeled with Roman numerals I, II, and III
         iii. Obtained by placing limb electrodes on the fleshy part of the upper outer arms and inner lower calves
      b. Next three leads are augmented (enlarged) leads called aVR, aVL, and aVF
      c. Six chest leads
         i. Precordial leads
         ii. Obtained by placing chest electrode(s) to recommended positions

## III. PERFORMING THE ECG

A. Preparing the equipment
B. Prepare the room—watch for electrical interference
C. Prepare patient
   1. Explain procedure
   2. Patient must be relaxed
   3. Any movement can cause interference
   4. Conduct patient education
D. Standardization
   1. Enables a provider to judge deviations from the standard

2. Usual standardization mark is 2 mm wide and 10 mm high
   a. Mark should begin each lead to provide a reliable reading with the sensitivity dial at 1 (normal)
   b. If mark too large, turn sensitivity dial down to 1/2 to produce mark 5 mm high and 2 mm wide
   c. If mark too small, turn sensitivity dial up to 2 to produce mark 20 mm high and 2 mm wide
3. Stylus should be centered on paper
4. Tracing paper run at speed of 25 mm/sec
   a. If ECG cycles are too close together, run at 50 mm/sec to separate and spread out the tracing, making it easier to read
   b. Note this adjustment in pen on the tracing

E. Artifacts
1. Somatic tremor
2. Minimize patient movement
3. AC (alternating current)—power cords should be kept away from the patient
4. Wandering baseline caused by electrodes improperly applied or on improperly cleaned skin
5. Interrupted baseline caused by the wire becoming separated from the electrode

F. Cardiac arrythmias
1. Premature atrial contractions
2. Paroxysmal atrial tachycardia
3. Atrial fibrillation
4. Premature ventricular contractions
5. Ventricular tachycardia
6. Ventricular fibrillation

## /. HOLTER MONITORING (PROCEDURE 47–2)

A. 24-hour, or ambulatory, ECG
B. Patient wears electrodes to monitor heart activity for 24 hours and returns for analysis by provider
C. Patient keeps diary of all activities and symptoms experienced while monitor is worn
D. Often reveals undetected problems at office visits to provider

## . STRESS TEST

A. Determines patients at high risk for developing heart disease
B. Test is performed while patient is exercising

## I. DEFIBRILLATOR

A. Designed to provide countershock to convert arrhythmias into regular rhythm
B. Should have routine check for proper working condition

# HAPTER ACTIVITIES

1. Invite a cardiologist to the class to explain cardiac conditions and procedures.
2. Have students role-play the medical assistant, explaining cardiac diagnostic tests and procedures to a patient.

3. Have students practice placing chest leads on several different-sized classmates. This will assist students with learning how to place electrodes properly on a variety of patients, including those with larger beasts, which can be more difficult.
4. Invite a speaker from the American Heart Association to discuss the various types of heart conditions and explain th importance of heart health and living a heart-healthy lifestyle.
5. Invite a sales representative to come out and discuss a variety of cardiac equipment used in the field and give a demonstration of some of his or her company's products such as Holter monitors and ECG machines.
6. Practice placing chest leads on male classmates and discuss what might need to be done if they have hairy chests to allow for proper contact between the skin and the electrodes.
7. Have students pair up and demonstrate proper hookup of a Holter monitor as well as provide patient education on th equipment and the activity diet along with dos and don'ts.
8. Have students search the Web for a national organization that focuses on cardiac disorders and have them pick a topic to present to the class.
9. Assign students various artifacts and arrhythmias; have them make creative poster boards with information regardin these and present them to the class. Be sure to have them discuss the causes.
10. Have students research the effects of smoking and alcohol consumption on the heart and write a paper about it.

## ANSWERS TO CHECK YOUR KNOWLEDGE QUESTIONS

1. A heated pen-like instrument that produces a printed representation on the ECG paper is known as a/an:

   a. galvanometer.

   **b. stylus.**

   c. amplifier.

   d. electrode.

2. Each large square on the ECG paper measures 5 mm by 5 mm and represents ____ seconds.

   **a. 0.2**

   b. 0.04

   c. 0.1

   d. 1.0

3. Which of the following wave(s) on the graph paper represents the repolarization of the ventricles or the time of recovery before another contraction?

   a. P

   b. QRS

   c. ST

   **d. T**

4. What can you do with the sensitivity dial if the ECG tracing is too small?

   a. Turn down to 1

   b. Turn down to 1/2

   c. Turn up to 5

   **d. Turn up to 2**

5. The routine ECG consists of how many leads?
   **a. 12**
   b. 10
   c. 6
   d. 4
6. The **augmented** leads are also known as:
   a. leads I, II and III.
   b. chest leads.
   **c. aVL, aVR, aVF.**
   d. precordial leads.
7. What kind of interference is caused by improperly applied electrodes?
   a. Somatic tremor
   **b. Wandering baseline**
   c. Interrupted baseline
   d. AC interference
8. The following is a diagnostic tool that tests the structure and function of the heart through the use of sound waves reflected through the heart:
   a. defibrillator.
   b. Holter monitor.
   **c. echocardiography.**
   d. treadmill.

# HAPTER 48 Radiology Procedures

## BHES Curriculum

| | |
|---|---|
| M.A.A.1.2.c | Assist the provider with the regimen of diagnostic and treatment modalities as they relate to each body system |
| M.A.A.1.4.a | Document accurately |
| M.A.A.1.9.k | Prepare and maintain examination and treatment area |
| M.A.A.1.9.l | Prepare patient for examinations and treatments |
| M.A.A.1.9.m | Assist provider with routine and specialty examinations and treatments |
| M.A.A.1.9.r | Teach patients methods of health promotion and disease prevention |

## AAHEP Core Curriculum

| | |
|---|---|
| I.P.6 | Perform patient screening using established protocols |
| I.P.10 | Assist provider with patient care |
| I.A.2 | Use language and verbal skills that enable patients' understanding |
| I.A.1 | Apply critical thinking skills in performing patient assessment and care |
| IV.P.2 | Report relevant information to others succinctly and accurately |
| IV.P.5 | Instruct patients according to their needs to promote health maintenance and disease prevention |
| IV.P.6 | Prepare a patient for procedures or treatments |
| IV.P.8 | Document patient care |
| IX.P.7 | Document accurately in the patient chart |

## ESSON OUTLINE

### RADIOLOGICAL STUDIES

A. Aid in diagnosis, screening, and therapy
   1. Your role
   2. Off-site testing
B. X-rays
   1. X-ray photograph is taken for permanent record
      a. Known also as roentgen rays
      b. High-energy electromagnetic radiation produced by the collision of a beam of electrons with a metal target in an X-ray tube
   2. Patients must follow preparation instructions except for X-rays of the chest and extremities
   3. Aid in diagnosis of tumors, fractures, and other disorders and diseases
   4. Therapeutic X-rays used in treatment of cancer
      a. Teletherapy
      b. Brachytherapy

C. Safety
   1. Radiation exposure risk for employees
      a. Dosimeter or film badge
      b. Lead shielding
   2. Risk for patients
      a. Precautions if possibility of pregnancy should be determined prior to testing because it is seriously damaging to the fetus, especially in the first trimester of pregnancy
      b. Clear explanation for patients
D. Preparing patients for X-rays
   1. Patient support and reassurance
   2. Explain expectations and procedure
   3. Special considerations with children
   4. Clear instructions and understanding
E. Radiological procedures
   1. Cholecystogram
      a. X-ray study of the gallbladder
      b. Contrast media make gallbladder visible
   2. Upper GI series—barium swallow
      a. Patient drinks (flavored) contrast medium during examination while radiologist observes flow of substance directly by means of fluoroscope at different angles (positions)
      b. Patient preparation is critical
      c. Films taken for a permanent record
      d. Performed to observe the functioning of the patient's esophagus, stomach, duodenum, and small intestine
      e. Detects disorders and diseases such as hiatal hernias, peptic (duodenal) ulcers, and tumors
   3. Lower GI series—barium enema
      a. Patient has barium sulfate contrast medium introduced into the colon by an enema tube
      b. Radiologist observes flow of barium into lower bowel
      c. Patient preparation is critical
      d. Provider often orders a barium enema with air contrast
         i. Procedure distends barium-filled colon with air to make structures more visible
         ii. Causes some discomfort and pain
         iii. Tell patient to take deep breaths through mouth to help relax abdominal muscles
         iv. Patient may have a strong urge to defecate, which is normal (some patients cannot resist urge)
      e. Encourage patient to drink plenty of liquids over the first few days following the procedure to help evacuate the residual barium
      f. Permanent films are made
      g. Helpful in diagnosing lesions, tumors, and other diseases of the colon
   4. Intravenous pyelogram (IVP)
      a. Study of genitourinary system, requiring patient to prepare with laxatives, enemas, and fasting
      b. Intravenous injection of iodine, the contrast medium, defines structures of urinary system

   c. Retrograde pyelogram
      i. Study of urinary tract by inserting sterile catheter into urinary meatus, through bladder, and up into ureters
      ii. Radiopaque contrast medium flows upward into kidneys
      iii. Usually done in conjunction with cystoscopy
      iv. Patient should have iodine sensitivity testing prior to this procedure to determine possibility of allergic reaction
      v. Voiding cystogram might be ordered in conjunction with this also (no special patient preparation needed)
5. KUB (kidneys, ureters, bladder)
   a. X-ray of patient's abdomen, termed *flat plate of the abdomen*
   b. Requires no patient preparation
   c. Aids in diagnosing urinary system diseases and disorders, in determining the position of an IUD, or locating foreign bodies in the digestive tract (surgery indicated if an object blocks the normal digestive flow, especially in young children)
6. Mammography
   a. X-ray of the breast tissue to detect cancerous tumors
   b. Patient education and preparation critical
   c. May detect tumors as small as 1 cm or less in size
   d. Early detection is critical (remind patients of their responsibility)
   e. See Chapter 40 for BSE instructions and advise reporting any lump or other abnormality STAT
   f. American Cancer Society recommends baseline mammography at age of 40 years then every one to two years thereafter
   g. Procedure requires patient to move into various positions so that different angles of the breast tissue can be X-rayed
   h. X-ray pictures called mammograms
7. Body scans
   a. Rapid scanning of single-tissue planes performed by a process that generates images of the tissues in slices about 1 cm thick
      i. Computerized axial tomography CAT scan (CT scan)
      ii. Computerized transverse axial tomography (CTAT) scan (CT scan)
   b. Performed in seconds
   c. Scans aid in diagnosis of disorders and diseases of breasts or internal organs
8. Nuclear medicine
   a. Branch of medicine that uses radionuclides in the diagnosis and treatment of disease
   b. Almost any organ can be viewed and recorded
      i. Patient ingests, or is injected with, radioactive material
      ii. Uptake study
   c. Procedure requires radioactive substance with careful supervision
   d. Return of patient in 24 hours to measure amount of radioactivity in a particular organ, e.g., radioactive thyroid uptake to determine function of thyroid gland

E. Sonographic studies
    1. Ultrasonography is a technique in which internal structures are made visible by recording reflections of ultrasonic sound waves directed into tissues
    2. Handheld instrument called transducer changes waves into electrical energy
    3. Energy transformed into image on monitor or printed out on paper in wavy lines
        a. Picture formed represents cross section of organ
        b. Photos taken for permanent record
    4. Abdominopelvic cavity ultrasonography
        a. Gel or lotion used to promote better conduction and easier movement of transducer across skin
        b. Used to locate aneurysms of the aorta and other blood vessel abnormalities
        c. Can determine size and shape of internal organs
    5. Used for identification of cysts and tumors of eye
    6. Used to detect and identify masses and obstructions of the urinary tract
    7. Obstetrical and gynecological ultrasonography
        a. Useful in determining size, maturity, and position of fetus without radiation
        b. Instruct patients to avoid foods that produce gas and to drink plenty of fluids
    8. Used in treatments to relieve inflammation and pain with sound waves vibrating into tissues and producing heat
F. Magnetic resonance imaging (MRI)
    1. Technique to view structures inside human body
    2. Noninvasive with no radiation exposure
    3. Patient lies on padded table and is placed into tunnel-like or open structure for 30 to 60 minutes
    4. Becomes invasive when intravenous contrast media is administered to patient under certain conditions
        a. Done during last series of images of examination
        b. Used to detect certain pathologies
    5. Patient resumes normal activity following procedure
    6. No known harmful effects
    7. Radio signals are sent from scanner that is influenced by strong magnetic fields to which the body responds
        a. Advise patient to remove all metallic objects
        b. Female patients should be advised not to wear mascara because it contains flakes of metal
    8. Interview patient about claustrophobia for tunnel-like structure—open-sided MRI possible
    9. Advise patient that machine makes lots of banging and whirring noises
    10. Technician should observe patient during test (microphone in tunnel so patient can be heard)
    11. Contraindications for patient use
        a. Pacemakers
        b. Metallic implants
        c. First trimester of pregnancy
        d. Severe claustrophobia
        e. Obesity
G. Patient education

## HAPTER ACTIVITIES

1. Have students practice communication skills by role playing with one student being a child, the other the MA. Be sure to face patient at eye level and use simple terms. Ask the child to explain in his or her own words what you have said. This can also be performed on children if they are available.
2. Using role-playing techniques, practice instructing patients about the various radiological procedures and any prep or dietary factors they need to follow.
3. Ask students to prepare an information sheet that can be given to the patient prior to leaving the office when an X-ray procedure has been scheduled.
4. Using role-playing techniques, act as if you are training in a new employee on preparing a patient for a cholecystogram. Go over the required prep and explain the procedure thoroughly to the patent, ensuring complete understanding.
5. Have students practice documenting the preparation of a patient for an X-ray procedure in a mock patient chart or an EHR. When finished, have them do the same with an X-ray procedure that is scheduled at an outside facility.
6. Have students make a set of flash cards with the name of a radiological procedure on one side and patient prep instructions on the other. Have them use the cards to study and to quiz their classmates.
7. Invite a radiologist to class to discuss common reasons for radiologic procedures and conditions that might warrant an X-ray.
8. Contact a local radiological center and arrange for the students to observe for part of the day. Have them try to see as many special procedures (barium enema, barium swallow, fluoroscopy, IVP, and so on) as they can. Have them take notes and write a paper about their experience to present to the class.
9. Have students research the Internet to find information regarding new imaging techniques. Have them discuss their findings in small groups and then compile a list to compare with other groups and have large group discussion on what they found.

## NSWERS TO CHECK YOUR KNOWLEDGE QUESTIONS

1. In this type of therapeutic radiation, radioactive implants are placed by the radiologist close to or into the cancerous tissue.
   a. Teletherapy
   **b. Brachytherapy**
   c. Physical therapy
   d. None of the above
2. A dosimeter can last up to:
   a. 1 month.
   b. 2 months.
   **c. 3 months.**
   d. 6 months.
3. Sonograms can be very useful in diagnosing:
   a. gallstones.
   b. tumors.

c. heart defects.

**d. all of the above**

4. Which of the following studies does not require special preparation?

**a. Chest X-ray**

b. Cholecystogram

c. Upper GI

d. Barium enema

5. This method of radiology generates images of the tissue in slices about 1 cm thick:

**a. CT scan.**

b. MRI.

c. mammogram.

d. sonogram.

# UNIT 16 MINOR SURGICAL PROCEDURES
# CHAPTER 49 Preparing for Surgery

## BHES Curriculum

| | |
|---|---|
| MA.A.1.4. c | Follow established policies when initiating or terminating medical treatment |
| MA.A.1.9. b | Apply principles of aseptic techniques and infection control |
| MA.A.1.9. d | Recognize and understand various treatment protocols |
| MA.A.1.9. | Use Standard Precautions |
| MA.A.1.9.k | Prepare and maintain examination and treatment area |
| MA.A.1.9. l | Prepare patient for examinations and treatments |
| MA.A.1.9. n | Assist provider with minor office surgical procedures |
| MA.A.1.9.o (4) | Sterilization techniques |
| MA.A.1.9. p | Advise patients of office policies and procedures |

## CAAHEP Core Curriculum

| | |
|---|---|
| I.P.10 | Assist provider with patient care |
| I.A.2 | Use language and verbal skills that enable patients' understanding |
| III.C.2 | Define asepsis |
| III.C.3 | Discuss infection control procedures |
| III.C.8 | Differentiate between medical and surgical asepsis used in ambulatory care settings, identifying when each is appropriate |
| III.P.2 | Practice Standard Precautions |
| III.P.3 | Select appropriate barrier and personal protective equipment (PPE) for potentially infectious situations |
| III.P.4 | Perform hand washing |
| III.A.2 | Explain the rationale for performance of a procedure to the patient |
| III.A.3 | Show awareness of patients' concerns about the procedure being performed |

## ESSON OUTLINE

### SCHEDULING MINOR OFFICE SURGERY

A. Medical assistant usually schedules minor procedures

B. Give pre- and postop instructions to patient

### . PREPARING THE ROOM FOR SURGERY

A. Instruments

1. Each instrument used in minor surgery has specific function
2. Instruments are costly
3. Instruments must be carefully maintained
4. Follow manufacturer's recommendations for cleaning, sterilization, and storage
5. All surgical instruments must be autoclaved

B. Instrument care

1. Most instruments cared for in same manner
2. General rules to follow when cleaning and caring for instruments (see list in text)

C. Instrument components
   1. Ring handle
   2. Thumb handle
   3. Ratchet
   4. Serrations
   5. Teeth

D. Instrument classification (Table 49–1)

E. Supplies
   1. Preparing surgical instruments and supplies a day in advance
   2. Check disposable equipment for length of sterility

F. Tray setup (Procedure 49–1)
   1. Know provider's preference
   2. Maintain written information

## III. PREPARING YOURSELF FOR SURGERY

A. Perform a surgical hand washing (Procedure 49–2)

B. Don appropriate PPE

C. Gowning

D. Don sterile gloves (Procedure 49–3)

## IV. PREPARING PATIENT FOR SURGERY

A. Consent form
   1. Explain and ensure understanding
   2. Obtain signature
   3. Authorized person must sign for minor or incompetent

B. Patient preparation
   1. Measure patient's vital signs and record
   2. Have patient empty bladder
   3. Position and drape patient for procedure

C. Skin preparation (Procedure 49–4)
   1. Remove body hair to discourage microbial accumulation
   2. Area shaved
   3. Antiseptic used
   4. Careful not to nick patient's skin and treat if occurs

# CHAPTER ACTIVITIES

1. Arrange a tour of the local hospital and ask to have a person working in central supply, or surgical supply, show the instruments, explain their operation and care, and discuss their use in procedures.
2. Obtain a catalog of medical and surgical supplies. Have students look up the operation, care, and costs of various instruments and supplies to gain a general knowledge of commonly used items.
3. Obtain disposable skin prep sets for students to practice with each other.

# NSWERS TO CHECK YOUR KNOWLEDGE QUESTIONS

1. A fenestrated sheet is one that has a(n):
   a. fold.
   b. pleat.
   c. stain.
   **d. opening.**
2. Autoclaved items remain sterile for ____________ if they have been properly processed and protected from moisture.
   a. 3 days
   **b. 30 days**
   c. 3 weeks
   d. 3 months
3. To reduce the possibility of infection from a surgical procedure, skin preparation includes:
   a. cleaning the site with a soapy solution.
   b. shaving the skin.
   c. applying antiseptic solution.
   **d. all of the above.**
4. Before a surgical procedure can be performed, you must obtain a:
   **a. signed consent form.**
   b. verbal authorization.
   c. medical history.
   d. medication list.
5. The sterile tray should be set up:
   a. just before the provider enters the room.
   **b. prior to the patients entering the room.**
   c. 30 minutes before the procedure.
   d. while the patient is gowning.
6. The Mayo stand should be adjusted to:
   **a. waist level.**
   b. hip level.
   c. be level with the countertop.
   d. be level with the exam table.
7. During skin prep, avoid nicking the skin because this could cause a(n):
   a. rough surface.
   **b. infection.**
   c. irritation.
   d. redness.

# HAPTER 50 Assisting with Minor Surgery

## BHES Curriculum

| | |
|---|---|
| MA.A.1.9. b | Apply principles of aseptic techniques and infection control |
| MA.A.1.9. d | Recognize and understand various treatment protocols |
| MA.A.1.9. e | Recognize emergencies and treatments and in-office minor surgical procedures |
| MA.A.1.9. k | Prepare and maintain examination and treatment area |
| MA.A.1.9. l | Prepare patient for examinations and treatments |
| MA.A.1.9.n | Assist provider with in-office minor surgical procedures |
| MA.A.1.9. r | Teach patients methods of health promotion and disease prevention |
| MA.A.1.10.d (3) | Perform wound collection procedures |

## AAHEP Core Curriculum

| | |
|---|---|
| I.P. 10 | Assist provider with patient care |
| I.A. 2 | Use language and verbal skills that enable patients' understanding |
| III.P. 3 | Select appropriate barrier and personal protective equipment (PPE) for potentially infectious situations |
| III.P. 7 | Obtain specimens for microbiological testing |
| III.A. 1 | Display sensitivity to patients' rights and feelings in collecting specimens |
| III.A. 2 | Explain the rationale for performance of a procedure to the patient |
| III.A. 3 | Show awareness of patients' concerns about the procedure being performed |

# ESSON OUTLINE

## GENERAL INFORMATION

A. Maintain sterile technique

B. Common procedures (Table 50–1)

## . ASSISTING PROVIDER AS APPROPRIATE (PROCEDURE 50–2)

A. Anesthetics
   1. Common anesthetic agents
      a. Xylocaine
      b. Novocain
   2. Provider or anesthesiologist administers anesthetic
   3. Caution with hemophilia
      a. Mark this information with red ink on patient's chart
      b. Must have surgery *only* in hospital

B. Specimen collection
   1. Biopsy
      a. Careful labeling and handling of specimen required
      b. Formalin preservative
      c. Specimen transferred with forceps
      d. Lab request must accompany tissue specimen

2. Electrocautery
    a. Used following removal of warts or polyps
    b. Controls bleeding
    c. Care of tips
3. Cryosurgery
    a. Uses subfreezing temperature to remove or destroy tissue
    b. Usually with carbon dioxide or liquid nitrogen

C. Bandaging
1. Advise patient to keep dressing clean and dry
2. Keep bandage dry during showers and baths
    a. Sponge bath preferred until bandage comes off
    b. Important in minimizing possibility of infection
3. If infection occurs, MA might be asked to obtain a specimen for laboratory analysis

D. Wound collection (Procedure 50–1)

E. Postoperative instructions
1. Confirm follow-up appointment with patient
2. Specific instructions given by provider in certain cases
3. Providers might prescribe analgesic for minor pain

### III. APPLYING SUTURES

A. Thread that joins skin of a wound

B. Most offices have policy for treatment of lacerations

C. Assist provider in suturing laceration (Procedure 50–3)
1. Record number of sutures provider inserts and anatomical location
2. Provide patient education after procedure

### IV. SUTURE REMOVAL (PROCEDURE 50–4)

A. Remove the same number of sutures as were inserted

B. Suture not removed can become infected

C. Ask provider to inspect healing wound—provider might order additional closure materials

## CHAPTER ACTIVITIES

1. Arrange to have students observe minor surgery (one or two at a time) in a general or surgical practice. Request a facility tour if possible.
2 Have students practice with the Instruments Review games on the Premium Website.
3. Have students make flash cards for the surgical procedures discussed in this chapter with a description of the procedure and the tray setup for each.
4. Review the types and sizes of suture materials.

# ANSWERS TO CHECK YOUR KNOWLEDGE QUESTIONS

1. Which of the following types of anesthesia is not used in minor surgical procedures performed in the office?
   a. Local
   b. Nerve block
   c. Topical
   **d. General**
2. The method used to remove skin tags and warts is:
   **a. electrocautery.**
   b. cryosurgery.
   c. laser surgery.
   d. biopsy.
3. Local anesthesia begins to numb an area in:
   a. 30 minutes.
   **b. 5–15 minutes.**
   c. 1 hour.
   d. 3 hours.
4. A serious blood-clotting disease in which the absence of one of the necessary blood-clotting factors prevents blood from coagulating is:
   a. coagulitis.
   **b. hemophilia.**
   c. hemophilitis.
   d. angiocoagulitis.
5. A type of suture that does not need to be removed is made from:
   a. silk.
   b. nylon.
   **c. catgut.**
   d. all of the above.

# UNIT 17 MEDICATION ADMINISTRATION PROCEDURES
# CHAPTER 51 Pharmacology Fundamentals

## ABHES Curriculum

| | |
|---|---|
| MA.A.1.4.f | Comply with federal, state, and local health laws and regulations |
| MA.A.1.6.b | Properly use PDR, drug handbook, and other drug references to identify a drug's classification, usual dosage, usual side effects, and contraindications |
| MA.A.1.6.e | Comply with federal, state, and local health laws and regulations |
| MA.A.1.10.c | Dispose of biohazardous materials |

## CAAHEP Core Curriculum

| | |
|---|---|
| I.C.11 | Identify the classifications of medications, including desired effects, side effects, and adverse reactions |
| IX.C.13. | Discuss all levels of governmental legislation and regulation as they apply to medical assisting practice, including FDA and DEA regulations |
| X.C.1. | Differentiate between legal, ethical, and moral issues affecting health care |

## LESSON OUTLINE

### I. DRUG CATEGORIES AND CLASSIFICATIONS

A. It is helpful to include interesting or unusual tidbits about the different medication classes that act as memory aids for students. For example, students might remember that a vasopressor "presses the vessel smaller" to raise blood pressure or that a serious adverse effect of Lasix overdose is ototoxicity and that aspirin can cause ringing in the ears.

B. Commonly prescribed medications (Table 51–1)

### II. DRUG ACTIONS

A. Chemotherapeutic

B. Pharmacodynamic

  1. Agonists and antagonists
  2. Synergistic drugs

C. Miscellaneous

D. Considerations of drug actions

E. Drug effects

  1. Local
  2. Remote
  3. Systemic

### III. DRUG FORMS (TABLE 51–2)

A. Drugs can come in a single form or be available in a variety of forms

  1. Capsules
  2. Drops
  3. Inhalants
  4. Liquids

5. Powders
6. Skin preparations
7. Suppositories
8. Tablets
9. Transdermal patches

## IV. DRUG NAMES

A. Generic/official
B. Trade
C. Chemical
D. Look-alike/sound-alike drug names
E. Prescription drugs
   1. FDA
   2. DEA
F. Controlled substances
   1. Schedule drugs
   2. Storing controlled substances
   3. Controlled substances and the medical assistant
G. Nonprescription drugs
   1. Over-the-counter drugs
   2. Vitamins, herbal supplements, alternative remedies

## V. HANDLING MEDICATIONS IN THE MEDICAL OFFICE

A. Proper storage
B. Stock medications
C. Samples
D. Refrigerated medications
   1. Temperature logs
   2. MSDS
E. Disposing of drugs

## VI. PHARMACEUTICAL REFERENCES

A. PDR—prescription drugs
B. PDR—nonprescription drugs
C. Product inserts
D. Professional drug handbooks
E. Electronic and online resources

# CHAPTER ACTIVITIES

1. Have drills or games that involve recognizing and categorizing many of the most commonly used prescription and nonprescription medications, including desired effects, side effects, and adverse reactions.

2. List and identify the most common drug forms.
3. Have students make up flash cards of the Words to Know in class and review them with their classmates in pairs.
4. Write a generic or trade name on the board and ask the students to look up the corresponding name or classification.

# ANSWERS TO CHECK YOUR KNOWLEDGE QUESTIONS

1. Which of the following is NOT one of the three main groups used to describe actions of drugs?
   a. Miscellaneous
   b. Pharmacodynamic
   **c. Narcotic**
   d. Chemotherapeutic
2. Drugs may be used to do which of the following EXCEPT:
   **a. restore lost function of an irreparably damaged organ.**
   b. enhance remaining function of a damaged organ.
   c. replace hormones no longer being made by the body.
   d. reverse allergic reactions.
3. Upon learning that a patient is taking herbal supplements, the MA's most appropriate response is to:
   a. advise the patient to stop taking all herbal supplements at once.
   b. advise the patient to stop taking any prescription medications that interact with the herbal supplements.
   **c. record the herbal supplements, doses and the reasons the patient is taking them in the patient's chart and alert the physician.**
   d. this is not of concern because herbal supplements are not really medications.
4. Which of the following is correct?
   a. Schedule IV drugs have no legal or medicinal purpose.
   **b. Schedule I drugs include street drugs.**
   c. Schedule III drugs cannot be refilled.
   d. All schedule drugs require a prescription.
5. Drugs are more likely to enter the sewer and water systems through:
   a. flushing unused medication down the toilet.
   b. excesses released from manufacturing plants.
   c. illegal suppliers disposing of excess inventory.
   **d. natural excretion of drug not completely absorbed by the body.**
6. Which of the following best describes a pharmacodynamic drug?
   a. Treatment for allergies
   b. Remedy for metabolic disorders
   c. Cures cancer
   **d. Inhibits the action of an enzyme**
7. What is required to store controlled substances legally?
   a. DEA license
   b. Current medical credentials of provider prominently displayed
   **c. Double-lock system of access**
   d. Refrigerator with temperature log

8. Which of the following comments is true?
   a. A medication can fall into only one category.
   **b. Over-the-counter medications do not require a prescription but can still be harmful if used incorrectly.**
   c. Schedule I drugs require a handwritten prescription.
   d. If a medication allergy does not manifest after the first exposure to a drug, there is no need to be concerned about an allergy in the future.

## PROCEDURE SCENARIO

The following scenario is provided for use with the Procedure 51–1 Competency Checklist. It is optional; instructors may choose to modify the scenarios or make up their own.

### PROCEDURE 51–1

This procedure requires students to use the PDR to locate information about certain drugs. Two drugs are provided for competency testing.

| | Trade Name | Generic Name | Recommended Dose or Route | Common Side Effects |
|---|---|---|---|---|
| 1. | Singulair | Montelukast sodium | 4 mg po | Upper respiratory infection, fever, headache, pharyngitis |
| 2. | Reglan | Metoclopramide Hydrochloride | 10 mg IM, IV, po | Restlessness, drowsiness, fatigue, dizziness |

# CHAPTER 52 Measurement Systems, Basic Mathematics, and Dosage Calculations

## ABHES Curriculum

| | |
|---|---|
| MA.A.1.6.a | Demonstrate accurate occupational math and metric conversions for proper medication administration |

## CAAHEP Core Curriculum

| | |
|---|---|
| II.C.1 | Demonstrate knowledge of basic math computations |
| II.C.2 | Apply mathematical computations to solve equations |
| II.C.3 | Identify measurement systems |
| II.C. 4 | Define basic units of measurements and equivalents in metric, apothecary, and household systems |
| II.C.5 | Convert among measurement systems |
| II.C.6 | Identify both abbreviations and symbols used in calculating medication dosages |

# LESSON OUTLINE

## I. SYSTEMS OF MEASUREMENT

A. The metric system

B. Household measures (Figure 52–1)

C. The apothecary system

## II. REVIEW OF BASIC MATH

A. Placement of whole numbers and decimals (Figure 52–2)

B. Review examples of math problems (Table 52–1)

C. General rules for working with decimals (Table 52–2)

D. Working with fractions (Table 52–3)

E. Working with percentages

F. Ratio and proportion

## III. DOSAGE CALCULATIONS

A. Basic formula—(Needed/Available) × Vehicle = Dose

B. Ratio and proportion method

1. Dosage on hand:amount on hand = dosage desired:*amount desired* ($x$)
2. Solve for $x$
3. Calculating dosages for tablets and capsules

C. Converting between units of measurement

1. Identify the equivalent
2. Set up a proportion of two equivalent ratios
3. Solve for $x$

D. Calculating dosages for liquid medications

E. Calculating dosages by weight—Conversion factor: 1 kg = 2.2 lbs

## CHAPTER ACTIVITIES

1. Students can review the "Systems of Measurement" tutorial on the StudyWARE™ Software for more practice
2. Students can review the "Fractions and Decimals" tutorial on the StudyWARE™ Software for more practice
3. Students can review the "Ratio, Percents, and Equations" tutorial on the StudyWARE™ Software for more practice
4. Students can review the "Conversions" tutorial on the StudyWARE™ Software for more practice
5. Students can review the "Oral Dosages" and "Parenteral Dosages" tutorials on the StudyWARE™ Software for more practice

## ANSWERS TO CHECK YOUR KNOWLEDGE QUESTIONS

1. Which system of measurement is most commonly used in health care?
   a. Apothecary
   **b. Metric**
   c. Standard
   d. Household
2. Drop, cup, and pint are measurements in which system?
   a. Apothecary
   b. Metric
   c. Standard
   **d. Household**
3. The prefix centi- means what?
   a. 1/10 of a unit
   **b. 1/100 of a unit**
   c. 10 units
   d. 100 units
4. In the basic formula method, the prescribed amount would be inserted into what place in the formula?
   **a. Needed**
   b. Available
   c. Vehicle
   d. Dose
5. What are the three steps used in finding the correct amount of medication in the ratio and proportion method?
   a. Calculate, convert, confirm
   b. Convert, calculate, confirm
   **c. Convert, construct, calculate**
   d. Construct, calculate, convert
6. What is the conversion factor for converting pounds into kilograms?
   a. 1 lb = 2 kg
   b. 1 lb = 2.2 kg
   c. 2 lb = 1 kg
   **d. 2.2 lb = 1 kg**

# CHAPTER 53 Administering Oral and Non-Injectable Medications

## ABHES Curriculum

| | |
|---|---|
| MA.A.1.4.a | Document accurately |
| MA.A.1.4.f | Comply with federal, state, and local health laws and regulations |
| MA.A.1.6.c | Identify and define common abbreviations that are accepted in prescription writing |
| MA.A.1.6.d. | Understand legal aspects of writing prescriptions, including federal and state laws |
| MA.A.1.6.e | Comply with federal, state, and local health laws and regulations |
| MA.A.1.9.i | Use standard precautions |
| MA.A.1.9.j | Prepare and administer oral and parenteral medications as directed by provider |
| MA.A.1.8.aa | Be attentive, listen, and learn |
| MA.A.1.8. cc | Communicate on the recipient's level of comprehension |
| MA.A.1.8. dd | Serve as liaison between provider and others |
| MA.A.1.8. ii | Recognize and respond to verbal and nonverbal communication |
| MA.A.1.9. j | Prepare and administer oral and parenteral medications as directed by provider |
| MA.A.1.11.b (9) | Demonstrate professionalism by conducting work within scope of education, training, and ability |

## CAAHEP Core Curriculum

| | |
|---|---|
| I.P.8 | Administer oral medications |
| I.P.9 | Administer parenteral medications, excluding IV medications |
| I.P. 10 | Assist provider with patient care |
| I.A. 1 | Apply critical thinking skills in performing patient assessment and care |
| I.A. 2 | Use language and verbal skills that enable patients' understanding |
| IV.P.8 | Document patient care |
| IV.A. 7 | Demonstrate recognition of the patient's level of understanding in communications |
| IX.C.1 | Discuss legal scope of practice for medical assistants |
| IX.C.13 | Discuss all levels of governmental legislation and regulation as they apply to medical assisting practice, including FDA and DEA regulations |
| IX.C.14 | Describe the process to follow if an error is made in patient care |
| IX.P. 2 | Perform within scope of practice |
| IX.P.7 | Document accurately in the patient record |
| IX.P.8 | Apply local, state, and federal health care legislation and regulation appropriate to the medical assisting practice setting |
| IX.A.2 | Demonstrate awareness of the consequences of not working within the legal scope of practice |
| IX.A.3 | Recognize the importance of local, state, and federal legislation and regulations in the practice setting |

## LESSON OUTLINE

### I. ROUTES OF MEDICATION ADMINISTRATION—IDENTIFY ROUTES THAT MEDICAL ASSISTANTS DO NOT PERFORM

## II. PRESCRIPTIONS

A. Define

B. Elements of a prescription

C. Appropriate way to handle an incomplete or incorrect prescription

D. Preparing prescriptions (Procedure 53–1)

  a. Identify steps

  b. Calling in a prescription to a pharmacy (Procedure 53–2)

  c. E-prescribing

## III. MEDICATION ORDERS (PROCEDURE 53–3)

A. How does this differ from a prescription?

B. Elements of a medication order

## IV. THE SEVEN RIGHTS OF MEDICATION ADMINISTRATION

A. Right: patient, medication, dose, route, technique, time, documentation

B. Medication errors

  1. Different elements that define a medication error

  2. What to do if an error is made

## V. MEDICATION DOCUMENTATION (PROCEDURE 53–4)

A. Who, what, when, where, why

B. Elements required for appropriate documentation

C. Abbreviations used in documenting medications (Table 53–1)

  1. Joint Commission's DO NOT USE list

  2. Institute of Safe Medication Practice's list of error-prone abbreviations (Figure 53–7)

D. Documenting medication and immunization side effects and adverse events

  1. Information required for documentation

  2. Manufacturer, lot number, serial number, container's expiration date

  3. Discuss CDC, IAC, NCVIA, VAERS

  4. Vaccination registries

  5. Signing off the order

## VI. ADMINISTERING ORAL AND NON-INJECTABLE MEDICATIONS

A. Oral administration (Procedure 53–5)

B. Sublingual and buccal administration

C. Parenteral – non-injectables

  1. Nasal, ophthalmic, and otic (Procedures 53–6, 53–7)

  2. Inhalation administration

  3. Topical administration

4. Rectal administration (Procedure 53–8)
5. Vaginal administration (Procedure 53–9)

# CHAPTER ACTIVITIES

1. Prepare a prescription for the provider's signature, using the information provided.
2. Student should demonstrate calling a prescription in to another student who has correct answer. The "pharmacist" can prompt student for missing information and intentionally provide an incorrect read back to be corrected by student calling prescription in.
3. Discuss and compare different routes of administration and the pros and cons of each.
4. Demonstrate accurately recording a medication entry on whiteboard or blackboard.
5. Set out various types of oral and parenteral (non-injectable) medication delivery materials, and in a timed assessment, have students correctly identify each component, that is, patches, tablets, capsules, suppositories, ointments, and so on.
6. Have students describe proper patient education prior to administering the medications listed in this chapter.
7. Practice applying mock transdermal patches to each other, using appropriate technique and disposal procedures.

# ANSWERS TO CHECK YOUR KNOWLEDGE QUESTIONS

1. A prescription is best described as:
   a. instructions for administering medications in the office.
   b. labeling of a drug container.
   c. whether a generic medication may be substituted for the trade name.
   **d. a written order that authorizes the dispensing of a medication to a patient.**
2. The prescription abbreviation "DAW" stands for:
   a. Do As you Wish.
   b. Don't Authorize When (followed by date).
   **c. Dispense as Written.**
   d. none of the above.
3. If the prescribing practitioner leaves out a minor part of the prescription, the MA's most appropriate action should be to:
   a. fill in the information if it is minor.
   b. ask another person in the office what should be included.
   **c. return the prescription to the prescriber to be completed.**
   d. nothing; the pharmacist will know what to put there.
4. Which of the following is an advantage of e-prescriptions?
   a. Reduces the possibility of forgery
   b. Helps maintain a running record of patient medications
   c. Prevents handwriting errors
   **d. All of the above**
5. A medication order should contain the following elements EXCEPT:
   a. patient name.
   b. signature of prescriber.

**c. site where the medication should be given.**

d. amount of medication to be given.

6. Which of the following list best describes the Seven Rights?

**a. Checklist of criteria to help prevent medication errors**

b. The MA's entitlements while working for a provider

c. Patient's entitlements under HIPAA

d. None of the above

7. Which of the following criteria is NOT required in documenting immunizations?

a. Pharmaceutical company name

**b. Color of contents**

c. Expiration date

d. Serial number of container

# PROCEDURE SCENARIOS

The following scenarios are provided for use with the competency checklists for Procedures 53–1 through 53–4. They are optional; instructors may choose to modify the scenarios or make up their own. The following referenced forms can be downloaded by the student from the Premium Website.

## Procedures 53–1 through 53–4

On the Premium Website, students can view the Media Link for this chapter on "Preparing Prescriptions and Medication Orders." Based on this video, complete the following procedures:

- **Procedure 53–1:** Correctly prepare a prescription for Sarah Edmonson for an Advair inhaler, based on the information given by the provider. Procedure Form 53–1 is a mock prescription blank.
- **Procedure 53–2:** After the prescription has been completed from Procedure 53–1, students can role-play, calling the prescription into a pharmacy, ensuring that you give the "pharmacist" all necessary information. Document the call in the patient's chart.
- **Procedure 53–3:** Correctly prepare a medication order for Edward Robinson for ibuprofen 600 mg, based on the information given by the provider.
- **Procedure 53–4:** After the medication is administered to Edward Robinson, per the provider's medication order, correctly document the oral medication administration in the patient's chart.

# CHAPTER 54 Administering Injections and Immunizations

## ABHES Curriculum

| | |
|---|---|
| MA.A.1.4. a | Document accurately |
| MA.A.1.6.e | Comply with federal, state, and local health laws and regulations |
| MA.A.1.9.b | Apply principles of aseptic techniques and infection control |
| MA.A.1.9.g | Maintain medications and immunization records |
| MA.A.1.9.i | Use standard precautions |
| MA.A.1.9.j | Prepare and administer oral and parenteral medications as directed by physician |

## CAAHEP Core Curriculum

| | |
|---|---|
| I.P.7 | Select proper sites for administering parenteral medication |
| I.P.9 | Administer parenteral medications, excluding IV |
| I.A.1 | Apply critical thinking skills in performing patient assessment and care |
| I.A. 2 | Use language and verbal skills that enable patients' understanding |
| II.P. 1 | Prepare proper dosages of medication for administration |
| II.A. 1 | Verify ordered doses or dosages prior to administration |
| III.P. 2 | Practice Standard Precautions |
| III.A. 2 | Explain the rationale for performance of a procedure to the patient |
| III.A. 3 | Show awareness of patients' concerns regarding their perceptions of the procedure being performed |
| IV.P.8 | Document patient care |
| IX.P.7 | Document accurately in the patient record |
| IX.P.8 | Apply local, state, and federal health care legislation and regulation appropriate to the medical assisting practice setting |
| IX.A.2 | Demonstrate awareness of the consequences of not working within the legal scope of practice |
| IX.A.3 | Recognize the importance of local, state, and federal legislation and regulations in the practice setting |
| XI.C.2 | Identify safety techniques that can prevent accidents and maintain a safe work environment |

## LESSON OUTLINE

### I. PARENTERAL INJECTABLE MEDICATION

A. Reasons parenteral routes may be chosen
   1. When patient is unable to tolerate medications by mouth
   2. When other routes of administration do not provide the desired effect quickly or predictably enough
   3. When medication given by mouth would be destroyed by the gastrointestinal tract
   4. When continuous delivery is required to achieve the desired outcome

B. Discuss injections given by medical assistants: intradermal, subcutaneous, intramuscular
   1. Briefly mention the kinds of injections MAs are not permitted to administer: IV, intraosseous, intrathecal, etc.; their uses; and the reasons they should never be attempted by MAs.
   2. Discuss legal implications involved in acting beyond a medical assistant's scope of practice

3. Intravenous medications Clinical Pearl Box
    a. MAs are not permitted to provide direct IV injections or initiate an IV
    b. MAs should be able to recognize a problem and report it to the physician immediately

## II. PREPARING TO ADMINISTER INJECTIONS

A. Needles and syringes
    1. Identify needle and syringe parts
    2. Sizes of syringes: 3 mL, tuberculin, insulin
    3. Reading the amount of medication in a syringe
B. Medication containers
    1. Ampules (Procedure 54–1)
    2. Vials (Procedure 54–2)
    3. Cartridge units
    4. Single-dose, prefilled disposable syringe, and cartridge units
    5. Powdered medication that must be reconstituted before use (Procedure 54–3)
C. Safety Considerations
    1. Handling needles safely
    2. Disposing of needles safely
    3. What to do in the event of a needlestick
    4. Needle safety devices (see Table 54–1)
    5. Other safety considerations
D. Preparing the patient
    1. Explaining the procedure
    2. Authorization forms for immunizations
    3. Skin preparation
    4. Giving injections to children
        a. Parent education
        b. Reassuring parents and child

## III. ADMINISTERING INJECTIONS

A. Angles of injection
B. Intradermal injections (Procedure 54–4)
    1. Purpose
    2. Syringe size
    3. Needle size
    4. Angle of injection
    5. Other notes
C. Subcutaneous injections (Procedure 54–5)
    1. Purpose
    2. Syringe size
    3. Needle size

4. Angle of injection
5. Other notes

D. Intramuscular injections (Procedure 54–6)

1. Purpose
2. Syringe size
3. Needle size
4. Angle of injection
5. Other notes

E. Z-Track IM method (Procedure 54–7)

F. Injections for infants and small children—Preferred site is vastus lateralis

G. Assisting with IV injections

## V. IMMUNIZATIONS AND SCHEDULES

A. Types of vaccines

1. Live
2. Pathogenic toxin
3. Killed

B. Immunization schedules

C. Patient preparation and documentation

1. Why immunize? Discuss advantages.
2. Discuss common illnesses reduced by immunizations, method of spreading, complications associated with contracting disease
3. Vaccination information sheets (VIS) and other authorization forms

D. Common illnesses reduced by immunizations

1. Influenza
2. Pneumonia
3. Haemophilus influenza type B (Hib, HIB)
4. Measles, mumps, and rubella (MMR)
5. Diphtheria
6. Pertussis (whooping cough)
7. Rabies
8. Tetanus
9. Rotavirus
10. Varicella zoster (chicken pox)
11. Hepatitis A
12. Hepatitis B
13. Human papillomavirus (HPV)
14. Meningitis (bacterial)
15. Polio

## CHAPTER ACTIVITIES

1. Set out various types of medication delivery materials and, in a timed assessment, have students correctly identify each component, e.g., different types of syringes, gauge needles, and so on.
2. Have students describe proper patient education prior to administering injections and immunizations.
3. Have students practice drawing up water into different types of syringes in an ordered amount.
4. Have students go to the VAERS Website and prepare a complete and accurate VIS form. Instructors may use this as a hand-in for extra credit to assess appropriate use of Internet resources and accurate completion of standardized forms. All fields should be completed legibly and completely. Missing information should have an explanation.
5. Have students go to www.immunize.org/catg.d/p2022.pdf and download a vaccine administration record. Using the current vaccination schedule, enter possible dates of vaccinations up to age 15 for patient John Smith, born January 1 of next year. (*Do not simply transfer dates and data from example provided.*) Instructors can have this turned in also as an extra-credit opportunity or use as a discussion in class. They can also assign this to teams who divide up by ages or by vaccinations and fill in appropriate data.

## ANSWERS TO CHECK YOUR KNOWLEDGE QUESTIONS

1. What is an *anaphylactic* reaction?
   a. The patient faints as a result of the medication administration.
   **b. The patient has an allergic reaction as a result of the medication administration.**
   c. The patient has a needlestick injury.
   d. The patient develops a wheal.
2. When is the intradermal route of injection used?
   a. To administer medication directly into a vein.
   b. To give immunizations.
   **c. To administer small doses of medication.**
   d. For allergy testing.
3. All the following are reasons parenteral routes are indicated instead of oral routes, except for which?
   a. The patient is unable to tolerate medications by mouth.
   b. The medication would be destroyed by the GI tract.
   **c. There is less risk involved with parenteral routes than with oral routes.**
   d. The medication needs to be effective more quickly.
4. Which document should always be signed before an immunization is given?
   **a. VIS**
   b. HIB
   c. MMR
   d. CDC
5. Which of these sites is not used for intramuscular injections?
   **a. Anterior forearm**
   b. Gluteus medius
   c. Deltoid
   d. Vastus lateralis

6. In the _________ category of vaccine, the pathogenic organism is rendered inactive and then injected into the body, which stimulates antibody production.
   a. pathogenic toxin
   b. live attenuated pathogen
   **c. killed pathogen**
   d. passive toxin
7. What do the initials MMR represent?
   a. Mumps, meningitis, rotavirus
   b. Measles, meningitis, rabies
   c. Measles, mumps, rubeola
   **d. Measles, mumps, rubella**

# NIT 18 FIRST AID AND RESPONDING TO EMERGENCIES
# HAPTER 55 Emergencies in the Medical Office

## BHES Curriculum

M.A.A.1.4.a Document accurately

M.A.A.1.9.b Apply principles of aseptic techniques and infection control

M.A.A.1.9.d Recognize and understand various treatment protocols

M.A.A.1.9.e Recognize emergencies and treatments and minor office surgical procedures

M.A.A.1.9.i Use standard precautions

M.A.A.1.9.k Prepare and maintain examination and treatment area

M.A.A.1.9.l Prepare patient for examinations and treatments

M.A.A.1.9.o (3) Perform telephone and in-person screening

M.A.A.1.9.o (5) Perform first aid and CPR

## AAHEP Core Curriculum

I.P.6 Perform patient screening, using established protocols

I.P.10 Assist provider with patient care

I.A.1 Apply critical thinking skills in performing patient assessment and care

III.C.11 Describe Standard Precautions

III.C.12 Discuss the application of Standard Precautions

III.P.2 Practice Standard Precautions

III.P.3 Select appropriate barrier and personal protective equipment (PPE) for potentially infectious situations

IV.P.2 Report relevant information to others succinctly and accurately

IV.P.6 Prepare a patient for procedures and treatments

IV.P.8 Document patient care

IX.P.2 Perform within scope of practice

IX.P.6 Complete an incident report

IX.P.7 Document accurately in the patient chart

XI.C.5 State principles and steps of professional and provider CPR

XI.C.13 Discuss potential roles of the medical assistant in emergency preparedness

# ESSON OUTLINE

## HANDLING EMERGENCIES IN THE MEDICAL OFFICE

A. Emergency is any situation requiring decided action
   1. Medical emergency is
   2. Important to know appropriate response and provider assistance
   3. Provide care at level of competence equal to training and experience

B. Office policy manual and documentation
   1. Emergency guidelines
   2. Emergency plan and assignments
   3. All staff members prepared to administer first aid and CPR

4. Goal to get patient stable and released

C. Documenting emergency procedures
    1. Identify individual responsible for recording incidents
    2. Patient's record documentation
    3. Usual required information
    4. Document office staff injury as well

D. Crash carts and emergency kits
    1. Collect and maintain in a special place
    2. Purchase prepared kit
    3. Equipment available
    4. Medications stocked on it
    5. Check on regular schedule for items and expiration dates

E. Other emergency equipment
    1. Defibrillation unit and automated external defibrillator (AED)
    2. Oxygen tank
    3. Ambu bag

## II. RECOGNIZE AND RESPOND TO AN EMERGENCY

A. Emergency situations that demand immediate medical intervention

B. If witnessing an emergency, victim's actions can alert you that something is happening, check for universal emergency medication identification

C. Activating EMS
    1. Advantages of trauma and critical care facilities
    2. Critical first hour
    3. EMS and 911 availability
    4. Know how to summon assistance
    5. Importance of emergency number list posted by phone
    6. Purpose of number list with emergency supplies

D. Documenting emergencies when life-saving measures fail
    1. Notifying local law enforcement agencies
    2. Removal of body
    3. Documentation of death

E. Telephone screening in an emergency
    1. If emergency is called into provider's office, MA must be prepared to respond
        a. Listen to caller
        b. Ask questions
        c. Follow office policy
        d. Get assistance if needed
        e. Activate EMS
    2. If caller states there is an emergency, do not put on hold

## I. CPR AND AED PROCEDURES

A. Definition of sudden cardiac arrest

B. Life-saving procedure that can double or triple rate of survival

C. All MAs should take approved CPR and standard first aid course

D. Responding to cardiac arrest: American Heart Association guidelines

E. Basic life-saving and CPR procedures: ABCs of CPR (airway, breathing, circulation)

F. AED procedure

  1. Steps to operate
  2. Necessity to have training in use
  3. Cautions with use
  4. Essential to provide patient chance of survival
  5. Chart specific information regarding use
  6. Ensure equipment is in operating order at all times

G. Documenting CPR and AED procedures

H. CPR for children and infants

I. CPR safety

  1. Concern with disease transmission
  2. Use of barrier device when CPR job-related

## V. COMMON EMERGENCIES IN THE MEDICAL OFFICE

A. Distinguishing severity of illness

  1. Chronic
  2. Insidious
  3. Urgent
  4. Sudden
  5. Severe
  6. Life threatening

B. Diabetic ketoacidosis or insulin shock

  1. Diabetic ketoacidosis
     a. Increased amount of sugar in blood
     b. Consumption of excess carbohydrates
     c. Infection
     d. Fever
     e. Emotional stress
     f. Failure to take insulin
     g. Symptoms: confusion, dizziness, weakness, nausea, dry and flushed skin, and a fruity breath odor
  2. Insulin shock
     a. Excess amount of insulin in blood
     b. Lack of food
     c. Vomiting

d. Excess exercise
e. Too much insulin taken
f. Symptoms consist of anxiety, confusion, pounding heartbeat, hunger, diaphoresis, pale and moist skin, and possibility of seizures

C. Fainting
1. Temporarily diminished supply of blood to the brain
2. Called syncope
3. Pale, perspiring, clammy skin
4. Treat with aromatic spirits of ammonia and prone positioning
5. Monitor vital signs

D. Heart attack
1. Medical term is myocardial infarction
2. Severe chest pain, radiating down left arm or left shoulder and jaw
3. Rapid, weak pulse
4. Profuse perspiration
5. Cyanotic lips and nails
6. Position on examination table
7. Prepare for medication and ECG
8. Initiate CPR if required
9. Symptoms for women

E. Heat and cold exposure
1. Heatstroke
a. Red, dry face
b. Skin hot and dry
c. Elevated temperature
d. Rapid pulse with deep and slow respiration
e. Dilated pupils and muscle cramps
f. Treat with bed rest, elevated head, and ice bags
2. Heat exhaustion
a. Face pale, cool, and moist
b. Skin cool and clammy with profuse perspiration
c. Headache, confusion, and giddiness
d. Pulse weak and rapid and respirations quiet and shallow
e. Thirst, nausea, and vomiting
f. Treat with recumbent position with head lowered, maintain warmth
3. Heat cramps
a. From long-time exposure to heat
b. Diaphoresis, causing depletion of water
c. Complaints of muscle cramps, faintness, and exhaustion
d. Treat with salt intake, balanced electrolyte drink, and rest in cool site

4. Freezing temperatures
    a. Called hypothermia
    b. Frostbite affects hands, feet, ears, and nose most often
    c. Symptoms are tingling, numbness, and pain, and later redness of skin
    d. Treat by slowly warming and hot liquids to drink
    e. Never rub areas or smoke
    f. Apply dressing and avoid pressure

F. Hemorrhage

1. Arterial
    a. Bright red blood in spurts
    b. Death possible if large artery
2. Venous
    a. Dark red blood in steady flow
    b. Control quickly with direct pressure and elevation
    c. Pressure points to control bleeding
3. Capillary: steady oozing that often clots spontaneously
4. Internal bleeding
    a. Shock symptoms
    b. Surgical intervention
    c. Symptoms suggest location of bleeding
    d. Ruptured organs or an aneurysm
5. Nosebleed
6. Vaginal bleeding

G. Poisoning

1. Ingested, absorbed, inhaled, injected, acquired from bites or stings
2. Poison control center assistance
    a. What was taken
    b. How much
    c. Time taken
3. Oxygen or resuscitation for inhalation poisoning
4. Hospitalization if injection

H. Seizures

1. Also called convulsions
2. Severe involuntary contraction of muscles that first causes patient to become rigid and then to have uncontrollable movements
3. Characteristics
4. Aspiration prevention
5. Need for rest and emotional support

I. Obstructed airway

1. Food aspiration
2. Toys or toy parts
3. Buttons, candy, filmy plastic, and balloons

4. Universal distress signal
5. Abdominal thrust (Procedure 54–1)
6. Chest thrust maneuver with pregnancy or obese patients
7. Finger sweep with jaw thrust
8. Special considerations for infants

J. Accidental, allergic, and drug-induced distress
1. Edema of vocal cords resulting from allergic reaction
2. Drowning
3. Toxic gas or suffocation
4. Asthmatic attack
5. Reaction to medication

K. Shock
1. Serious depressor of body functions
    a. Rapid, thready, weak pulse
    b. Shallow, rapid respirations
    c. Dilated pupils
    d. Ashen color
    e. Cool, clammy skin
2. Maintain body warmth
3. Causes
    a. Heart attack
    b. Respiratory collapse
    c. Following trauma and physical injury
        i. Extensive burns
        ii. Electrical shock
        iii. Hemorrhage
        iv. Near drowning
        v. Severe infection
        vi. Anaphylactic shock

L. Stroke
1. Stroke or apoplexy
2. Ruptured artery or occlusion
3. Symptoms include sagging facial muscles, one-sided paralysis or inability to use arm or leg, unequal pupils, confusion, slurred speech, loss of bladder and bowel control
4. Considered emergency
5. American Heart Association recommendations
    a. Initial field evaluation
    b. Rapid transport
    c. Medical evaluation
    d. CT scan
    e. Use of fibrinolytics or treat hemorrhage

M. Shock

## HAPTER ACTIVITIES

1. Invite an EMT to share emergency experiences.
2. Have students interview a medical assistant currently working in a family practice office. Ask how many emergencies he or she has personally been involved with and whether he or she has had experience with AED use or oxygen administration. Write a summary and present it to the class.
3. Have students visit the American Heart Association or American Red Cross Websites and obtain any recent changes in CPR certification for health care workers.
4. Invite a speaker from the American Heart Association to discuss the various types of heart conditions and explain the importance of heart health and living a heart-healthy lifestyle.
5. Invite a sales representative to discuss a variety of emergency equipment used in the field and give a demonstration on some of the products, such as AEDs and oxygen equipment.
6. Practice placing pads for the AED on classmates and discuss troubleshooting and how to operate the machine. Also discuss the differences for adults, children, and infants.
7. Have students pair up and demonstrate proper use of oxygen equipment as well as provide patient education on the equipment with any dos and don'ts.
8. Have students search the Web for a national organization that focuses on cardiac disorders; have them pick a topic and present the information to the class.
9. Assign students various arrhythmias; have them make creative poster boards with information regarding the condition and present the posters to the class. Be sure to have the students discuss the causes.
10. Have students research the effects of smoking and alcohol consumption on the heart and write a paper about it.
11. Telephone different ambulance services and your local fire departments to determine whether patients are charged for ambulance transportation and how much. Report to the class.
12. Have students make posters reflecting the differences of the symptoms of a heart attack between males and females. Also have them discuss emergency care for heart attack victims.

## NSWERS TO CHECK YOUR KNOWLEDGE QUESTIONS

1. This unit is computerized and can analyze the heart rhythm of a person in fibrillation or arrest, recognize a shockable rhythm, and advise the operator through lights and voice prompts if a shock is indicated.
   a. ECG
   **b. AED**
   c. EMS
   d. Ambu bag
2. The most immediate information you need to relay to EMS includes:
   **a. the nature of the situation and the address of the victim's location.**
   b. the victim's name.
   c. the caller's name and phone number in case the connection is lost.
   d. when the problem started.
3. When distinguishing the severity and length of time for onset of disease or illness, which of the following common terms describes having rapid onset, severe symptoms, and a short course?
   a. Chronic
   b. Subtle

**c. Acute**

d. Life threatening

4. In which of the following emergency situations should the patient be given some form of sugar to help alleviate the situation?

a. Diabetic ketoacidosis

b. Hyperglycemia

c. Diaphoresis

**d. Hypoglycemia**

5. The signs of a patient having heat exhaustion would be:

**a. pale, cool, and moist skin and normal body temperature.**

b. hot and dry skin and body temperature possibly above 40°C/104°F.

c. a weak pulse and shallow breathing, body temperature dropping lower than 35°C/95°F.

d. white or grayish-yellow skin waxy in appearance.

6. Symptoms that might include shortness of breath; a burning sensation in the chest; nausea and vomiting; unexplaine fatigue or weakness; and/or pain in the jaw, neck, shoulder, back, or ear could indicate:

**a. heart attack.**

b. stroke.

c. shock.

d eizure.

7. If an obstructed airway is complete, the object must be removed immediately, within ________, to prevent brain damage from lack of oxygen.

a. 30 seconds

b. 2 minutes

**c. 4 minutes**

d. 6 minutes

8. Coughing up what appears to be coffee grounds can indicate:

a. lung hemorrhage.

**b. a chronic slow bleed of the stomach.**

c. epistaxis.

d. an ulcer has started bleeding.

# HAPTER 56 First Aid for Accidents and Injuries

## BHES Curriculum

| | |
|---|---|
| M.A.A.1.4.a | Document accurately |
| M.A.A.1.9.b | Apply principles of aseptic techniques and infection control |
| M.A.A.1.9.d | Recognize and understand various treatment protocols |
| M.A.A.1.9.e | Recognize emergencies and treatments and minor office surgical procedures |
| M.A.A.1.9.i | Use standard precautions |
| M.A.A.1.9.k | Prepare and maintain examination and treatment area |
| M.A.A.1.9.l | Prepare patient for examinations and treatments |
| M.A.A.1.9.o | Perform first aid and CPR |

## AAHEP Core Curriculum

| | |
|---|---|
| I.P.10 | Assist provider with patient care |
| I.A.1 | Apply critical thinking skills in performing patient assessment and care |
| III.C.11 | Describe Standard Precautions |
| III.C.12 | Discuss the application of Standard Precautions |
| III.P.2 | Practice Standard Precautions |
| III.P.3 | Select appropriate barrier and personal protective equipment (PPE) for potentially infectious situations |
| IV.P.2 | Report relevant information to others succinctly and accurately |
| IV.P.6 | Prepare a patient for procedures or treatments |
| IV.P.8 | Document patient care |
| IX.P.2 | Perform within scope of practice |
| IX.P.6 | Complete an incident report |
| IX.P.7 | Document accurately in the patient chart |

## ESSON OUTLINE

### . ACCIDENTS AND INJURIES

A. Knowing basic first aid important

B. Seek medical assistance if unsure

C. Phone screening

### I. COMMON INJURIES

A. Foreign bodies

1. In the eye

    a. Remove with fold of tissue or moistened cotton

    b. Turn upper lid over swab and remove

    c. Flush with water

    d. Embedded material requires medical intervention

    e. Cover both eyes with compresses
    f. Advise not to rub
  2. In the ear
    a. Instill warm oil; then drain
    b. Avoid oil with smooth objects
    c. Irrigate out objects that will not swell with water
  3. In the nose, irrigate or reach with forceps
  4. Swallowed items will move through system and be eliminated
  5. Splinters
    a. Use needle or thumb forceps
    b. Area washed and covered with adhesive bandage
  6. Fish hook
    a. Removal techniques
    b. Clean and dress wound
    c. Tetanus and antibiotic
B. Strains and sprains
  1. Treatment for strains
    a. Rest in comfortable position
    b. Ice then heat
    c. Analgesic or muscle relaxers
  2. Treatment for sprain
    a. Elevate
    b. Apply ice first 48–72 hours
    c. Elastic bandage for support
C. Dislocations
  1. Usually severe pain and deformity at joint
  2. Immobilize and get medical attention
D. Fractures
  1. Closed or simple
  2. Open or compound
    a. Control bleeding
    b. Splint as is
  3. Treat for shock
  4. Check pulse, motor and sensory reflexes (PMS)
  5. Medical attention as soon as possible

## III. BITES AND STINGS

A. Come from humans, animals, and insects
B. Can be superficial or break the skin

C. Animal bites and danger of rabies
   1. Cleanse thoroughly
   2. Provider examination
   3. Report bite to authorities
   4. Observe animal
   5. Anti-rabies serum if rabid or animal not available
   6. Snake bites
D. Human bites and HIV or hepatitis B infection
   1. Skin surface breaks and biter has bleeding gums
   2. Give hepatitis B immunization
   3. Tetanus injection
E. Stings
   1. Number of stings is factor
   2. Allergic responses critical
      a. Restlessness
      b. Shortness of breath with cyanotic skin
      c. Nausea, vomiting, diarrhea
      d. Need for emergency kit
   3. Removal of stinger by scraping

## V. BURNS

A. Types of burns
   1. Thermal burns as result of fires, matches, gasoline, space heater, firecrackers, scalding, curling irons, stoves, hot irons, and sunburn
   2. Chemical burns from acids or alkalines contact, ingestion, inhalation, or injection
   3. Electrical burns from faulty wiring, chewing electrical cords, power lines, and lightning
B. Classification of burns
   1. Percentage of body surface area (BSA)
   2. Degree of skin involvement
      a. First-degree (superficial), primarily involves epidermis
      b. Second-degree (partial-thickness), involves epidermis and part of dermis
      c. Third- and fourth-degree (full-thickness), involves epidermis, dermis, and subcutaneous, extends through all skin into muscle and bone
   3. Classified by combination of BSA and depth of burn
      a. Minor burn has third-degree covering less than 2 percent BSA; second-degree covering less than 15 percent for adults and 10 percent for children
      b. Moderate burn has third-degree covering 2 percent to 10 percent BSA; second-degree covering from 15 percent to 25 percent adults or more than 10 percent for child
      c. Major burn has third-degree over more than 10 percent of BSA; second-degree over more than 25 percent for adults or move than 20 percent for child
      d. Also major are burns of hands, feet, genitalia; burns with fractures; poor-risk patients; electrical burns

C. Treatment

1. Minor burn treated with cold water
    a. No butter or ointment
    b. Ice prohibited due to frostbite possibility
    c. Photosensitive drugs increase sunburn risk
2. Second-degree burn
    a. Can involve prevention of shock
    b. Removal of jewelry due to edema
    c. Force fluids
    d. Cover area with sterile dressing
    e. Provider break blisters
3. Third- and fourth-degree burn
    a. Immediate medical treatment
    b. Surgical intervention possible
    c. Replacement fluids by IV
    d. Pain medication and tetanus
    e. No cleaning, cover with sterile dressing
    f. Treat for shock
    g. Tetanus injection
4. Electrical burns
    a. Remove victim from electrical source
        i. Electrical shut-off
        ii. Water conduction danger
    b. Administer CPR if arrest
    c. Treat burn as non-electrical
    d. Damage along conduction path
5. Chemical burns
    a. Remove clothing from area
    b. Brush off dry chemical first
    c. Flood with water
    d. Cover with sterile dressing
    e. Flush eye for 20 minutes and have provider examine

## V. USE OF HEAT AND COLD

A. Disposable packs

B. Activate and reuse

C. Place in covering or towel

D. Use on 20 minutes, off 10, if not ordered differently

E. Cold applications

1. Decreases local circulation
2. Provides local anesthetic
3. Relieves inflammation
4. Controls bleeding and swelling

F. Heat applications

1. Increase tissue temperature
2. Increase circulation
3. Increase healing
4. Decrease pain
5. Relieve congestion in deep tissues

## VI. WOUNDS

A. Abrasions are scrapes of epidermis: treat by cleaning and applying dressing

B. Avulsion: clean and replace flap of torn skin

C. Incision is clean cut by a sharp object might require Steri-Strips or sutures to close

D. Laceration is a tearing of tissue hard to clean and close

E. Puncture is from pointed object or bite: clean thoroughly

F. Cleaning wounds (Procedure 56–1)

1. Cleaning and assessing
2. Wash (Betadine) or other antibacterial agent
3. Apply disinfectant
4. With severe bleeding, initial cleaning delayed until medical care
5. Pressure bandage applied
6. Prepare suture setup
7. Question about wound and tetanus situation

G. Dressings and bandaging wounds

1. Apply nonstick dressing
2. Bandage with appropriate material
   a. Tubular gauze and cylinder (Procedure 56–2)
   b. Open or closed spiral (Procedure 56–3)
   c. Figure-eight (Procedure 56–4)
   d. Cravat from triangular bandage (Procedure 56–5)

## CHAPTER ACTIVITIES

1. Supply students with a picture of skin and have them label it and indicate which layers are involved in burn classifications.
2. Assign wound areas, such as the internal aspect of the calf, for students to clean or bandage.
3. As a class, list the steps for wound cleansing on the board and then practice on a partner.
4. Invite a speaker from the American Red Cross to discuss the first aid training they provide and the various types of injuries that might need first aid response.
5. Assign students various types of wounds and burns and have them make creative poster boards with information regarding the types and present them to the class. Be sure to have students discuss the causes.
6. Have students role play in pairs, one being the MA and the other being the patient, and provide patient education about bandage care and signs of infection to watch for.
7. Have students search the Web for a national organization that focuses on muscular skeletal conditions that need first aid care, such as sprains, strains, dislocations, and fractures; have them pick a topic and present the information to the class.

## ANSWERS TO CHECK YOUR KNOWLEDGE QUESTIONS

1. With all human bites, a tetanus injection must be administered to the patient if he or she has not received one within:
   a. one year.
   **b. five years.**
   c. seven years.
   d. ten years.
2. At least half of all dislocations involve which of the following body parts?
   **a. Shoulder**
   b. Wrist
   c. Ankle
   d. Knee
3. A ________ leaves the stinger in the skin, and it should be removed immediately by scraping it out carefully with a credit card or other rigid object.
   a. wasp
   b. hornet
   c. yellow jacket
   **d. honeybee**
4. Partial thickness burns are also referred to as:
   a. first-degree burns.
   **b. second-degree burns.**
   c. third-degree burns.
   d. fourth-degree burns.

5. When using the PRINCE method on a strain or sprain, the injury should be treated with a cold pack for the first __________ hours.
   a. 12–24
   b. 24–36
   c. 24–48
   **d. 48–72**
6. Which of the following types of wounds involves the skin being torn off and the wound bleeding profusely?
   a. Laceration
   **b. Avulsion**
   c. Abrasion
   d. Puncture
7. This type of fracture involves an open wound.
   a. Simple
   b. Closed
   **c. Compound**
   d. Both a and b are correct

# UNIT 19 REHABILITATION AND HEALTHY LIVING
# CHAPTER 57 Rehabilitation

## ABHES Curriculum

| | |
|---|---|
| M.A.A.1.4.a | Document accurately |
| M.A.A.1.5.b | Identify and respond appropriately when working or caring for patients with special needs |
| M.A.A.1.9.d | Recognize and understand various treatment protocols |
| M.A.A.1.9.l | Prepare patient for examinations and treatments |
| M.A.A.1.9.m | Assist provider with routine and specialty examinations and treatments |
| M.A.A.1.9.q | Instruct patients with special needs |
| M.A.A.1.9.r | Teach patients methods of health promotion and disease prevention |

## CAAHEP Core Curriculum

| | |
|---|---|
| I.P.10 | Assist provider with patient care |
| IV.P.5 | Instruct patients according to their needs to promote health maintenance and disease prevention |
| IV.P.6 | Prepare a patient for procedures or treatments |
| IV.P.8 | Document patient care |
| IV.P.9 | Document patient education |
| IX.P.7 | Document accurately in the patient record |
| XI.C.10 | Identify principles of body mechanics and ergonomics |
| XI.P.11 | Use proper body mechanics |

## LESSON OUTLINE

### I. BODY MECHANICS

A. Reduce injury to self and others

B. Practice at work and home

C. Proper posture

D. Techniques for lifting and moving

E. Ergonomics

### II. TRANSFERRING PATIENTS TO AND FROM WHEELCHAIR

A. For patient unable to ambulate

B. Enlist help to move patient from chair if necessary

C. Remember safety precautions (lock wheels)

D. Refer to Chapter 39 for procedures regarding helping patients into and out of wheelchair

E. Use gait belt for assistance with moving

## III. LEARN HOW TO ASSIST PATIENT TO THE FLOOR WHEN FALLING

## IV. INDICATIONS FOR MOBILITY DEVICES

A. After accident or injury
B. Following stroke
C. After surgery
D. Severe medical condition
E. Arthritis
F. Older adult
G. Physically challenged

## V. TYPES OF MOBILITY DEVICES

A. Safety at home
  1. Floor free of spills and clutter
  2. Remove loose or damaged floor coverings
  3. Avoid using slippery products on floor
  4. Appropriate, properly fitting footwear
B. Arm sling
  1. Supports arm after fracture or injury
  2. Hand higher than elbow
  3. Refer to Procedure 57–2
C. Cane
  1. Fitting guidelines
  2. Regular or quad base
  3. Refer to Procedure 57–3
D. Crutches
  1. To permit healing of foot, ankle, knee, or leg
  2. Fitting guidelines
  3. Different styles of crutches
  4. Gait patterns shown in text
  5. Refer to Procedure 57–4
E. Walker
  1. Supports patient unable to use crutches
  2. Fitting guidelines
  3. Instruct in proper use
  4. Types of walkers
  5. Refer to Procedure 57–5
F. Wheelchair
  1. Standard
  2. Motorized

## 'I. RANGE OF MOTION

A. Passive exercise to improve circulation and promote muscle tone

B. Abduction, adduction, flexion, extension, rotation, and pronation

# ;HAPTER ACTIVITIES

1. Invite a physical therapist to the class to explain rehabilitative conditions and procedures.
2. Have students roleplay the medical assistant, explaining patient education on the various rehabilitation modalities to a patient.
3. Have students practice instructing each other in crutch fitting and have each practice the various gait walks and standing and sitting with them.
4. Have students use the instructions and diagrams in the text to practice the range-of-motion exercises to become familiar with the movements.
5. Invite a sales representative to come out and discuss a variety of rehabilitative equipment used in the field and give a demonstration of some of their products such as arm slings, canes, and walkers.
6. Have students practice walking with a cane and a walker to get a general idea of what the patient will encounter.
7. Have students pair up and demonstrate proper application of arm slings. Be sure to have them cover checking for circulation impairment.
8. Have students search the Web for a national organization that focuses on rehabilitative disorders; have them pick a topic and present the information to the class.
9. Assign students various reasons mobility devices are used; have them make creative poster boards with information regarding such devices and present them to the class. Be sure to have students discuss the causes for such devices to be necessary.
10. Ask students to practice putting a sling on a patient who is standing, sitting, and lying down.
11. Have students role-play in pairs to practice adjusting crutches.
12. Assign students to use crutches, a walker, and a wheelchair for a day.

# NSWERS TO CHECK YOUR KNOWLEDGE QUESTIONS

1. When using proper body mechanics, which of the following statements is true?
   a. Always bend from the waist to allow the largest muscles of the legs to do the hard work.
   b. Hold heavy objects far away from the body.
   **c. Check your posture by reminding yourself to keep your chin and chest up.**
   d. Check your posture by keeping shoulders forward and pelvis tilted slightly inward.
2. An example of a situation when the use of a mobility device would be needed includes:
   a. arthritis sufferers.
   b. after a stroke.
   c. physically challenged.
   **d. all of the above.**
3. When using a cane for support, the arm should hang naturally at the side with the elbow flexed at about a _______-degree angle.
   a. 10–15
   b. 20–25

**c. 25–30**

d. 30–45

4. When adjusting crutches for the correct height, adjust them so that the underarm pad is _______ below the axilla.

   a. 1 inch

   **b. 2 inches**

   c. 4 inches

   d. 6 inches

5. Which of the following crutch gaits positions both crutches and the left foot forward and then brings up the right foot?

   **a. Three-point**

   b. Four-point

   c. Two-point

   d. Swing-through

# CHAPTER 58 Nutrition, Exercise, and Healthy Living

## ABHES Curriculum

| | |
|---|---|
| MA.A.1.2.a | Comprehend and explain to the patient the importance of diet and nutrition; effectively convey and educate categories of patients who require special diets or diet modifications regarding proper diet and nutrition guidelines; identify categories of patients who require special diets or diet modifications |
| MA.A.1.4.a | Document accurately |
| MA.A.1.8.y | Effective communication (aa–ll below) |
| MA.A.1.9.l | Prepare patient for examinations and treatments |
| MA.A.1.9.m | Assist provider with routine and specialty examinations and treatments |
| MA.A.1.9.r | Teach patients methods of health promotion and disease prevention |

## CAAHEP Core Curriculum

| | |
|---|---|
| I.P.10 | Assist provider with patient care |
| I.A.1 | Apply critical thinking skills in performing patient assessment and care |
| I.A.3 | Demonstrate respect for diversity in approaching patients and families |
| IV.P.5 | Instruct patients according to their needs to promote health maintenance and disease prevention |
| IV.P.6 | Prepare a patient for procedures or treatments |
| IV.P.8 | Document patient care |
| IV.P.9 | Document patient education |
| IX.P.7 | Document accurately in the patient chart |
| X.A.3 | Demonstrate awareness of diversity in providing patient care |

# LESSON OUTLINE

## I. HEALTHY LIVING

A. Health

B. Guidelines for good health (see Table 58–1)

## II. NUTRITION

A. The processes involved in taking in, assimilating, and using nutrients

B. Nutrients

1. Body best able to function with adequate nutrients, exercise, and rest
2. Poor diet and sedentary lifestyle lead to many health issues

C. Calories

1. Carbohydrates, proteins, and fats have calorie values
2. A calorie is a unit of heat

D. Vitamins and minerals

1. Vitamins are organic substances found in foods; essential to good health and growth
    a. Fat-soluble vitamins are A, D, E, and K
    b. Water-soluble vitamins are C and B complex
2. Minerals are naturally occurring inorganic, homogeneous, solid substances, 13 said to be essential

## III. HEALTHY EATING

A. Dietary Guidelines for Americans
  1. Updated every five years
  2. Four major priority action steps for Americans from 2010 report
  3. Basis for all government programs relating to nutrition, including MyPlate

B. MyPlate Food Guidance Systems
  1. Introduced in 2011
  2. No longer one-size-fits-all; customized for each person
  3. Involves making smart food choices and exercise
  4. Includes other meal planning, food tracker, and interactive tools

## IV. NUTRITION FACTS LABELS

A. Nutritional Labeling and Education Act requires manufacturers to put nutritional facts labels on all foods
  1. Serving size
  2. Servings per container
  3. Amount per serving
  4. Listing of food nutrients with respective gram amounts

B. Help patients understand the components of food labels

## V. FOODS THAT PROMOTE HEALTH

A. Fruits and vegetables
B. Whole grains
C. Ginger
D. Garlic
E. Walnuts

## VI. MEAL SUPPLEMENTS: LIQUIDS AND POWDERS

## VII. HERBAL PRODUCTS AND DIETARY SUPPLEMENTS

A. Differentiate between OTC and dietary supplements

B. FDA regulations
  1. Label statement
  2. Popular herbs
    a. St. John's wort
    b. Black cohosh
    c. Melatonin
    d. Willow bark
    e. Echinacea
    f. Saw palmetto
    g. Glucosamine
    h. Ginseng
    i. Ginkgo biloba

## ʼIII. WEIGHT CONTROL

A. Diet should be nutritionally sound and contain foods from the food guide pyramid
   1. Many weight-control plans, organizations, and products available
   2. No all-purpose diet for weight loss
B. 30 percent above ideal body weight considered obese: associated health problems with overweight and obesity
C. Therapeutic diets
   1. Clear liquid diet
   2. BRAT diet
   3. Soft
   4. Low calorie
   5. Specialized therapeutic diets
D. Popular diets
   1. Diets promising rapid weight loss
   2. Only proven long-term and safe method is burn more calories than you consume
E. Cultural influences on diet
F. Health concerns in adolescents
   1. Anorexia nervosa—psychoneurotic disorder: patient refuses to eat over a period of time
      a. Performs rigorous exercise
      b. Patient has self-image of being overweight
      c. Problems include emaciation and amenorrhea
      d. Poor self-image and has fear of gaining weight
      e. May be result of emotional stress or conflict
      f. Symptoms: personality change, irritability, refusal to eat, weight loss
   2. Bulimia nervosa—binge eating and purging behavior
      a. Eats very large quantities of food at a time
      b. Eats regular meals to conceal disorder
      c. Poor self-image and feelings of inadequacy
      d. Symptoms: dark circles under eyes, muscle wasting, dental cavities (damage to tooth enamel from vomiting stomach acid often)
   3. Promote and establish good health habits
      a. Discuss problems in private
      b. Be understanding and supportive
      c. Give printed information about smoking, teen pregnancy, etc.
      d. Bring problems to provider's attention
      e. Might need referral for counseling

### IX. EXERCISE

A. Physical exertion for improvement of health or correction of physical deformity

B. Must be approved by provider to safeguard patient from overextension and stress

C. Benefits

1. Fosters a positive outlook and coping behavior
2. Improves circulation and muscle tone and relieves tensions
3. Walking is safest form of exercise

D. Stretching exercises

### X. HEALTHY SPIRIT: MEDITATION

### XI. SLEEP

A. Natural way for the body to rest and restore itself

B. Average number of hours in 24-hour period is 6 to 8

C. Insomnia

1. Trouble sleeping
2. Should seek medical attention

## CHAPTER ACTIVITIES

1. Have students research popular diet programs and give the pros and cons of each.
2. Ask a registered dietitian to give a presentation regarding nutrition, meal planning, cooking tips, or whatever you fee the class might be interested in. You might also ask the presenter to explain special diets.
3. Encourage students to bring in newspaper and magazine articles regarding diet and exercise to share with the class. Keep a file or notebook for this purpose.
4. Invite a gastroenterologist, or a medical assistant employed by one, to speak to the class about eating disorders and treatments for various digestive tract disorders.
5. Have students make posters with health tips about diet and exercise.
6. Have students make large drawings or posters of the food guide pyramid and select the best ones to display in the classroom or school cafeteria.
7. Have students keep track of their daily diet and exercise routines for two weeks and then discuss them in class.
8. Encourage students to list the priorities in their lives such as activities, assignments, and social functions. Give them blank calendars to record all their important dates, for instance, when assignments are due or when they should study for tests. This activity will help start them in managing their own personal time and stress by helping them plan their time and avoid the last-minute rush in getting things done. It should show them the basic steps in reducing stress.
9. Ask students to bring in articles about stress-related illnesses to share with other class members and have group discussions on how to eliminate some of the stressors of life.

## ANSWERS TO CHECK YOUR KNOWLEDGE QUESTIONS

1. The body gets energy from:

   **a. fats.**

   b. water.

c. electrolytes.

d. vitamins.

2. A gram of fat has approximately ___________ calories.

a. four

b. five

c. seven

**d. nine**

3. The basic amount of calories required to maintain an average-sized adult expending a low level of energy is ___________ per day.

a. 1200–1500

**b. 1500–1800**

c. 70

d. 150

4. Which of the following is a water-soluble vitamin?

**a. Vitamin C**

b. Vitamin D

c. Vitamin K

d. Vitamin E

5. Which of the following disorders is characterized by bingeing and purging?

a. Anorexia

b. Gluttony

**c. Bulimia**

d. Obesity

6. Which of the following is considered a vitamin C deficiency disease?

a. Rickets

**b. Scurvy**

c. Beriberi

d. Spongy bones

7. Which of the following are protective elements found in fruits and vegetables?

a. Hydro-proteins

**b. Phytochemicals**

c. Amino acids

d. Tryptophan

8. This dietary supplement is a hormone produced naturally in the pineal gland within the brain. It plays a part in regulating sleep patterns.

a. St. John wort

b. Echinacea

**c. Melatonin**

d. Ginseng

9. Regular exercise is known to:

a. improve circulation.

b. improve muscle tone.

c. relieve tension.

**d. all of the above.**

10. Which of the following cultural or religious groups have dietary laws that prohibit eating pork and drinking alcohol?

a. Hindu

**b. Islamic**

c. Jewish

d. Catholic

# UNIT 20 WORKPLACE READINESS
# CHAPTER 59 Practicum and the Job Search

## ABHES Curriculum

| | |
|---|---|
| MA.A.1.11.a | Perform the essential requirements for employment such as résumé writing, effective interviewing, dressing professionally, and following up appropriately |
| MA.A.1.11.b | Demonstrate professionalism (1–9) |

## CAAHEP Core Curriculum

| | |
|---|---|
| IV.C.8 | Recognize elements of fundamental writing skills |
| IV.C.12 | Organize technical information and summaries |
| IV.P.10 | Compose professional and business letters |
| IV.A | Concepts of effective communication |

## LESSON OUTLINE

### I. THE PRACTICUM EXPERIENCE

A. Applying skills learned in the classroom

B. 160 hours for accredited program (ABHES/CAAHEP)

C. The purpose of practicum

1. Meet performance objectives
2. Gain experience

D. Practicum policies

1. Philosophy and goals of the externship experience
2. The role of the school
3. The role of the health facility
4. The on-site supervisor's role
5. The student's obligation

E. Practicum evaluations

1. Appearance
2. Attitude
3. Maturity
4. Dependability
5. Initiative
6. Administrative tasks
7. Clinical tasks
8. Interpersonal relationships

## II. SELF-ASSESSMENT AND CAREER ENTRY

A. Everyone has personal characteristics that affect his or her way of doing things
   1. Strong points
   2. Weak points
   3. Get a good idea about who you are
B. Desirable skills
   1. Communication skills
   2. Computer proficiency
   3. Critical thinking and analytical skills
   4. Teamwork and interpersonal skills
   5. Time management
C. Desirable qualities
   1. Positive attitude
   2. Strong work ethic
   3. Dependability
   4. Honesty and integrity
   5. Punctuality
   6. Flexibility
   7. Motivated—takes initiative
D. At work and on time
   1. Attendance is most important
   2. Leaving early is not advised
E. Taking care of yourself—Good health will keep you productive and energized

## III. PREPARING YOUR RÉSUMÉ (PROCEDURE 59–1)

A. Develop a personal résumé
B. Complete, accurate, and neatly organized
C. Informs the prospective employer of how qualified you are
D. One page is preferred length
E. Elements of a résumé
   1. Contact information
   2. Objective (optional)
   3. Education
   4. Experience
   5. Professional affiliations
   6. Professional achievements and awards
   7. Community service
   8. Professional memberships, achievements, and volunteer activities
F. Résumé styles
   1. Functional
   2. Targeted

3. Chronological
4. Skills

G. Keeping your résumé current

1. Update regularly
2. Maintain on a single page

## V. PREPARING YOUR COVER LETTER (PROCEDURE 59–2)

A. States why you should be hired for position

B. Personalized

C. Error free

## . STARTING YOUR JOB SEARCH

A. Job descriptions

1. Title of the position
2. Person(s) to whom responsible
3. Summary of the position
4. Primary duties of the job
5. Expectations of the person in the job
6. Requirements of the position
7. Qualifications for the job
8. Additional criteria per facility

B. Resources for finding jobs

1. The Internet
    a. Listed and updated regularly
    b. Quick and easy
2. Classified advertisement
    a. Request for qualified applicant
    b. Customary to write a cover letter
3. Public employment services
    a. Job openings on file
    b. No fee for service
4. Private employment agencies
    a. Cover letter and résumé both used
    b. Fee paid
5. Other contacts
    a. Offices in which no position is available
    b. Public libraries
    c. Periodicals and books
    d. Membership in professional associations
    e. Industry-sponsored job fairs

### VI. COMPLETING AN APPLICATION FORM (PROCEDURE 59–3)

A. Simple to complex

B. Use résumé

C. Transcribe dates and information correctly

D. Must be complete, neat, and legible

E. Use black ink only

### VII. INTERVIEWING FOR THE JOB

A. Face-to-face meeting

B. Dos and don'ts

C. Personal appearance

1. Extremely important
2. Dress for success
3. Nonverbal messages speak loudly
4. Personal cleanliness is vital

D. Preparing for the interview

1. Plan your time beforehand
2. Arrive 10–15 minutes early
3. Call to explain any delays

E. During the interview

1. Remember your body language
2. Maintain eye contact
3. Prepare to answer questions regarding career goals
4. Prepare list of references and other documents
5. An interviewer will appreciate openness
6. A firm handshake at the conclusion of the interview

F. Interview follow-up letter (Procedure 59–4)

### VIII. AFTER YOU ARE EMPLOYED

A. Where your work history begins

B. Chances of advances

C. Continuing education

1. Keep up with changes
2. Read
3. Courses related to area of interest
4. Professional organizations
5. Educational seminars

## CHAPTER ACTIVITIES

1. Have students choose from one of the four styles of résumés discussed in the chapter and write their own résumé. Make copies to share with the class and have a class discussion about each résumé.

2. Have students find a classified ad for a medical assisting position from their local paper and then write a cover letter responding to the ad.
3,. Have students complete the application forms provided in their textbooks, making sure to follow directions accurately.
4. Have students role-play interviewing each other. Have them make a list of questions to ask each other as the interviewer and the interviewee.
5. Have students make a list of their personal strengths and weaknesses and what they feel they should do to improve themselves.

## NSWERS TO CHECK YOUR KNOWLEDGE QUESTIONS

1. A practicum should be treated:
   a. as a work experience.
   **b. as a learning experience.**
   c. as a possible job lead.
   d. as a regular school day.
2. What is the goal of a résumé?
   a. To present a personal profile
   b. To get a job
   c. To show off your achievements
   **d. To receive an interview**
3. All of the following are personal qualities except:
   **a. critical thinking skills.**
   b. initiative.
   c. dependability.
   d. positive attitude.
4. A résumé style that highlights your previous work experiences related to the position you are seeking is which type of résumé?
   a. Skills
   b. Chronological
   **c. Targeted**
   d. Functional
5. When should you arrive at an interview?
   a. Right on time
   b. 5 minutes early
   **c. 10 minutes early**
   d. 20 minutes early
6. All of the following are background checks may be performed on an applicant except:
   a. credit rating.
   b. criminal record.
   c. drug screen.
   **d. marital status.**

# Part 3

# INSTRUCTOR TOOLS

| An introduction and review of the program curricular component includes: | | Graduates: | |
|---|---|---|---|
| **1. General Orientation** | **Reference** | **1. General Orientation** | **Reference** |
| a. Employment conditions | Ch 1 | a. Comprehend the current employment outlook for the medical assistant | Ch 1 |
| b. The allied health professions | Ch 1, 22 | b. Compare and contrast the allied health professions and understand their relation to medical assisting | Ch 2, 22 |
| c. Credentialing of the medical assistant | Ch 1 | c. Understand medical assistant credentialing requirements and the process to obtain the credential; comprehend the importance of credentialing | Ch 1 |
| d. General responsibilities of the medical assistant | Ch 1 | d. Have knowledge of the general responsibilities of the medical assistant | Ch 1 |
| e. The scope of practice within the state of employment | Ch 1, 5 | e. Define scope of practice for the medical assistant, and comprehend the conditions for practice within the state that the medical assistant is employed | Ch 1, 5 |
| **2. Anatomy and Physiology** | **Reference** | **2. Anatomy and Physiology** | **Reference** |
| a. Diet and nutrition | Ch 58 | a. Comprehend and explain to the patient the importance of diet and nutrition; effectively convey and educate categories of patients who require special diets or diet modifications patients regarding the proper diet and nutrition guidelines; identify categories of patients who require special diets or diet modifications modifications | Ch 58 |
| b. Introduction to anatomy and physiology | Ch 23–35, 36 | b. Identify and apply the knowledge of all body systems; their structure and functions; and their common diseases, symptoms, and etiologies | Ch 23–35, 36 |
| c. Body systems | Ch 23–35, 38, 40, 41 | c. Assist the physician with the regimen of diagnostic and treatment modalities as they relate to each body system | Ch 23–35, 38, 40, 41; *all clinical and lab proc* |
| d. Common diseases, diagnoses, and treatments | Ch 23–35 | | |
| **3. Medical Terminology** | **Reference** | **3. Medical Terminology** | **Reference** |
| a. Basic structure of medical words | Ch 3, 4 | a. Define and use entire basic structure of medical words and be able to accurately identify in the correct context; i.e., root, prefix, suffix, combinations, spelling, and definitions | Ch 3, 4 |
| b. Word element combinations | Ch 3, 4 | b. Build and dissect medical terms from roots/suffixes to understand the word element combinations that create medical terminology | Ch 3, 4 |
| c. Medical terms for specialties | Ch 4, 23–36 | c. Understand the various medical terminology for each specialty | Ch 4, 23–36 |
| d. Medical abbreviations | Ch 4 | d. Recognize and identify acceptable medical abbreviations | Ch 4 |

| **4. Medical Law and Ethics** | **Reference** | **4. Medical Law and Ethics** | **Reference** |
|---|---|---|---|
| a. Documentation | Ch 5, 9, 13, 37; *throughout* | a. Document accurately | Ch 5, 9, 13, 37; Ch 13 WB Comp Practice 1; *throughout* |
| b. Federal and state guidelines | Ch 5, 6, 13 | b Institute federal and state guidelines when releasing medical records or information | Ch 5, 6, 13 |
| c. Established policies | Ch 5, 49 | c. Follow established policies when initiating or terminating medical treatment | Ch 5, 49 |
| d. Liability coverage | Ch 22 | d. Understand the importance of maintaining liability coverage once employed in the industry | Ch 22 |
| e. Risk management | Ch 21, 36 | e. Perform risk management procedures | Ch 21, 36; Proc 36-1 |
| f. Health laws and regulations | Ch 5, 36, 42, 43, 51, 53 | f. Comply with federal, state, and local health laws and regulations | Ch 5, 36, 42, 43, 51, 53; Proc 36-1 |
| **5. Psychology of Human Relations** | **Reference** | **5. Psychology of Human Relations** | **Reference** |
| a. Abnormal behavior patterns | Ch 21 | a. Define and understand abnormal behavior patterns | Ch 21; Ch 21 WB Video Case Study |
| b. Patients with special needs | Ch 42, 57 | b. Identify and respond appropriately when working/caring for patients with special needs | Ch 5, 7, 8, 42 |
| c. Empathy for terminally ill patients | Ch 8 | c. Use empathy when treating terminally ill patients; identify common stages that terminally ill patients go through family members of patients struggling with terminal illness and list organizations/support groups that can assist patients | Ch 8 |
| d. Support groups for terminally ill patients | Ch 8 | d. Identify common stages that terminally ill patients go through and list organizations/support groups that can assist struggling with terminal illness patients and family members of patients | Ch 8 |
| e. Being a patient advocate | Ch 1, 8 | e. Advocate on behalf of family/patients, having ability to deal and communicate with family | Ch 1, 8; Proc 8-2 |
| f. Developmental stages of life | Ch 42 | f. Identify and discuss developmental stages of life | Ch 42 |
| g. Heredity, culture, and environment | Ch 6, 8 | g. Analyze the effect of hereditary, cultural, and environmental influences | Ch 6, 8 |
| **6. Pharmacology** | **Reference** | **6. Pharmacology** | **Reference** |
| a. Math and metric conversions | Ch 52 | a. Demonstrate accurate occupational math and metric conversions for proper medication administration | Ch 52; Workbook Ch 52 |
| b. Use of drug references | Ch 51 | . Properly utilize PDR, drug handbook, and other drug references to identify a drug's classification, usual dosage, usual side effects, and contraindications | Ch 51; Proc 51-1 |
| c. Common abbreviations | Ch 53 | c. Identify and define common abbreviations that are accepted | Ch 53; Proc 53-1 |

| d. Legal aspects | Ch 53 | d. Understand legal aspects of writing prescriptions, including federal and state laws in prescription writing. | Ch 53; Proc 53-1 |
|---|---|---|---|
| e. Laws and regulations | Ch 51, 53 | e. Comply with federal, state, and local health laws and regulations | Ch 51, 53; Proc 53-1, 53-2, 53-3, 53-4 |
| **7. Basic Keyboarding/Computer Concepts** | **Reference** | **7. Basic Keyboarding/Computer Concepts** | **Reference** |
| a. Keyboarding skills | Ch 10 | a. Perform basic keyboarding skills including: | Ch 10; Proc 10-1 |
| | | (1) Locating the keys on a keyboard | Ch 10; Proc 10-1 |
| | | (2) Typing medical correspondence and basic reports | Ch 10; Proc 10-1 |
| b. Office systems and software | Ch 10, 11 | b. Identify and properly utilize office machines, computerized systems, and medical software such as: | Ch 10, 11; Proc 10-1, 11-1, 11-2 |
| | | (1) Efficiently maintain and understand different types of medical correspondence and medical reports | Ch10; Proc 10-1 |
| | | (2) Apply computer application skills using variety of different electronic programs including both practice management software and EMR software | Ch 10, 16, 18; Proc 10-1 |
| **8. Medical Office Business Procedures/Management** | **Reference** | **8. Medical Office Business Procedures/Management** | **Reference** |
| a. Clerical duties | Ch 9, 10, 11 | a. Perform basic clerical functions | Ch 9, 10, 11; Proc 9-4, 9-5, 10-1, 11-2 |
| b. Medical records | Ch 12, 13 | b. Prepare and maintain medical records | Ch 12, 13; Proc 12-3 |
| c. Appointments | Ch 12 | c. Schedule and manage appointments | Ch 12 |
| d. Office procedures | Ch 12, 13 | d. Apply concepts for office procedures | Ch 12, 13 |
| e. Information and resources | Ch 9, 22 | e. Locate resources and information for patients and employers | Ch 9, 22; Proc 9-4, 9-5, 22-2 |
| f. Admissions scheduling | Ch 12 | f. Schedule inpatient and outpatient admissions | Ch 12 |
| g. Bank statements and deposits | Ch 19 | g. Prepare and reconcile a bank statement and deposit record | Ch 19; Proc 19-2, 19-3 |
| h. Day sheets | Ch 16 | h. Post entries on a day sheet | Ch 16; Proc 16-1 |
| i. Billing | Ch 16, 17, 18 | i. Perform billing and collection procedures | Ch 16, 17, 18 |
| j. Accounts payable | Ch 19, Ch 20 | j. Perform accounts payable procedures | Ch 19; Proc 19-1; Ch 20 |
| k. Accounts receivable | Ch 16 | k. Perform accounts receivable procedures | Ch 16; Proc 16-1 |
| l. Petty cash | Ch 20 | l. Establish and maintain a petty cash fund | Ch 20; Proc 20-1 |
| m. Adjustments | Ch 16 | m. Post adjustments | Ch 16; Proc 16-1 |
| n. Credit balance | Ch 18 | n. Process credit balances | Ch 18; Proc 18-2 |
| o. Refunds | Ch 18 | o. Process refunds | Ch 18; Proc 18-2 |
| p. Non-sufficient funds | Ch 18 | p. Post non-sufficient funds (NSF) | Ch 18; Proc 18-1 |
| q. Collections | Ch 18 | q. Post collection agency payments | Ch 18; Proc 18-1 |
| r. Third parties | Ch 14, 17 | r. Apply third-party guidelines | Ch 14, 17; Proc 17-1 |
| s. Referrals | Ch 14 | s. Obtain managed care referrals and pre-certification | Ch 14; Proc 14-1 |
| t. Coding | Ch 15 | t. Perform diagnostic and procedural coding | Ch 15; Proc 15-1, 15-2 |

| u. Insurance claims | Ch 15 | u. Prepare and submit insurance claims | Ch 15; WB Competency Practice |
|---|---|---|---|
| v. Fee schedules | Ch 14 | v. Use physician fee schedule | Ch 14 |
| w. Bookkeeping systems | Ch 16 | w. Use manual or computerized bookkeeping systems | Ch 16; Proc 16-1 |
| x. Office management duties (y–z below) | Ch 21, 22, 43 | x. Maintain medical facility | Ch 21, 22; Proc 21-1, 21-2, 21-3 |
| | | y. Perform routine maintenance of administrative and clinical equipment | Ch 11, 43; Proc 11-1, 11-3, 43-1 |
| | | z. Maintain inventory equipment and supplies | Ch 21; Proc 21-4 |
| y. Effective communication (aa–ll below) | Ch 1, 2, 7, 9, 12, 15, 22, 37, 38 39 40 41, 42, 53, 58 | aa. Are attentive, listen, and learn | Ch 1, 7, 8, 37; Proc 7-1, 8-1, 9-1, 9-2, 37-1, 37-2; *throughout* |
| | | bb. Are impartial and show empathy when dealing with patients | Ch 1, 7, 8, 37; Proc 7-1, 8-1, 9-1, 37-1, 37-2 |
| | | cc. Communicate on the recipient's level of comprehension | Ch 7, 8, 37, 38, 42; Proc 7-1, 8-1, 37-1, 37-2; *throughout* |
| | | dd. Serve as liaison between physician and others | Ch 2, 8, 9, 10, 15, 22, 37, 38, 39, 40, 41, 42, 53; Proc 8-1, 8-2, 9-3, 101 222 3 1 3 2; *throughout* |
| | | ee. Use proper telephone techniques | Ch 9; Proc 9-1, 9-2, 9-3 |
| | | ff. Interview effectively | Ch 9, 12, 37; Proc 9-1, 12-3, 12-4, 37-1, 37-2 |
| | | gg. Use pertinent medical terminology | Ch 10, 37; Proc 10-1, 37-1, 37-2 |
| | | hh. Receive, organize, prioritize, and transmit information expediently | Ch 9, 37; Proc 9-1, 9-3, 37-1, 37-2 |
| | | ii. Recognize and respond to verbal and non-verbal communication | Ch 7, 8, 37; Proc 7-1, 8-1, 37-1, 37-2; *throughout* |
| | | jj. Perform fundamental writing skills including correct grammar, spelling, and formatting techniques when writing prescriptions, documenting medical records, etc. | Ch 9, 10, 37, 38; Proc 9-4, 9-5, 10-1 37 1, 37-2; *throughout* |
| | | kk. Adapt to individualized needs | Ch 7, 8, 37; Proc 7-1, 8-1, 37-1, 37-2; *throughout* |
| | | ll. Apply electronic technology | Ch 8, 10, 11, 12; Proc 8-2, 10-1, 11-2 |
| **9. Medical Office Clinical Procedures** | **Reference** | **9. Medical Office Clinical Procedures** | **Reference** |
| a. Patient history | Ch 37 | a. Obtain chief complaint, recording patient history | Ch 37; Proc 37-1, 37-2 |

| | | | |
|---|---|---|---|
| b. Aseptic technique | Ch 36, 39, 49 | b. Apply principles of aseptic techniques and infection control | Ch 36, 39, 49; Proc 36-2, 36-5, 36-6, 36-8, 39-1, 49-2, 49-3, 49-4; *throughout* |
| c. Vital signs | Ch 38 | c. Take vital signs | Ch 38; Proc 38-1, 38-2, 38-3, 38-4, 38-5, 38-6, 38-7, 38-8 |
| d. Treatment protocols | Ch 49, 50, 57 | d. Recognize and understand various treatment protocols | Ch 49, 50, 57; Proc 49-5, 50-1, 50-2, 50-3, 50-4 |
| e. Emergencies and office surgical procedures | Ch 50, 54, 55, 56 | e. Recognize emergencies and treatments and minor office surgical procedures | Ch 50, 55, 56; Proc 50-1, 50-2, 50-3, 50-4, 55-1 |
| f. Test results | Ch 45, 46, 47 | f. Screen and follow up patient test results | Ch 45, 46, 47; Proc 45-8, 46-5, 47-1, 47-2 |
| g. Records for medications and immunizations | Ch 37, 42 | g. Maintain medication and immunization records | Ch 37, 42 |
| h. Wrapping for sterilization | Ch 36 | h. Wrap items for autoclaving | Ch 36; Proc 36-7 |
| i. Standard precautions | Ch 21, 36, 40, 49, 55 | i. Use standard precautions | Ch 21, 36, 49, 55; Proc 21-4, 36-2, 36-3, 36-4, 49-3, 49-4; *throughout* |
| j. Parenteral medications | Ch 53, 54 | j. Prepare and administer oral and parenteral medications as directed by physician | Ch 53; Proc 53-2, 54-1, 54-2, 54-4, 54-5, 54-6, 54-7 |
| k. Maintenance of treatment and examination area | Ch 39, 40, 41, 42, 45, 46, 49, 50, 55 | k. Prepare and maintain examination and treatment area | Ch 39, 42, 45, 46, 49, 50, 55; Proc 39-1, 49-1, 50-1, 50-2, 50-3, 50-4 |
| l. Patient preparation | Ch 39, 40, 41, 42, 45, 46, 47, 49, 50, 55, 57, 58 | l. Prepare patient for examinations and treatments | Ch 39, 40, 41, 42, 45, 46, 47, 49, 50, 55, 57, 58; Proc 39-1, 49-5, all Proc in Ch 40, 41, 42, 47, 50 |
| m. Assisting the physician with examinations and treatments | Ch 39, 40, 41, 42, 47, 49, 57, 58 | m. Assist physician with routine and specialty examinations and treatments | Ch 39, 40, 41, 42, 47, 49, 57, 58; Proc 39-1, all Proc in Ch 40, 41, 47; Proc 42-3, 49-5 |
| n. Assisting the physician with minor surgical procedures | Ch 49, 50 | n. Assist physician with minor office surgical procedures | Ch 49, 50; Proc 49-5, 50-1, 50-2, 50-3, 50-4 |
| o. Electrocardiograms, respiratory testing, screening, sterilization, first aid, and CPR | Ch 37, 40, 47, 49 | o. Perform: | |
| | | (1) Electrocardiograms | Ch 47; Proc 47-1, 47-2 |
| | | (2) Respiratory testing | Ch 40; Proc 40-7, 40-8, 40-9 |
| | | (3) Telephone and in-person screening | Ch 37, 55; Proc 37-1 |
| | | (4) Sterilization techniques | Ch 49; Proc 49-2 |
| | | (5) First aid and CPR | Ch 55, 56 |
| p. Patient instructions (p–r below) | Ch 40, 41, 42, 46, 49, 50, 57, 58 | p. Advise patients of office policies and procedures | Ch 46, 49, 50; Proc 46-1, 46-6, 46-8 |

| | | | |
|---|---|---|---|
| | | q. Instruct patients with special needs | Ch 57 |
| | | r. Teach patients methods of health promotion and disease prevention | Ch 36, 40, 41, 42, 49, 50, 57, 58; Proc 41-1, 50-1, 50-2, 50-3, 50-4 |
| **10. Medical Laboratory Procedures** | **Reference** | **10. Medical Laboratory Procedures** | **Reference** |
| a. Quality control | Ch 44 45, 46 | a. Practice quality control | Ch 45, 46; Proc 45-1, 45-2, 46-2, 46-7, 46-11 |
| b. CLIA-waived tests | Ch 45 | b. Perform selected CLIA-waived tests that assist with diagnosis and treatment: | |
| | | (1) Urinalysis | Ch 46; Proc 46-3, 46-4 |
| | | (2) Hematology testing | Ch 45; Proc 45-1, 45-2, 45-3, 45-4, 45-5 |
| | | (3) Chemistry testing | Ch 45; Proc 45-6 |
| | | (4) Immunology testing | Ch 45; Proc 45-7 |
| | | (5) Microbiology testing | Ch 46; Proc 46-7 |
| | | (6) Kit testing: | |
| | | (a) Pregnancy | Ch 46; Proc 46-2 |
| | | (b) Quick strep | Ch 46; Proc 46-11 |
| | | (c) Dip sticks | Ch 46; Proc 46-3 |
| c. Biohazards | Ch 21, 36, 51, *throughout* | c. Dispose of biohazardous materials | Ch 21, 36, 51; Proc 21-4, 36-3 *throughout* |
| d. Specimens | Ch 43, 44, 45, 46, 50 | d. Collect, label, and process specimens: | |
| | | (1) Perform venipuncture | Ch 43; Proc 43-2, 43-3, 43-4 |
| | | (2) Perform capillary puncture | Ch 43, 45, 46; Proc 43-1 |
| | | (3) Perform wound collection procedures | Ch 46, 50; Proc 46-9, 50-1 |
| | | (4) Obtain throat specimens for microbiologic testing | Ch 46; Proc 46-10, 46-11 |
| e. Patient instructions (collection of urine and feces) | Ch 46 | e. Instruct patients in the collection of a clean-catch mid-stream urine specimen | Ch 46; Proc 46-1 |
| | | f. Instruct patients in the collection of a fecal specimen | Ch 46; Proc 46-6 |
| **11. Career Development** | **Reference** | **11. Career Development** | **Reference** |
| a. Essentials for employment | Ch 1, 59 | a. Perform the essential requirements for employment such as résumé writing, effective interviewing, dressing professionally, and following up appropriately | Ch 59; Proc 59-1, 59-2, 59-3 |
| b. Professionalism | Ch 1; *throughout* | b. Demonstrate professionalism by: | Ch 1, 37; *throughout* |
| | | (1) Exhibiting dependability, punctuality, and a positive work ethic | Ch 1, 7, 59; Proc 1-1 |
| | | (2) Exhibiting a positive attitude and a sense of responsibility | Ch 1, 21; Proc 1-1, 21-6, Ch 21 WB Video Case Study |

| | | | |
|---|---|---|---|
| | | (3) Maintaining confidentiality at all times | Ch 1, 5, 8, 9, 37; Proc 1-1, 9-2, 37-1, 37-2, 38-3 |
| | | (4) Being cognizant of ethical boundaries | Ch 1, 6, 7, 8, 37; Proc 1-1, 7-1, 8-1, 37-1, 37-2; Ch 8 WB Video Case Study |
| | | (5) Exhibiting initiative | Ch 1, 15; Proc 1-1, 15-1, 15-2 |
| | | (6) Adapting to change | Ch 1, 21; Proc 1-1, 21-6, Ch 21 WB Video Case Study |
| | | (7) Expressing a responsible attitude | Ch 1, Proc 1-1 |
| | | (8) Being courteous and diplomatic | Ch 1, 6, 37; Proc 1-1, 37-1, 37-2 |
| | | (9) Conducting work within scope of education, training, and ability | Ch 1, Proc 1-1 |

| Cognitive | | Psychomotor | | Affective | |
|---|---|---|---|---|---|
| I.C Anatomy & Physiology | Reference | I.P Anatomy & Physiology | Reference | I.A Anatomy & Physiology | Reference |
| 1. Describe structural organization of the human body | Ch 23–35 | 1. Obtain vital signs | Ch 38; Proc 38-1, 38-2, 38-3, 38-4, 38-5, 38-6, 38-7, 38-8 | 1. Apply critical thinking skills in performing patient assessment and care | Ch 8, 23–35, 36, 37, 55; Proc 37-1, 37-2; *All clinical and lab procedures* |
| 2. Identify body systems | Ch 23–35 | 2. Perform venipuncture | Ch 43; Proc 43-2, 43-3, 43-4 | 2. Use language/verbal skills that enable patients' understanding | Ch 12, 37; Proc 12-4, 37-1, 37-2; *All clinical and lab procedures* |
| 3. Describe body planes, directional terms, quadrants, and cavities | Ch 23–35 | 3. Perform capillary puncture | Ch 43, 45; Proc 43-1 | 3. Demonstrate respect for diversity in approaching patients and families | Ch 8, 37, 58; Proc 8-1, 37-1, 37-2 |
| 4. List major organs in each body system | Ch 23–35, 38 | 4. Perform pulmonary function testing | | | |
| 5. Describe the normal function of each body system | Ch 23–35, 45, 46 | 5. Perform electrocardiography | Ch 47; Proc 47-1, 47-2 | | |
| 6. Identify common pathology related to each body system | Ch 23–35, 36 | 6. Perform patient screening using established protocols | Ch 37, 55; Proc 37-1, 37-2 | | |
| 7. Analyze pathology as it relates to the interaction of body systems | Ch 23–35 | 7. Select proper sites for administering parenteral medication | Ch 54; all Proc in Ch 54 | | |
| 8. Discuss implications for disease and disability when homeostasis is not maintained | Ch 23–35, 38, 46, 47 | 8. Administer oral medications | Ch 53; Proc 53-5 | | |
| 9. Describe implications for treatment related to pathology | Ch 23–35, 45, 46 | 9. Administer parenteral (excluding IV) medications | Ch 53, 54; Proc 53-6, 53-7, 53-8, 53-9, 54-1, 54-2, 54-3, 54-4, 54-5, 54-6, 54-7 | | |
| 10. Compare body structure and function of the human body across the life span | Ch 23–35 | 10. Assist physician with patient care | Ch 39, 40, 41, 42, 46, 49, 50, 53, 54, 55, 57, 58; Proc 39-2, 39-3, 39-4, 49-1, 49-5, all in Ch 40, 41, 42, 50, 53 | | |
| 11. Identify the classifications of medications, including desired effects, side effects and adverse reactions | Ch 23–36, 51 | 11. Perform quality control measures | Ch 45, 46; Proc 45-1, 45-2, 46-2, 46-7, 46-11 | | |
| 12. Describe the relationship between anatomy and physiology of all body systems and medications used for treatment in each | Ch 23–35 | 12. Perform hematology testing | Ch 45, 46; Proc 45-1, 45-2, 45-3, 45-4, 45-5 | | |
| | | 13. Perform chemistry testing | Ch 45; Proc 45-6 | | |

| | | | | | |
|---|---|---|---|---|---|
| | | 14. Perform urinalysis | Ch 46; Proc 46-3, 46-4 | | |
| | | 15. Perform immunology testing | Ch 45; Proc 45-7 | | |
| | | 16. Screen test results | Ch 45, 46, 47; Proc 45-8, 47-1, 47-2 | | |
| **Cognitive** | | **Psychomotor** | | **Affective** | |
| **II.C Applied Mathematics** | **Reference** | **II.P Applied Mathematics** | **Reference** | **II.A Applied Mathematics** | **Reference** |
| 1. Demonstrate knowledge of basic math computations | Ch 52 | 1. Prepare proper dosages of medication for administration | Ch 53, 54; Proc 53-5, all Proc in Ch 54 | 1. Verify ordered doses/dosages prior to administration | Ch 53, 54; Proc 53-5, all Proc in Ch 54 |
| 2. Apply mathematical computations to solve equations | Ch 52 | 2. Maintain laboratory test results using flow sheets | Ch 45; Proc 45-5 | 2. Distinguish between normal and abnormal test results | Ch 40, 45, 46, 47; Proc 40-9, 45-8, 46-5; 47-1, 47-2 |
| 3. Identify measurement systems | Ch 52 | 3. Maintain growth charts | Ch 42; Proc 42-1, 42-2 | | |
| 4. Define basic units of measurement in metric, apothecary and household systems | Ch 52 | | | | |
| 5. Convert among measurement systems | Ch 52 | | | | |
| 6. Identify both abbreviations and symbols used in calculating medication dosages | Ch 52 | | | | |
| 7. Analyze charts, graphs and/or tables in the interpretation of healthcare results | Ch 42, 45 | | | | |
| **Cognitive** | | **Psychomotor** | | **Affective** | |
| **III.C Applied Microbiology/Infection Control** | **Reference** | **III.P Applied Microbiology/Infection Control** | **Reference** | **III.A Applied Microbiology/Infection Control** | **Reference** |
| 1. Describe the infection cycle, including the infectious agent, reservoir, susceptible host, means of transmission, portals of entry, and portals of exit | Ch 36 | 1. Participate in training on Standard Precautions | Ch 36 | 1. Display sensitivity to patient rights and feelings in collecting specimens | Ch 43, 45, 46, 50; Proc 43-2, 43-3, 43-4, all in Ch 45-46, 50-1, 50-2 |
| 2. Define asepsis | Ch 36, 49 | 2. Practice Standard Precautions | Ch 36, 43, 45, 46, 49, 55; Proc 36-2, 36-3, 36-4, 49-3, 49-4; *All clinical and lab procedures* | 2. Explain the rationale for performance of a procedure to the patient | Ch 40, 41, 43, 45, 46, 50; Proc 41-1, 43-2, 43-3, 43-4; *All clinical and lab procedures* |

| 3. Discuss infection control procedures. | Ch 36, 39, 49 | 3. Select appropriate barrier/personal protective equipment (PPE) for potentially infectious situations | Ch 36, 45, 46, 49, 50, 55; Proc 36-4, 36-5, 36-6, 49-3, 49-4, all in Ch 45, 46, 50 | 3. Show awareness of patients' concerns regarding their perceptions related to the procedure being performed | Ch 40, 41, 42, 43, 45, 46, 47, 50, 53, 54; Proc 40-1, 41-1, 42-1, 47-1, 53-5, all in Ch 43, 45, 46, 50, 54 |
|---|---|---|---|---|---|
| 4. Identify personal safety precautions as established by the Occupational Safety and Health Administration (OSHA) | Ch 36, 44 | 4. Perform handwashing | Ch 36, 49; Proc 36-2, 49-2 | | |
| 5. List major types of infectious agents | Ch 36 | 5. Prepare items for autoclaving | Ch 36; Proc 36-5, 36-7 | | |
| 6. Compare different methods of controlling the growth of microorganisms | Ch 36 | 6. Perform sterilization procedures | Ch 36; Proc 36-6, 36-8 | | |
| 7. Match types and uses of personal protective equipment (PPE) | Ch 36, 44 | 7. Obtain specimens for microbiological testing | Ch 43, 46, 50; Proc 43-2, 43-3, 43-4, 46-6, 46-9, 46-10, 46-11, 50-1, 50-2 | | |
| 8. Differentiate between medical and surgical asepsis used in ambulatory care settings, identifying when each is appropriate | Ch 36, 49 | 8. Perform CLIA waived microbiology testing | Ch 46; Proc 46-7, 46-11 | | |
| 9. Discuss quality control issues related to handling microbiological specimens | Ch 44, 45, 46 | | | | |
| 10. Identify disease processes that are indications for CLIA waived tests | Ch 45, 46 | | | | |
| 11. Describe Standard Precautions, including: | Ch 36, 55 | | | | |
| a. Transmission based precautions | Ch 36 | | | | |
| b. Purpose | Ch 36 | | | | |
| c. Activities regulated | Ch 36 | | | | |
| 12. Discuss the application of Standard Precautions with regard to: | Ch 36, 55 | | | | |
| a. All body fluids, secretions and excretions | Ch 36 | | | | |
| b. Blood | Ch 36 | | | | |
| c. Non intact skin | Ch 36 | | | | |
| d. Mucous membranes | Ch 36 | | | | |
| 13. Identify the role of the Center for Disease Control (CDC) regulations in healthcare settings. | Ch 5, 36 | | | | |

| Cognitive | | Psychomotor | | Affective | |
|---|---|---|---|---|---|
| **IV.C Concepts of Effective Communication** | **Reference** | **IV.P Concepts of Effective Communication** | **Reference** | **IV.A Concepts of Effective Communication** | **Reference** |
| 1. Identify styles and types of verbal communication | Ch 7 | 1. Use reflection, restatement and clarification techniques to obtain a patient history | Ch 37; Proc 37-1, 37-2 | 1. Demonstrate empathy in communicating with patients, family and staff | Ch 7, 8, 9, 37; Proc 7-1, 8-1, 9-1, 37-1, 37-2 |
| 2. Identify nonverbal communication | Ch 7 | 2. Report relevant information to others succinctly and accurately | Ch 9, 10, 22, 37, 53, 55; Proc 9-1, 9-3, 10-1, 22-2, 37-1, 37-2, 53-2 | 2. Apply active listening skills | Ch 7, 8, 9, 37; Proc 7-1, 8-1, 9-1, 9-2, 37-1, 37-2 |
| 3. Recognize communication barriers | Ch 7 | 3. Use medical terminology, pronouncing medical terms correctly, to communicate information, patient history, data and observations | Ch 10, 37; Proc 10-1, 37-1, 37-2 | 3. Use appropriate body language and other nonverbal skills in communicating with patients, family and staff | Ch 7, 8, 37; Proc 7-1, 8-1, 37-1, 37-2 |
| 4. Identify techniques for overcoming communication barriers | Ch 7, 9, 37 | 4. Explain general office policies | Ch 12; Proc 12-4 | 4. Demonstrate awareness of the territorial boundaries of the person with whom communicating | Ch 7, 8, 37; Proc 7-1, 8-1, 37-1, 37-2 |
| 5. Recognize the elements of oral communication using a sender-receiver process | Ch 7 | 5. Instruct patients according to their needs to promote health maintenance and disease prevention | Ch 8, 40, 41, 57, 58; Proc 8-1, 40-8, 41-1 | 5. Demonstrate sensitivity appropriate to the message being delivered | Ch 9; Proc 9-1 |
| 6. Differentiate between subjective and objective information | Ch 13, 37 | 6. Prepare a patient for procedures and/or treatments | Ch 39, 40, 41, 42, 47, 55, 57; all Proc in Ch 40, 41, 42, 47 | 6. Demonstrate awareness of how an individual's personal appearance affects anticipated responses | Ch 7; Ch 7 WB Video Case Study |
| 7. Identify resources and adaptations that are required based on individual needs, i.e., culture and environment, developmental life stage, language, and physical threats to communication | Ch 8, 37 | 7. Demonstrate telephone techniques | Ch 9, 53, 55; Proc 9-1, 9-2, 9-3, 53-2 | 7. Demonstrate recognition of the patient's level of understanding in communications | Ch 8, 9, 37, 53; Proc 8-1, 9-3, 37-1, 37-2, 53-2 |
| 8. Recognize elements of fundamental writing skills | Ch 10 | 8. Document patient care | Telephone documentation: Ch 9; *Included in all appropriate procedures* | 8. Analyze communications in providing appropriate responses/feedback | Ch 8, 9, 37; Proc 8-1, 9-1, 37-1, 37-2 |
| 9. Discuss applications of electronic technology in effective communication | Ch 9, 10, 11 | 9. Document patient education | Ch 8, 58; Proc 8-1 | 9. Recognize and protect personal boundaries in communicating with others | Ch 8, 37; Proc 37-1, 37-2; Ch 8 WB Video Case Study |
| 10. Diagram medical terms, labeling the word parts | Ch 3, 4 | 10. Compose professional/business letters | Ch 10; Proc 10-1 | 10. Demonstrate respect for individual diversity, incorporating awareness of one's own biases in areas including gender, race, religion, age and economic status | Ch 7, 8, 37; Proc 7-1, 8-1, 37-1, 37-2; Ch 8 WB Video Case Study |

| | | | | | |
|---|---|---|---|---|---|
| 11. Define both medical terms and abbreviations related to all body systems | Ch 3, 4 | 11. Respond to nonverbal communication | Ch 7, Proc 7-1 | | |
| 12. Organize technical information and summaries | Ch 10, 11 | 12. Develop and maintain a current list of community resources related to patients' healthcare needs | Ch 9; Proc 9-4 | | |
| 13. Identify the role of self boundaries in the health care environment | Ch 7, 8 | 13. Advocate on behalf of patients | Ch 8; Proc 8-2 | | |
| 14. Recognize the role of patient advocacy in the practice of medical assisting | Ch 8 | | | | |
| 15. Discuss the role of assertiveness in effective professional communication | Ch 8 | | | | |
| 16. Differentiate between adaptive and nonadaptive coping mechanisms | Ch 7 | | | | |
| **Cognitive** | | **Psychomotor** | | **Affective** | |
| **V.C Administrative Functions** | **Reference** | **V.P Administrative Functions** | **Reference** | **V.A Administrative Functions** | **Reference** |
| 1. Discuss pros and cons of various types of appointment management systems | Ch 12 | 1. Manage appointment schedule, using established priorities | Ch 12; Proc 12-1 | 1. Consider staff needs and limitations in establishment of a filing system | Ch 13 |
| 2. Describe scheduling guidelines | Ch 12 | 2. Schedule patient admissions and/or procedures | Ch 12; Proc 12-2 | 2. Implement time management principles to maintain effective office function | Ch 9, 37; Proc 9-1, 37-1, 37-2 |
| 3. Recognize office policies and protocols for handling appointments | Ch 12 | 3. Organize a patient's medical record | Ch 13; Proc 13-1 | | |
| 4. Identify critical information required for scheduling patient admissions and/or procedures | Ch 12 | 4. File medical records | Ch 13; Proc 13-2, 13-3 | | |
| 5. Identify systems for organizing medical records | Ch 13 | 5. Execute data management using electronic healthcare records such as the EMR | Ch 12; Proc 12-3 | | |
| 6. Describe various types of content maintained in a patient's medical record | Ch 13 | 6. Use office hardware and software to maintain office systems | Ch 11, Proc 11-1, 11-2 | | |
| 7. Discuss pros and cons of various filing methods | Ch 13 | 7. Use internet to access information related to the medical office | Ch 8, 9; Proc 8-2, 9-4, 9-5 | | |
| 8. Identify both equipment and supplies needed for filing medical records | Ch 13 | 8. Maintain organization by filing | Ch 13; Proc 13-2, 13-3 | | |
| 9. Describe indexing rules | Ch 13 | 9. Perform routine maintenance of office equipment with documentation | Ch 11, 44; Proc 11-3, 44-1 | | |
| 10. Discuss filing procedures | Ch 13 | 10. Perform an office inventory | Ch 21, Proc 21-2 | | |

| 11. Discuss principles of using Electronic Medical Record (EMR) | Ch 11,13 | | | | |
|---|---|---|---|---|---|
| 12. Identify types of records common to the healthcare setting | Ch 13 | | | | |
| 13. Identify time management principles | Ch 1, 9 | | | | |
| 14. Discuss the importance of routine maintenance of office equipment | Ch 11, 44 | | | | |
| **Cognitive** | | **Psychomotor** | | **Affective** | |
| **VI.C Basic Practice Finances** | **Reference** | **VI.P Basic Practice Finances** | **Reference** | **VI.A Basic Practice Finances** | **Reference** |
| 1. Explain basic bookkeeping computations. | Ch 16, 20 | 1. Prepare a bank deposit | Ch 19; Proc 19-2 | 1. Demonstrate sensitivity and professionalism in handling accounts receivable activities with clients | Ch 16, 18 |
| 2. Differentiate between bookkeeping and accounting | Ch 16, 20 | 2. Perform accounts receivable procedures, including: | | | |
| 3. Describe banking procedures | Ch 19 | a. Post entries on a daysheet | Ch 16; Proc 16-1 | | |
| 4. Discuss precautions for accepting checks. | Ch 19 | b. Perform billing procedures | Ch 16, 17, 18 | | |
| 5. Compare types of endorsement | Ch 19 | c. Perform collection procedures | Ch 18; Proc 18-1 | | |
| 6. Differentiate between accounts payable and accounts receivable | Ch 20 | d. Post adjustments | Ch 16; Proc 16-1 | | |
| 7. Compare manual and computerized bookkeeping systems used in ambulatory healthcare | Ch 16 | e. Process a credit balance | Ch 18; Proc 18-2 | | |
| 8. Describe common periodic financial reports | Ch 20 | f. Process refunds | Ch 18; Proc 18-2 | | |
| 9. Explain both billing and payment options. | Ch 16, 18 | g. Post non-sufficient fund (NSF) checks. | Ch 18; Proc 18-1 | | |
| 10. Identify procedure for preparing patient accounts | Ch 16 | h. Post collection agency payments. | Ch 18; Proc 18-1 | | |
| 11. Discuss procedures for collecting outstanding accounts | Ch 18 | 3. Utilize computerized office billing systems | Ch 16; Proc 16-1 | | |
| 12. Describe the impact of both the Fair Debt Collection Act and the Federal Truth in Lending Act of 1968 as they apply to collections | Ch 18 | | | | |
| 13. Discuss types of adjustments that may be made to a patient's account | Ch 16, 17, 18, 20 | | | | |

| Cognitive | | Psychomotor | | Affective | |
|---|---|---|---|---|---|
| **VII.C Managed Care/Insurance** | **Reference** | **VII.P Managed Care/Insurance** | **Reference** | **VII.A Managed Care/Insurance** | **Reference** |
| 1. Identify types of insurance plans | Ch 14 | 1. Apply both managed care policies and procedures | Ch 14, 17; Proc 17-1 | 1. Demonstrate assertive communication with managed care and/or insurance providers | Ch 14 |
| 2. Identify models of managed care | Ch 14 | 2. Apply third party guidelines | Ch 14, 17; Proc 17-1 | 2. Demonstrate sensitivity in communicating with both providers and patients | Ch 14 |
| 3. Discuss workers' compensation as it applies to patients | Ch 14 | 3. Complete insurance claim forms | Ch 14, 17; Proc 17-1 | 3. Communicate in language the patient can understand regarding managed care and insurance plans | Ch 14 |
| 4. Describe procedures for implementing both managed care and insurance plans | Ch 14 | 4. Obtain precertification, including documentation | Ch 14; Proc 14 | | |
| 5. Discuss utilization review principles. | Ch 12, 14 | 5. Obtain preauthorization, including documentation | Ch 14; Proc 14 | | |
| 6. Discuss referral process for patients in a managed care program | Ch 14 | 6. Verify eligibility for managed care services | Ch 12, 14; Proc 12 | | |
| 7. Describe how guidelines are used in processing an insurance claim | Ch 14, 17 | | | | |
| 8. Compare processes for filing insurance claims both manually and electronically | Ch 17 | | | | |
| 9. Describe guidelines for third-party claims | Ch 17 | | | | |
| 10. Discuss types of physician fee schedules | Ch 14 | | | | |
| 11. Describe the concept of RBRVS | Ch 14 | | | | |
| 12. Define Diagnosis-Related Groups(DRGs) | Ch 14 | | | | |

| Cognitive | | Psychomotor | | Affective | |
|---|---|---|---|---|---|
| **VIII.C Procedural and Diagnostic Coding** | **Reference** | **VIII.P Procedural and Diagnostic Coding** | **Reference** | **VIII.A Procedural and Diagnostic Coding** | **Reference** |
| 1. Describe how to use the most current procedural coding system | Ch 15 | 1. Perform procedural coding | Ch 15; Proc 15-1 | 1. Work with physician to achieve the maximum reimbursement | Ch 15; Proc 15-1, 15-2 |
| 2. Define upcoding and why it should be avoided | Ch 15 | 2. Perform diagnostic coding | Ch 15; Proc 15-2 | | |
| 3. Describe how to use the most current diagnostic coding classification system | Ch 15 | | | | |
| 4. Describe how to use the most current HCPCS coding | Ch 15 | | | | |

| Cognitive | | Psychomotor | | Affective | |
|---|---|---|---|---|---|
| **IX.C Legal Implications** | **Reference** | **IX.P Legal Implications** | **Reference** | **IX.A Legal Implications** | **Reference** |
| 1. Discuss legal scope of practice for medical assistants | Ch 1, 5, 53 | 1. Respond to issues of confidentiality | Ch 12; Proc 12-3, 12-4 | 1. Demonstrate sensitivity to patient rights | Ch 12, 37, 43; Proc 12-4, 37-1, 37-2; *throughout* |
| 2. Explore issue of confidentiality as it applies to the medical assistant. | Ch 5 | 2. Perform within scope of practice | Ch 53 | 2. Demonstrate awareness of the consequences of not working within the legal scope of practice | Ch 5, 53 |
| 3. Describe the implications of HIPAA for the medical assistant in various medical settings | Ch 5, 11, 22 | 3. Apply HIPAA rules in regard to privacy/release of information | Ch 12; Proc 12-3, 12-4 | 3. Recognize the importance of local, state and federal legislation and regulations in the practice setting | Ch 2, 53 |
| 4. Summarize the Patient Bill of Rights | Ch 12 | 4. Practice within the standard of care for a medical assistant | Ch 5 | | |
| 5. Discuss licensure and certification as it applies to healthcare providers | Ch 2 | 5. Incorporate the Patient's Bill of Rights into personal practice and medical office policies and procedures | Ch 12; Proc 12-4 | | |
| 6. Describe liability, professional, personal injury, and third party insurance | Ch 22 | 6. Complete an incident report | Ch 36; Proc 36-1 | | |
| 7. Compare and contrast physician and medical assistant roles in terms of standard of care | Ch 5 | 7. Document accurately in the patient record | Ch 5, 37; Proc 37-1, 37-2; *all clinical and lab procedures* | | |
| 8. Compare criminal and civil law as it applies to the practicing medical assistant. | Ch 5 | 8. Apply local, state and federal health care legislation and regulation appropriate to the medical assisting practice setting | Ch 36, 53; Proc 36-1, 53-1, 53-3 | | |
| 9. Provide an example of tort law as it would apply to a medical assistant | Ch 5 | | | | |
| 10. Explain how the following impact the medical assistant's practice and give examples | Ch 5 | | | | |
| a. Negligence | Ch 5 | | | | |
| b. Malpractice | Ch 5 | | | | |
| c. Statute of Limitations | Ch 5 | | | | |
| d. Good Samaritan Act(s) | Ch 5 | | | | |
| e. Uniform Anatomical Gift Act | | | | | |
| f. Living will/Advanced directives | Ch 5 | | | | |
| g. Medical durable power of attorney | Ch 5 | | | | |
| 11. Identify how the Americans with Disabilities Act (ADA) applies to the medical assisting profession | Ch 5 | | | | |

| | | | | | |
|---|---|---|---|---|---|
| 12. List and discuss legal and illegal interview questions | Ch 59 | | | | |
| 13. Discuss all levels of governmental legislation and regulation as they apply to medical assisting practice, including FDA and DEA regulations | Ch 1, 5, 44, 51, 53 | | | | |
| 14. Describe the process to follow if an error is made in patient care | Ch 53 | | | | |
| **Cognitive** | | **Psychomotor** | | **Affective** | |
| **X.C Ethical Considerations** | **Reference** | **X.P Ethical Considerations** | **Reference** | **X.A Ethical Considerations** | **Reference** |
| 1. Differentiate between legal, ethical, and moral issues affecting healthcare | Ch 6, 51 | 1. Report illegal and/or unsafe activities and behaviors that affect health, safety and welfare of others to proper authorities | Ch 6; Ch 6 WB Critical Thinking | 1. Apply ethical behaviors, including honesty/integrity in performance of medical assisting practice | Ch 6; Ch 6 WB Critical Thinking |
| 2. Compare personal, professional and organizational ethics | Ch 6 | 2. Develop a plan for separation of personal and professional ethics | Ch 6; Ch 6 WB Critical Thinking | 2. Examine the impact personal ethics and morals may have on the individual's practice | Ch 6; Ch 6 WB Critical Thinking |
| 3. Discuss the role of cultural, social and ethnic diversity in ethical performance of medical assisting practice | Ch 6 | | | 3. Demonstrate awareness of diversity in providing patient care | Ch 6, 58; Ch 6 WB Critical Thinking |
| 4. Identify where to report illegal and/or unsafe activities and behaviors that affect health, safety and welfare of others. | Ch 6 | | | | |
| 5. Identify the effect personal ethics may have on professional performance | Ch 6 | | | | |
| **Cognitive** | | **Psychomotor** | | **Affective** | |
| **XI.C Protective Practices** | **Reference** | **XI.P Protective Practices** | **Reference** | **XI.A Protective Practices** | **Reference** |
| 1. Describe personal protective equipment | Ch 36, 44 | 1. Comply with safety signs, symbols and labels. | Ch 21; Ch 21 WB Critical Thinking | 1. Recognize the effects of stress on all persons involved in emergency situations | Ch 21; Ch 21 WB Video Case Study |
| 2. Identify safety techniques that can be used to prevent accidents and maintain a safe work environment | Ch 21, 36, 44, 54 | 2. Evaluate the work environment to identify safe vs. unsafe working conditions. | Ch 21; Proc 21-1, 21-3 | 2. Demonstrate self awareness in responding to emergency situations | Ch 21; Ch 21 WB Video Case Study |
| 3. Describe the importance of Materials Safety Data Sheets (MSDS) in a healthcare setting | Ch 21 | 3. Develop a personal (patient and employee) safety plan. | Ch 21; Proc 21-6 | | |
| 4. Identify safety signs, symbols and labels | Ch 21 | 4. Develop an environmental safety plan. | Ch 21; Proc 21-6 | | |
| 5. State principles and steps of professional/provider CPR | Ch 55 | 5. Demonstrate proper use of the following equipment: | | | |

| 6. Describe basic principles of first aid | Ch 55, 56 | a. Eyewash | Ch 21 | | |
|---|---|---|---|---|---|
| 7. Describe fundamental principles for evacuation of a healthcare setting | Ch 21 | b. Fire extinguishers | Ch 21, Proc 21-5 | | |
| 8. Discuss fire safety issues in a healthcare environment | Ch 21 | c. Sharps disposal containers | Ch 21, 43, 54 | | |
| 9. Discuss requirements for responding to hazardous material disposal | Ch 21, 36 | 6. Participate in a mock environmental exposure event with documentation of steps taken. | Ch 21; Proc 21-4 | | |
| 10. Identify principles of body mechanics and ergonomics. | Ch 11, 57 | 7. Explain an evacuation plan for a physician's office | Ch 21; Proc 21-6 | | |
| 11. Discuss critical elements of an emergency plan for response to a natural disaster or other emergency | Ch 21 | 8. Demonstrate methods of fire prevention in the healthcare setting | Ch 21, Proc 21-5 | | |
| 12. Identify emergency preparedness plans in your community | Ch 21 | 9. Maintain provider/professional level CPR certification. | | | |
| 13. Discuss potential role(s) of the medical assistant in emergency preparedness | Ch 21, 55 | 10. Perform first aid procedures | Ch 55, 56 | | |
| | | 11. Use proper body mechanics | Ch 40, 41, 57; Proc 40-1, 41-1, 57-1 | | |
| | | 12. Maintain a current list of community resources for emergency preparedness | Ch 9; Proc 9-5 | | |

# CONCEPTS AND PRINCIPLES OF TEACHING AND LEARNING

## Vhat is Teaching?

he word *teaching* implies that a person with knowledge in some area is assisting another person in *learning,* or acquiring that ame information or capability. The teaching–learning process has been in progress since the beginning of time. Teaching volves the imparting of information and insight from one's own experiences as well as one's areas of knowledge.

Philosophically, is it possible to teach if there is not a learner? Unless someone learns, has teaching taken place? The nswer is "no." Knowing the subject matter well does not automatically ensure that it can be taught to others. Instructors must lan their own activities as well as those for their students. It is an instructor's responsibility to plan the experiences or activities which the learner will take part; it is the student's responsibility to learn.

You cannot *give* learners any skills or knowledge. Learners must be engaged in active experiences that will change the ay they think or act. Not only must they receive information, but they also must attempt to use new ideas and put them into ractice. It is the teacher's responsibility to lead students as quickly as possible to the mastery of the skills and knowledge, ithout having them experience random trial-and-error efforts to learn.

Teaching involves guiding the learners through planned experiences in such a way that they make steady progress in erfecting skills or understanding new ideas. Failing to provide for learners in a way that is appropriate for their learning styles ill usually result in disappointment for the teacher as well as the students. Students will be unable to do what they have been hown or to understand what they have been told. In other words: telling is not teaching, listening is not learning, and watching is ot learning. But, all three may need to be used to assist learning.

Thus, the ways and means of teaching (teaching methods) have a profound effect on how students learn, and they annot be selected at random. Methods must be selected on the basis of knowing how learners learn.

## Iow do Students Learn?

he way in which a person learns something is called the person's learning style. Not all people learn the same way. Each style is ot exclusive and we all use a combination styles. Nonetheless, one method usually provides more success than another when it matched to what needs to be learned.

### isual Learners

ome people are visual learners; they learn best by looking at or watching something. For example, these people have little ifficulty perceiving information from books, projected material, or other written materials. They can watch a demonstration of a kill and return the demonstration fairly accurately.

### uditory Learners

ome people may be auditory learners; they learn best from hearing information. They respond well to directions from audio, resentations, discussions, and verbal instructions.

### inesthetic Learners

inally, other people may be kinesthetic/tactile learners; they learn best by touching or participating in an activity. They must erform a skill to learn it, or use somewhat different approaches to learning. For example, a student who has difficulty mastering medical terminology by studying the words or spelling them orally may be successful by tracing the words on the desktop with a finger.

### Learning Preferences

In addition to the visual, auditory, and kinesthetic/tactile styles are learning preferences. Self/individual learners do best alone and in quiet surroundings, since they are distracted by others and by interferences in their environment. These learners like to study independently and are usually self-motivated. They may have difficulty sharing information. Group learners, on the other hand, enjoy working on team activities, as well as studying and sharing their findings with others.

There are no good or bad learning styles, only differences that influence the way we perceive, process, and learn new information and behaviors. An instructor who develops the ability to understand how individual students learn best will be able to provide them with the alternative methods they need to master information and achieve great success.

**Clinical Pearl:** As an instructor, it is important to consider how you learn new information. Outside the formal classroom, think of how you have learned from written, audio, or visual materials without the presence of an instructor. Realizing your own preferences for learning will help you understand why you select certain methods of instruction. You may learn best by listening to information and taking notes, but your teaching methods should be varied so all learning styles can be accommodated. Your students' learning will be nurtured when you use a variety of teaching methods, provide a choice of activities, and accept results that are not necessarily exactly what you expected.

## Basic Learning Principles

The following information is included to give you a basis for understanding the learning process and how it affects attempts of individuals to learn new things. An instructor should consider some of the principles before planning learning experiences for students, including the following:

1. *We learn best when we are ready to learn.* With a strong purpose and a well-fixed reason, it is easier to receive instruction and make progress in learning.
2. *The more often we use what we have learned the better we can perform or understand it.* Long disuse can result in forgetting.
3. *If the things we have learned are useful and beneficial to us so that we are satisfied with what we have accomplished, we better retain what we have learned.* We are also more likely to desire to learn more.
4. *Learning something new is easier when we build upon something we already know.* It is best to start with simple steps that are related to things we can do or already understand and then proceed to new and more difficult tasks or ideas.
5. *Learning has to be accomplished step by step.* Every new thing we learn needs to be connected in as many ways as possible with things we already know. This can only be done if learning proceeds in an orderly way, one step at a time.
6. *Learning takes place by doing.* Before learning can become complete, we must put into practice what we are attempting to learn.
7. *Successful learning stimulates more learning.* Failure to learn or to understand discourages further learning. As far as possible, the teacher needs to plan instruction so that successful learning is ensured each step of the way.
8. *It is important that both the teacher and the learner know that the learner has really learned—that there is no pretending to please the instructor that something has been learned.* Knowing that one has learned is one way of reinforcing learning so that further learning is made easier.

9. *Generally speaking, the sooner the learner can have the satisfaction of knowing that something has been learned, the more ready the learner is for additional learning.* (Adapted from Leighbody, G.B. and Kidd, D.M. *Methods of Teaching Shop and Technical Subjects.* Delmar, Cengage Learning, Clifton Park, NY: 2000.)

Another text, *Learning System Design: An Approach to the Improvement of Instruction* by Davis et al., cites nine other eneral principles of learning and motivation:

1. *Meaningfulness: Students are likely to be motivated to learn things that are meaningful to them.* Meaningfulness is personal; something that is meaningful to you is apt to be important to you personally. Students are motivated by what they can relate to their experiences, their future, their interests, and their values. For example, when you are trying to explain how a person's temperature rises, remind students of when they may have had chills and fever with the flu.
2. *Prerequisites: Students are more likely to learn something new when they have all the prerequisites.* A student's past learning is probably the most important factor determining success or failure in learning. For example, a student who has learned to add, subtract, and multiply has the prerequisites to learn to divide, and is more likely to learn. In medical assisting, a student cannot be expected to convert a temperature from one scale to another without prerequisite math skills.
3. *Modeling: Students are more likely to acquire new behavior when presented with a model performance to watch and imitate.* Behave in the same fashion you want your students to behave. Rather than just telling them how to do something correctly, show them. Be aware that students are likely to imitate anything you do. Students who are taught by modeling are more likely to learn than students who are taught by telling. This is especially relevant to skill instruction. The importance and accuracy you demonstrate will be imitated by the students.
4. *Open Communication: Students are more likely to learn when the presentation is structured so that the instructor's messages are open to the students' inspection.* State all messages in a way that will ensure their reception by students. Stimulate as many of their senses as possible. Tell students exactly what is expected of them so that the open communication principle is not violated. For instance, course requirements, information, and examples should not be unclear, leading students to believe they are secrets.
5. *Novelty: Students are more likely to learn when their attention is attracted by relatively novel presentations.* Consider what students usually see and hear. Vary your style and means of presentation from the usual. For example, when teaching grooming, present the lesson attired and groomed in a totally unacceptable fashion. The students will never forget your message.
6. *Active Appropriate Practice: Students are more likely to learn when they take an active part in practice geared toward an instructional objective.* To learn, students should be given the opportunity to respond as they would in an actual setting. In other words, you cannot learn to paint by listening to a lecture or by taking notes while watching an artist. In the medical assisting field, it is absolutely essential that students participate actively in the practice of skills and procedures in a realistic simulated situation, with clearly stated performance objectives to be achieved.
7. *Distributed Practice: Students are more likely to learn when practice is scheduled in short periods distributed over time.* Excessively long practice sessions lead to fatigue, unpleasant associations with the subject matter, and mistakes in practice. To ensure that practice is productive, the teacher must have it well structured, meaningful, and vary the tasks to be accomplished. Very few students would become fatigued at a three-hour party.
8. *Fading: Students are more likely to learn when instruction prompts are withdrawn gradually.* Providing hints and prompting is important at the beginning, but these should be withdrawn systematically as learning occurs. If withdrawal does not occur, students begin to rely on the prompts. If it occurs too rapidly, students make errors. For example, the

need to protect oneself with gloves when performing particular procedures is essential. If you continue to tell the student this step, the behavior will not be learned.

9. *Pleasant Conditions and Consequences: Students are more likely to continue learning when instructional conditions are made pleasant.* To do this, you must eliminate the negative aspect of instruction and accentuate the positive aspects. For instance, you would eliminate the possibility of being bored by providing challenges and variety; frustrated from being placed in a situation where unattainable demands are made; or having an unpleasant experience, such as harsh comparison of a student's work or threat of failure.

**Clinical Pearl:** The following are some best practices when teaching:

- *Set challenging tasks during training.* A task with a 90% probability of success is too easy. One with only a 10% chance is too difficult. Neither is a challenge. Try to achieve about a 50% likelihood of success on the first attempt.
- *Give students knowledge of results.* Students should be told what they have done well and what they have done poorly. With poor results, students should be told how to improve their performance. Knowledge of results serves to improve performance and provide an incentive. Remember, the unsuccessful student needs feedback the most, but make it a helpful learning experience.
- *Reward students' efforts.* Unfortunately, many desirable student behaviors go unrewarded and many undesirable behaviors are rewarded simply by the amount of time and attention paid to them. Reward a desirable action as soon as it is detected. The action immediately preceding the reward is the one that will continue.

## Steps in the Learning Process

The first step in learning occurs when we receive a new impression or perceive a new stimulus. We have learned something when we do something that we could not do before or understand something we previously did not understand. If learning begins with perceptions or impressions, then the teacher needs to know how to send these messages to learners.

We receive impressions through our senses: sight, hearing, smell, touch, and taste. The most important way we receive impressions is through the eyes. If so much of what we learn comes from what we visualize, then it is very important that the teacher effectively provide students with visual impressions. We receive visual impressions from:

- Activities of people and things we observe
- Illustrations, art, video images, and television
- Written materials

The second way in which we receive most impressions is through our sense of hearing. The trained ear of an engine mechanic can identify particular sounds and diagnose problems. The physician learns to identify disease conditions based on sounds heard through a stethoscope. Learning occurs in the classroom and lab from hearing the lesson and explanations of procedures. We also learn from hearing questions and their answers, participating in discussions, and listening to videos, movies, and audiotapes.

The sense of touch is very important in some types of work. It ensures the quality of the finish on a product, for instance, or permits the fine adjustments of gauges to inspect a machined part. Again, physicians use the sense of touch to palpate the body and interpret findings.

To a somewhat lesser degree, the senses of smell and taste provide avenues for learning. We certainly learn from experience to identify substances based on their odor and taste. In the medical field, abnormal odors of the breath or urine can ave diagnostic significance. In other fields, chemists and food service personnel (for example) rely heavily on their senses of mell and taste.

It is wise to use as many senses as possible to present information, to ensure the best possible chance for learning. emember, some senses are more appropriate for conveying information than others. It would make little sense to teach students ) measure blood pressure by observing a manometer without first helping them to learn what to listen for with the stethoscope.

After a concept, fact, or skill is learned, it must be reinforced and used so it can develop into a behavior. We often say, I just do it from force of habit." What this really means is that the behavior we learned has been repeated so many times that ctive thinking is no longer required. Simple examples of this would be tying shoes or buttoning a coat (yet think how hard a )ddler struggles to learn these actions!). In medical assisting, you perform many procedures so frequently that you are not onscious of the steps you go through. Using the measurement of blood pressure as an example, think of all the steps required to erform this procedure accurately. When teaching students, you must demonstrate the way you wish to have them perform each dividual step, in the correct sequence. This will help them to develop quality skills.

Students will develop good skill habits when they learn from precise information, accurate demonstrations, skill ractice, reinforcement and correction, and repetition. Step by step, newly learned behaviors become habits.

Leighbody and Kidd also list facts that are important to the matter of habit formation:

1. *The first impression that the learner receives is a long-lasting impression.* This means the teacher's first demonstration must be clear and accurate. Mistaken ideas that are received by the student during the first demonstration are difficult to correct later. It is always a good idea to practice a procedure before you demonstrate it to your students. If the students are to follow a written procedure during a demonstration, you should also follow it just as it is written. It is often beneficial to have a student read the steps out loud as you perform the procedure; then you will neither omit nor add anything. In addition, since written materials are not always within your requirements, you will have the opportunity to make changes before the students begin practice.
2. *The sooner the student can attempt to practice a skill after seeing it demonstrated, the easier it will be to perform correctly and the sooner it will become a habit.* Remember, one of the principles of learning is that students are more likely to learn when they take an active part in practice geared toward an instructional objective.
3. *It is important that a skill be practiced as accurately as possible the first time it is attempted by the learner. The first practice determines, to a large extent, the manner in which the work will be performed in succeeding attempts.* One way to enhance a student's ability to perform a procedure correctly is to have students work in pairs with one reading and the other performing the steps in their correct sequence. However, it is the teacher's responsibility to closely observe new performers so that errors can be corrected promptly.
4. *The more often a skill is practiced, the sooner it will become a fixed habit.* If it is practiced incorrectly, it will become a habit that will have to be broken.
5. *Practice with the intent of improving is essential for the development of skill proficiency.*
6. *It is not possible to learn many skills at one time.* If a process involves many skills of a varied nature, it is better to divide the process into groups of skills and learn one group at a time.
7. *A skill that is learned well tends to be retained well.*
8. *For most skill learning, a number of short practice periods are more effective than a few long ones.*

Think of the learning process as a flight of stairs. Each step is a part of the total staircase. Individually, each step presents a portion of the whole and has a relationship to the one that precedes it and to the one that follows. A good lesson tep) is planned so that it continues from the preceding lesson and carries the learner forward naturally to the next one. The person who is climbing stairs can only reach the next step by using the one below. If any step is too high (difficult), the learner may find it impossible to reach.

**Clinical Pearl:** It is important to remember that students climb "stairs" at different rates. In your class, you may well have individuals standing on several steps at one time. You also should remember that climbing steps more slowly does not mean that the top will not be reached.

Put into practice what you have learned about teaching, learning, learning principles, perceiving information, and the steps in the learning process. Use methods to involve the various senses, vary your presentations, be alert to different learning styles, and make adjustments to meet your students' individual needs, and they will learn.

# DESIGNING LESSON PLANS

## Lesson Plan Organization

TITLE—Stated at the beginning of the instruction.

OBJECTIVES—Identify what the student should know or be able to do upon completion of this lesson. (These may be similar to the chapter objectives in the text, but will cover smaller segments of information.)

REFERENCES—Appropriate portion of the text from which the lesson will be taken. Also includes other sources from which information to be presented has been obtained. (Provide identification of sources of information.)

VISUAL AIDS—Software, video clips, illustrations, charts, models, etc to be utilized in the presentation of the lesson. (Noting the time required for videos, etc. is very helpful when planning lessons.)

EQUIPMENT/MATERIALS—Items that aid in lesson presentation, such as handouts, reference books, supplies, and demonstration equipment.

ESSENTIAL INSTRUCTIONAL COMPONENTS—Preparation, Presentation, Application, Evaluation, and Assignment.

## Essential Instructional Components

### PREPARATION

This step is actually two-fold. First, it identifies preparation of the instructor by describing what needs to be ready before the lesson can be taught (e.g., room arrangement, demonstration setup, review of text, demonstration volunteer). It is often advisable to practice a skill presentation to be certain all necessary materials are ready and the demonstration will be smooth. Second, it identifies the preparation of the students to receive the lesson. Any gimmick that secures their attention or arouses curiosity about the lesson will produce questions and ensure interest in what follows. For example, if you are presenting a lesson on proper office appearance, come to class dressed very inappropriately, wearing heavy cologne odor and chewing gum. The students' comments will lead directly to the content to be discussed, and they will always remember your presentation.

### PRESENTATION

This is the actual delivery of the material to be learned. Different types of information require different strategies. For instance, having students read a chapter would not be the best or only method to use in teaching them to perform a venipuncture. Some examples of instructional strategies and appropriate applications are as follows:

- **Lecture:** Presents information with which the student has little or no previous knowledge or experience; information goes from the teacher to the students. Appropriate for knowledge acquisition.
- **Discussion:** Presents information and requests input from students relative to the topic based on their knowledge of the subject matter; information goes from the teacher to the students and from the students to the teacher and other students. Appropriate for knowledge acquisition.
- **Panel Discussion:** Presents information by a group of people; provides variety and supplements the teacher's areas of knowledge. Presenters are usually considered knowledgeable in their fields. Appropriate for knowledge acquisition.
- **Guest Speaker:** Presents information by a person considered knowledgeable in the area being discussed; provides a variety of instruction and supplements the teacher's areas of knowledge. Appropriate for knowledge acquisition.

- **Role-Playing:** Portrays the position of another to make a concept or situation realistic. Very appropriate for the presentation of material dealing with attitudes and values. Also very appropriate for skill acquisition when portraying medical assistant/patient in laboratory practice.
- **Questioning:** Determines understanding. Appropriate for knowledge and skill acquisition.
- **Demonstration:** Presents procedure methods. Performed by the teacher for the instruction of the students. Appropriate for skill acquisition.
- **Visual Aid:** Supplements text illustrations and laboratory demonstrations to provide additional information. Appropriate for knowledge and skill acquisition.
- **Simulation:** Provides a safe environment for students to practice skills and behaviors, without the risk of making error "in real life." Appropriate for knowledge and skill acquisition.
- **Field Trip:** Supplements instructional program capabilities and provides additional information. Appropriate for knowledge, skill attitude, and value acquisition depending on the location visited.
- **Case Study:** Provides information from real-life situations that supplements the text and the instructor's areas of knowledge. Appropriate for knowledge, attitude, and value acquisition.
- **Independent Study:** Supplements text and adds to students' information. Can benefit other students if oral reports are given. Appropriate for knowledge, attitude, and value acquisition.
- **Testing:** Measures learning; gives students and the instructor information regarding the acquisition of knowledge.
- **Performance Procedure:** Measures learning; gives students and the instructor information regarding the acquisition of knowledge and skill.

There are many more examples that you can think of. The point is to vary your presentation of the lesson content with different strategies that will, according to the principles of learning, increase success. Successful teaching involves systematic, step-by-step presentation and includes periodic pauses to reinforce content and ask questions. Skill demonstration must follow the procedure as outlined in the text, or you must provide a written substitute.

## APPLICATION

Students should immediately apply the knowledge and/or skill that has just been presented. If the lesson was on related content, use situational examples to apply the concepts, assign Workbook exercises to reinforce the material, and utilize additional resources as appropriate. A skill presentation should be followed by an opportunity to practice the procedure that was demonstrated, following the steps as identified in the text. The students should be carefully observed so that errors in performance can be identified and corrected before they become learned. Following the written procedures should lead to proper technique.

## EVALUATION

This component can be formative or summative in nature. Evaluation should reflect the lesson's objectives. Evaluation strategies deal with determining whether learning has occurred. Some examples of evaluation strategies involve the following:

- **Questioning:** To assess understanding; usually used as formative evaluation and is done orally. Appropriate at any time throughout a course.
- **Quizzes:** To assess understanding; usually used as formative evaluation at the end of a small segment of instruction.
- **Tests:** To assess the acquisition of knowledge; usually used as summative evaluation at the ends of chapters, sections of instruction, or final examinations.

- **Checklists:** To assess acquisition of procedure skills; usually used as summative evaluation of performance. May also be used as a guide to self-evaluation during practice.
- **Progress Chart:** To display position in relation to total that is to be achieved. Provides input to students and teacher regarding progress.

Summative evaluation is usually the basis for determining grades. It can take various forms, such as a quiz, a test, a idterm, a final, as well as combination performance evaluations (taking vital signs, for example). Normally, the scores achieved n these performances result in the one grade earned for the course. In particular, it is these evaluations that are linked to the erformance objectives. The computerized test bank that accompanies the text will provide a means for summative evaluation of e material, since the test bank reflects the objectives of the text. The Competency Checklists in the Workbook provide a means f determining the evaluation of procedure performance; the Task is stated and each step is assessed a value that can be computed r a grade. The student knows all this information prior to performance.

Evaluation also provides the instructor with feedback as to the effectiveness of the presentation. If many students do not ccessfully demonstrate competence of either the related or skill information, then the method of presentation should be revised.

### SSIGNMENT

ssignments involve what the student should prepare, read, or study for the next class session.

## ample Lesson Plan

esson No. __________

| | ______________________________ |
|---|---|
| | (Title) |
| BJECTIVES: | (A brief, concise list of desired outcomes) |
| EFERENCES: | (Text pages to be covered, sources of information) |
| ISUAL AIDS: | (Identify by name, type, time, etc.) |
| QUIPMENT/MATERIALS: | (Lists items required to present lesson) |
| REPARATION: | (Teacher readiness and student readiness, three to five minutes; opening statement/activity that leads into presentation) |
| RESENTATION: | (30 to 45 minutes, covers content of lesson in logical sequence reflecting text or resource; if skill demonstration, presents each step and key point in a clear and concise manner) (Attach extra sheets as required to accommodate lesson outline.) |
| PPLICATION: | (Identifies method(s) to be used) |
| VALUATION: | (Lists oral questions; indicates written test or skill evaluation instrument) |
| SSIGNMENT: | (Optional: Identifies what the student should do to prepare for the next lesson or a future assignment) |

# 'UGGESTED CLASS ACTIVITIES

ʌs discussed, people acquire information best by different methods, so the more variety the better the chances to ensure the naterial is learned.

- **Buddy System**—One method of dealing with material missed by an absent student is to establish a *buddy system.* One person a week is assigned to be the "buddy" for those who are absent. This person is responsible for recording assignments, collecting handouts and other materials, and taking notes when appropriate. These are placed in a *buddy box,* which the absent student is responsible for checking when returning to class. This system frees the teacher for other duties and also teaches the students to assume responsibility.
- **Scrapbook**—If you enjoy photography and wish to have a record of students' achievements and activities, consider starting a "Photo Scrapbook" with the beginning of each new class. Besides pictures, you can include letters, activity programs, invitations, class events, and news items. The students will take a great deal of interest in having pictures and information about them included in the book.
- **Clinical Experience Reports**—If you have a clinical "observation" experience for students or a practicum program, take time during class to allow them to share what types of things they did, the kinds of patients they cared for, any problems they experienced, and what they learned. This allows students to talk about their activities, permits you to reinforce information and/or correct misconceptions, and encourages students to learn from one another's experiences. This can be in the form of an assignment with a structured sheet to complete and share or just an informal discussion if the students participate freely.
- **Review Bingo**—You can make a bingo game for any unit or chapter in the text that has sufficient new terminology to learn. If made from strong stock and perhaps laminated, the cards will last for many years. To play the game, place all cards in a box, shake, and pull out one piece. Read the definition only. Remember, since there are no column headings, you should allow enough time for students to search all squares for the term.
- **Mini-Health Clinic**—A mini-health clinic presents an excellent opportunity for students to demonstrate skills and obtain experience with people other than their classmates. Set up several screening stations and invite students from other programs, family members, school personnel, and friends to come to the clinic. Develop a health checkup sheet listing the stations with a space for each finding. Prepare a statement at the bottom declaring the health clinic to be an educational event for students and not to be considered as a physical examination. Have a space for the participant's signature indicating understanding and agreement to participate. This can be a great health education opportunity. For example, with pulse—a brief explanation of what pulse is and the "normal" ranges; with blood pressure—an explanation of what causes blood pressure and a chart of "normal ranges"; with visual screening—an explanation of what the numbers refer to, etc. With proper instruction, students can explain many of the assessments, giving them an excellent opportunity to practice patient teaching. Common screenings could include visual (Snellen), height/weight, pulse, blood pressure, urine testing, vital capacity, audiometer, temperature, Ishihara, Jaeger, and blood glucose.
- **Tray Setups**—Students are divided into teams and seated around a large table or work area. Instruments and materials are placed in the center of the table. In turn, students draw a card with a specific tray setup to prepare. The items are to be placed on the tray *in the order of use.* The first student to guess what the tray is used for earns a point for the team.
- **Word Identification**—This game is played with teams. The instructor gives a word (terminology or equipment), and the student must spell, define, or give the purpose of the term or equipment. A correct answer earns points for that student's team.

- **Increasing Student Response**—To get students to respond in class, use calling cards. Make a card for each student and place the cards within easy reach. Ask a question, then draw a card. (Calling the name first permits other students to let their minds wander.) To avoid having a student relax after being called, put the student's name back into the pack. If you should call a student's name three times, retire the card for this session.
- **When There Is Time Left Over**—When you finish presenting the lesson and there is still time before the class ends, use a copy of the workbook and ask students, at random, to give you their answers to a question. This tells you if the workbooks are up-to-date and provides motivation for students to be prepared for the *next* time.

# NSTRUCTOR NOTES FOR THE COMPETENCY CHALLENGE 2.0

## bout the Competency Challenge 2.0

the Competency Challenge 2.0, students will simulate a "week in the life" of an externship through 26 activities and a mprehensive patient case study, which are arranged on a Weekly Planner. Each activity corresponds to several general, lministrative, and clinical curriculum competencies.

On the Weekly Planner, Monday through Thursday focuses on specific medical assisting skills. Once an activity is lected on the Weekly Planner (Monday through Thursday), the student begins by watching a video or animation relating to the pic area. Then, the student will be required to complete a variety of questions and simulations in order to finish the activity.

The Friday activity is a capstone event, in which students follow a new patient through an office visit for a physical xam. This applies the competencies practiced on the previous days to a realistic patient case study.

## omputer Use and Log In Names

tudents must use the same computer each time using the Competency Challenge. Individual scores and competency information saved locally on the first computer used, and does not transfer between computers. So, students should always use the same omputer every time the Competency Challenge is accessed.

It is very important to note that when logging into the Competency Challenge program, students must use the same log name every time. Scores and competency information will be associated with this log in name. So, a different name is used, core and competency information will not appear in the program. Different names should only be used in the instance that more an one individual is using the program on the same computer.

## Jsing the Competency Challenge 2.0 with the Text

chapter correlation is included on the next page, to identify the activities that correspond to chapter content in *Medical ssisting: Administrative and Clinical Competencies, Seventh Edition*. Additional "How to Use" and "Help" file information is cluded within the software itself as well as on the Instructor Companion Site (www.cengage.com/login). Log in with your engage instructor password.

## coring the Competency Challenge 2.0

he Scores area keeps a record of all the activities completed, the time taken, and scores. If the student achieves a score of 75% r better on an activity (Monday through Thursday), the associated competencies will be "checked off" on the Competency hecklist. If the student scores less than 75%, the activity can be re-done until the threshold is met.

After all the activities are completed (Monday through Thursday) at the 75% score threshold, the Competency hecklist is completed. Students can print the Competency Checklist to hand in to the instructor, or to keep for their own records. ndividual activity scores can be printed as well.

## Weekly Planner Chapter Correlation

| | Monday | Tuesday | Wednesday | Thursday | Friday |
|---|---|---|---|---|---|
| **8:00** | Manage the Telephone and Make Appointments<br>Chapters 9, 12 | Perform General Clinical Practices<br>Chapter 36 | Perform Hematology Testing<br>Chapter 45 | Respond to Written Communication<br>Chapter 10 | Capstone<br>Patient Case Study |
| **9:00** | | Obtain Vital Signs<br>Chapter 38 | Perform Chemistry Testing<br>Chapter 45 | | |
| **10:00** | Manage the Medical Record<br>Chapter 13 | Prepare Patients for Exams<br>Chapter 39 | Perform Immunology Testing<br>Chapter 45 | Complete Inventory and Maintenance<br>Chapter 21 | |
| **11:00** | Perform Accounts Receivable Procedures<br>Chapter 16 | Prepare and Assist with Procedures, Treatments, and Minor Office Surgeries<br>Chapters 40, 50 | Perform Microbiology Testing<br>Chapter 46 | Prepare for Emergencies<br>Chapter 21 | |
| **12:00** | (Lunch) | | | | |
| **1:00** | Perform Billing and Collection Procedures and Post Accounting Transactions<br>Chapter 18 | Perform an Electrocardiogram<br>Chapter 47 | Perform Respiratory Testing<br>Chapter 40 | Respond to Legal and Ethical Issues<br>Chapters 5, 6 | |
| **2:00** | Perform Procedural and Diagnostic Coding<br>Chapter 15 | Perform a Venipuncture<br>Chapter 43 | Instruct in Urine Specimen Collection and Perform Urinalysis<br>Chapter 46 | | |
| **3:00** | Process Insurance Claims<br>Chapter 17 | Perform a Capillary Puncture<br>Chapter 43 | Instruct in Fecal Specimen Collection<br>Chapter 46 | Provide Patient Instructions<br>Chapter 8 or 40 | |
| **4:00** | | | Administer Medications<br>Chapter 54 | | |

# INSTRUCTOR NOTES FOR THE CRITICAL THINKING CHALLENGE 2.0

## About the Critical Thinking Challenge 2.0

The student is a character in each situation in the game, which simulates a 3-month externship in Dr. Conner's medical office. Students will be confronted with a series of situations in which critical thinking skills must be used to select the most correct action in response to the situation. Each situation is a video presented from the student's point of view. In some cases, the student will be directly involved in the situation, interacting with other staff members or patients; in other instances, the student will be a witness to the situation. However, in every situation presented, students must use critical thinking skills to respond.

## Using the Critical Thinking Challenge 2.0 with the Text

The Critical Thinking Challenge 2.0 can be used at any time throughout the medical assisting curriculum; it is not correlated to specific chapter skill content. Some programs use the Critical Thinking Challenge 2.0 as a capstone, or before students go out on externship or practicum. Additional "How to Use" information is included within the software itself as well as on the Instructor Companion Site (www.cengage.com/login). Log in with your Cengage instructor password.

## Scoring and Feedback

After each situation, students will receive positive and negative feedback discussing the merits of the decision made and the outcome of the situation, and then awarded points for overall decision-making skills.

Students receive points per situation according to the merits of the action chosen:

- Students receive 10 points for selecting the best action.
- Students receive 5 points for selecting a good action to take, but not the best action.
- Students do not receive any points for selecting the least-desirable action.

At the end of the game:

- If the score is *above 85 points*, the student will receive a certificate of completion as well as a "job offer" to work in Dr. Conner's office.
- If the score is *between 70 and 85 points*, the student will receive a certificate of completion as well as a letter of recommendation from Dr. Conner's office.
- If the score is *below 70 points,* game play is terminated and the student needs to start over. There is no certificate of completion at this level.
- The game is also terminated early if the least-desirable action is chosen by the student three times in a row at any point during game play.

The student completes the challenge successfully if he or she is able to print a certificate of completion, indicating a score of 70 or better. You may collect these certificates for grading purposes, and ultimately the students may keep the certificates in their portfolios.

## Scenario Synopses and Answer Keys

The following section summarizes each scenario and indicates correct answer choices. Correct answer choices are in **boldface** type.

**Scenario 1: Staph Infection**

| | |
|---|---|
| Objective of the scenario | Protecting the health and safety of the patients and medical staff |
| Synopsis of scenario | One of the medical assistants has been recently diagnosed with methicillin-resistant *Staphylococcus aureus* (MRSA) in a wound on the back of her hand. The medical assistant asks you not to say anything about her diagnosis because she needs the work. |
| Choices | 1) Tell your patients that staph is going around and they should take appropriate precautions like washing their hands, etc.<br>2) Assure the medical assistant that if she will cover her wound when working with patients, you will keep her secret.<br>3) **Tell the doctor what you have seen and what you know about this person.** |
| Follow-up | If the user does not select the most appropriate response (#3), the user receives a follow-up scenario: The medical assistant with MRSA continues to treat patients. The next week, Ms. Hunter, a patient, presents with what looks to be a staph infection, asking to see the doctor without an appointment. When you ask around, you find that this is the third patient that week that has come into the office with a staph infection. |
| Follow-up Choices | 1) Tell Ms. Hunter the office is really busy now and it would be better for her to come back in a few hours when things calm down.<br>2) Tell Ms. Hunter it doesn't look too serious and that she should try some OTC medications and call back if it doesn't resolve in a few days<br>3) **Explain to Ms. Hunter that you will put her chart in the queue although she may have to wait a little while around the regularly scheduled patients** |

**Scenario 2: Patient Confidentiality**

| | |
|---|---|
| Objective of the scenario | Observing HIPAA regulations with regard to electronic medical records and patient confidentiality |
| Synopsis of scenario | The office has an electronic health record system, and has computer laptops in each exam room; it is the responsibility of the medical assistant to ensure that previous patients' records are no longer displayed on the monitor. You escort Mr. Haskell to an exam room and ask him to disrobe in preparation for the exam. Back at the front desk, Mr. Haskell's cell phone is discovered. When you return to the exam room with Mr. Haskell's cell phone, you find him at the computer monitor reading the previous patient's medical history and diagnosis. |
| Choices | 1) Become angry with the patient for not following instructions and reading the other patient's record.<br>**2) Report the violation to the practice security officer.**<br>3) Tell the patient that is private information and he shouldn't tell anyone. Continue prepping for the exam. |

**Scenario 3: Dealing with Difficult Patients**

| | |
|---|---|
| Objective of the scenario | Emphasizing maintenance of composure and professionalism when confronted by an irate person |

| Synopsis of scenario | At the completion of the patient's visit, she comes to your window to schedule a follow-up appointment. You ask the patient to make her $20 co-payment, which is a policy posted in the office that co-payments are due at the time of service. She becomes angry, belligerent, and loud in reference to your request. |
|---|---|
| Choices | **1) Stay calm and explain the office policy.**<br>2) Ask the office manager to take control of the situation.<br>3) Yell back at the patient. Tell her she is being rude and unreasonable. |

**Scenario 4: Unauthorized Treatment**

| Objective(s) of the scenario | Making the correct moral/ethical decision and working within scope of practice |
|---|---|
| Synopsis of scenario | Cynthia Mason, another MA in the office, routinely brings her grandmother to the office to perform lab tests at no charge, also gets drug samples without asking the physician. Her grandmother is in poor health and does not have medical insurance. |
| Choices | 1) Tell your coworker that her secret is safe with you.<br>**2) Tell the doctor what this medical assistant has been doing behind her back.**<br>3) Ignore the incident and say nothing to anyone. |

**Scenario 5: Duty to Patients**

| Objective(s) of the scenario | Confronting coworkers who are acting inappropriately |
|---|---|
| Synopsis of scenario | Mr. Diaz, a Spanish-speaking patient, presents in the office with his daughter Maria to translate for him. Later, after the patient is roomed, you find Maurice Wallace, the MA, in the break room. He tells you that he's been invited to a party with Maria, but that he hasn't taken Mr. Diaz's vitals yet. |
| Choices | 1) Say "It's not OK to try to get a date with Mr. Diaz's daughter. Your responsibility is to Mr. Diaz, your patient."<br>2) Say "I guess there's no problem."<br>**3) Say, "It's not OK to try to get a date with Mr. Diaz's daughter." Report the incident to the office manager.** |
| Follow-up | If the user does not select the most appropriate response (#3), the user receives a follow-up scenario: Mr. Diaz becomes angry at Maurice for fraternizing with his daughter. He comes back to the front desk and demands to see the doctor. |
| Follow-up Choices | 1) Get the doctor.<br>2) Tell Mr. Diaz to calm down, and refrain from reporting the incident.<br>**3) Apologize to Mr. Diaz and get the office manager.** |

**Scenario 6: Overheard Conversation**

| Objective of the scenario | Demonstrating the need for empathy for all patients |
|---|---|

| | |
|---|---|
| Synopsis of scenario | One of the medical assistants, Cynthia Mason, has preconceived notions about disabled and obese patients. Cynthia sees Mr. Merrick in the waiting room, and starts telling another medical assistant how disgusting she thinks the patient is. She thinks that he is young enough that if he exercised, he wouldn't be obese and in a wheelchair, saying, "he's not disabled, he's just fat." Both you and the patient overhears the entire conversation. |
| Choices | **1) Console the patient. Later, report the incident to the office manager.**<br>2) Apologize for the conduct of your colleagues.<br>3) Pretend that nothing happened, and tell Mr. Merrick that the doctor will see him in a minute. |

**Scenario 7: Quality Controls**

| | |
|---|---|
| Objective of the scenario | CLIA '88 compliance |
| Synopsis of scenario | You perform a blood sugar test on a patient at the request of the nurse practitioner, who says the test is all set up. You don't run a control prior to performing the test. It's the end of the day, so you've assumed that the controls must have already been run. The results of the blood test are posted on the patient's medical record; the results are very low at 44 mg/dL. |
| Choices | 1) Tell the nurse practitioner the patient is ready to be seen.<br>**2) You consult the EMR's global log.**<br>3) Tell the nurse practitioner that the results seemed a little low. |

**Scenario 8: Child Abuse or Not?**

| | |
|---|---|
| Objective of the scenario | Emphasis on not jumping to conclusions |
| Synopsis of scenario | A parent brings injured child to the office for treatment of a bruised and swollen foot. During the in-person screening, the medical assistant notes other bruises on the child and suspects that the child is a victim of child abuse, not accidental injury. |
| Choices | 1) Call child protective services to report your suspicions.<br>**2) Discuss your observations with the nurse practitioner.**<br>3) Confront the parent about what you believe to be child abuse. |

**Scenario 9: Drug Samples**

| | |
|---|---|
| Objective of the scenario | Demonstrating ethical and moral judgment with close coworkers |
| Synopsis of scenario | A drug rep gives samples of an expensive and hard-to-find medication that Dr. Conners has requested. Cynthia Mason, an MA, sees the samples that the drug rep has left, and takes them. Later, you overhear Dr. Conners ask Cynthia if she has seen the samples, and her response that she says she doesn't know anything about it. You know that Cynthia has taken the medication. |
| Choices | 1) Tell the doctor what you saw.<br>2) Confront the medical assistant about the situation.<br>**3) Tell the office manager what you saw.** |

| | |
|---|---|
| Follow-up | If the user does not select response #1 or #3, the user receives a follow-up scenario: You confront Cynthia about the situation. You tell her you know she took the samples. She tells you that her sister is in a lot of pain. She also tells you that she could help you out, if you need samples for someone in your family. She asks you to keep it just between the two you. |
| Follow-up Choices | 1) Don't share the medications, but honor her request to keep quiet. You'd probably do the same thing if you were in her situation.<br>2) Say nothing—it's not your place. Agree to share the medications.<br>3) **Tell the office manager what you saw.** |

**Scenario 10**

| | |
|---|---|
| Objective of the scenario | The importance of scope of practice and first aid care. |
| Synopsis of scenario | A person enters the office with obvious physical injuries—bleeding from the head, compound fracture of the forearm. The doctor does not have the facilities to treat these types of injuries due to the nature of the practice. Maurice Wallace, the other MA in the office, goes to get the doctor. |
| Choices | 1) Consult the Triage section of the Policy & Procedure manual.<br>**2) Stabilize the patient where he is, and call 911.**<br>3) Go see where the medical assistant and doctor are. |
| Follow-up | If the user does not select the best response (#2), the user receives a follow-up scenario: You start to ask the patient questions from the Triage manual. The patient is only able to tell you his first name when he goes into shock. |
| Follow-up Choices | **1) Stabilize the patient where he is, and call 911.**<br>2) Move the patient to the clinical treatment room.<br>3) Call 911. |